Brain Tumors

Brain Tumors
Practical Guide to Diagnosis and Treatment

edited by

Joachim M. Baehring
Yale University School of Medicine
New Haven, Connecticut, U.S.A.

Joseph M. Piepmeier
Yale University School of Medicine
New Haven, Connecticut, U.S.A.

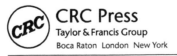

CRC Press
Taylor & Francis Group
Boca Raton London New York

CRC Press is an imprint of the
Taylor & Francis Group, an **informa** business

CRC Press
Taylor & Francis Group
6000 Broken Sound Parkway NW, Suite 300
Boca Raton, FL 33487-2742

First issued in paperback 2019

© 2007 by Taylor & Francis Group, LLC
CRC Press is an imprint of Taylor & Francis Group, an Informa business

No claim to original U.S. Government works

ISBN-13: 978-0-8493-3616-4 (hbk)
ISBN-13: 978-0-367-39022-8 (pbk)

This book contains information obtained from authentic and highly regarded sources. While all reasonable efforts have been made to publish reliable data and information, neither the author[s] nor the publisher can accept any legal responsibility or liability for any errors or omissions that may be made. The publishers wish to make clear that any views or opinions expressed in this book by individual editors, authors or contributors are personal to them and do not necessarily reflect the views/opinions of the publishers. The information or guidance contained in this book is intended for use by medical, scientific or health-care professionals and is provided strictly as a supplement to the medical or other professional's own judgement, their knowledge of the patient's medical history, relevant manufacturer's instructions and the appropriate best practice guidelines. Because of the rapid advances in medical science, any information or advice on dosages, procedures or diagnoses should be independently verified. The reader is strongly urged to consult the relevant national drug formulary and the drug companies' and device or material manufacturers' printed instructions, and their websites, before administering or utilizing any of the drugs, devices or materials mentioned in this book. This book does not indicate whether a particular treatment is appropriate or suitable for a particular individual. Ultimately it is the sole responsibility of the medical professional to make his or her own professional judgements, so as to advise and treat patients appropriately. The authors and publishers have also attempted to trace the copyright holders of all material reproduced in this publication and apologize to copyright holders if permission to publish in this form has not been obtained. If any copyright material has not been acknowledged please write and let us know so we may rectify in any future reprint.

A CIP record for this book is available from the British Library.

Library of Congress Cataloging-in-Publication Data available on application

Visit the Taylor & Francis Web site at
http://www.taylorandfrancis.com

and the CRC Press Web site at
http://www.crcpress.com

Preface

The last decade has dramatically changed the field of neurooncology. A new classification system has been put in place by the World Health Organization. New imaging techniques make possible early diagnosis of brain tumors and decreased morbidity from surgical intervention or irradiation. Classical therapeutic strategies have been refined and the standard of care for many tumors has changed. Knowledge of molecular mechanisms leading to brain cancer has grown exponentially and serves as the basis for novel more or less targeted treatment strategies.

This book is intended for clinicians who care for patients with primary and metastatic brain tumors and neurological complications of cancer. The book, largely written by clinical neurooncologists, provides a concise and up-to-date review of epidemiology, molecular pathogenesis—to the extent that is needed for the clinician to establish an accurate diagnosis and provide risk-stratified treatment, clinical presentation, diagnosis, therapy, and prognosis. The most essential information is presented in a format that is readable from "cover to cover." The book may serve as an introduction into the topic for the subspecialist in training and early career, as well as a concise review for the experienced neurooncologist, general neurosurgeon, neurologist, radiation oncologist, and medical oncologist. The reader is provided with contributions from experts in the field, who reflect their personal experience and interpretation of published studies.

Neurological complications of cancer and its treatment are becoming increasingly common as patients survive longer and are treated with new drugs or therapeutic modalities affecting the central as well as peripheral nervous system. As these problems are commonly encountered by any subspecialist involved in the care of patients with brain cancer, they are addressed in a major section.

We are committed to providing an up-to-date and readable resource on neurooncology. This will require further refinement in future editions. Comments from our colleagues are welcome.

Joachim M. Baehring
Joseph M. Piepmeier

Acknowledgments

We thank everyone who has helped us in the preparation of this book. Most importantly, we thank our contributing authors whose work provides the substance of this volume. It has been a privilege working with them and reading their chapters "first hand." We are grateful to the staff at Informa Healthcare USA, whose efforts assured timely completion. We thank our assistants Alienne Morrione, Susan Warnstedt, and Elizabeth D'Andrea whose support was instrumental in this undertaking.

Contents

PART II: PRIMARY NERVOUS SYSTEM TUMORS

Contributors

Lauren E. Abrey Department of Neurology, Memorial Sloan-Kettering Cancer Center, New York, New York, U.S.A.

Joachim M. Baehring Yale University School of Medicine, New Haven, Connecticut, U.S.A.

Serguei Bannykh Department of Pathology and Laboratory Medicine, Yale University School of Medicine, New Haven, Connecticut, U.S.A.

Antony Béhin Service de Neurologie Mazarin, Hôpital de la Salpêtrière, Paris, France and Service de Médecine Interne, Institut Jules Bordet, ULB, Bruxelles, Belgium

Jan C. Buckner Department of Oncology, Mayo Clinic College of Medicine, Rochester, Minnesota, U.S.A.

Marc Chamberlain Department of Interdisciplinary Oncology, H. Lee Moffitt Cancer Center, University of South Florida, Tampa, Florida, U.S.A.

Lawrence M. Cher Department of Oncology, Austin Health, Heidelberg, Victoria, Australia

Sajeel Chowdhary Department of Interdisciplinary Oncology, H. Lee Moffitt Cancer Center, University of South Florida, Tampa, Florida, U.S.A.

William T. Couldwell Department of Neurosurgery, University of Utah School of Medicine, Salt Lake City, Utah, U.S.A.

Mark Dannenbaum   Department of Neurosurgery, Baylor College of Medicine, and Department of Neurosurgery, The University of Texas M.D. Anderson Cancer Center, Houston, Texas, U.S.A.

Evanthia Galanis   Mayo Clinic College of Medicine, Rochester, Minnesota, U.S.A.

Oren N. Gottfried   Department of Neurosurgery, University of Utah School of Medicine, Salt Lake City, Utah, U.S.A.

Jeanine T. Grier   Department of Neurology, Massachusetts General Hospital, Boston, Massachusetts, U.S.A.

Jerzy Hildebrand   Service de Neurologie Mazarin, Hôpital de la Salpêtrière, Paris, France and Service de Médecine Interne, Institut Jules Bordet, ULB, Bruxelles, Belgium

Fred H. Hochberg   Pappas Center for Neuro-Oncology, Massachusetts General Hospital, Boston, Massachusetts, U.S.A.

Robert Jenkins   Department of Laboratory Medicine, Mayo Clinic College of Medicine, Rochester, Minnesota, U.S.A.

Evert C. A. Kaal   Department of Neurology, Medical Center Haaglanden, The Hague, The Netherlands

Kleopas A. Kleopa   Department of Clinical Neurosciences, The Cyprus Institute of Neurology and Genetics, Nicosia, Cyprus

Jonathan P. S. Knisely   Department of Therapeutic Radiology, Yale Medical School and Yale Cancer Center, New Haven, Connecticut, U.S.A.

Wilhelm Küker   Department of Neuroradiology, The Radcliffe Infirmary, Oxford, U.K.

Theodoros Kyriakides   Department of Clinical Neurosciences, The Cyprus Institute of Neurology and Genetics, Nicosia, Cyprus

Anita Lal   Departments of Neurological Surgery, Radiation Oncology, and The Brain Tumor Research Center, University of California, San Francisco, California, U.S.A.

Vanda A. Lennon   Departments of Immunology, Neurology and Laboratory Medicine and Pathology, Mayo Clinic College of Medicine, Rochester, Minnesota, U.S.A.

Tobey MacDonald Department of Oncology, Children's National Medical Center, and Department of Pediatrics, The George Washington University, Washington, D.C., U.S.A.

Masao Matsutani Department of Neurosurgery, School of Medicine, Saitama Medical University, Moroyamamachi, Irumagunn, Saitama, Japan

Michael W. McDermott Departments of Neurological Surgery, Radiation Oncology, and The Brain Tumor Research Center, University of California, San Francisco, California, U.S.A.

Nimish Mohile Department of Neurology, Memorial Sloan-Kettering Cancer Center, New York, New York, U.S.A.

Thomas Nägele Department of Neuroradiology, University Hospital Tuebingen, School of Medicine, Tuebingen, Germany

Terry Neill Department of Neurology, University of California at San Francisco, San Francisco, California, U.S.A.

Eylem Öcal Yale University School of Medicine, New Haven, Connecticut, U.S.A.

Ed Olson Department of Neurology, Feinberg School of Medicine, Northwestern University, Chicago, Illinois, U.S.A.

Roger J. Packer Departments of Neurology and Pediatrics, Children's National Medical Center, The George Washington University, Washington, D.C.; Department of Neurosurgery, University of Virginia, Charlottesville, Virginia; and Department of Neurology, Georgetown University, Washington, D.C., U.S.A.

Joseph M. Piepmeier Yale University School of Medicine, New Haven, Connecticut, U.S.A.

Sean J. Pittock Departments of Neurology and Laboratory Medicine and Pathology, Mayo Clinic College of Medicine, Rochester, Minnesota, U.S.A.

Scott R. Plotkin Department of Neurology, Massachusetts General Hospital, Boston, Massachusetts, U.S.A.

Jeffrey J. Raizer Department of Neurology, Feinberg School of Medicine, Northwestern University, Chicago, Illinois, U.S.A.

Ravi D. Rao   Department of Oncology, Mayo Clinic College of Medicine, Rochester, Minnesota, U.S.A.

Amyn M. Rojiani   Departments of Interdisciplinary Oncology and Pathology, H. Lee Moffitt Cancer Center, University of South Florida, Tampa, Florida, U.S.A.

James T. Rutka   Division of Neurosurgery, The Hospital for Sick Children, The University of Toronto, Toronto, Ontario, Canada

Raymond Sawaya   Department of Neurosurgery, Baylor College of Medicine, and Department of Neurosurgery, The University of Texas M.D. Anderson Cancer Center, Houston, Texas, U.S.A.

Vineeta Singh   Department of Neurology, University of California at San Francisco, San Francisco, California, U.S.A.

Akira Teramoto   Department of Neurosurgery, Nippon Medical School, Tokyo, Japan

Ty Thaiyananthan   Yale University School of Medicine, New Haven, Connecticut, U.S.A.

Tarik Tihan   Neuropathology Unit, UCSF School of Medicine, San Francisco, California, U.S.A.

Martin J. van den Bent   Neuro-Oncologie Unit, Daniel den Hoed Cancer Center/Erasmus University Medical Center, Rotterdam, The Netherlands

Charles J. Vecht   Department of Neurology, Medical Center Haaglanden, The Hague, The Netherlands

Gilbert Vezina   Department of Neuroradiology and Radiology, Children's National Medical Center, The George Washington University, Washington, D.C., U.S.A.

James Waldron   Department of Neurological Surgery, UCSF School of Medicine, San Francisco, California, U.S.A.

Marcus L. Ware   Departments of Neurological Surgery, Radiation Oncology, and The Brain Tumor Research Center, University of California, San Francisco, California, U.S.A.

Adrienne C. Weeks   Division of Neurosurgery, The Hospital for Sick Children, The University of Toronto, Toronto, Ontario, Canada

Martin H. Weiss   Department of Neurological Surgery, University of Southern California, Los Angeles, California, U.S.A.

Michael Weller   Department of General Neurology, Hertie Institute for Clinical Brain Research, University of Tuebingen, School of Medicine, Tuebingen, Germany

Wolfgang Wick   Department of General Neurology, Hertie Institute for Clinical Brain Research, University of Tuebingen, School of Medicine, Tuebingen, Germany

Daizo Yoshida   Department of Neurosurgery, Nippon Medical School, Tokyo, Japan

1

Principles of Neurosurgical Therapy

Eylem Öcal, Ty Thaiyananthan, and Joseph M. Piepmeier
Yale University School of Medicine,
New Haven, Connecticut, U.S.A.

Neurooncology has evolved into a multidisciplinary collaborative specialty that combines the expertise from radiation oncologists, neuroradiologists, neurologists, pathologists, and medical oncology. Each of these specialties provides important components of comprehensive care. Current management strategies can optimize outcomes by integrating not only the standard of care, but also novel and investigative therapies.

The challenge of surgical neurooncology is to reduce the tumor burden, minimize symptoms, preserve functional abilities, and manage the initial stages of treatment. In the surgical management of brain tumors, there have been dramatic improvements that help to achieve these goals. These improvements have reduced morbidity and increased the possibility for aggressive tumor resection. Significant advances in our understanding of the biology of primary brain tumors are on the verge of increasing survival for most malignant glioma patients. However, there has never been a randomized clinical trial to evaluate the relationship between the extent of surgery and outcome in gliomas. The survival benefits of aggressive surgery have been supported by retrospective reviews of clinical series. But surgery also has other goals including improvement in symptoms, reduction in seizures, and relief from steroid dependency as well as tissue for accurate diagnosis. All of these are important considerations (1).

This chapter will address current surgical strategies and illustrate how these can improve outcome. In addition, the limitations of surgery will be addressed to illustrate where advances are needed. Surgeons can play an

increasingly important role in tumor management as new therapies emerge
that include direct application of therapy into the tumor. As these improvements become the new standard of care, neurosurgeons will have important
roles in bringing new therapies into use.

PRESURGICAL PLANNING

Clinical Evaluation

Traditionally, brain tumors reach medical attention because they create progressive neurological symptoms that can persist over days to weeks. The
rapidity of progression is commonly associated with the growth rate of
the tumor; more aggressive tumors generate more rapid progression. For
primary malignant gliomas, focal or regional symptoms evolving over days
to a few weeks are typical. However, low-grade primary brain tumors most
commonly cause the new onset of seizures and it is this ictal event that leads
to a diagnosis. Benign extra-axial tumors (meningiomas and schwannomas)
can cause more subtle findings that may be present for years prior to diagnosis. Although these generalizations are helpful, it must be remembered
that the clinical presentation of patients with central nervous system tumors
can be variable. A careful history and physical examination remain a very
important initial steps in raising the suspicion of a progressive mass lesion
and directing whether investigation with imaging studies are warranted (2).

Corticosteroids are the most commonly used medications in perioperative management. While the most appropriate dose is patient dependent,
rapid and dramatic improvement in neurological symptoms are commonly
seen. It should be remembered that steroid use can also change the preoperative imaging findings. One benefit of steroid utilization is improvement in
tightening the blood–brain barrier. As a consequence, significant reduction
in areas of contrast enhancement can change the operative target. This can
be of critical importance when intraoperative images are utilized (Fig. 1).

The use of prophylactic anticonvulsants (AC) remains controversial.
The American Neurological Association has published a position on this
practice and recommended that prophylactic AC be avoided (3). There is no
benefit in reducing the frequency of a first seizure with this practice. Also, AC
can cause allergic reactions and debilitating side effects and significantly
reduce the bioavailability of systemic chemotherapy agents. Certainly, if a
patient has experienced a seizure, AC should be strongly considered; however,
in the absence of a seizure, AC should not be recommended.

Neurosurgeons are frequently the first physician examining and counseling patients with a brain tumor. It is unlikely that the patient will have
sufficient background that will enable them to understand the complexity
of brain tumor management. There are national support and advocacy
groups that can offer additional information and guidance. Many of these
groups provide World Wide Web–based counseling and information to help

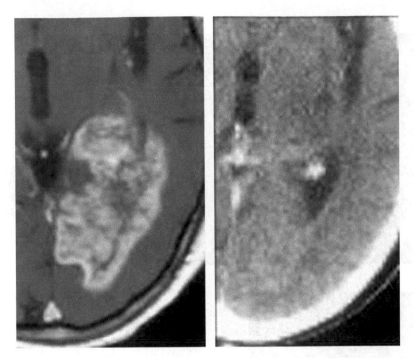

Figure 1 Preoperative T1-weighted MRI with gadolinium (*left*) shows a large heterogeneously enhancing mass lesion within the left temporo-occipital area (glioblastoma multiforme). Prebiopsy-enhanced CT (*right*) after dexamethasone therapy. Note the dramatic decrease in contrast enhancement as a result of steroid use.

patients come to terms with their diagnosis [for example, American Brain Tumor Association (4) and National Brain Tumor Foundation (5)]. In addition, academic medical centers often offer patient and family support groups. These resources are underutilized. It is not uncommon for patients to arrive for an evaluation with folders of pages downloaded from the Web. Because most of this information is unregulated, it is helpful for both the patient and the physician to direct the patient's search to reputable sources.

Preoperative Imaging

Modern imaging tools and recent advances in imaging techniques now serve as the basis of early diagnosis of brain tumors. This technology has moved into the operating room (OR). Magnetic resonance imaging (MRI) continues to be the most sensitive and preferred diagnostic study for identifying these lesions (6,7). All imaging sequences from preoperative MRIs should be carefully reviewed (Fig. 2).

Anatomical location of a tumor, size and distribution of tumor, and edema are often delineated on T1 and T2 sequences; potential cell density

(A)   **(B)**

(C)

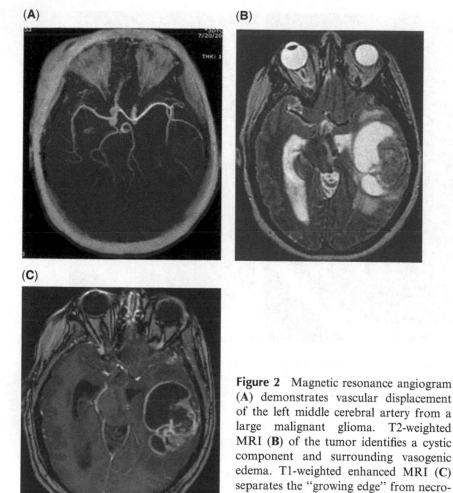

Figure 2 Magnetic resonance angiogram (**A**) demonstrates vascular displacement of the left middle cerebral artery from a large malignant glioma. T2-weighted MRI (**B**) of the tumor identifies a cystic component and surrounding vasogenic edema. T1-weighted enhanced MRI (**C**) separates the "growing edge" from necrotic and cystic areas. All of these sequences are useful for surgical planning.

can estimated from diffusion-weighted images (DWI); loss of blood–brain barrier and contrast enhancement help to estimate aggressiveness on T1-enhanced sequences (8). Subtle areas of tumor involvement or small metastatic tumors can be found with flair sequences. Gyral and vascular displacement, arterial encasement, ventricular extension, and obstruction are typically easily seen with careful review of these images (Fig. 3).

In addition to anatomical imaging, alternative imaging techniques, such as functional MRI (fMRI), magnetic resonance spectroscopy, and magnetic-source imaging (MSI), have become important tools to help the physician obtain information about the lesion itself and define its

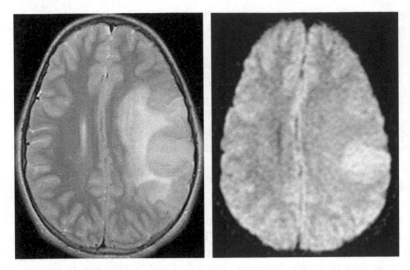

Figure 3 T2-weighted MRI (*left*) of a diffusely infiltrative glioma. Diffusion-weighted MRI (*right*) reveals restricted diffusion in the angular gyrus region, suggesting high cell density and optimal site for biopsy.

relationship to eloquent areas of the brain (6). This information can be critical for determining the goals of surgery and the relative risks of impairment with intervention. For example, fMRI offers a noninvasive alternative to obtain an understanding of the functional cortical regions of the brain that serve as primary areas for speech, motor, and visual function (8–11). Tumor infiltration into these regions may preclude aggressive resection, whereas displacement of critical cortical areas by tumor mass may indicate that resection of the lesion may be feasible with preservation of function (Fig. 4). Primary language cortex can be variable in location and is rarely predictable beyond the region of the dominant frontal and temporal operculum. When the orientation of the signal is perpendicular to the brain surface, the region of interest may reside in a sulcus and thus it cannot be easily stimulated with traditional brain-mapping techniques.

Proton magnetic resonance spectroscopy allows clinicians to measure the relative concentration of metabolites in defined regions of interest. The information gathered from this study can be used to plan biopsies and monitor patients after treatment (8,12). While these techniques are still in development, new data suggest that metabolic imaging may be a powerful tool for determining tumor infiltration into regions that anatomic imaging may miss.

MSI is a technique that fuses megnetoencephalography with anatomical MRI. Magnetoencephalography employs a biomagnetometer system to allow for simultaneous bihemispheric recordings. Various stimuli are applied and magnetoencephalograpic signals are recorded. This data is

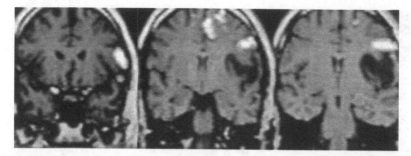

Figure 4 Functional MRI of primary language region in the frontal lobe superior to a glioma.

then coregistered with a high-resolution MRI image sequence (fluid-attenuated inversion recovery (FLAIR), T2-weighted, or T1 with contrast) to help identify if tumor is located within functional areas of the brain (8).

A new tool that can determine the relationship between tumor and white matter pathways is diffusion tensor imaging (DTI) (8,13). DTI is a modification of DWI that is able to visualize the preferential diffusion of water along white matter fibers. Image contrast is based upon the principle of diffusion anisotropy: diffusion of water molecules parallel to white matter tracts is less restricted than water diffusion perpendicular to them. This information can then be used to create color-coded maps that identify white matter tracts in areas where a tumor is located (8,13).

Integration of imaging into operative management with frameless stereotaxis and coregistration of anatomic, functional, and metabolic data have provided surgeons with detailed information that can direct surgical strategies. Intraoperative imaging with computed tomography (CT) and MRI has brought these diagnostic tools into the surgical suite. This merger of technology and surgery provides the surgeon with powerful tools and real-time information to enhance patient outcome.

INTRAOPERATIVE PATIENT CARE

Neuroanesthesia

An experienced neuroanesthesiologist is a very important collaborator in brain tumor surgery to maintain cerebral perfusion pressure (CPP), provide the neurosurgeon with optimal brain relaxation, and to maintain hemodynamic stability throughout the procedure (14,15). The appropriate choice of anesthetics can optimize CPP, intracranial pressure (ICP), cerebral blood flow (CBF), and cerebral metabolic rate for oxygen ($CMRO_2$), and ensure compatibility with neurophysiological monitoring (14). Propofol and thiopental are often used because of their beneficial effects on reducing $CMRO_2$ and ICP. Isoflurane's nominal effect on CBF and its ability to decrease $CMRO_2$ while offering a cerebral protective effect make it an agent of choice for the neuroanesthesiologist (15). Sevoflurane, a new agent with similar properties of isoflurane with a low lipid solubility allowing for faster recovery from anesthesia, may provide significant advantages in neurosurgical patients (15).

Routine use of mannitol is not necessary for most cases when brain relaxation can be attained with patient positioning and hyperventilation. When additional brain relaxation is required, rapid infusion of mannitol (0.5–1.0 g/kg) can achieve measurable effect within 20 to 30 minutes. On occasion, other diuretics may be needed, and the dose and selection can be performed by an experienced anesthesiologist.

Invasive arterial line monitoring and electrocardiography are used to monitor blood pressure and assess for dysrhythmias, which can affect CPP (14,16). Central venous pressure, pulmonary artery catheterization, and precordial Doppler sonography are performed on a case-specific basis if the patient's medical condition warrants and if the surgical approach is associated with a high risk of air embolism. Pulse oximetry, core temperature measurement with an esophageal stethoscope, and capnography are routine measurements for virtually all neurosurgical patients (15).

Intraoperative Neurophysiological Monitoring

Intraoperative neurophysiologic monitoring is used to assess the integrity of neuronal pathways and to identify functional cortical areas. These monitoring modalities include computer-processed electroencephalography, recording of somatosensory-evoked potentials (SEP), motor-evoked potentials (MEP), brain stem auditory-evoked potentials, or visual-evoked potentials, and monitoring of cranial nerve function (17). These techniques are commonly used for procedures in the proximity of the motor or language cortex and during resection of brain stem tumors. Sensory pathways from the peripheral nerve to the sensory cortex can be assessed by SEP monitoring, while MEPs can be used to assess the integrity of descending motor pathways (Fig. 5).

Primary language cortex mapping is frequently required for resection of lesions in the dominant frontal and temporal lobes with "awake" surgery and intravenous sedation. Identification of the primary cortical areas that control speech is performed with bipolar stimulation (60 Hz, single pulse 1 msec at an amplitude 2–10 mA), resulting in speech arrest. In approximately 20% of patients, no specific primary language area can be found using this method. It is believed that cortical targets in these patients reside within a sulcus and are not generally reached by this technique. Localization of subcortical language pathways is less well defined. Preliminary experience suggests the existence of a main ventral pathway connecting the temporal and frontal lobes in the inferior fronto-occipital fasciculus (18). Subcortical

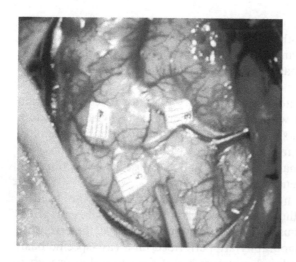

Figure 5 Intraoperative view of cortical mapping with bipolar electrodes.

stimulation parameters are less well defined and as a rule, frequent stimulation is required for the resection of deep tumors in this region.

SURGICAL TECHNIQUES

Tumor Surgery

The continued drive to improve the accuracy and reduce the morbidity of brain tumor procedures has forced an evolution of surgical technology (17). Neurosurgeons commonly have a dedicated OR environment to perform surgery on disorders of the brain and spine, designed to accommodate stereotactic brain biposies, resection of tumors involving eloquent brain tissue, transsphenoidal procedures, intraoperative monitoring of cranial nerves, along with guidance and imaging systems that produce reliable feedback during the procedure.

Video cameras can be linked to microscopes or fixed to movable light sources in order to aid in teaching and allowing OR personnel to view the surgery and participate more efficiently (Fig. 6) (15). The operating microscope is a common tool for tumor surgeons. Improved illumination and magnification aid in defining the tumor margin as well as control of bleeding. High-grade tumors are commonly identified by their color, consistency, and vascularity. Low-grade gliomas can be indistinguishable from white matter. This is particularly true for oligodendrogliomas. The use of stereotaxis or intraoperative imaging can be essential for identifying the surgical margins.

Surgical Morbidity

The risk of neurological injury is primarily the result of tumor location including proximity to critical cortical areas, vascular and white matter

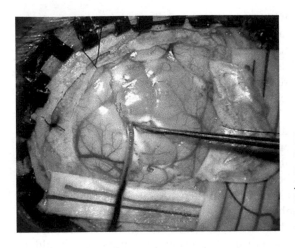

Figure 6 Intraoperative view of removal of a high-grade glioma. This image is projected onto several video monitors so the staff and students can follow the progress of the surgery.

anatomy. Infiltrated cortical regions, stretched fiber tracts, and encased vascular anatomy can present challenges even to experienced surgeons. The ability to anticipate these findings and to consider contingency plans is mandatory to prevent unintended harm. Elevated ICP from cerebral edema and tumor mass can result in dramatic brain herniation requiring rapid decompression. Sacrifice of a dominant cortical vein also will result in swelling and loss of control of the surgical field. When these events occur, the surgeon must be prepared to act quickly, often with the help of the anesthesiologist. Confirming the status of the CO_2, head elevation, rapid infusion of mannitol, and aspiration of CSF (ventricular catheter) can often salvage a patient from a potentially disastrous complication. Anticipation of significant brain swelling and preemptive action can be critical to success. For example, Figure 2 illustrates a large glioblastoma with mass effect and compression of the diencephalon. Uncontrolled herniation of the dominant temporal lobe is a significant risk upon opening the dura. Hyperventilation and mannitol were insufficient to reverse this at the time of surgery. Review of the preoperative MRI also showed that this tumor contained a large cystic component. Aspiration of the fluid from the cyst prior to opening the dura prevented herniation and resulted in a controlled operative field.

Some surgical procedures are associated with anticipated transient deficits. For example, resection of the supplementary motor region often results in transient contralateral hemiparesis. Forewarning the patient of this can reduce anxiety and help prepare the patient for rehabilitation. Resections that extend to primary motor and language cortex can interrupt function. As long as the primary regions are not injured, recovery commonly occurs with time. Resection of large tumors in the nondominant frontal lobe will cause problems with processing information and impairment in visual-spatial orientation. Although these deficits may be acceptable to many patients and not interfere with their normal daily activities, these issues should be discussed preoperatively.

The most common cause of symptomatic postoperative bleeding is a subtotal tumor removal. The fragility of neovascularity from the tumor is often difficult to control and more likely to be the source of postoperative problems. This requires special attention during surgery to prevent subsequent problems.

Deep vein thrombosis and pulmonary embolism remain common complications in the brain tumor population. Prophylactic therapy can reduce their occurrence but not in all patients. A plegic leg in an obese, dehydrated and immobile patient may be sufficient risk to consider prophylactic insertion of a filter in the inferior vena cava to preclude fatal embolism. Routine monitoring of venous thrombosis with lower extremity Doppler studies also may help identify problems before they become emergencies. There are no firm guidelines in these cases; however, preventative measures should be considered when the patient is at risk.

Endoscopic Neurosurgery

Minimally invasive surgery is gaining popularity among neurosurgeons. New techniques and surgical equipment are being modified to minimize iatrogenic injury to normal structures when approaching a lesion. These advances aim to decrease patient discomfort, shorten hospital stay, improve cosmetic results, and allow patients to return to their normal activities as soon as possible (19).

Endoscopy has become an essential tool in minimally invasive surgery. Endoscopes provide a wide variety of viewing angles and magnified visualization of the surrounding structures through a narrow corridor. Two major categories of endoscopes are currently used in neurosurgery. Rigid endoscopes offer superior image resolution while flexible fiberoptic systems provide more adaptability for navigation (19).

Endoscopy is commonly applied in the management of intraventricular tumors, cysts, transnasal approaches to pituitary tumors, and skull base tumors. Endoscopic third ventriculostomy and septostomy are being performed commonly for noncommunicating and compartmentalized hydrocephalus (Fig. 7).

Frameless and Frame-Based Stereotaxy

Stereotactic guidance is a common technology in the neurosurgical OR. There are several commercially available systems that integrate surface recognition or fixed fiducial registration for guidance. Most systems are highly reliable and accurate. Intraoperative use has become commonplace and user-friendly. The major disadvantage of frameless and frame-based systems is their susceptibility to changes in the brain as a result of surgery that cannot be updated into the surgical planning. Significant shifts in location of

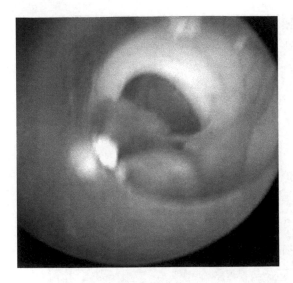

Figure 7 View through an endoscope of the foramen of Monro. Note the choroids plexus and septal vein.

pathology and normal anatomy can make these systems less reliable. While it is possible to accommodate these problems by experience, newer updated systems are required to address this issue. The problem of target shifting is most commonly seen with cystic lesions where removal of fluid volume can change target location in reference to surface anatomy. These systems are very reliable for stereotactic biopsy. Most stereotactic techniques enable the surgeon to place a probe within a few millimeters of the desired target region (Fig. 8).

Intraoperative Imaging

Real-time visualization of brain anatomy can overcome the issue of brain shift changes, which degrade the information obtained from preoperative images. Ultrasound offers real-time imaging, but does not clearly show a tumor's definite margins. Tumors are typically hyperechoic and difficult to distinguish from surgical changes at the margins. Although intraoperative CT does provide better tissue resolution and creates three-dimensional displays from datasets, intraoperative MRI (iMRI) continues to be considered superior in all regards. By providing multiplanar and high-resolution images, iMRI has become a popular modality in differentiating normal and abnormal tissue densities as well as accounting for brain shifts. One limitation of iMRI is the leakage of gadolinium at the edges of resection margins, which can be difficult to distinguish form residual tumor.

Many new open configuration MR scanner designs allow for maximum patient access with high signal-to-noise ratio. Variations in mechanical designs account for differences in the amount of surgical access during the imaging and in the field strength, which impacts the image quality. The "double

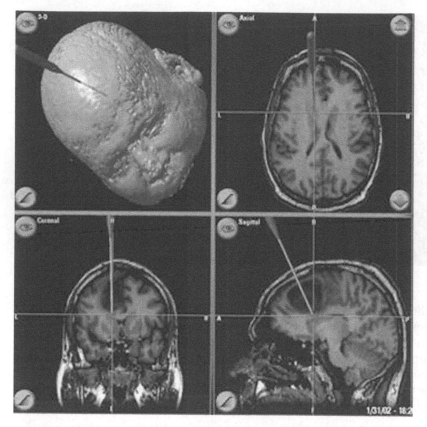

Figure 8 Frameless stereotactic view during resection of a glioma. Note the probe is at the inferior margin of the lesion marking the extent of resection.

doughnut" design was the first MR scanner to be integrated into the surgical suite and utilizes a 0.5-T magnet system. However, this design requires MR-compatible instrumentation. The "lateral aperture" system places fewer restrictions on instrument compatibility but has the disadvantages of requiring the patient to be moved from the OR table to a scanner table and has a low magnetic field of 0.2 T. Finally, the "pit" and "crane" systems provide a high magnetic field of 1.5 T, which allows better resolution abilities (Fig. 9) (17,20,21).

SURGICAL ADJUNCTS

Stereotactic Radiosurgery

Stereotactic radiosurgery (SRS) is a noninvasive treatment modality and an option for certain types of benign and malignant brain tumors and vascular lesions. It uses multiple beams of ionizing radiation to provide a single, high

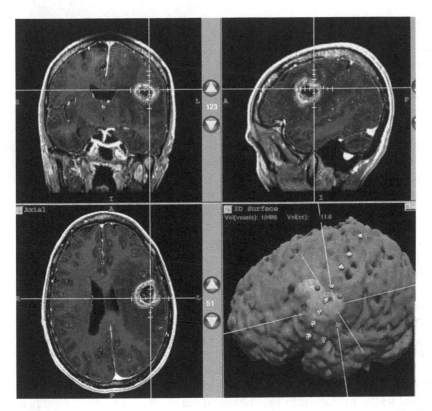

Figure 9 Operative image of frameless stereotactic view with tumor outlined and functional motor/language mapping. Precise localization of the tumor and its relationship to the primary motor region and language are shown. *Source*: Courtesy of Alexandra Golby.

dose to a defined target in the brain (22). Radiosurgery capitalizes on the radiobiologic effect of the radiation on cells and the subsequent resulting vasculopathy. The aim of SRS is to minimize radiation exposure of the surrounding normal brain tissue while maximizing the dose applied to the target. It can be performed on an outpatient basis. Its application extends from benign and malignant intracranial masses to arteriovenous malformations and functional diseases (23). The SRS treatment can be used as a primary therapy, for recurrent disease, as an adjuvant therapy in combination with surgery, or as an alternative to conventional radiotherapy (22). Tumors less than 2.5 to 3 cm or surgically inaccessible solitary or single metastatic lesion represent the most common indication for SRS. Results with pituitary tumors, acoustic neuromas, and craniopharyngiomas are also promising. It may serve as an appealing option for patients whose medical condition or age would increase morbidity of open surgery.

INVESTIGATIVE STUDIES

The application of new technology and devices in the surgical management of brain tumor patients has significantly improved operative care. Tumor resections and biopsies can be performed with greater accuracy and safety and in a setting where the surgeon can be provided with real-time updated imaging data to direct operative procedures. However, these improvements have not been sufficient to significantly improve long-term survival for malignant glioma patients. Investigative therapies continue to search for better results and many of these research strategies also involve surgery as a component of treatment.

Local and regional application of chemotherapy, radiation sources, and targeted agents that selectively bind to tumor cells present the advantage of increasing the concentration of therapeutic agent at the site of tumor infiltration, bypassing the blood–brain barrier and reducing the toxicity of systemic administration. Biodegradable substrates have been utilized to deliver chemotherapy at the resection margin by diffusion into the surrounding brain. This strategy can reduce systemic toxicity and circumvent the blood–brain barrier, but the distribution of active agent is limited to within a few millimeters and dependent on the concentration of agent at the source (24,25).

Better distribution can be achieved with convection-enhanced delivery. This strategy utilizes catheters to infuse an agent by pressure and distribute to a wider region based on the pressure wave generated by a pump. Drug distribution by this strategy is limited by fluid dynamics and the propensity for fluid waves to track into the subarachnoid space, ventricles, or surgical resection cavity, thus limiting access to the tumor. Optimal future strategies will utilize both techniques by convection delivery of biodegradable nanoparticles to eliminate the obstacles found with current technique.

Surgeons will continue to be among the pioneers of future therapy. Precise access to target regions with stereotactic placement of therapy offered in an environment of maximal reduction of residual tumor burden will keep surgeons in the lead of finding and developing better therapies. Surgeons can offer access to tumor specimens and encourage their patients to participate in clinical trials. This is an important responsibility. As leaders in neurooncology, surgeons can continue to be important members of the multidisciplinary team.

REFERENCES

1. Vives K, Piepmeier J. Complications and expected outcomes of glioma surgery. J Neurooncol 1999; 42:289–302.
2. Piepmeier J, Baehring J. Surgical resection for patients with benign primary brain tumors and low grade gliomas. J Neurooncol 2004; 69:55–65.
3. Glantz MJ, Cole BF, Forsyth PA, Recht LD, Wen PY, Chamberlain MC, Grossman SA, Cairncross JG. Practice parameter: anticonvulsant prophylaxis

in patients with newly diagnosed brain tumors. Report of the Quality Standards Subcommittee of the American Academy of Neurology. Neurology 2000; 23:54(10):1886–1893.

4. www.hope.abta.org.
5. www.braintumor.org.
6. Keles EG, Berger M. Advances in neurosurgical technique in the current management of brain tumors. Semin Oncol 2004; 31:659–665.
7. Byrne T, Piepmeier J, Yoshida D. Imaging and clinical features of gliomas. In: Tindall G, Cooper P, Barrow D, (eds) The Practice of Neurosurgery. Lippincott, Williams and Wilkins, 1996; 637–648.
8. Rees J. Advances in magnetic resonance imaging of brain tumor. Curr Opin Neurol 2003; 16:643–650.
9. DeYoe EA, Bandettini P, Neitz J, Miller D, Winans P. Functional magnetic resonance imaging (fMRI) of the human brain. J Neurosci Methods 1994; 54:171–187.
10. Toronov V, Walker S, Gupta R, Choi JH, Gratton E, Hueber D, Webber A. The roles of changes in deoxyhemoglobin concentration and regional cerebral blood volume in the fMRI BOLD signal. Neuroimage 2003; 19:1521–1531.
11. Vlieger EJ, Majoie CB, Leenstra S, den Heeten GJ. Functional magnetic resonance imaging for neurosurgical planning in neurooncology. Eur Radiol 2004; 14:1143–1153.
12. Lecler X, Huisman AGM, Sorensen AG. The potential of proton magnetic resonance spectroscopy in the diagnosis and management of patients with brain tumors. Curr Opin Oncol 2002; 14:292–298.
13. Pajevic S, Pierpaoli C. Color schemes to represent the orientation of anisotropic tissues from diffusion tensor data: application to white matter fiber tract mapping in the human brain. Magn Res Med 1999; 42:526–540.
14. Toms S, Ferson D, Sawaya R. Basic surgical techniques in the resection of malignant gliomas. J Neurooncol 1999; 42:215–226.
15. Whittle IR. Surgery for gliomas. Curr Opin Neurol 2002; 15:663–669.
16. Chang SM, Parney IF, Huang W, Anderson FA, Asher AL, Bernstein M, Lillehei KO, Brem H, Berger M, Laws E. Patterns of care for adults with newly diagnosed malignant glioma. JAMA 2005; 293(5):557–564.
17. Barnett GH, Nathoo N. The modern brain tumor operating room: from standard essentials to current state-of-the-art. J Neurooncol 2004; 69:25–33.
18. Daffau H, Gattignol P, Mandonnet E. New insights into the anatomo-functional connectivity of the semantic system: a study using cortico-subcortical electrostimulations. Brain 2005; 128(4):797–810.
19. Badie B, Brooks N, Souweidane MM. Endoscopic and minimally invasive microsurgical approaches for treating brain tumor patients. J Neurooncol 2004; 69:209–219.
20. Lipson AC, Gargollo PC, Black P. Intraoperative magnetic resonance imaging: considerations for the operating room of the future. J Clin Neurosci 2001; 8(4):305–310.
21. Randa Z, Keles EG, Berger MS. Intraoperative imaging techniques in the treatment of brain tumors. Curr Opin Oncol 1999; 11(3):152–160.
22. Suh J, Vogelbaum MA, Barnett G. Update of stereotactic radiosurgery for brain tumors. Curr Opin Neurol 2004; 17(6):681–686.

23. Gerosa M, Nicolato A, Foroni R, The role of gamma knife radiosurgery in the treatment of primary and metastatic brain tumors. Curr Opin Oncol 2003; 15(3): 188–196.
24. Guerin C, Olivi A, Weomgart J, Lawson C, Brem H. Recent advances in brain tumor therapy: local intracerebral drug delivery by polymers. Invest New Drugs 2004; 22:27–37.
25. Prins RM, Liau LM. Immunology and immunotherapy in neurosurgical disease. Neurosurgery 2003; 53:144–153.

2

Principles of Radiation Therapy

Jonathan P. S. Knisely

*Department of Therapeutic Radiology, Yale Medical School and
Yale Cancer Center, New Haven, Connecticut, U.S.A.*

INTRODUCTION

Ionizing radiation, surgical resection, and systemically delivered drugs and
molecules are all commonly used for the treatment of solid tumors. All three
modalities may be used for tumors anywhere in the body, but there are few
sites for which radiation therapy plays such a vital role in disease management as the central nervous system (CNS). Radiation therapy is a locoregional treatment, and it occupies a position intermediate between surgery
and chemotherapy in its ability to treat intensively a portion of the body
that cannot be safely resected while at the same time very effectively sparing
the rest of the body from treatment-related side effects.

The importance of radiation therapy for tumors that arise in or around
the CNS or metastasize to the brain is because of the difficulty that exists in
surgically extirpating tumors in the CNS, despite recent advances in stereo-
taxic procedures that may incorporate functional imaging and intraoperative
mapping or may even be performed under magnetic resonance guidance (1).
The small number of effective drugs for CNS tumors and the relative difficulty that the blood–brain barrier presents to effective drug delivery have
made systemic approaches less than optimal for controlling most tumors
in the CNS (2). Many primary CNS tumors have little or no chance of metastatic spread within or outside the CNS. Locoregional control of tumors

arising in or metastatic to the CNS is critical. The spatially disparate localization of highly specialized functions in the brain and the inability to regenerate brain cells in any significant fashion after injury to the brain makes avoidance of iatrogenic damage in the treatment of CNS tumors and the prevention of tumor-induced CNS damage pivotal in the selection of interventions and the timing of these interventions.

When treatments are chosen, the treating oncologists must have a clear understanding of the potential for harm induced by any chosen treatments. Attention must be paid to not only the short term, but also the potential for lifelong morbidity associated with the treatments selected. Given its importance in management of CNS tumors, it must be acknowledged by radiation oncologists and by those caring for patients with CNS tumors that incautious or inappropriate use of ionizing radiation can have such profoundly adverse sequelae in few, if any, other tumor sites.

GENERAL PRINCIPLES

Radiotherapy is relatively straightforward—aim the radiation where the tumor is, and do not exceed the tolerance of the normal tissues adjacent to the tumor. The effectiveness of radiotherapy is largely limited by the potential for normal tissue injury. Routinely fractionated radiation therapy, delivered five days/wk for between approximately two and seven weeks, can treat radiographically normal brain tissue with acceptable morbidity that contains infiltrating tumor cells or subclinical metastatic foci at the same time that the tumor is treated with acceptable morbidity. Irradiating normal tissues at the same time that the tumor is treated is one of the particular attributes that may be regarded as being both an asset and a liability of radiation therapy in the treatment of CNS tumors. Stereotactic radiosurgical (SRS) treatment, where all the radiation is delivered in a single large dose, decreases the volume of normal tissues incidentally included with the tumor in the high-dose volume to the maximum extent feasible, and the dose delivered to the tumor can then be maximized. In SRS, doses approximately an order of magnitude higher than the usual single fraction daily dose can be delivered with acceptable normal tissue complication rates.

Knowledge of the tolerance of normal tissues that are adjacent to or infiltrated by the tumor tissue that is to be treated is essential. The tolerance of normal tissues to radiation is a function of the volume that will be treated, the daily dose that will be used, and, if the treatment is divided into fractions, the total dose that will be delivered and the total time period over which this therapy will be delivered. This is true no matter how irradiation is delivered. It is important to be cognizant of what is safe and what is of uncertain safety as different radiotherapy fractionation schemes are prescribed and delivered to varying volumes that include different amounts and types of normal tissues.

Radiation management of neurooncologic problems also involves a critical assessment of the appropriateness of the use of radiation therapy in one or another fashion for each individual patient. A patient who presents with leptomeningeal and parenchymal brain metastases has a very different set of conditions that govern the appropriate use of radiation therapy than a patient with a benign skull base tumor, such as a meningioma or vestibular schwannoma, and this differs again from a patient with a primary intracranial low- or high-grade glioma. Some patients will be better served by deferring radiation therapy until more definite knowledge of the behavior of the tumor in question can be assessed by reimaging for evidence of growth that may have occurred in the intervening months. Some patients need radiation treatment on an urgent basis to prevent loss of function from occurring. Some patients would be better served with a neurosurgical approach or with systemic management, and this should be recommended, when appropriate. The decision for a radiation oncology intervention is based on a complex set of clinical and imaging data, and the value of multidisciplinary tumor boards in reviewing therapeutic options is generally accepted (3).

A radiation oncologist's ability to target intracranial tumors has improved significantly over the past several decades. The use of high-resolution cross-sectional volumetric imaging studies [computed tomography (CT) and magnetic resonance imaging (MRI)] and computerized software that allows radiation therapy treatment planning to be performed in a virtual reality mode is nearly universal. Subtle tweaking of radiotherapy treatment parameters can be performed at a computer workstation to visualize the effects of these changes on the radiation doses being delivered to normal tissues and to the target in near "real time." Additional incorporated software algorithms allow the calculation of the radiation doses being delivered to discrete volumes of tissues within the CNS and objective comparisons to be made between different radiotherapy treatment plans.

This improved ability to target intracranial tumors has perhaps increased the radiation oncologist's responsibility as regards what should be treated, using what daily dose, and to what total dose to achieve control of the pathologic process being treated. Simply put, not everything should be treated the same way.

Radiobiology

Radiotherapy evolved empirically over the past century to be a five days/wk discipline. A course of curative radiation treatment will go on for approximately five to seven weeks, most commonly with doses of 1.8 to 2.0 Gray being administered daily. Palliative treatments are also usually administered on a five days/wk basis, but with fewer and larger daily radiation fractions given over a one- to three-week time period. It has been pointed out that tumor cells do not take weekends off, but the tolerance of normal tissues for fractionated irradiation in the doses that are commonly given has been a very important consideration as these empirically derived regimens evolved. Investigations into radiotherapy regimens that use multiple daily treatments, different doses, and schedules that do not halt for weekends have been performed (4,5). The results for tumors in the CNS have not been dramatically improved beyond what is achieved with more conventional radiotherapy treatment schedules and some unanticipated toxicities have been identified that relate to normal tissue tolerance of the CNS (5).

Developments in radiobiology and physics have been the foundation for all the rational advances in radiation oncology over the past century. Radiobiology is the study of how ionizing radiation interacts with biological molecules in living systems. The probability of cell survival after single doses of ionizing radiation is a function of absorbed dose, which in radiation oncology is measured in units called "Grays" (Fig. 1). The biological molecules that are the primary target for inactivation in radiation therapy are the chromosomal DNA molecules. Cellular repair processes that protect the integrity of the genome may make certain nonspecific radiogenic perturbations more or less likely to result in the desired effect of tumor eradication or control when a course of fractionated irradiation is given. The effects of fractionated radiation on a tissue are dependent on the total dose, the size of each dose fraction, the interval between fractions, and the total time

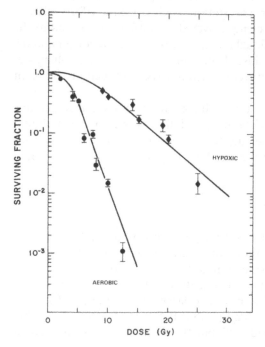

Figure 1 Mammalian cell survival curves after irradiation in aerobic conditions or after maintenance under hypoxic conditions for one hour prior to and through irradiation. Cell survival was assayed immediately after irradiation with a colony formation assay.

of treatment. Four separate radiobiological processes have been grouped together as central dogmas to organize thinking about how to improve clinical radiation oncology by altering these parameters. They are known as the "Four R's," and are, respectively: repopulation, reoxygenation, repair, and redistribution (6–9).

The process of repopulation is clearly important in the ability of a course of radiation or any repetitively administered therapy to eliminate a tumor. If the tumor regrows or repopulates faster than a treatment can eliminate the tumor's clonogenic stem cells, the treatment will never eradicate the tumor. Tumors of different origins have different propensities to "repopulate" over a course of radiation treatment, and in some cases may require an accelerated pace of radiation delivery, called altered fractionation.

Tumor oxygenation is also critical. Oxygen molecules present in tissues are a source of oxygen free radicals that augment the damage done by the electrons scattered by the incident radiation. A dose of radiation given to cells that have the ambient oxygen tension of capillary venous blood is approximately threefold more lethal than the same dose given to cells that are transiently anoxic during the moment when irradiation is given (Fig. 2). The spatially and temporally chaotic blood flow within the inadequate tumor neovasculature is a source of both chronic and intermittent hypoxia within tumors. This hypoxia is not a feature of normal tissues and preferentially protects the hypoxic tumor cells from radiation injury (10). Oxygen delivery to hypoxic cells will be augmented by the eradication of well oxygenated tumor cells with the first fractions in a course of radiotherapy, and an increased radiation sensitivity will result for those cells that were protected by hypoxia during these same treatments, facilitating their eradication by subsequent treatments. There is also evidence that the hypoxic microenvironment is a selection force that acts in concert with the inherent genetic instability of tumor cells to select for more adverse and aggressive phenotypes, including those with *p53* mutations (11–13).

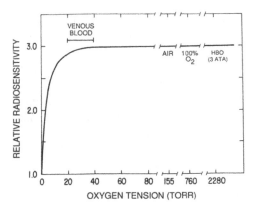

Figure 2 Effect of oxygen tension on tumor cell radiosensitivity. Response to irradiation was normalized to the response for maximally hypoxic cells. Oxygen tensions found in venous capillary blood provide maximal radiation sensitization; no augmentation is seen for supraphysiologic oxygen tensions.

Experiments conducted to assess the sensitivity of cells at certain points in the cell cycle have determined that cells in the G2M phase are the most sensitive to the effects of irradiation, and that cells in the S phase are most resistant (9). More and less radioresistant and radiosensitive phases in the cell cycle are thought to relate to the temporal expression of genes that detect and respond to DNA damage (14). After exposure to ionizing radiation, the progression of cells through the cell cycle is typically delayed at G1S and G2M. These delays, or checkpoints, allow surveillance of the genome and repair of chromosomal abnormalities to occur before they are irrevocably incorporated into the genome. Deficiencies in the repair of radiation damage in tumor cells relative to normal cells may be related to problems with appropriately pausing at these checkpoints, and should allow deletion of tumor cells and sparing of normal tissue. The temporal progression through the cell cycle postirradiation will result in the redistribution of cells from more radioresistant to more radiosensitive phases as successive fractions of radiation are delivered, called "redistribution." Factors other than the four R's of radiobiology that modulate cellular radiosensitivity include a number of things that are not directly related to DNA damage, such as presence and activation state of numerous interconnected and complementary membrane bound and intracellular signaling pathways (15,16).

The intrinsic radiation sensitivity of different cell lines is known to differ in controlled experimental conditions (17), and can also apparently be altered by interactions between the stroma and the tumor cells (18). The probabilities of tumor control and of damage to normal tissue both increase with increasing radiation dose. These probabilities mapped against dose describe sigmoid curves (Fig. 3), but the exact shapes of the sigmoid curves and the relative positions of these curves to each other for any given patient or tumor are unknown; empirical clinical evidence has governed the treatment techniques that have developed for treating most tumors. In radiotherapy, the relative position of these curves defines the therapeutic ratio. This is simply expressed as the ratio of the probability of tumor control to the probability of a complication.

Some tumors, such as CNS germinomas, are easily cured with well-tolerated doses of fractionated irradiation, while others (gliomas) are so seldom cured by tolerable doses of radiation that it may be reasonably considered to "never" occur. Experimental data shows that cellular responses to individual radiation doses vary. It is well recognized and acknowledged that no matter what type of cell is being irradiated, large doses will kill proportionately more cells than small doses. Radiosurgical treatments may be more effective than fractionated irradiation for eradicating certain tumors for this reason (19,20). The shape of the dose–response curves shown in Figure 1 is attributed to the ability of cells to repair small amounts of genomic radiation damage. The "shoulder" of the curve represents the repairable damage. In clinical radiation therapy, the small amount of damage done in a single

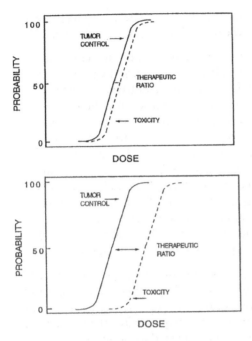

Figure 3 The therapeutic ratio may be increased by increasing the effect of a treatment such as radiation on a tumor or by decreasing the effect on normal tissues. Increasing the separation between the curves increases the chance of an uncomplicated and successful treatment. The relative position and inflection of these curves is unknown, and for certain tumors, the curve for toxicity may lie to the left of the curve for tumor control.

treatment is repeated numerous times to provide durable tumor control without unacceptable normal tissue toxicity.

The use of larger fraction sizes to increase the damage to the tumor appears to be a simple method for increasing the antitumor effect for a given total dose of fractionated radiation. Unfortunately, the effect on slowly proliferating normal tissues (such as the brain) is increased as well (21,22). Treatment of normal brain cells with high daily doses of radiation is likely to cause unacceptable delayed side effects such as leukoencephalopathy, atrophy, and even frank tissue necrosis if the patient lives long enough (23). Treatment techniques that use large daily fractions and include significant volumes of normal nerve cells in the volume receiving high doses of irradiation are to be discouraged except in the palliative treatment of patients with very limited survivals. Any additional tumor cell kill that can be achieved with the use of radiation sensitizers or other substances that do not concomitantly increase normal tissue damage will increase the therapeutic ratio (Fig. 3).

Radiotherapy Physics

A variety of methods have been used since the discovery of radioactivity by Becquerel and X rays by Röntgen to treat CNS tumors with ionizing radiation. Most of these efforts were made to try to increase the therapeutic ratio using the relatively primitive equipment of the time. These may have started with Alexander Graham Bell's provocative observation in 1903 that ...

the Röntgen X-rays, and the rays emitted by radium, have been found to have a marked curative effect upon external cancers, but that the effects upon deep seated cancers have not thus far proved satisfactory. It has occurred to me that one reason for the unsatisfactory nature of these latter experiments arises from the fact that the rays have been applied externally, thus having to pass through healthy tissues of various depths in order to reach the cancerous matter. The Crookes's tube from which the Röntgen rays are emitted is, of course, too bulky to be admitted into the middle of a mass of cancer, but there is no reason why a tiny fragment of radium sealed up in a fine glass tube should not be inserted into the very heart of the cancer, thus acting on the diseased material. Would it not be worth while making experiments along this line? (24)

The vast majority of present day radiation therapy for CNS tumors uses specialized particle accelerators developed for medical applications (linear accelerators, or linacs) to direct high-energy X rays at the tumor. Nearly all currently used linacs are interfaced with computers that help monitor their functioning and ensure that complicated treatments are delivered as prescribed.

A linac's deeply penetrating photon beams can be precisely positioned so as to allow uniform radiation treatment of the entire CNS or of a very small target within the CNS. A linac's gantry (which points the radiation beam at the target) pivots about a point in space called the "isocenter." The size of the isocenter for most medical linacs is of the order of approximately 1 to 2 mm, and the planning process usually locates the isocenter in or near the center of the volume being treated with irradiation. The collimator, which shapes the radiation beams coming from the gantry, can rotate to improve the conformality of the shaping that is performed, and the couch, upon which the patient lies to receive treatment, has the ability to carry out translations in all three primary axes and rotations in the plane of the table-top (yaw). Specialized couches can also correct for pitch and roll, but these are not commonly available. These specialized features for positioning the patient and aiming the radiation therapy are necessary to reproducibly direct the radiation therapy to the exact volume to which the radiation oncologist has prescribed treatment.

The relative amount of radiation energy deposited by a photon beam at various depths in tissue is directly related to the energy of the photons. Low photon energy was a major shortcoming of all external irradiation equipment until well after World War II. Whereas kilovoltage X rays will deposit the highest doses in the skin, megavoltage beams from a linac do not deposit their maximum amount of energy until a depth of up to several centimeters has been reached. The development of linacs has permitted doses to be delivered to tissues CNS that would previously have been limited by the tolerance of the scalp. For a given dose being delivered to an intracranial target, the use of higher energy beams will deliver lower doses to normal tissues than will lower energy beams; this simple factor can improve the therapeutic ratio.

Several significant differences exist between the various types of ionizing radiation that are used in radiation therapy today and how the energy from these sources is deposited in tissue. High-energy X rays and gamma rays are attenuated, but not completely stopped by the tissues through which they pass. Doses of externally administered radiation are thus delivered to normal tissues on entry and exit. Charged particles such as electrons, protons, and heavy nuclei deposit some energy en route to the target, but very little energy is deposited deep to the target (25). Encapsulated radionuclide sources may be implanted into tumors (brachytherapy) and unsealed radioactive sources such as ^{90}Y or ^{32}P may be placed into cystic tumors such as craniopharyngiomas or cystic gliomas (26). These radionuclides emit very low energy radiation, which does not penetrate deeply, and thus must be put directly in contact with the tumor. Boron–neutron capture therapy uses epithermal neutron irradiation of boron containing compounds that will undergo a radioactive decay if a neutron is captured by the boron nucleus. Preferential accumulation of the boronated compounds within the tumor nuclei is required to maximally improve the therapeutic ratio with this technique, as the charged particles produced from the radioactive decay have very limited penetration in tissue (27). These specialized methods of delivering radiation therapy are used at a limited number of centers for a limited subset of treatments, but are employed because their special physical radiation dose distribution characteristics can increase the therapeutic ratio between the tumor and adjacent normal tissues.

As stated above, the vast majority of radiation therapy for tumors in the CNS is linac based, and the vast majority of treatments are administered using fractionation to protect normal tissues. Current-day cross-sectional imaging can accurately identify the spatial location of tumors in the CNS and a course of radiation therapy can be appropriately planned using fractionated or SRS techniques.

Single fraction SRS, despite its ability to target lesions with submillimeter accuracy, is generally limited to intracranial targets less than or equal to 3.5 cm in maximal diameter because of concerns about the tolerance of adjacent tissues to incidental irradiation that occurs as photon beams enter and exit the targeted tissue as well as from internally scattered radiation (28,29). A tumor at the upper size limit or larger should only rarely be treated with stereotactic radiosurgery in preference to fractionated radiotherapy or resection, and great care must be taken when considering stereotactic radiosurgery for tumors close to the optic nerves and chiasm (30,31).

The process of planning stereotactic radiosurgery is generally based upon an imaging study obtained immediately after the placement of a minimally invasive stereotactic headframe, and a presumption is made that there will be no shift of coordinates between any targeting performed on the basis of that scan and the time of treatment delivery later that day, given that the localization equipment (the stereotactic frame) is rigidly attached to the outer table of the patient's skull.

Submillimeter localization is not possible with fractionated irradiation. If all other aspects of imaging and planning are assumed to be of the same quality as for radiosurgery, the treatment accuracy is limited primarily by the accuracy of daily treatment positioning (32). In developing a radiotherapy treatment plan, the anticipated positioning changes that may occur during the delivery of that planned course of radiation therapy should be incorporated into the planning process (33).

For CNS irradiation, a custom-fitted thermoplastic mask is frequently used to help with immobilization and daily localization. This mask is made with the patient positioned as specified for daily radiation treatment, and a treatment planning CT scan of the cranium (or occasionally the entire craniospinal axis) is done to identify bony anatomic landmarks, air filled structures, and soft tissues. After developing a radiation therapy plan, these images can be used to generate digitally reconstructed radiographs that will show the setup positioning and the anatomy that will be directly traversed by any radiation beams aimed at the targeted tissues. These can be compared to the films that are obtained with the patient in the treatment position on the linac to ensure that the patient is correctly positioned to treat the tumor as prescribed (33). The accuracy of reproducing positioning with a well-made custom formed thermoplastic mask is generally felt to be on the order of approximately 2 mm (34).

For CNS tumors, MR imaging is often incorporated into the radiotherapy treatment planning process. Various algorithms can rigidly register an MR imaging study to a CT imaging study, reformat the MRI study, and redisplay its voxels within the CT scan's geometric parameters. From the registered, reformatted, redisplayed MRI scan, the determination of the intracranial location of tumors not readily visualized on a CT scan is facilitated. Different MRI pulse sequences (e.g., FLAIR, T1 post gadolinium administration with or without fat saturation techniques, etc.) can be used to help clearly identify the location of pathology and normal tissues (35).

The process of planning radiation therapy is only started with the acquisition of these various imaging studies and their cross-registration. The target that is to be treated must be identified and segmented out, or contoured on a slice-by-slice basis using specialized software on a dedicated workstation. Relevant normal tissues must also be contoured so that a calculation of the radiation doses delivered to the tumor and normal structures can be calculated.

For the past century, radiation therapy has been planned by experts who were familiar with commonly used techniques of aiming radiation beams from various directions at the tumor, and who could calculate the doses of radiation received by normal tissues and by the tumor if uniformly intense X-ray beams of certain energies were applied in certain relative proportions. Only coplanar beams could be used and determining the dose on planes other than those that passed the isocenter was rarely if ever done because of the difficulty of the calculations involved. This dosimetric process of calculation has been speeded by the advent of high-speed computers and specialized software programs (33). High-speed computer calculations allowed noncoplanar beams to be used routinely, and multiple iterations of a plan could be calculated to compare various approaches in treatment delivery. The use of coplanar or noncoplanar beams that are precisely shaped to match the tumor's configuration from angle from which the beam is incident upon the tumor is called three-dimensional conformal radiation therapy (3DCRT). This approach, through the careful selection of radiation beam directions and energies can frequently allow critical structures near the tumor to receive doses of radiation low enough to avoid injury while generating dosimetrically uniform treatment plans that neither underdose the tumor nor overdose contiguous normal tissues.

In the past decade, computers and software programs have been developed that have allowed this planning process to be turned on its head. This is known as intensity-modulated radiation therapy (IMRT) (36,37). In IMRT, the target and normal tissues are identified for the computer, and beam energies, entry points and dose constraints are given for the tumor and for normal tissues. Relative rankings of importance are provided to algorithmically prioritize conflicting dosimetric goals (e.g., a high dose to the tumor and a low dose to immediately adjacent normal tissue). The computer then selects beamlets (subdivisions of the X-ray beams that have been chosen) of varying intensity and calculates how closely these summed beamlets will come to achieving the goals that have been set. These beamlets may be as small as 3 to 5 mm in dimension, depending on the hardware that has been installed on the linac to deliver IMRT. The intensity of the radiation being delivered will vary from beamlet-to-beamlet, which is a very significant difference from the uniform radiation beams that have been a foundation of conventionally planned radiation therapy. This great sensitivity to position of a target or a normal tissue with relationship to beam delivery (because of the great heterogeneity of dose delivery that is possible with IMRT) has heightened concern about reproducible positioning for IMRT treatment of CNS and other tumors (38).

Multiple iterations are commonly required to obtain an acceptable IMRT plan; the instructions given to the computer must be adjusted with each iteration to refine the process so as to more closely approach the desired dosimetric goals. IMRT has not been shown to be able to dramatically alter any of the parameters that affect the tolerance of CNS irradiation for the vast majority of clinical settings; even cochlear protection during posterior fossa irradiation is not clearly improved with IMRT compared to 3DCRT (39). Adequately powered clinical trials with appropriately designed instruments to quantify the benefits that may follow from treatment with IMRT still need to be performed for all CNS tumors (38).

Treatment of benign tumors close to critical structures may be one potential use for IMRT, where the sculpting of dose distributions with IMRT may allow a lowering of long-term treatment-related morbidity. It may be that IMRT will be used instead of 3DCRT because of the ability to automatically generate plans that meet specific dosimetric goals across a broad range of intracranial tumor locations. Preferential dosimetric sparing of eloquent cortex may become a routine therapeutic goal with IMRT. Determination of whether the parameters that will be most appropriate for IMRT are the same as for 3DCRT may be clearer as further experience is gained with this treatment technique (38).

No matter how simple or complex a plan, once it has been generated and approved and any physical confirmation of plan parameters that may be required for safety and quality assurance purposes has been completed, the patient returns to the department for films to be taken on the linac to document the accuracy of positioning for treatment. Once these portal films have been approved, daily treatment can start. For treatment devices such as the Gamma Knife, that do not permit portal films to be done, the radiation oncologist's approval of both the radiosurgery treatment plan (following a review of the dosimetry on the treatment planning computer) and the accuracy of the patient positioning must be obtained prior to starting treatment.

APPLICATIONS

Involved Field

This is one of the commonest ways that radiation therapy is used in the CNS. In the planning process, the tumor is localized in space, and beams are chosen to treat the volume that includes the tumor. The treatment is usually given with two or more beams; consideration should be given to shaping the radiation beams to protect normal tissues that are not at risk because of physical barriers (such as a dural surface) to tumor spread. Thought must be given to the uniformity of the radiation dose distribution and the location of any volumes that may be getting more or less dose than that delivered to the isocenter. Underdosing tumor is likely to result in poorer tumor control; overdosing adjacent normal brain tissue may cause radiation injury to develop. The location of critical normal tissues (such as the optic nerves and chiasm and the brainstem) to the radiation beams merits consideration during the planning process, so as to minimize the risk of a potentially avoidable treatment-related complication. These normal tissues are relatively hardy, though and may be anticipated to tolerate doses that are 85% to 90% of what is being delivered to a tumor in an aggressive radiation therapy treatment program.

Involved field radiation therapy is effectively used for all manner of benign and malignant intracranial primary tumors. Daily doses of 1.8 to 3 Gray or more may be used, with a total dose delivered of up to 63 Gray (in seven weeks) to 45 Gray (in three weeks). 3DCRT and IMRT techniques can be sued to deliver fractionated irradiation to involved fields.

Whole Brain Radiation Therapy

Whole brain radiation therapy (WBRT) is supposed to uniformly irradiate the entire intracranial contents. Care must be taken, as the treatment is planned, to not accidentally exclude tissues that should be treated or include tissues that should not be irradiated. The prototype field for this treatment treats the CNS contents from the right and left sides with a rectangular portal that has its inferior border located along the skull base. Blocks can be introduced to prevent direct irradiation of the eyes. A modification of WBRT includes the uppermost cervical spine within the radiotherapy treatment volume. This modification of the radiotherapy portal facilitates safe junctioning of radiotherapy portals to treat the spine, either as separate palliative fields, or as part of combined treatment for craniospinal irradiation.

WBRT is useful when the entire CNS is felt to be potentially involved with tumor cells. WBRT is most commonly used for the treatment of metastatic cancer to the brain, either as a treatment of known disease or as a prophylactic treatment for presumed disease, but has been used to treat other conditions that affect the entire CNS, such as primary CNS lymphoma. Doses between 1.8 and 3.0 to 4.0 Gray are commonly used with total doses that range from 45 to 50.4 Gray (in 5–5.5 weeks to 30 Gray in 2 weeks or 20 Gray in 1 week). Prophylactic treatment delivers lower total doses, as the presumed burden of disease is smaller and the risk–benefit ratio for higher dose treatment is unfavorable. Some clinicians have developed IMRT techniques to treat the cranial contents while decreasing the dose to the scalp, and lessening radiotherapy-related alopecia (40).

It does not appear that one fractionation scheme is superior to another in controlling macroscopic brain metastases—habits and reimbursement incentives may play a more significant role in management decisions (41). It appears that the neurocognitive effects of uncontrolled tumor progression in the CNS are much more significant than the morbidities of CNS irradiation (42,43).

Craniospinal

Craniospinal radiotherapy matches the radiotherapy portals being used to treat the cranial contents with one or more radiation therapy portals to treat the spine. It is used to treat diseases such as medulloblastoma and primary CNS germinoma, when there is a risk of cerebrospinal fluid dissemination throughout the neuraxis. Technical improvements in radiation delivery are responsible for a significant portion of the increases in cures for these malignancies compared to only a few decades ago. Great care must be taken in the planning and delivery of these treatments to ensure that there is no component of the spine that receives successive daily treatment by two sets of radiation fields. Such an occurrence could lead to radiation injury to the spinal cord that would result in paralysis from that level down. Similarly, incomplete coverage of the CNS at the skull base or at the junction between radiation portals or at the distal end of the thecal sac in the sacrum may lead to recurrence of disease (44,45). Craniospinal radiotherapy is one of the most exacting radiation therapy treatments performed; there are probably good indications for this being done at larger centers when such a referral is feasible (46). There appear to possibly be advantages to proton therapy for craniospinal treatment, but long-term follow-up is still lacking with this treatment technique (25,47).

The homogeneous irradiation of the craniospinal axis is nearly always combined with a more intense localized (involved field) treatment to the primary tumor site (e.g., the posterior fossa or the tumor bed for medulloblastoma or the ventricular ependymal surfaces or the suprasellar/pineal region for germinoma) (48,49). One of the major acute toxicities of craniospinal irradiation is cytopenias that can be lifethreatening or even fatal. Halting craniospinal irradiation and administering treatment to the smaller involved field (or "conedown") portals is often required when platelet or granulocyte counts are profoundly low. Once counts have recovered, the craniospinal treatment can often be completed without further interruption.

Stereotactic

Stereotactic treatment, by virtue of its extremely focal nature, demands the best possible patient immobilization, target localization, and treatment delivery. The foundation of the discipline has been rigid, frame-based immobilization, but the term is now being applied to noninvasive immobilization techniques that approach submillimeter positioning accuracy. In single session stereotactic radiosurgery, tumors less than or equal to 3.5 cm in diameter can be targeted and treated in a single session with acceptable acute and delayed toxicities and with very good tumor control rates.

For metastatic disease to the brain, there is a survival benefit for delivering SRS after whole brain irradiation for single metastases (50). There are a number of reports of SRS used in the absence of whole brain irradiation for metastatic disease to the CNS, but no phase III trials have been completed to evaluate whether or not it is safe to omit the fractionated irradiation as part of the initial management of brain metastases (51). Guidelines have been promulgated to try to guide appropriate use of radiosurgery for brain metastases (52). Some investigators have detected what they believe may be neurocognitive sequelae from radiosurgery delivered to one to three brain metastases without whole brain irradiation (53).

Some clinicians have reported series in which a radiosurgical approach was essayed, but because of tumor conformation or concerns about normal tissue toxicity, the entire tumor was not treated. This has resulted in high rates of local recurrence of tumor (54,55). Other clinicians' concerns regarding the dose of scattered radiation delivered in some situations to adjacent normal tissues (such as the optic nerves or brain stem) in single dose radiosurgery and regarding the accuracy of their linacs in delivering treatment to very small targets led to the development of what has been termed fractionated stereotactic radiation therapy (FSRT). There is a premium on reproducible immobilization that approaches that possible with SRS for FSRT. How often it is actually achieved is dependent upon a host of patient, equipment, and facility-dependent factors.

FSRT loses the physical accuracy of dose delivery and the high logs of cell kill that can be achieved with SRS, but it can exploit radiobiological processes that will increase the therapeutic ratio for certain clinical scenarios. Although FSRT approaches started at the time when IMRT was not clinically used, this approach does not prevent IMRT from being used to try to further increase the therapeutic ratio. Geometrically complex tumors can be treated with plans that include volumes of normal brain tissue that could not be treated with single fraction stereotactic radiosurgery; the volumes of normal brain tissue treated to high doses are much smaller than would be treated with conventional 3DCRT or IMRT. This approach should improve the therapeutic ratio, as long as the doses that irradiated normal tissues can tolerate are not exceeded.

As yet, there are only a limited number of series of patients treated with FSRT reported in the medical literature. Not unexpectedly, there are no phase III comparisons to surgical intervention, single fraction stereotactic radiosurgery, or conventionally planned and delivered radiation therapy. Reviews of results for stereotactic approaches appear to vary slightly from center-to-center, probably based upon selection criteria, differences in target delineation, or dose prescription (56–60). Lower complication rates for normal tissues might be anticipated for tumors that are immediately adjacent to critical normal tissues through the use of fractionated treatment approaches, and this may be true for vestibular schwannomas (61–63). It is unlikely that a phase III trial comparing FSRT and SRS will ever be performed for vestibular schwannomas to determine the comparative advantages for the equally important endpoints of tumor control and the preservation of CN V, VII, and VIII function.

Perhaps not surprisingly, some initial reports of FSRT for parasellar meningiomas and pituitary adenomas have a high rate of visual and other toxicity (64–66). It is possible that these complications may have stemmed from problems with inaccurate reproduction of patient positioning set up and a lack of dose homogeneity that occurred as treatment conformality was emphasized. Doses of radiation to the optic nerves and chiasm were delivered that were greater than the recognized tolerance of these structures. Also, just as in single fraction radiosurgery, inadequate dosimetric coverage of the tumors may have led to high local recurrence rates, which certainly should be considered among treatment-related toxicities. The morbidities detailed in these pioneering reports of high-precision, highly conformal fractionated irradiation for intracranial tumors are interesting, and should serve as signals to guide those who follow on how to improve the therapeutic outcome with these treatment approaches.

Brachytherapy

This treatment technique relies upon radioactive sources being placed into the tissues to be treated with ionizing radiation. It allows differential irradiation and relative sparing of normal tissue. The energy spectrum of the radioactive emissions from brachytherapy sources is generally low enough that the dose delivered to normal tissues is much attenuated by the tumor tissue into which the sources are placed. Historically, radiation sources such as ^{227}Ra or ^{137}Cs were used. Sources more commonly used at present, such as ^{125}I or ^{192}Ir, are encapsulated in metal to avoid environmental contamination and to filter out the lowest energy radiation. The gamma rays produced by these radioactive elements are not so powerful as those from historically used sources. At the time of a neurosurgical procedure, these radiation sources are placed into the tumor to deliver treatment. The sources may be removed in a few days time or may be left there permanently.

Brachytherapy techniques have been used as a way of delivering a higher dose of radiation after external beam irradiation to the site felt to be at highest risk of local progression of tumor. Several randomized trials of brachytherapy for malignant gliomas have been carried out, and none were able to show an increased survival with the addition of this specialized radiation (67,68). Brachytherapy in conjunction with hyperthermia has been shown to prolong the survival of patients with recurrent malignant gliomas (69). Brachytherapy has also been used for low-grade gliomas (70,71).

A novel FDA approved brachytherapy device has recently been brought into clinical practice. This balloon-like device is placed within a surgical resection cavity and is subsequently filled with an ^{125}I containing solution to deliver uniform radiation to the margin of the resection cavity. Following the delivery of the prescribed dose of radiation, the radioactive solution is removed, with a subsequent surgical procedure required to remove the device. Broad experience with this system is still lacking (72).

Radiation-Sensitizing Agents

Increasing the ratio of tumor cell to normal tissue toxicity for a given dose of CNS irradiation, be it WBRT, involved field irradiation, or treatment with focal techniques, has been a major research interest in radiation biology for decades. Based on radiobiological principles, clinical trials have been mounted that have attempted to increase the therapeutic ratio by delivering the radiation faster (by giving more than one fraction per day or more than five days/wk—essentially, by using radiation as the radiation sensitizer) (3,4,73), by changing oxygen delivery parameters to the tumor (74), and by using standard chemotherapy drugs and agents that are known from bench research to be radiation sensitizers (75), hypoxic cell cytotoxins (76), antiangiogenesis drugs (77), etc. A large number of strategies and agents have been evaluated over the years, and newly developed agents are still being tested for activity (74,78). There are, as yet, despite decades of investigation, no generally recognized clinically useful radiation-sensitizing agents (41). The desire to increase the cytotoxicity of radiation by adding compounds to increase tumor cell kill in the CNS has not been able to favorably and decisively increase the therapeutic ratio. It is hoped that novel compounds expressly designed to take advantage of gene expression and repression by hypoxia-responsive signaling pathways will be better able to achieve this goal (79,80).

Molecular biological advances have been applied to evaluate the causes of varying radiation responses in various tissues. A detailed understanding is still far from at hand, but studies elucidating important pathways in radiation response and toxicity are being conducted (79–81). Knowledge gained from radiobiological investigations will undoubtedly benefit patients through novel strategies that will increase the therapeutic ratio for the use of ionizing radiation to treat tumors.

Complications of CNS Irradiation

The clinical complications of CNS irradiation may be described using several different classification schemes. One commonly used scheme is to separate early from late complications, where early (usually reversible) complications occur during or immediately after a course of treatment, and late (usually irreversible) complications are those that may occur several months to years after a course of treatment (82). Radiation-related complications may occur because of incidental or direct irradiation of normal tissues in the treatment of CNS tumors and may occur as a systemic, or "abscopal" side effect. Some sequelae may be lifethreatening or fatal (83). Others, such as alopecia or fatigue may seem to border on the trivial to a physician, but may have devastating effects upon quality of life. The patient and his or her family are entitled to be apprised of possible radiotherapy related side effects that may arise, and should be provided assistance with coping with any treatment-related sequelae to the maximum extent possible. Using a temporospatial approach to describe side effects will help organize a complete description of possible side effects to patients. Describing anticipated and possible side effects, with an assessment of the likelihood of its occurrence, and a statement of whether it may be temporary or permanent will help the patient identify what he or she may want to hear about in more detail.

During the planning process, consideration of possible acute toxicities that might be minimized or avoided by changing the angle of entry of a radiation beam is good medicine, as it will make both the patient's treatment and the management of treatment-related toxicities easier. During the course of radiation therapy, the radiation oncologist will monitor the acute side effects of treatment and intervene appropriately to treat radiation-related symptoms. It is most important to monitor and appropriately adjust dexamethasone doses for treatment-related edema that worsens any presenting neurologic signs. The lowest doses that maintain the highest possible level of function should be used. The metabolism of anticonvulsant agents may be affected by medications such as dexamethasone, so as steroid doses changes, the serum levels of any required anticonvulsant agents should be monitored.

Radiotherapy almost always causes alopecia in the incidentally irradiated scalp. Places where the skin is tangentially irradiated may develop some hyperpigmentation and dry desquamation, because a higher physical dose is delivered to superficial tissues by a glancing beam than by a beam that is orthogonal to the skin surface. Dry skin may take several weeks to remit, and it may take several months before new hair growth starts. Hair that regrows may be sparser, darker, and more curly than the hair that grew before irradiation. General alopecia is expected after whole brain irradiation, and focal irradiation will lead to focal alopecia. Radiosurgical treatment of a meningioma or metastasis adjacent to the calvarial surface will cause alopecia overlying the tumor. Alopecia from radiotherapy is generally temporary, but the extent and timing of the recovery of hair follicles is related to the delivered follicular radiotherapy dose.

The skull and nondividing tissues such as the connective tissue of the scalp and meninges tolerate radiation without difficulty, but these tissues may not heal as promptly as unirradiated tissues if a postirradiation craniotomy is required. Irradiation of the meninges is generally asymptomatic, though occasionally patients develop minor meningeal irritation that results in headaches. Acetaminophen is generally able to alleviate these headaches. Auditory sequelae are common enough to merit description. Treatment that involves the ear may occasionally cause occlusion of the external auditory canal with desquamated debris. Irradiation of the middle ear may lead to fluid accumulation that may require an α-agonist to facilitate drainage through the Eustachian tube. Occasionally the placement of a grommet in the tympanic membrane by an otorhinolaryngologist is required. Irradiation of the cochlea may cause high-frequency hearing loss, and this may be exacerbated by platinum-based chemotherapy. Hearing loss from cochlear damage will be permanent, but the other auditory side effects will remit shortly after irradiation ceases.

Marrow irradiation that occurs as part of cranial irradiation usually only causes some minor abnormalities in the hematologic laboratory profile. The larger proportion of the marrow volume that is treated in craniospinal irradiation will cause a significant risk of cytopenias (thrombocytopenia and leukopenia) that may be lifethreatening or fatal. The effects of this marrow irradiation will not be reversed immediately upon cessation of craniospinal radiotherapy, necessitating twice weekly monitoring of the blood counts in the middle and later parts of a course of craniospinal treatment so that treatment may be stopped before cytopenias require a medical intervention with transfusions or cytokine therapies.

No specific complaints are associated with therapeutic radiation to brain and nervous tissues. This is probably because of the absence of brain-specific innervation. Headaches from meningeal irritation or exacerbation of preexisting tumor-related deficits may develop and are generally responsive to dexamethasone therapy. Radiation treatment may be associated with general side effects such as fatigue or loss of appetite. Occasionally the sense of taste will change so that some foods or flavors are less appetizing. This side effect is not secondary to irradiation of the oral cavity, but is an abscopal effect. Treatment-related fatigue and any change experienced in the sense of taste will improve on a week-by-week basis after irradiation ends.

There can be a period of time, after radiotherapy has finished, in which a profound drowsiness can occur (84). This "somnolence syndrome" is generally temporary. It is assumed to be linked to the apoptosis of CNS and endothelial cells that occurs with therapeutic irradiation (80). A patient can lose physical conditioning as a result of the fatigue experienced during the irradiation; experiencing the somnolence syndrome will further worsen any remaining physical reserves that a patient may have for carrying out self-care or other usual activities of daily life. Similarly, L'Hermitte's syndrome will be experienced for several months by some proportion of patients who receive radiotherapy treatment that includes the cervicothoracic spinal cord, and it, too is felt to be related to radiation-related early changes in oligodendroglial cell populations (80).

Treatment of the hypothalamus and pituitary can lead to an early menopause or other symptoms or signs of anterior pituitary insufficiency (85,86). This generally takes several years to a decade or more to become manifest, but if it occurs, it will require ongoing medical management on a lifelong basis. It is surpassingly unusual to have water balance derangement from irradiation or to have hypothalamic injury that results in bizarre somatic syndromes (86).

Radiation treatment of the brain will lead, over time, to problems with neurocognitive functioning. The problems appear to be dose and volume related, and the deficits that are induced by radiotherapy appear to have a course that waxes and wanes over time (87). Even radiosurgery can apparently induce some subtle deficits (53). There is no useful data to guide clinicians counseling patients regarding the likelihood of adverse sequelae on quality of life with early versus late WBRT for brain metastases or for low grade gliomas. Careful use of ionizing radiation when treating the tumor so as to minimize tumor-related or iatrogenic sequelae will result in the best possible outcomes for patients who receive radiation as part of the management of their brain tumors.

Radiotherapy's adverse effects on the CNS are related to dose, volume, treatment duration, and fraction size. Molecular tools and better neurobiological insight have permitted experiments to be done in rodent models and in cellular systems that are elucidating the similarities and differences between radiation damage to the CNS and other types of damage (80). The manifestations of radiation damage in the CNS is not merely endothelial cell or oligodendroglial cell injury being expressed, but is a dynamic continuum after the initial injury that is modulated by a number of interacting processes.

The nonspecific stress response elicited by injury from CNS irradiation modifies gene expression profiles, with different genes expressed over time (88,89). Postirradiation endothelial cell apoptosis initiates blood–brain barrier disruption within hours, and irradiation also triggers a brisk apoptotic response in oligodendroglial cells (90–92). The relationship of these early events to late radiation changes has not yet been sorted out. The limited responses that the CNS is capable of manifesting to injury means that the reactions of the CNS to ionizing radiation damage overlap with those for inflammation, ischemia, and other injuries. It is theorized that the overlapping cytokine cascades that are initiated by the original radiation injury combined with radiation's ability to inhibit normal neural stem cell regeneration may lead to the microenvironmental changes of hypoxia and inflammation that ultimately result in the late cell loss that is perhaps unique to radiation injury (93). The elucidation of these molecular pathways in greater detail may provide clear targets for molecular interventions to decrease radiation related morbidity for the CNS (79,94).

REFERENCES

1. McPherson CM, Sawaya R. Technologic advances in surgery for brain tumors: tools of the trade in the modern neurosurgical operating room. J Natl Compr Canc Netw 2005; 3(5):705–710.
2. Kesari S, Ramakrishna N, Sauvageot C, et al. Targeted molecular therapy of malignant gliomas. Curr Neurol Neurosci Rep 2005; 5(3):186–197.
3. Sawaya R. Chairman's reflection on the past, present and future of neurosurgical oncology. J Neurooncol 2004; 69(1–3):19–23.
4. Simpson WJ, Platts ME. Fractionation study in the treatment of glioblastoma multiforme. Int J Radiat Oncol Biol Phys 1976; 1(7–8):639–644.
5. Dische S, Saunders MI. The CHART regimen and morbidity. Acta Oncol 1999; 38(2):147–152.

6. Withers HR. In: Lett J, Adler H, eds. Advances in Radiation Biology. Vol. 5. New York: Academic Press, 1975:241–271.
7. Bentzen SM. Quantitative clinical radiobiology. Acta Oncol 1993; 32(3):259–275.
8. Shrieve DC, Klish M, Wendland MM, et al. Basic principles of radiobiology, radiotherapy, and radiosurgery. Neurosurg Clin N Am 2004; 15(4):467–479.
9. Hall EJ. Radiobiology for the Radiobiologist. Philadelphia: Williams & Wilkins, 2000.
10. Carmeliet P, Jain RK. Angiogenesis in cancer and other diseases. Nature 2000; 407(6801):249–257.
11. Graeber TG, Osmanian C, Jacks T, et al. Hypoxia-mediated selection of cells with diminished apoptotic potential in solid tumours. Nature 1996; 379(6560): 88–91.
12. Vaupel P, Mayer A. Hypoxia and anemia: effects on tumor biology and treatment resistance. Transfus Clin Biol 2005; 12(1):5–10.
13. Bindra RS, Glazer PM. Genetic instability and the tumor microenvironment: towards the concept of microenvironment-induced mutagenesis. Mutat Res 2005; 569(1–2):75–85.
14. Li L, Zou L. Sensing, signaling, and responding to DNA damage: organization of the checkpoint pathways in mammalian cells. J Cell Biochem 2005; 94(2):298–306.
15. Dewey WC, Ling CC, Meyn RE. Radiation-induced apoptosis: relevance to radiotherapy. Int J Radiat Oncol Biol Phys 1995; 33(4):781–796.
16. Connell PP, Kron SJ, Weichselbaum RR. Relevance and irrelevance of DNA damage response to radiotherapy. DNA Repair (Amst). 2004; 3(8–9):1245–1251.
17. Taghian A, Ramsay J, Allalunis-Turner J, et al. Intrinsic radiation sensitivity may not be the major determinant of the poor clinical outcome of glioblastoma multiforme. Int J Radiat Oncol Biol Phys 1993; 25(2):243–249.
18. Moeller BJ, Cao Y, Li CY, et al. Radiation activates HIF-1 to regulate vascular radiosensitivity in tumors: role of reoxygenation, free radicals, and stress granules. Cancer Cell 2004; 5(5):429–441.
19. Flickinger JC, Loeffler JS, Larson DA. Stereotactic radiosurgery for intracranial malignancies. Oncology (Williston Park). 1994; 8(1):81–86.
20. Larson DA, Flickinger JC, Loeffler JS. The radiobiology of radiosurgery. Int J Radiat Oncol Biol Phys 1993; 25(3):557–561.
21. Lee AW, Foo W, Chappell R, et al. Effect of time, dose, and fractionation on temporal lobe necrosis following radiotherapy for nasopharyngeal carcinoma. Int J Radiat Oncol Biol Phys 1998; 40(1):35–42.
22. Sheline GE, Wara WM, Smith V. Therapeutic irradiation and brain injury. Int J Radiat Oncol Biol Phys 1980; 6(9):1215–1228.
23. Marks JE, Baglan RJ, Prassad SC, et al. Cerebral radionecrosis: incidence and risk in relation to dose, time, fractionation and volume. Int J Radiat Oncol Biol Phys 1981; 7(2):243–252.
24. Bell AG. Correspondence. Nature, 6 August 1903.
25. Levin WP, Kooy H, Loeffler JS, et al. Proton beam therapy. Br J Cancer 2005; 93(8):849–854.
26. Blackburn TP, Doughty D, Plowman PN. Stereotactic intracavitary therapy of recurrent cystic craniopharyngioma by instillation of 90Yttrium. Br J Neurosurg 1999; 13(4):359–365.

27. Gupta N, Gahbauer RA, Blue TE, et al. Common challenges and problems in clinical trials of boron neutron capture therapy of brain tumors. J Neurooncol 2003; 62(1–2):197–210.
28. Luxton G, Petrovich Z, Jozsef G, et al. Stereotactic radiosurgery: principles and comparison of treatment methods. Neurosurgery 1993; 32(2):241–259.
29. Flickinger JC. Dosimetry and dose-volume relationships in radiosurgery. In: Alexander E III, Loeffler JS, Lunsford LD, eds. Stereotactic Radiosurgery. New York: McGraw-Hill, 1993:31–41.
30. Suh JH, Vogelbaum MA, Barnett GH. Update of stereotactic radiosurgery for brain tumors. Curr Opin Neurol 2004; 17(6):681–686.
31. Tishler RB, Loeffler JS, Lunsford LD, et al. Tolerance of cranial nerves of the cavernous sinus to radiosurgery. Int J Radiat Oncol Biol Phys 1993; 27(2): 215–221.
32. Lightstone AW, Benedict SH, Bova FJ, et al. American Association of Physicists in Medicine Radiation Therapy Committee. Intracranial stereotactic positioning systems: Report of the American Association of Physicists in Medicine Radiation Therapy Committee Task Group no. 68. Med Phys 2005; 32(7):2380–2398.
33. Fraass B, Doppke K, Hunt M, et al. American Association of Physicists in Medicine Radiation Therapy Committee Task Group 53: quality assurance for clinical radiotherapy treatment planning. Med Phys 1998; 25(10):1773–1829.
34. Thornton AF Jr., Ten Haken RK, Gerhardsson A, et al. Three-dimensional motion analysis of an improved head immobilization system for simulation, CT, MRI, and PET imaging. Radiother Oncol 1991; 20(4):224–228.
35. Knisely JPS, Yue N, Chen Z, et al. Automatic three dimensional co-registration of diagnostic MRI and treatment planning CT for brain tumor radiotherapy treatment planning. Int J Radiat Oncol Biol Phys 1999; 45:3(suppl 1):190.
36. Fraass BA, Kessler ML, McShan DL, et al. Optimization and clinical use of multisegment intensity-modulated radiation therapy for high-dose conformal therapy. Semin Radiat Oncol 1999; 9(1):60–77.
37. Webb S. The physical basis of IMRT and inverse planning. Br J Radiol 2003; 76(910):678–689.
38. Knisely JPS. Intensity Modulated Radiation Therapy, Brain Talk, Vol. 7–2, Harrisburg, PA: International Radiosurgery Support Association 2002.
39. Breen SL, Kehagioglou P, Usher C, et al. A comparison of conventional, conformal and intensity-modulated coplanar radiotherapy plans for posterior fossa treatment. Br J Radiol 2004; 77(921):768–774.
40. Roberge D, Parker W, Niazi TM, OliVares M. Treating the contents and not the container: dosimetric Study of hair-sparing whole brain intensity modulated radiation therapy. Technol Cancer Res Treat, 2005 Oct; 4(5):567–70.
41. Tsao MN, Lloyd NS, Wong RK, et al. Supportive Care Guidelines Group of Cancer Care Ontario's Program in Evidence-based Care. Radiotherapeutic management of brain metastases: a systematic review and meta-analysis. Cancer Treat Rev 2005; 31(4):256–273.
42. Meyers CA, Smith JA, Bezjak A, et al. Neurocognitive function and progression in patients with brain metastases treated with whole-brain radiation and motexafin gadolinium: results of a randomized phase III trial. J Clin Oncol 2004; 22(1):157–165.

43. Klein M, Heimans JJ, Aaronson NK, et al. Effect of radiotherapy and other treatment-related factors on mid-term to long-term cognitive sequelae in low-grade gliomas: a comparative study. Lancet 2002; 360(9343):1361–1368.
44. Miralbell R, Bleher A, Huguenin P, et al. Pediatric medulloblastoma: radiation treatment technique and patterns of failure. Int J Radiat Oncol Biol Phys 1997; 37(3):523–529.
45. Scharf CB, Paulino AC, Goldberg KN. Determination of the inferior border of the thecal sac using magnetic resonance imaging: implications on radiation therapy treatment planning. Int J Radiat Oncol Biol Phys 1998; 41(3):621–624.
46. Michalski JM, Klein EE, Gerber R. Method to plan, administer, and verify supine craniospinal irradiation. J Appl Clin Med Phys 2002; 3(4):310–316.
47. St Clair WH, Adams JA, Bues M, et al. Advantage of protons compared to conventional X-ray or IMRT in the treatment of a pediatric patient with medulloblastoma. Int J Radiat Oncol Biol Phys 2004; 58(3):727–734.
48. Wolden SL, Dunkel IJ, Souweidane MM, et al. Patterns of failure using a conformal radiation therapy tumor bed boost for medulloblastoma. J Clin Oncol 2003; 21(16):3079–3083.
49. Kocsis B, Szekely G, Pap L, et al. Effects of radiation treatment planning and patient fixation on the results of postoperative radiotherapy of childhood medulloblastoma. Strahlenther Onkol 2003; 179(12):854–859.
50. Andrews DW, Scott CB, Sperduto PW, et al. Whole brain radiation therapy with or without stereotactic radiosurgery boost for patients with one to three brain metastases: phase III results of the RTOG 9508 randomised trial. Lancet 2004; 363(9422):1665–1672.
51. Sneed PK, Suh JH, Goetsch SJ, et al. A multi-institutional review of radiosurgery alone vs. radiosurgery with whole brain radiotherapy as the initial management of brain metastases. Int J Radiat Oncol Biol Phys 2002; 53(3):519–526.
52. Mehta MP, Tsao MN, Whelan TJ, et al. The American Society for Therapeutic Radiology and Oncology (ASTRO) evidence-based review of the role of radiosurgery for brain metastases. Int J Radiat Oncol Biol Phys 2005; 63(1):37–46.
53. Chang EL, Wefel JS, Meyers CA, et al. Prospective neurocognitive evaluation of patients with 1 to 3 newly diagnosed brain metastases treated with stereotactic radiosurgery alone. Int J Radiat Oncol Biol Phys 2004; 60(suppl):S164–S165.
54. Iwai Y, Yamanaka K, Ishiguro T. Gamma knife radiosurgery for the treatment of cavernous sinus meningiomas. Neurosurgery 2003; 52(3):517–524.
55. Malik I, Rowe JG, Walton L, et al. The use of stereotactic radiosurgery in the management of meningiomas. Br J Neurosurg 2005; 19(1):13–20.
56. Loeffler JS, Barker FG, Chapman PH. Role of radiosurgery in the management of central nervous system metastases. Cancer Chemother Pharmacol 1999; 43(suppl):S11–S14.
57. Sperduto PW. A review of stereotactic radiosurgery in the management of brain metastases. Technol Cancer Res Treat 2003; 2(2):105–110.
58. Pollock BE, Foote RL. The evolving role of stereotactic radiosurgery for patients with skull base tumors. J Neurooncol 2004; 69(1–3):199–207.
59. Regis J, Delsanti C, Roche PH, et al. Functional outcomes of radiosurgical treatment of vestibular schwannomas: 1000 successive cases and review of the literature. Neurochirurgie 2004; 50(2–3 Pt 2):301–311.

60. Sheehan JP, Niranjan A, Sheehan JM, et al. Stereotactic radiosurgery for pituitary adenomas: an intermediate review of its safety, efficacy, and role in the neurosurgical treatment armamentarium. J Neurosurg 2005; 102(4):678–691.
61. Andrews DW, Suarez O, Goldman HW, et al. Stereotactic radiosurgery and fractionated stereotactic radiotherapy for the treatment of acoustic schwannomas: comparative observations of 125 patients treated at one institution. Int J Radiat Oncol Biol Phys 2001; 50(5):1265–1278.
62. Williams JA. Fractionated stereotactic radiotherapy for acoustic neuromas. Acta Neurochir (Wien) 2002; 144(12):1249–1254.
63. Combs SE, Volk S, Schulz-Ertner D, et al. Management of acoustic neuromas with fractionated stereotactic radiotherapy (FSRT): long-term results in 106 patients treated in a single institution. Int J Radiat Oncol Biol Phys 2005; 63(1):75–81.
64. Uy NW, Woo SY, Teh BS, et al. Intensity-modulated radiation therapy (IMRT) for meningioma. Int J Radiat Oncol Biol Phys 2002; 53(5):1265–1270.
65. Paek SH, Downes MB, Bednarz G, et al. Integration of surgery with fractionated stereotactic radiotherapy for treatment of nonfunctioning pituitary macroadenomas. Int J Radiat Oncol Biol Phys 2005; 61(3):795–808.
66. Milker-Zabel S, Zabel A, Schulz-Ertner D, et al. Fractionated stereotactic radiotherapy in patients with benign or atypical intracranial meningioma: long-term experience and prognostic factors. Int J Radiat Oncol Biol Phys 2005; 61(3): 809–816.
67. Laperriere NJ, Leung PM, McKenzie S, et al. Randomized study of brachytherapy in the initial management of patients with malignant astrocytoma. Int J Radiat Oncol Biol Phys 1998; 41(5):1005–1011.
68. Selker RG, Shapiro WR, Burger P, et al. The Brain Tumor Cooperative Group NIH Trial 87–01: a randomized comparison of surgery, external radiotherapy, and carmustine versus surgery, interstitial radiotherapy boost, external radiation therapy, and carmustine. Neurosurgery 2002; 51(2):343–355.
69. Sneed PK, Stauffer PR, McDermott MW, et al. Survival benefit of hyperthermia in a prospective randomized trial of brachytherapy boost +/− hyperthermia for glioblastoma multiforme. Int J Radiat Oncol Biol Phys 1998; 40(2): 287–295.
70. Kreth FW, Faist M, Rossner R, et al. The risk of interstitial radiotherapy of low-grade gliomas. Radiother Oncol 1997; 43(3):253–260.
71. Mehrkens JH, Kreth FW, Muacevic A, et al. Long term course of WHO grade II astrocytomas of the Insula of Reil after I-125 interstitial irradiation. J Neurol 2004; 251(12):1455–1464.
72. Chan TA, Weingart JD, Parisi M, et al. Treatment of recurrent glioblastoma multiforme with GliaSite brachytherapy. Int J Radiat Oncol Biol Phys 2005; 62(4):1133–1139.
73. Packer RJ, Prados M, Phillips P, et al. Treatment of children with newly diagnosed brain stem gliomas with intravenous recombinant beta-interferon and hyperfractionated radiation therapy: a Childrens Cancer Group phase I/II study. Cancer 1996; 77(10):2150–2156.
74. Knisely JP, Rockwell S. Importance of hypoxia in the biology and treatment of brain tumors. Neuroimaging Clin N Am 2002; 12(4):525–536.

75. McGinn CJ, Kinsella TJ. The experimental and clinical rationale for the use of S-phase-specific radiosensitizers to overcome tumor cell repopulation. Semin Oncol 1992; 19(4 suppl 11):21–28.
76. Halperin EC, Herndon J, Schold SC, et al. A phase III randomized prospective trial of external beam radiotherapy, mitomycin C, carmustine, and 6-mercapto-purine for the treatment of adults with anaplastic glioma of the brain. CNS Cancer Consortium. Int J Radiat Oncol Biol Phys 1996; 34(4):793–802.
77. Knisely JP, Berkey BA, Chakravarti A, et al. RTOG 0118: a phase III study of conventional radiation therapy alone vs. conventional radiation therapy plus thalidomide for multiple brain metastases. J Clin Oncol (Meeting Abstracts) 2005; 23(16S):1500.
78. Langer CJ, Mehta MP. Current management of brain metastases, with a focus on systemic options. J Clin Oncol 2005; 23(25):6207–6219.
79. Leo C, Giaccia AJ, Denko NC. The hypoxic tumor microenvironment and gene expression. Semin Radiat Oncol 2004; 14(3):207–214.
80. Wong CS, Van der Kogel AJ. Mechanisms of radiation injury to the central nervous system: implications for neuroprotection. Mol Interv 2004; 4(5): 273–284.
81. Haffty BG, Glazer PM. Molecular markers in clinical radiation oncology. Oncogene 2003; 22(37):5915–5925.
82. Boldrey E, Sheline G. Delayed transitory clinical manifestations after radiation treatment of intracranial tumors. Acta Radiol Ther Phys Biol 1966; 5:5–10.
83. Engenhart R, Kimmig BN, Hover KH, et al. Stereotactic single high dose radiation therapy of benign intracranial meningiomas. Int J Radiat Oncol Biol Phys 1990; 19(4):1021–1026.
84. Rider WD. Radiation damage to the brain—a new syndrome. J Can Assoc Radiol 1963; 14:67–69.
85. Littley MD, Shalet SM, Beardwell CG. Radiation and hypothalamic-pituitary function. Baillieres Clin Endocrinol Metab 1990; 4(1):147–175.
86. Pai HH, Thornton A, Katznelson L, et al. Hypothalamic/pituitary function following high-dose conformal radiotherapy to the base of skull: demonstration of a dose-effect relationship using dose-volume histogram analysis. Int J Radiat Oncol Biol Phys 2001; 49(4):1079–1092.
87. Armstrong CL, Gyato K, Awadalla AW, et al. A critical review of the clinical effects of therapeutic irradiation damage to the brain: the roots of controversy. Neuropsychol Rev 2004; 14(1):65–86.
88. Hong JH, Chiang CS, Campbell IL, et al. Induction of acute phase gene expression by brain irradiation. Int J Radiat Oncol Biol Phys 1995; 33(3):619–626.
89. Chiang CS, Hong JH, Stalder A, et al. Delayed molecular responses to brain irradiation. Int J Radiat Biol 1997; 72(1):45–53.
90. Li YQ, Chen P, Haimovitz-Friedman A, et al. Endothelial apoptosis initiates acute blood-brain barrier disruption after ionizing radiation. Cancer Res 2003; 63(18):5950–5956.
91. Li YQ, Jay V, Wong CS. Oligodendrocytes in the adult rat spinal cord undergo radiation-induced apoptosis. Cancer Res 1996; 56(23):5417–5422.
92. Kurita H, Kawahara N, Asai A, et al. Radiation-induced apoptosis of oligodendrocytes in the adult rat brain. Neurol Res 2001; 23(8):869–874.

93. Nordal RA, Nagy A, Pintilie M, et al. Hypoxia and hypoxia-inducible factor-1 target genes in central nervous system radiation injury: a role for vascular endothelial growth factor. Clin Cancer Res 2004; 10(10):3342–3353.
94. Nordal RA, Wong CS. Molecular targets in radiation-induced blood-brain barrier disruption. Int J Radiat Oncol Biol Phys 2005; 62(1):279–287.

3

Principles of Chemotherapy

Lauren E. Abrey and Nimish Mohile

Department of Neurology, Memorial Sloan-Kettering Cancer Center, New York, New York, U.S.A.

INTRODUCTION

Modern cancer chemotherapy originated with the development of chemicals that were used as weapons in World War I. In the 1940s, a team of scientists led by Goodman and Gilman initiated the first cancer chemotherapy trial. While investigating chemical warfare agents, they found that nitrogen mustard, known to induce leukopenia in exposed soldiers, had cytotoxic effects in animals. Believing that these agents could have the same effect on the uncontrolled growth of lymphoid cells, they applied this to a patient in the terminal stages of non-Hodgkin's lymphoma. The result was a dramatic, although short lived, response (1). Their success and subsequent trials in individual patients heralded the beginning of a new era in cancer treatment. In the same decade, researchers noted that the recently discovered vitamin, folic acid, enhanced cell proliferation in children with acute lymphoblastic leukemia (ALL). Sydney Farber at Harvard Medical School developed methotrexate (MTX), a folic acid antagonist and the first drug to induce remission in a hematologic neoplasm (2). These steps led to a major congressionally funded effort by the National Cancer Institute (NCI) to research and develop chemotherapy (3). Over the next 60 years, thousands of researchers developed scores of new agents for clinical use. Ongoing pharmacological discoveries continue to change the ways in which cancer is treated.

In neuro-oncology, the impact of chemotherapy has been limited by the persistently dismal prognoses of our patients. The history of brain tumor chemotherapy began in the 1970s when Wilson and Walker independently published their reports of the treatment of malignant brain tumors with BCNU, a nitrosurea. Although no increase in survival could be accurately measured, in both published series patients had noticeable clinical benefit. Wilson described a 45-year-old detective with severe headaches and profound hemiplegia. After treatment, he was able to walk independently, his headaches had remitted, and he was asked to return to work. Improving or maintaining neurologic function remains one of the major goals of chemotherapy administration in brain tumor patients (4,5).

BASIC PRINCIPLES

Cancer cells are characterized by their limitless growth. They evade the normal homeostatic mechanisms that control a normal cell's life, growth, differentiation, and death. Cancer cells have a unique ability to invade surrounding tissues and to form foci of tumor at distant sites. At the molecular level, chemotherapy seeks to undercut a tumor cell's ability to do these tasks.

Chemotherapy can interfere with a cell's function in division and replication or it can directly damage the cell's genetic machinery. The former method exerts its activity on the cell cycle. The cell cycle consists of five phases, G_0, G_1, S, G_2, and M (Fig. 1). It regulates a cell's departure from a quiescent state into a proliferative state. Each phase has a set function related to DNA and RNA synthesis, replication, and cell mitosis. Cell

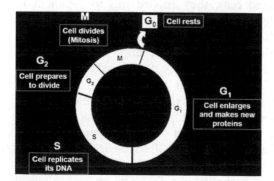

Figure 1 G_0, the resting phase, can last for years depending on the cell type. When the cell needs to replicate, it is signaled to enter G_1, a phase of preparation for DNA synthesis. This is followed by the S phase, where actual DNA synthesis and replication occur. G_2 follows and gives the cell time to prepare for mitosis. Finally, the M phase is when mitosis occurs and two identical daughter cells are created. The cell can then reenter G_1 or lay dormant in G_0.

cycle–specific drugs are agents that interfere with a particular phase or subphase of the cell cycle (Table 1). Tumor cells need to be in these phases in order for the drug to have an effect. For this reason, these agents are typically given in divided doses or as a continuous infusion in order to maximize their effects on cells that are actively dividing. Cell cycle–specific agents are limited to killing those cells that are in the cell cycle—the growth fraction. Cell cycle–nonspecific agents directly damage DNA or enzymes that repair and regulate DNA. They are more toxic because they can affect cells in any state. These agents can be given as a bolus and reduce the actual number of cells in a tumor, thereby reducing the tumor burden (6).

Chemotherapy follows first-order kinetics. The number of cells killed is proportional to the dose administered. Higher doses are more effective because they kill more tumor cells. A single dose will, however, only kill a certain percentage of cells, depending on the properties of the drug. For this reason, successive doses are needed to continue killing a proportion of cells until only one cell remains.

Table 1 Classification of Chemotherapeutic Agents

Cell cycle–specific agents	Cell cycle–nonspecific agents
Vinca alkaloids	Alkylating agents
Vincristine	Nitrogen mustards
Vinblastine	Cyclophosphamide
Vinorelbine	Ifosfamide
Antimetabolites	Nitrosoureas
Antifolates	BCNU (carmustine)
Methotrexate	CCNU (lomustine)
Pyrimidine analogs	Procarbazine
5-FU	Temozolomide
Cytarabine (Ara-C)	Platinum compounds
Gemcitabine	Cisplatin
Capecitabine	Carboplatin
Purine analogs	Other
6-MP	Thiotepa
Thioguanine	Dacarbazine (DTIC)
Epipodophyllotoxins	Anthracycline antibiotics
Etoposide (VP-16)	Doxorubicin
Teniposide	Daunorubicin
Taxanes	Hormones
Paclitaxel	Tamoxifen
Docetaxel	Mifepristone
Camptothecins	Other agents
Topotecan	Hydroxyurea
Irinotecan (CPT-11)	Vitamin A compounds
	Thalidomide

Chemotherapy may be given to eradicate a tumor as a single agent or in combination with other drugs. It can be given before surgery to reduce the tumor burden or after surgery to destroy the remaining cells. Numerous terms are used to describe these different strategies and are defined in Table 2.

Two of the more significant advances in the administration of cytotoxic agents were the use of combination therapy and adjuvant therapy. Combination therapy, first used for the treatment of ALL in 1965, resulted in better cure rates and longer periods of remission. Using a cell cycle–specific and cell cycle–nonspecific agent together, for example, reduces both the growth fraction and the tumor burden of a cancer. Agents with different mechanisms of action are better able to target cancers that have a heterogeneous population of cells, as is often seen in highly malignant tumors. These cells may have different chemosensitivities and they may develop different forms of drug resistance. With combination therapy, they are vulnerable to the effects of multiple drugs. Perhaps the most significant advantage is our ability to use multiple agents with a better therapeutic index. That is, using drugs at doses that in combination are effective, while limiting some of the more significant toxicities (7). Adjuvant chemotherapy, a course of treatment given after surgery or radiotherapy to kill residual tumor cells, was found to be effective in the early 1970s (8). In brain tumors that are initially treated with surgery or radiotherapy, adjuvant chemotherapy plays a critical role in maintaining quality of life and, in some cases, prolongs survival.

Table 2 Chemotherapy Terms and Definitions

Terms	Definitions
Induction	The use of a high-dose regimen to induce a cure. Commonly used for hematologic malignancies
Consolidation	Chemotherapy given after induction with the goal of increasing the possibility of a cure or to prolong survival
Maintenance	Low-dose therapy used when patients are in remission, to delay recurrence
Adjuvant therapy	Chemotherapy given in addition to surgery or radiotherapy to kill remaining tumor cells
Neoadjuvant therapy	Chemotherapy is given preoperatively or postoperatively to help reduce the tumor burden or to reduce tumor size enough to allow for a more feasible resection
Palliative therapy	Chemotherapy given, typically at low doses, to provide relief from pain or to improve function, when cure is not possible
Salvage regimens	Chemotherapy given at time of recurrence or progression. It may be given at high or low doses and is potentially curative

Table 3 Single Agent and Combination Chemotherapy Regimens for Common CNS Tumors

Aggressive or malignant meningioma (51)
  Hydroxyurea 500 mg PO bid
  Cyclophosphamide, adriamycin, and vincristine (1-mo cycle)
    Cyclophosphamide 500 mg/m^2 IV days 1–3
    Adriamycin 15 mg/m^2 IV day 1
    Vincristine 1.4 mg/m^2 day 1
  Dacarbazine and adriamycin (1-mo cycle)
    Dacarbazine 900 mg/m^2 IV days 1–4
    Adriamycin 90 mg/m^2 IV days 1–4
  Ifosfamide 200 mg/m^2 days 1–5 with mesna 1200 mg/m^2 IV per month
Recurrent and anaplastic glial tumors
  Recurrent and anaplastic oligodendroglioma
  PCV (8-wk cycle)
    PCB 60 mg/m^2 days 8–21
    CCNU 110 mg/m^2 day 1
    VCR 1.4 mg/m^2 day 8 and 29
  Intensive PCV (6-wk cycle)
    PCB 75 mg/m^2
    CCNU 130 mg/m^2
    VCR 1.4 mg/m^2
  TMZ (28-day cycle) 150–200 mg/m^2 days 1–5
  Anaplastic astrocytoma
  BCNU 150–200 mg/m^2 q8 wk
  PCV (see above)
  TMZ (28-day cycle) 150–200 mg/m^2 days 1–5
Glioblastoma multiforme
  TMZ: 75 mg/m^2 daily with concurrent XRT
  TMZ (28-day cycle) 150–250 mg/m^2 days 1–5
  BCNU 150–200 mg/m^2 q8 wk
  PCV
  Intensive PCV
  Second line therapies
  CPT-11: 225 mg/m^2 IV weekly for 4 wk with 2 wk off
  TMZ + CPT-11 (28-day cycle)
    TMZ 150 mg/m^2 and CPT-11 50 mg/m^2 IV days 1–5
  Platinum/etoposide (28-day cycle)
    Etoposide 150 mg/m^2 days 2 and 3 with cisplatin 90 mg/m^2 IV day 1 or
      carboplatin 350 mg/m^2 day 1
Primary CNS lymphoma
  HD-MTX 1.8–8.0 g/m^2
  HD-Ara-C 3 g/m^2 × 2 (post-WBRT)

Abbreviations: PCB, procarbazine; VCR, vincristine; TMZ, temozolomide; XRT, external beam radiation therapy; CPT-11, irinotecan; HD, high dose; MTX, methotrexate; Ara-C, cytarabine; WBRT, whole brain radiation therapy.

Table 4 Toxicities of Chemotherapeutic Agents Commonly Used in Neuro-Oncology

Chemotherapy	Systemic toxicity	Neurotoxicity	Measures to lessen toxicity
Cyclophosphamide and ifosfamide	Myelosuppression, N/V, hemorrhagic cystitis	Acute encephalopathy (ifosfamide)	Mesna to prevent hemorrhagic cystitis
CCNU and BCNU	Myelosuppression, N/V, pulmonary fibrosis		
Procarbazine	Myelosuppression, N/V, rash		
Temozolomide	Myelosuppression, N/V, headache, constipation		
Cisplatin/carboplatin	Myelosuppression, nephrotoxicity	PN and ototoxicity (cisplatin)	Aggressive hydration
Vinca alkaloids		PN, cranial nerve palsies, seizures, myopathy	Use maximum of 2.8 mg vincristine per dose to lessen PN
Paclitaxel	Myelosuppression, hypersensitivity reaction, cardiac conduction block	PN	Diphendydramine prevents hypersensitivity reaction
Etoposide (VP-16)	Myelosuppression, N/V	Mild PN	
Methotrexate	Myelosuppression, mucositis, nephrotoxicity	Acute chemical arachnoiditis, subacute or chronic encephalopathy	Leucovorin and aggressive hydration to lessen nephrotoxicity with HD-MTX
5-Fluorouracil, capecitabine	Myelosuppression, mucositis, skin reaction	Ataxia, confusion, seizures, leukoencephalopathy	
Cytarabine, gemcitabine	Myelosuppression, flu-like syndrome, mucositis	Cerebellar syndrome, encephalopathy	Vitamin B_6 to lessen skin symptoms
Irinotecan	N/V, myelosuppression, diarrhea		

Abbreviations: N/V, nausea and vomiting; PN, peripheral neuropathy; MTX, methotrexate; HD, high dose.

UNIQUE ASPECTS LIMITING CHEMOTHERAPY IN BRAIN TUMORS

There are several variables that render brain tumors particularly resistant to the effects of chemotherapy. As in other cancers, the successful use of chemotherapy depends on understanding drug delivery, drug interactions, and drug resistance. The brain's inherent protective mechanisms present obstacles to treatment not encountered in other organs.

The Blood–Brain Barrier

In the early decades of chemotherapy, intracranial metastases were noted to have poor responses to the same agents that were effective against the systemic tumor. Clinicians postulated that brain metastases of chemosensitive tumors failed to respond to systemic agents due to the presence of the blood–brain barrier (BBB) (9). Although the true impact of the BBB continues to be debated, the importance of BBB research in drug delivery and chemotherapeutics cannot be overstated (10).

While the BBB may be designed to protect the brain, it also acts as a barricade to potentially beneficial medications. The BBB lines the blood vessels of the brain and helps protect the brain from toxins. It consists of a layer of endothelial cells that are connected by tight junctions. The tight junctions form a seal that reinforces the barrier created by the lipophilic plasma membranes of the endothelial cells. Efflux transporters such as P-glycoprotein (Pgp) also line the BBB in an effort to jettison those toxins that are able to successfully pass through. The BBB prevents passive entry of water-soluble substances larger than 180 D. Even substances such as glucose and amino acids require active transport by specific proteins in order to enter the cerebral interstitium. Other compounds enter by receptor-mediated or adsorptive endocytosis. The majority of chemotherapeutic drugs are larger than 200 KD and are water soluble; the BBB precludes their entry. Early drugs that had success in the treatment of brain tumors were highly lipid soluble, e.g., CCNU, or were metabolized to a lipid-soluble intermediate as in the case of procarbazine (9,11).

The contrast enhancement of a high-grade intracranial tumor on magnetic resonance imaging (MRI) is essentially a radiographic demonstration of BBB disruption. The extent of disruption varies considerably among different tumors and within individual tumors. The BBB is most permeable in the center of the tumor. Permeability is patchy along the periphery, where the tumor is highly vascular and is actively proliferating (12). Achieving adequate levels of drug near the center, where disruption of the BBB is maximum, is usually insufficient. Drug diffuses outward from the center toward the ventricles, achieving suboptimal levels in the margins of the tumor. Thus, at the margins where rapidly dividing cells are most susceptible to chemotherapy that access is often most restricted. Another region that evades therapeutic doses of chemotherapy is the area of normal brain adjacent to the tumor. Here too, despite the presence of invading tumor cells, the BBB remains intact, and drug concentrations are much lower than at the center of the tumor (13).

Breaching the BBB

For the neuro-oncologist who wants to successfully use chemotherapy to eradicate brain tumors, the BBB constitutes an ongoing challenge. Few medications have been able to penetrate the BBB as effectively as L-dopa in the treatment of Parkinson's disease. The discovery of mechanisms to circumvent the BBB has been critical in improving drug delivery to intracranial tumors. These mechanisms include osmotic disruption of the BBB, alternate means of drug delivery, and methods of chemotherapy dose intensification.

Disruption of the BBB has been studied since the 1940s, with the goal of transiently "opening" the BBB to allow the entry of therapeutic agents. Hypertonic solutions and contrast agents used in radiological procedures, such as mannitol, had the most success. The osmotic effect of mannitol results in contraction of the endothelial cells lining the BBB, leading to opening of the tight junctions. Studies done in animals have demonstrated a marked increase in concentration of some chemotherapeutic drugs within the brain. In theory, osmotic BBB disruption allows for uniform delivery of agents to the entire central nervous system (CNS), thereby eliminating the discrepancy of drug concentrations between the center of the tumor, the periphery, and the adjacent normal brain tissue (12). This principle has been investigated in the treatment of primary CNS lymphoma (PCNSL), where osmotic BBB disruption is followed by intra-arterial MTX (14). Although the procedure is technically demanding with a risk of acute neurotoxicity, it is a feasible way to outmaneuver the BBB.

Intra-arterial administration of drug achieves higher levels of drug in the plasma than intravenous (IV) administration. This, in turn, leads to more drug that can diffuse across the BBB into the CNS. Ideally, this approach is used for drugs that are small, lipophilic, and do not require systemic activation. Although drug levels have been documented to be higher with intra-arterial administration, clinical benefit has yet to be shown. Intra-arterial therapy can be associated with local hemorrhage or infection related to arterial catheterization. More serious complications, including stroke and arterial dissection, have been observed (15).

Intrathecal delivery of drug is accomplished by direct injection into the cerebrospinal fluid (CSF). High CSF concentrations are achieved with minimal systemic toxicity. This approach is ideal for drugs that do not require systemic activation or that are degraded by systemic enzymes. Intrathecal injection necessitates access into either the lumbar cistern via a lumbar puncture or the surgical placement of a reservoir providing access to the frontal horn. Hemorrhage and infection are potential complications. The rapid turnover of CSF and the potential interference with CSF pathways by intracranial tumors can limit the effectiveness of this route. Blockage by tumor can result in higher drug levels in some areas leading to toxicity. Drugs commonly given by this route, usually for the treatment of leptomeningeal metastases, include MTX, Ara-C, and thiotepa (15).

Local delivery of chemotherapy circumvents the BBB. In theory, toxicity to the rest of the CNS is minimized. One approach involves the use of a biodegradable polymer that can provide controlled release of a drug. Animal studies using polymers demonstrated considerable increases in intracerebral drug concentrations compared to serum. In humans, the use of BCNU polymers has been studied and is in use in some centers for the treatment of recurrent glioblastoma multiforme (GBM). Limitations of this technique include erratic distribution of the drug and poor diffusion of the drug into nearby brain parenchyma. Clinically, there is a risk of local neurotoxicity (16). Convection-enhanced delivery employs a catheter to instill the drug into the tumor. This not only bypasses the BBB, but may also overcome the local diffusion barriers that are intrinsic to brain parenchyma (17). Other methods in development include the use of antibodies and viruses to deliver chemotherapy to specific sites (18).

Chemotherapy dose intensification, as used in regimens delivering high-dose chemotherapy with stem cell rescue, is theoretically attractive for use against brain tumors. Higher doses of unbound drug in the plasma increase the diffusion of drug across the BBB. Therefore, these regimens may be able to deliver sufficient doses of drug to all areas of the tumor and to the adjacent "normal" brain. In addition, higher doses may be able to overcome intrinsic drug resistance. High-dose regimens are frequently studied in the pediatric setting in an effort to avoid brain radiation. The limitation of a high dose is most commonly severe or longstanding myelosuppression. This complication necessitates the partnership of high-dose regimens with autologous bone marrow transplantation. Peripheral hematopoietic stem cells are harvested prior to administration of chemotherapy. Then, after chemotherapy is given, they are reinfused, retaining the ability of the body to reconstitute the immune and hematopoietic systems (19). Although this approach has been successful for some hematological malignancies, there has been limited benefit for solid tumors. In adults, Phase I and Phase II protocols have investigated its use against numerous brain tumors, with the most promising results so far limited to the treatment of anaplastic oligodendrogliomas. In children, both survival and quality of life are improved when high-dose chemotherapy and stem cell transplant are used for the treatment of medulloblastomas and recurrent germ cell tumors (20,21).

Drug Resistance

Chemotherapy treatment failure in brain tumors is, in part, attributed to drug resistance. In high-grade tumors, such as GBM, the considerable regional heterogeneity and diversity of cells within the tumor confer intrinsic resistance to chemotherapy (10). Cell populations from different areas in the same tumor have been demonstrated to have variable chemosensitivities (22). The rapid growth of high-grade tumors contributes to genetic instability that increases the ability of tumor cells to acquire resistance to chemotherapy. Knowledge of the different mechanisms of resistance is vital to understand ways in which such resistance can be overcome. Intrinsic resistance develops from within the tumor itself. Acquired resistance develops in response to chemotherapy. Tumors being treated with sublethal doses of chemotherapy tend to be more prone to developing resistance. Depending on the underlying molecular changes, resistance can be conferred to multiple drugs or to a single agent. Resistance to specific drugs or specific classes of drugs will be discussed along with individual drugs later in this chapter.

The hallmark of multiple drug resistance (MDR) is the ability of a tumor to be resistant to an array of drugs that are structurally dissimilar. MDR is accomplished by a number of mechanisms. Pgp, a member of the adenosine triphosphate (ATP)–binding cassette (ABC) family of transporter proteins, is encoded by the Mdr1 gene. This protein impairs the intracellular accumulation of drugs by actively transporting them out of the cytosol. Pgp is thought to have a protective role in normal endothelial cells in the brain by preventing the entry of toxic substances. Pgp is overexpressed in tumors, and the extent of expression correlates directly with tumor grade (23,24). However, the mechanism of the increase in Pgp expression is unclear.

Another protein, called the multidrug resistance–associated protein (MRP), is also a member of the ABC family of proteins and works via ATP-driven efflux of chemotherapy. MRP is not thought to be expressed in normal brain, and its expression does not correlate with tumor grade. Of note, MRP's resistance to drugs such as etoposide and vincristine have been reversed in vitro by MRP inhibitors such as verapamil (25).

MDR can be conferred by intrinsic protective mechanisms and defects in target enzymes. Glutathione and a related group of enzymes protect cells from being damaged by free-radical systems. They are overexpressed in primary brain tumors and may play a role in resistance to a wide array of chemotherapeutic agents. Alterations in target enzymes found in cancer cells can make them resistant to drugs. An example of this is topoisomerase II, a target of numerous drugs. Alterations in this enzyme or reduced levels of the enzyme make tumor cells less susceptible to topoisomerase-inhibiting agents (23).

Drug Interactions

Drug interactions can be another cause of chemotherapy treatment failure. Antiepileptic drugs (AEDs) are the most problematic. The interaction between these two classes of drugs was highlighted in an early study of the use of paclitaxel in the treatment of malignant gliomas. Few of the patients in the study developed the toxicities that other cancer patients had previously reported at similar doses. In addition, drug levels of paclitaxel were 30% less than expected. The decrease in drug levels and side effects was related to their concurrent use of P450 enzyme-inducing AEDs (26).

Seizures are relatively common in patients with brain tumors and can have significant effects on a patient's quality of life. Choosing an appropriate AED is a challenge for the clinician. Almost all traditional AED's induce the metabolism of other drugs that utilize the cytochrome P450 system, mostly through the specific isozyme, CYP3A4. Many of these AED's have real or theoretical interactions with commonly used chemotherapeutic agents such as carboplatin, BCNU, etoposide, irinotecan, CCNU, procarbazine, tamoxifen, temozolomide, and vincristine (27). These interactions can make dosing and administration of cytotoxic therapy more complicated and may compromise the antineoplastic effects of therapy. Valproic acid, though not an enzyme inducer, has been found to inhibit the glucuronidation of an intermediate metabolite of irinotecan that is required for antitumor activity (28). In turn, chemotherapeutic medications can affect the metabolism of some AED's. Decreased serum concentrations of AED's due to drug interactions are thought to be a significant contributor to the refractory nature of tumor-associated epilepsy (29). Furthermore, carbamazepine, phenytoin, valproate, and phenobarbital can all cause hematological suppression, which can contribute to the toxicities of myelosuppressive chemotherapy. Only lamotrigine, gabapentin, and levetiracetam are thought to have no significant interactions with common chemotherapeutic medications (27).

Dexamethasone, commonly used in the management of cerebral edema, is hypothesized to play a role in reconstituting the BBB after its disruption by an intracranial tumor (30). In theory, this may prevent chemotherapy from effectively entering the intracerebral circulation and exerting its effects on tumor cells. The actual extent of this interaction and the effect on drug levels in the brain are not well understood. Additionally, enzyme-inducing AEDs can alter the metabolism of dexamethasone and interfere with the treatment of cerebral edema (31).

SPECIFIC CHEMOTHERAPEUTIC AGENTS

Alkylating Agents

The alkylating agents were the first drugs used clinically in humans as cancer chemotherapy. Originally developed for use in chemical warfare, nitrogen mustard was used experimentally in the early 1940s and found to induce brief remission in non-Hodgkin's lymphomas. Alkylating drugs work by forming highly reactive ions that bind to bases on DNA, leading to strand breaks, impaired DNA replication, and cross-linking of DNA that interferes with DNA unwinding. The ultimate result is impairment of DNA, RNA, and protein synthesis (Fig. 2).

Nitrogen Mustards

Nitrogen mustards form reactive carbonium ions that alkylate DNA. These drugs include mechlorethamine, melphalan, chlorambucil, cyclophosphamide, and ifosfamide. Cyclophosphamide and ifosfamide have been used in the treatment of malignant meningioma. They require hepatic activation, with ifosfamide being specifically metabolized by the hepatic P450 system. Their predominant toxicities include hematologic suppression and hemorrhagic cystitis (see Table 4 for a list of toxicities of commonly used chemotherapies). The latter can be lessened by IV hydration and the use of mesna, a compound that binds and prevents damage by the metabolic breakdown product, acrolein (15). Up to 30% of patients on ifosfamide will develop an acute encephalopathy hours to days after the onset of therapy. Neurological toxicity is more common after oral administration and with higher doses. Typically, the encephalopathy will resolve two to three days after discontinuation, but there are rare occasions where it has progressed to coma and death. Neurotoxicity can be minimized

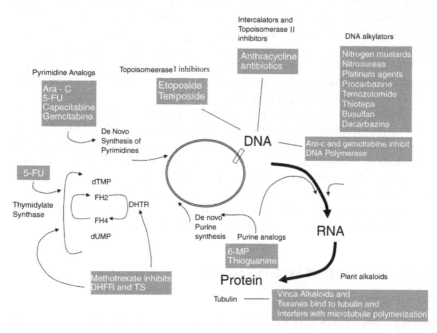

Figure 2 Schematic diagram showing mechanisms of action of chemotherapy. *Abbreviations*: 5-FU, 5-fluorouracil; dTMP, deoxythymidine monophosphate; DHFR, dihydrofolate reductase; dUMP, deoxyuracil monophosphate; 6-MP, mercaptopurine.

considerably with prophylactic and ongoing administration of methylene blue along with the ifosfamide regimen (32).

Nitrosoureas

The nitrosoureas are unique due to their high lipid solubility. Their ability to penetrate the BBB makes them well suited for use in the treatment of brain tumors. The drugs included in this class are BCNU, lomustine (CCNU), nimustine (ACNU), and semustine (MeCCNU). These drugs do not require hepatic or other enzymatic systems to convert them into their active intermediates. The most common adverse effects of these agents are myelosuppression, which can be dose limiting, and gastrointestinal (GI) side effects such as nausea and vomiting. Pulmonary fibrosis can also occur and is seen most commonly with cumulative doses of BCNU. BCNU and CCNU are used alone and in combination for the treatment of malignant glial tumors. BCNU can be given at a dose of $150-200 \, mg/m^2$ every eight weeks for up to six cycles before the risk of pulmonary fibrosis becomes significant. CCNU, as a single agent, can be given at $110-130 \, mg/m^2$ every six to eight weeks (4,5,15) (see Table 3 for a list of commonly used chemotherapy regimens in neuro-oncology).

Procarbazine

Procarbazine is administered orally as it is easily absorbed in the GI tract. It is enzymatically converted in the liver into an active metabolite (an azoxyprocarbazine derivative), which easily crosses the BBB. It acts by specifically alkylating the O_6 position of guanine on DNA. Procarbazine has pharmacologic activities similar to those of monoamine oxidase inhibitors and disulfiram. It has noteworthy interactions with many substances including tyramine, tricyclic antidepressants, sympathomimetic agents, and alcohol. Toxicities include nausea, vomiting, fatigue, and rash. Myelosuppression is uncommon but can be dose limiting. Procarbazine has been used alone or in combination with other agents for the treatment of various brain tumors. As a single agent, it can be given orally at $150 \, mg/m^2$ in 28-day cycles (15).

PCV

PCV is a combination regimen of procarbazine, CCNU, and vincristine, used for anaplastic and recurrent oligodendrogliomas and astrocytomas. It is considered a first-line agent against GBM, but there is controversy as to whether it is as efficacious as BCNU alone. Over an eight-week cycle, CCNU is given on day 1 at $110 \, mg/m^2$, procarbazine at $60 \, mg/m^2$ on days 8 to 21, and vincristine $1.4 \, mg/m^2$ on days 14 and 29. A more intense regimen, given every six weeks, with higher doses of CCNU and procarbazine, can be given. Vincristine is omitted by some practitioners in order to avoid peripheral nervous system toxicity. Overall, dominant side effects include myelosuppression, nausea, and fatigue (33).

Temozolomide

Temozolomide, an agent first used in the 1990s for melanoma and brain tumors, alkylates DNA at the N_7 and O_6 positions of guanine. It is orally administered, is easily absorbed, and spontaneously converts to an active metabolite at physiologic pH levels. Temozolomide's primary toxicities are nausea, headache, constipation, and myelosuppression (34); however, it is a well-tolerated drug. As an alkylating agent, temozolomide can theoretically lead to myelodysplastic syndromes and acute leukemias but, as long-term follow-up is limited, this has been rarely reported (35). It is currently being widely used in the treatment of malignant tumors of astrocytic and oligodendroglial lineage. Typically, it is administered in doses of 150–200 mg/m^2 for five days in a 28-day cycle. When given concurrently with external beam radiation therapy, temozolomide is given as 75 mg/m^2 daily.

Some alkylating agents, including temozolomide, are vulnerable to a particular type of resistance involving the DNA-repair enzyme, O_6-methylguanine-DNA methyltransferase (MGMT). MGMT repairs DNA by removing alkyl groups from the O_6 position on guanine, a critical site of DNA alkylation by temozolomide and procarbazine. If the tumor cell DNA is not repaired, cytotoxicity and apoptosis ensue. Tumor cells with high levels of MGMT are resistant to such manipulation due to their ability to continuously repair damaged DNA, thereby rendering alkylating agents ineffective. In tumors with low levels of MGMT (accomplished at the molecular level by methylation and subsequent inactivation of the MGMT promoter), cells have increased sensitivity to alkylating agents such as temozolomide. In future practice, tumor's "methylation status" may have prognostic implications and impact the clinician's choice of chemotherapy. This example highlights the importance of understanding mechanisms of drug resistance and the potential to aid in clinical and therapeutic decisions (36).

Platinum Compounds

The major platinum compounds in use are cisplatin and carboplatin. These drugs interfere with DNA and protein synthesis by forming DNA cross-links. They are water-soluble compounds and poorly penetrate the BBB; early studies demonstrated considerably lower levels of drug in the brain compared to the serum. Administration of cisplatin requires aggressive hydration to prevent nephrotoxicity and antiemetic therapy to prevent nausea and vomiting. Cisplatin can lead to myelosuppression. In the nervous system, complications include peripheral neuropathy and ototoxicity. Carboplatin can lead to considerable myelosuppression but is not significantly neurotoxic.

Metallothioneins form chelation complexes with platinum compounds and inactivate them, thereby imparting drug resistance. CNS germinomas are particularly chemosensitive to platinum-based agents. Both agents have been used in the treatment of malignant gliomas as single drugs or as part of multidrug regimens. They are commonly given in combination with etoposide in a 28-day cycle, where either cisplatin is given on day 1 at a dose $90 \, mg/m^2$ or carboplatin at $350 \, mg/m^2$ (15,37).

Other Alkylating Agents

Thiotepa is commonly used in high-dose regimens in conjunction with stem cell rescue or as a treatment for leptomeningeal metastases. It is an alkylating agent that easily crosses the BBB and has minimal neurotoxicity. Busulfan also crosses the BBB and is known to cause seizures at higher doses. Dacarbazine (DTIC) is used in the treatment of melanomas and malignant meningiomas; it has a mechanism of action and structure that is similar to temozolomide.

Plant Alkaloids

The first alkaloids were discovered from the plant, *Catharanthus roseus,* whose derivatives were initially used for the treatment of scurvy, diabetes, and chronic wounds. Studies of the plant led to the isolation of the alkaloids which were found to cause profound leukopenia. These agents, referred to as the vinca alkaloids, are cell cycle–specific antimitotic agents that act by binding to tubulin and interfering with the assembly of microtubules. The other alkaloids, also derived from plants, bind to tubulin, but have different mechanisms of actions. These include the taxanes and the podophyllins (38).

Vinca Alkaloids

The common vinca alkaloids include vincristine, vinblastine, and the more recently developed vinorelbine. They specifically prevent microtubule polymerization and induce depolymerization, thereby halting mitosis during metaphase. These drugs are water soluble, poorly penetrate the BBB, and rely on the liver for their metabolism. They have a considerable list of side effects to the peripheral and CNS including peripheral neuropathy, myopathy, cranial neuropathies, and seizures. Peripheral neuropathy, the most limiting toxicity, can be devastating and irreversible. Vincristine is used in the treatment of malignant gliomas as part of PCV or in combination with carboplatin for low-grade gliomas. Vinblastine is also used in the treatment of pediatric low-grade gliomas.

Taxanes

Paclitaxel, the first of the taxanes, is derived from the bark of *Taxus brevifolia*, the Pacific Yew, and was discovered in 1963 as part of an NCI plant-screening program for anticancer compounds. Docetaxel, a related compound, is derived from needles of the same tree. The taxanes bind to tubulin, but contrary to the action of the vinca alkaloids, they promote the assembly of microtubules. However, the microtubules formed are dysfunctional and interfere with cell division. Some tumor cells contain abnormal tubulins which do not normally polymerize into microtubules; this dysfunction is normalized by the taxanes, making these cells resistant. Both drugs are metabolized by the liver and poorly penetrate the BBB. Paclitaxel's metabolism and clearance is hastened by enzyme-inducing AEDs (39). Both drugs can lead to significant neutropenia that can be dose-limiting. Treatment with paclitaxel requires pretreatment with diphen-hydramine to prevent a hypersensitivity reaction. Other adverse effects of paclitaxel include cardiac conduction block and a distal sensory small- and large-fiber peripheral neuropathy. Early work on glioma cell lines suggested that paclitaxel may be promising, but clinical studies have not demonstrated it to be an effective agent against glial tumors (40).

Epipodophyllotoxins

The epipodophyllotoxins, etoposide and teniposide, originate from podophyl-lotoxin, which is a plant-derived inhibitor of microtubule assembly. Etoposide (VP-16) and teniposide bind to tubulin but do not affect microtubules. They are potent inhibitors of topoisomerase II, a DNA repair enzyme. The end result is the formation of single- and double-strand breaks in DNA that lead to cell cycle arrest in G_2. Although they are lipophilic, these drugs have difficulty crossing the BBB because of their large size. The most common adverse effects from these drugs are myelosuppression, nausea, and vomiting. In addition, etoposide is associated with a mild peripheral neuropathy (41). Etoposide is typically given as part of combination regimens to treat malig-nant gliomas, but it also has been used as a single agent.

Antimetabolites

The antimetabolites interfere with DNA synthesis. They include antifolates, pyrimidine analogs, and purine analogs. The antifolates, aminopterin and MTX, were the first agents to induce remission in ALL (2). MTX was later found to be active against solid tumors and to be curative treatment for choriocarcinomas. MTX continues to be used both as an anticancer agent and, more recently, for the treatment of some inflammatory conditions. In neuro-oncology, MTX is a first-line agent for the treatment of PCNSL.

Methotrexate

MTX inhibits dihydrofolate reductase (DHFR). This leads to depletion of folates, single carbon carriers that are necessary for pyrimidine, purine, and protein biosynthesis. It also inhibits thymidylate synthase, which results in mis-incorporation of uracil into DNA. Tumor cells with increased levels of DHFR can be resistant to MTX. MTX can be given intravenously, intra-arterially, or intrathecally. Adverse effects include myelosuppression, mucositis, and neph-rotoxicity. When given systemically in high doses, therapeutic levels in the

CSF can be attained. High-dose administration requires vigorous hydration and alkalinization of the urine with sodium bicarbonate to prevent precipitation of MTX in the urine. It can be associated with an acute or chronic encephalopathy. Intrathecal administration can also lead to myelosuppression and mucositis, but is more commonly associated with neurotoxicity. Patients can develop an acute chemical arachnoiditis, a subacute encephalopathy (after a few courses of treatment), or a chronic encephalopathy that can occur months to years after treatment. Toxicities can be alleviated but not eliminated by the administration of leucovorin, a reduced folate that does not require DHFR to work. It preferentially rescues purine and pyrimidine biosynthesis in nontumor cells. High-dose MTX is commonly used alone or as part of a multiagent regimen for the treatment of PCNSL. Due to its ability to penetrate the CNS, when delivered in high doses, it has been used for the treatment of brain and leptomeningeal metastases (42).

Pyrimidine Analogs

The pyrimidine analogs, 5-fluorouracil (5-FU) and cytarabine (Ara-c), have similar mechanisms of action. They ultimately interfere with the de novo synthesis of pyrimidines. Capecitabine and gemcitabine are also members of this drug class.

5-FU inhibits thymidylate synthase and gets incorporated into DNA and RNA. It also results in the misincorporation of uracil into DNA. The drug is catabolized to an inactive compound by dihydropyrimidine dehydrogenase (DPD). Patients who lack this enzyme are prone to developing severe toxicity. Conversely, increased expression of thymidylate synthase interferes with 5-FU's ability to halt DNA synthesis and confers resistance. 5-FU leads to myelosuppression, mucositis, skin reactions, and neurotoxicity. The dermatologic symptoms can be controlled with concurrent administration of vitamin B_6. Neurological manifestations are cerebellar ataxia, confusion, and seizures. An encephalopathy, with diffuse white matter changes, is seen rarely and is usually associated with lack of DPD (43). 5-FU is not currently a standard treatment, alone or in combination, for any primary brain tumor. Capecitabine is an oral analog of 5-FU and requires multiple steps to be activated. It is currently in use for refractory metastatic breast and colon tumors. It is known to have numerous drug interactions, including warfarin and phenytoin. It can lead to marked increases in phenytoin levels and drug toxicity. It, like 5-FU, is associated with mucositis and dermatologic toxicities. Leukoencephalopathy, similar to that seen with 5-FU, has also been reported (44).

Ara-C has been used in the treatment of PCNSL and leptomeningeal metastases from systemic cancers. Once activated, Ara-C is incorporated into DNA and inhibits the activity of DNA polymerase. Resistance to therapy is usually related to downregulation of activation enzymes or upregulation of catabolic enzymes. It is usually administered as a bolus or continuous infusion, but can be given intrathecally for the treatment of leptomeningeal metastases. Common toxicities include myelosuppression and mucositis. With higher doses, patients can develop a cerebellar syndrome, encephalopathy, or conjunctivitis (15). Gemcitabine has a mechanism of action similar to Ara-C and is used predominantly in the treatment of solid tumors.

Purine Analogs

The purine analogs are not active agents for brain tumors. Their discovery in the 1950s led to the Nobel Prize for George Hitchings and Gertrude Elion. The trademark agents of this class are 6-mercaptopurine and thioguanine. They are enzymatically activated in the cell by hypoxanthine guanine phosphoribosyltransferase (the same enzyme whose deficiency leads to the Lesch-Nyan syndrome) and then incorporated into DNA and RNA. Common toxicities include myelosuppression, mucositis, and hepatotoxicity. Other agents in this class, fludarabine and cladribine, have similar mechanisms of action and toxicities; they are active against some leukemias and lymphomas (45).

Camptothecins

The camptothecins were discovered when an extract from the wood of a Chinese tree, *Camptotheca acuminata,* investigated as part of an NCI screening program, was found to be active against a line of murine leukemia cells. Irinotecan (CPT-11) and topotecan are derivatives of the original extract. These agents bind to and inactivate topoisomerase I, leading to accumulation of DNA single strand breaks. Both drugs are associated with nausea, vomiting, and myelosuppression. Irinotecan can also lead to severe diarrhea, which can be dose-limiting. Although it is water soluble, irinotecan is able to cross the BBB and reach therapeutic levels in CSF. Unlike topotecan, irinotecan has demonstrated some activity against malignant gliomas as a single agent or in combination with temozolomide (46,47).

Anthracyclines

The anthracycline antibiotics were originally thought to interfere with cellular functions by intercalating into the DNA double helix. More recent work suggests that their cytotoxic activity derives from their function as a topoisomerase II inhibitor. The major drugs in this class are doxorubicin and daunorubicin, but a number of newer analogs with similar activity exist. These agents have a wide spectrum of activity against both solid and hematologic neoplasms. Resistance to this class of drugs can be significant and is usually due to drug efflux by MDR and MRP transporter proteins. Anthracyclines are associated with myelosuppression, mucositis, and alopecia, but the most concerning toxicity is to the heart. Cardiac toxicity develops with cumulative doses and can lead to arrhythmias, heart block, cardiomyopathy, and heart failure. Doxorubicin is used as part of combination regimens in the treatment of meningiomas. The novel development of liposomal delivery systems for doxorubicin and daunorubicin is under investigation for their potential role in the treatment of malignant gliomas and brain metastases. These agents may be more able to cross the BBB and may be associated with less cardiotoxicity (48,49).

Other Agents

Tamoxifen and Mifepristone

Tamoxifen is an antiestrogen compound that is typically used for the treatment of estrogen receptor–positive breast cancers and has a number of mechanisms of action. Tamoxifen has been studied in brain tumors in an effort to inhibit protein kinase C. Protein kinase C is expressed in glioma cell lines, and the expression is promoted by epidermal growth factors. Tamoxifen has been investigated as part of multiagent regimens against high-grade gliomas with only modest benefit. Side effects include dizziness and gait ataxia (15,50). Mifepristone, an antiprogestin, has been used for blockade of progesterone receptor and is under investigation for the treatment of meningiomas. It is associated with fatigue, hot flashes and gynecomastia. Tamoxifen and mifepristone have both been used in the treatment of recurrent meningiomas (51).

Hydroxyurea

Hydroxyurea works in a manner similar to the antimetabolites. It inhibits the enzyme ribonucleotide diphosphate reductase, which reduces ribonucleotides to form deoxyribonucleotides. This results in fewer available deoxyribonucleotides that are available for DNA synthesis. It is administered orally and readily crosses the BBB. It is used for the treatment of recurrent and unresectable meningiomas and is given at a dose of 500 mg twice a day (50). Its predominant toxicity is myelosuppression. It has also been used as a radiosensitizer in conjunction with other agents for the treatment of malignant gliomas.

Vitamin A Compounds

Vitamin A compounds such as *cis*-Retinoic acid (Accutane) have been traditionally used for the treatment of acne. Investigation of their use in neuro-oncology began with the discovery that they are active against glioma cell lines in vitro. They have only modest success in clinical investigations as a sole agent (33). Data is more promising when it is used in conjunction with temozolomide. Side effects include dry skin, rash, and photosensitivity.

Thalidomide

Thalidomide has been studied and continues to be under investigation for activity against malignant gliomas. Well known for causing birth defects when administered to pregnant women, it is currently being used and investigated for its antiangiogenic properties. It can lead to neuropathy, fatigue, and constipation. It, like Accutane, must be administered in conjunction with oral contraceptives in women of child-bearing age (33).

SUPPORTIVE CARE

Antiemetic Therapy

Chemotherapy-related side effects have a considerable impact on the quality of life for brain tumor patients. Nausea and vomiting are the most frequent complaints; they are caused by the release of emetogenic substances that bind to receptors in either the area postrema or the chemoreceptor trigger zone of the brainstem. Treatment is centered on receptor blockade. Antiemetics such as phenothiazines and metoclopramide block dopamine receptors; however, their use is limited by drowsiness, extrapyramidal features, and a lower seizure threshold.

Serotonin antagonists are newer antiemetics that specifically block $5HT_3$. They are extremely effective for acute emesis (emesis occurring during the first 24 hours of treatment) when given prior to chemotherapy. In this setting, oral therapy is as effective as IV. The treatment of delayed emesis, occurring at least 24 hours after chemotherapy, is more problematic. Corticosteroids are the mainstay of treatment and are given with either a dopamine antagonist or a $5HT_3$ antagonist (52). The mechanism of action of corticosteroids in this setting is not well understood. Dexamethasone is most often used and is also helpful in treating patients taking highly emetogenic chemotherapy. In general, the drugs with the highest emetogenic potential include platinum agents, anthracyclines, and carmustine. Drugs that bind the neurokinin type 1 receptor (substance P is the physiologic ligand for this receptor), such as Aprepitant, are particularly effective with platinum agents. Moderately emetogenic chemotherapies include irinotecan, MTX, procarbazine, thiotepa, temozolomide, and topotecan (53). Commonly used antiemetic regimens are listed in Table 5.

Colony-Stimulating Factors

Neutropenia is a significant concern for any patient taking myelotoxic chemotherapy. It can lead to hospitalization, the need for IV antibiotics, delay of chemotherapy, and, in severe cases, death. The advent of recombinant colony-stimulating factors has significantly minimized these complications. Granulocyte colony-stimulating fact (G-CSF), a growth factor that stimulates the proliferation of neutrophils, can be used prophylactically to prevent infection or to treat neutropenic patients. Although primary prophylaxis reduces hospitalization and morbidity, it has not been shown to reduce mortality (54). Therefore, G-CSF in the cancer patient is reserved to treat

Table 5 Pretreatment Antiemetic Regimens

Chemotherapy regimen	Antiemetic pretreatment
IV Carmustine	Palonosetron 250 mg IV
IV Irinotecan	Dexamethasone 12 mg PO/IV
HD-MTX	Metoclopramide 10 mg PO/IV prn
HD-Ara-C	Above regimen +
Etoposide/carboplatin	Aprepitant 125 mg PO on day 1; 80 mg
Etoposide/cisplatin	on subsequent days
PCV	Granisetron 1–2 mg PO
Intensive PCV	Dexamethasone 12 mg PO
Lomustine	Metoclopramide 10 mg PO/IV prn
Procarbazine	Granisetron 1 mg PO
Temozolomide	

Abbreviations: IV, intravenous; PO, by mouth; HD, high dose; MTX, methotrexate; Ara-C, cytarabine.

patients who are at higher risk for complications. This includes patients with a prior history of neutropenia-related hospitalization, neutropenia lasting more than 7 to 10 days, and absolute neutrophil count less than 500/mm^3. It is often given to the febrile, neutropenic patient as an adjunct to antibiotic therapy. Its use should not overlap with the use of cytotoxic agents because the stimulated progenitor cells may become susceptible to the effects of chemotherapy. G-CSF (Filgastrim) and pegylated G-CSF (Pegfilgastrim) are most commonly used. Filgastrim results in an immediate brief leukopenia followed by an increase in neutrophil count that can be sustained for several days before reaching a plateau. Administration should typically be stopped once the neutrophil count is adequate; this is usually between 5000 and 7000/mm^3. Pegfilgastrim has the advantage of being longer acting and can therefore be administered only one time during each chemotherapy cycle. Additionally, these agents are used to induce the mobilization of peripheral blood stem cells for high-dose chemotherapy regimens with stem cell rescue (54,55).

Diarrhea and Constipation

Chemotherapy-induced diarrhea can be life threatening, if severe. Even in milder cases, it should be taken seriously as it can lead to discomfort and noncompliance. Good supportive management depends on appropriate evaluation and treatment. A history of atypical features such as fevers, blood, or severe pain should prompt further evaluation to determine the exact etiology. Initial supportive care should consist of oral fluid intake to prevent dehydration and avoidance of foods containing lactose. Pharmacologic treatments are centered on the use of opioids, particularly loperamide.

If diarrhea persists despite standard doses of loperamide, higher doses can be used. When diarrhea is refractory to opioids, other medications such as octreotide can be tried. A more complete workup for etiology may be necessary and the patient may require hospitalization for IV hydration (56).

Although constipation is commonly encountered as a complication of opioid analgesic use, it can also be caused or exacerbated by chemotherapy. Constipation that is unrecognized and untreated can lead to bowel obstruction or perforation and may require surgical intervention. For those patients at risk, preventive treatment with a bowel regimen is usually very effective. A typical regimen includes a stool softener with a laxative. For refractory constipation, another laxative can be added or an enema can be administered. In some, manual disimpaction may be necessary (57).

Fertility Preservation

Issues related to infertility following cytotoxic chemotherapy are probably under-recognized. For cancer survivors, the ability to conceive their own children can significantly affect their quality of life. With continuing advances in reproductive technology, the cancer clinician will be increasingly obligated to be aware of and discuss these matters. Many chemotherapeutic agents cause gonadotoxicity. In men, the seminiferous epithelium can be damaged, leading to impaired spermatogenesis and subsequent oligospermia or azoospermia. Management involves cryopreservation of semen prior to chemotherapy. This is reserved for later use in in vitro fertilization (IVF). In women, chemotherapy can lead to premature ovarian failure and early menopause (58). The options for preserving fertility are more complicated. Oocytes can be obtained, fertilized in vitro and frozen. Due to the freezing and thawing process, successful pregnancy rates are only between 20% and 30%. At the moment, however, this is the most fruitful method. Other options are experimental, including oophorectomy followed by either cryopreservation and subsequent IVF or transplantation. For the interested patient, proper management requires appropriate referral to a specialist in the field (59).

REFERENCES

1. Gilman A. The initial clinical trial of nitrogen mustard. Am J Surg 1963; 105:574–578.
2. Chabner BA, et al. Timeline: Chemotherapy and the war on cancer. Nat Rev Cancer 2005; 5(1):65–72.
3. Frei E III. The national cancer chemotherapy program. Science 1982; 217(4560): 600–606.
4. Walker MD, et al. BCNU (1,3-bis(2-chloroethyl)-l-nitrosourea; NSC-409962) in the treatment of malignant brain tumor-a preliminary report. Cancer Chemother Rep 1970; 54(4):263–271.

5. Wilson CB, et al. 1,3-bis (2-chloroethyl)-1-nitrosourea (NSC-409962) in the treatment of brain tumors. Cancer Chemother Rep 1970; 54(4):273–281.
6. Chabner BA, Longo DL, eds. Cancer chemotherapy and biotherapy: principles and practices. 3rd ed. Lippincott, Philadelphia: Williams and Wilkins, 2001.
7. Frei E III, et al. The effectiveness of combinations of antileukemic agents in inducing and maintaining remission in children with acute leukemia. Blood 1965; 26(5):643–656.
8. Bonnadonna G, et al. Combination chemotherapy as an adjuvant treatment in operable breast cancer. N Engl J Med 1976; 294(8):405–410.
9. Levin VA. A pharmacologic basis for brain tumor chemotherapy. Semin Oncol 1975; 2(1):57–61.
10. Stewart DJ. A critique of the role of the blood-brain barrier in the chemotherapy of human brain tumors. J Neurooncol 1994; 20(2):121–139.
11. Neuwelt EA. Mechanisms of disease: the blood-brain barrier. Neurosurgery 2004; 54(1):131–140.
12. Kroll R, et al. Outwitting the blood-brain barrier for therapeutic purposes: osmotic opening and other means. Neurosurgery 1998; 42(5):1083–1099.
13. Donelli MG, et al. Do anticancer agents reach the tumor target in the human brain? Cancer Chemother Pharmacol 1992; 30(4):251–260.
14. Fortin D, et al. Enhanced chemotherapy delivery by intraarterial infusion and blood-brain barrier disruption in malignant brain tumors: the sherbrooke experience. Cancer 2005; 103(12):2606–2615.
15. Newton HB, et al. Clinical presentation, diagnosis, and pharmacotherapy of patients with primary brain tumors. Ann Pharmacother 1999; 33(7–8):816–832.
16. Ciordia R, et al. Cytotoxic chemotherapy: advances in delivery, pharmacology, and testing. Curr Oncl Rep 2000; 2(5):445–453.
17. Groothius DR, et al. Comparison of 14C-sucrose delivery to the brain by intravenous, intraventricular, and convection-enhanced intracerebral infusion. J Neurosurg 1999; 90(2):321–331.
18. Kraemer DF, et al. Chemotherapeutic does intensification for treatment of malignant brain tumors: recent developments and future directions. Curr Neurol Neurosci Rep 2002; 2(3):216–224.
19. Fine HA, et al. High-dose chemotherapy with autologous bone marrow transplantation in the treatment of high grade astrocytomas in adults: therapeutic rationale and clinical experience. Bone Marrow Transplant 1992; 10(4): 315–321.
20. Abrey LE, et al. High-dose chemotherapy with stem cell rescue as initial therapy for anaplastic oligodendroglioma. J Neurooncol 2003; 65(2):127–134.
21. Gardner SL. Application of stem cell transplant for brain tumors. Pediatr Transplant 2004; 8:28–32.
22. Shapiro WR, et al. Principles of brain tumor chemotherapy. Semin Oncol 1986; 13(1):56–69.
23. Bredel M. Anticancer drug resistance in primary human brain tumors. Brain Res Rev 2001; 35(2):161–204.
24. von Bossanyi P, et al. Immunohistochemical expression of P-glycoprotein and glutathione S-transferases in cerebral gliomas and response to chemotherapy. Acta Neuropathol 1997; 94(6):605–611.

25. Abe T, et al. Chemosensitisation of spontaneous multidrug resistance by a 1,4-dihydropyridine analogue and verapamil in human glioma cell lines overexpressing MRP of MDR1. Br J Cancer 1995; 72(2):418–423.
26. Fetell MR, et al. Preirradiation paclitaxel in glioblastoma multiforme: efficacy, pharmacology, and drug interactions. New Approaches to Brain Tumor Therapy Central Nervous System Consortium. J Clin Oncol 1997; 15(9):3121–3128.
27. Sirven JI, et al. Seizure prophylaxis in patients with brain tumors: a meta-analysis. Mayo Clin Proc 2004; 79(12):1489–1494.
28. Gupta E, et al. Modulation of glucuronidation of SN-38, the active metabolite of irinotecan, by valproic acid and phenobarbital. Cancer Chemother Pharmacol 1997; 39(5):440–444.
29. Gattis WA, et al. Possible interaction involving phenytoin, dexamethasone, and antineoplastic agents: a case report and review. Ann Pharmacother 1996; 30(5):520–526.
30. Galicich JH, et al. Use of dexamethasone in treatment of cerebral edema associated with brain tumors. J Lancet 1961; 81:46–53.
31. Vecht CJ, et al. Treating seizures in patients with brain tumors: Drug interactions between antiepileptic and chemotherapeutic agents. Semin Oncol 2003; 30(6): 49–52.
32. Nicolao P, et al. Neurological toxicity of ifosfamide. Oncology 2003; 65 (2):11–16.
33. Parney IF, et al. Current chemotherapy for glioblastoma. Cancer J 2003; 9(3): 149–156.
34. O'reilly SM, et al. Temozolomide: a new oral cytotoxic chemotherapeutic agent with promising activity against primary brain tumours. Eur J Cancer 1993; 29A(7):940–943.
35. Su YW, et al. Treatment-related myelodysplastic syndrome after temozolomide for recurrent high-grade glioma. J Neurooncol 2005; 71(3):315–318.
36. Hegi ME, et al. MGMT gene silencing and benefit from temozolomide in glioblastoma. N Engl J Med 2005; 352(10):997–1003.
37. Doz F, et al. Comparison of the cytotoxic activities of cisplatin and carboplatin against glioma cell lines at pharmacologically relevant drug exposures. J Neurooncol 1991; 11(1):27–35.
38. Zhou XJ, et al. Preclinical and clinical pharmacology of vinca alkaloids. Drugs 1992; 44(suppl 4):1–16.
39. Chang SM, et al. Phase I study of paclitaxel in patients with recurrent malignant glioma: a North American Brain Tumor Consortium report. J Clin Oncol 1998; 16(6):2188–2194.
40. Rowinsky EK, et al. Paclitaxel (taxol). N Engl J Med 1995; 332(15):1004–1014.
41. Van Maanen JM, et al. Mechanism of action of antitumor drug etoposide: a review. J Natl Cancer Inst 1988; 80(19):1526–1533.
42. Treon SP, et al. Concepts in use of high-dose Methotrexate therapy. Clin Chem 1996; 42(8):1322–1329.
43. Diasio RB. Clinical implications of dihydropyrimidine dehydrogenase on 5-FU pharmacology. Oncology 2001; 15(1):21–26.
44. Niemann B, et al. Toxic encephalopathy induced by capecitabine. Oncology 2004; 66(4):331–335.

45. Hitchings GH, et al. The chemistry and biochemistry of purine analogs. Ann NY Acad Sci 1954; 60(2):195–199.
46. Pipas JM, et al. A Phase II trail of paclitaxel and topotecan with filgrastim in patients with recurrent or refractory glioblastoma multiforme or anaplastic astrocytoma. J Neurooncol 2005; 71(3):301–305.
47. Slichenmyer WJ, et al. The current status of camptothecin analogues as antitumor agents. J Natl Cancer Inst 1993; 85(4):271–291.
48. Honig A, et al. Brain Metastases in breast cancer—an in vitro study to evaluate new systemic chemotherapeutic options. Anticancer Res 2005; 5(1):65–72.
49. Allen TM, et al. Advantage of liposomal delivery systems for anthracyclines. Semin Oncol 2004; 31(6):5–15.
50. Friedman ZY. Recent advances in understanding the molecular mechanisms of tamoxifen action. Cancer Invest 1998; 16(6):391–396.
51. Chamberlain MC. Intracerebral Meningiomas. Curr Treat Options Neurol 2004; 6(4):297–305.
52. Gralla R. New agents, new treatment, and antiemetic therapy. Sem Oncol 2002; 29(1):119–124.
53. Einhorn LH, et al. Antiemetic therapy for multiple-day chemotherapy and high-dose chemotherapy with stem cell transplant: review and consensus statement. Support Care Cancer 2005; 13:112–116.
54. Lieschke GJ, et al. Granulocyte colony-stimulating factor and granulocyte-macrophage colony-stimulating factor (2). NEJM 1992; 327(2):99–106.
55. Waladkhani AR, et al. Pegfilgrastim: a recent advance in the prophylaxis of chemotherapy-induced neutrupenia. Eur J Cancer Care 2004; 13:371–379.
56. Wadler S, et al. Recommended guidelines for the treatment of chemotherapy-induced diarrhea. J Clin Oncol 1998; 16(9):3169–3178.
57. Klaschik E, et al. Constipation–modern laxative therapy. Support Care Cancer 2003; 11:679–685.
58. Wallace WH, et al. Fertility preservation for young patients with cancer: who is at risk and what can be offered? Lancet Oncol 2005; 6:209–218.
59. Lobo R, et al. Potential options for preservation of fertility in women. NEJM 2005; 353:64–73.

4

New Approaches to Brain Tumor Therapy

Michael Weller and Wolfgang Wick

Department of General Neurology, Hertie Institute for Clinical Brain Research, University of Tuebingen, School of Medicine, Tuebingen, Germany

INTRODUCTION

Operative procedures, improved precision of irradiation, and adjuvant che-motherapy have slightly improved the survival of glioma patients in the past decades. A significant step ahead has not yet been accomplished. The reason for this failure is due to the biology of malignant gliomas. Deep infiltration of healthy and neurologically vulnerable brain structures prevents total tumor resection; there is inherent resistance to the radiotherapy and chemo-therapy that can be safely applied to the brain. Given the major steps that have been made in the last years in the understanding of genetic and cell biologic mechanisms that are involved in the initiation and progression of gliomas, this clearer understanding should be translated into approaches targeting the key molecular effectors of glioma malignancy. These novel therapeutic strategies are based on new pharmaceutical compounds that are designed to interfere with specific targets in glioma signal transduction pathways or focus on gene therapy to modify the tumor microenvironment. This chapter deals with preclinical or clinical stage developments in glioma therapy. Specifically, the novel tyrosine kinase inhibitors measures to influ-ence motility and angiogensis, proapoptotic strategies, and immunotherapy are discussed. It finishes with an outlook on glioma-initiating cells and cellular vectors as novel vehicles for glioma therapy.

FOCUS ON INHIBITION OF SURVIVAL PATHWAYS

Strategies to Target Tyrosine Kinases in Brain Tumor Therapy

Although more than 20 members of the receptor tyrosine kinase family have been identified (1), and a variety of these receptors have been implicated in glial tumorigenesis, previous studies have demonstrated that receptors for platelet-derived- and epidermal growth factor receptor (PDGFR and EGFR) may represent particularly important contributors to dysregulated proliferation. This is supported by recent observations that antibody- and antisense-mediated neutralization of PDGFR and EGFR can substantially inhibit glioma growth in vitro. However, significant limitations to the use of these strategies for the in vivo treatment of human gliomas have precluded their clinical application. Recently, pharmacological inhibitors of PDGFR (e.g., STI571) and EGFR (e.g., ZD1839) have been developed, which demonstrate potent inhibition of receptor-dependent signaling. However, the appropriate subgroups of gliomas to be treated with these agents remain to be defined, calling attention to the need for identifying biologically relevant surrogates that predict response. Because these agents will likely be independently effective in only a subset of tumors, optimal strategies for combining them with other therapeutic approaches need to be determined.

Tyrosine Kinase Regulation and Dysregulation

A current European Organization for Research and Treatment of Cancer (EORTC) glioblastoma trial analyzes vatalanib, a tyrosine kinase inhibitor and vascular endothelial growth factor receptor (VEGFR) kinase inhibitor (PTK787) added to concomitant and adjuvant radiochemotherapy with temozolomide (2). The standard setting for testing the toxicity and efficacy of novel substances is a phase I or phase I/II clinical study in progressive or recurrent tumors. As of August 2005, 10 clinical trials on tyrosine kinase inhibitors in malignant brain tumors were activated (3). Among the substances are AEE787, an antiangiogenic compound lapatinib (GW572016), an ErbB-2 and EGFR dual tyrosine kinase inhibitor everolimus, an immunosuppressive and antiangiogenic agent and EGFR antagonists that are discussed in this chapter in greater detail.

PDGFR/c-Kit

Imatinib Mesylate: Although a number of pharmaceutical companies have developed PDGFR inhibitors that are in various phases of clinical development, the agent that has progressed by far the furthest is STI571 (CGP57148B, also known as "Imatinib"). This compound is a low-molecular-weight synthetic 2-phenylaminopyrimidine that initially reached clinical interest, not because of its PDGFR inhibitory effects, but because of its potent inhibition of Bcr-Abl, a fusion protein produced by Philadelphia chromosome–positive leukemias (4–7). Significant activity of this agent was demonstrated in preclinical models of Bcr-Abl–positive tumors, which led to phase I and II studies in patients with Philadelphia chromosome–positive leukemias. A second target for STI571, based on its receptor inhibitory profile, was c-kit, which is mutated to a constitutively activated form in gastrointestinal stromal tumors. Early studies demonstrated striking efficacy in patients with advanced disease. Because subsequent studies also demonstrated that this agent was extremely potent in blocking PDGFR signaling by both the α- and the β-receptors and disrupting PDGF/PDGFR ligand–receptor autocrine and paracrine loops (8), this agent was tested in tumors with PDGFR-driven proliferation. Preliminary studies in glioma cell lines demonstrated inhibition of proliferation in vitro and delay of tumor growth in vivo. This was less striking than in leukemias, most likely relating to the fact that multiple pathways are known to contribute to glioma proliferation, rather than a single overriding pathway, not to the limitations of PDGFR as a target in general. Thus, despite the fact that the tyrosine kinase receptors targeted by STI571 are expressed on a variety of normal cells throughout the body, preclinical and clinical studies with this agent seemed to indicate that antiproliferative effects were mediated selectively on neoplastic cells, with relatively little systemic toxicity (9). The North American Brain Tumor Consortium (NABTC) and the Pediatric Brain Tumor Consortium initiated phase I studies in children and adults with malignant gliomas. An unexpected finding from several of these studies, which have yet to be fully analyzed, is that a subset of patients experienced intratumoral hemorrhage during treatment. This might be due to the known effects of this agent on perivascular cell permeability (7,9). Correlative imaging studies, including magnetic resonance spectroscopy and positron-emission tomography, have been performed on a subset of patients on the pediatric trial, and it is hoped that this will provide insights into this issue. Because objective responses and long-term survivors have been observed in the pediatric phase I trial, a phase II study has been opened for patients with brain stem malignant gliomas, although care has been taken to include stopping rules for an intolerable frequency of hemorrhagic events. In contrast to the experiences in North America, an intergroup study from Europe observed intratumoral hemorrhage in only 1 of 51 patients. Partial radiological responses were observed in 3 of 19 patients treated with 600 mg/day and 1 of 33 patients treated with 800 mg/day, and an additional one and four patients in these respective subsets had stable disease for more than six months (8). An intriguing observation from a second, smaller, study was that prolonged disease control was achieved in three of six high-grade glioma patients younger than 45 years of age, versus only one of nine older than 45 years (10). Combinations of STI571 and conventional chemotherapeutic agents have also been examined. Although the optimal agent to employ in this regard remains uncertain, promising results have been reported from Germany with hydroxyurea (1000 mg/day) combined with 400 mg/day of STI571, with objective disease regression in 5 of 26 patients (11). Currently, a randomized phase III study is active in several European countries to examine the activity of STI571 in recurrent glioblatoma. This study compares hydroxyurea with and without STI571. Tight imaging regimens every six weeks allow to very early add STI571 in the hydroxyurea-only arm or to dose escalate STI571 from 600 to 800 mg in the alternative arm.

Epidermal Growth Factor Receptor

Inhibition of EGFR is an important strategy because EGFR mediates anti-apoptotic effects and enhances survival of glioma cells in vivo. Accordingly, pharmacological inhibition of EGFR sensitizes glioma cells to CD95L- and Apo2L/TRAIL–induced apoptosis. In some cell lines, the inhibition of EGFR may be compensated for by signaling through other receptor tyrosine kinases such as insulin-like growth factor receptor I. The combination of EGFR inhibitors with inhibitors of other receptor tyrosine kinases may therefore improve the efficacy of this approach. Recent work has offered an explanation for the efficacy of coinhibition: the kinase c-Src downstream of the EGFR phosphorylates and inhibits the tumor suppressor phosphatase and tensin homolog deleted on chromosome ten (PTEN). Inhibition of EGFR may thus restore the function of PTEN and thus put a break on PI3K signaling.

Gefitinib

ZD1839 (Gefitinib), a low-molecular-weight synthetic quinazoline, was designed as a potent and selective inhibitor of the EGFR tyrosine kinase. It is active against EGFR at nanomolar concentrations in cell-free systems, with 100-fold less activity against other EGFR family members, such as ErbB-2, and has little or no enzyme inhibitory activity against other tyrosine and serine–threonine kinases (12). It is effective in blocking EGFR autophosphorylation and inhibiting EGFR-dependent cell signaling in cell lines that rely heavily on EGFR activation for proliferative stimulation, but has virtually no effect on EGFR-independent proliferation. Tumor growth inhibition is associated with cell cycle arrest in the G1 phase of the cell cycle. ZD1839 has also demonstrated antitumor activity in vivo in a number of human tumor xenograft models after oral administration, particularly in model systems in which proliferation is dependent on EGFR-mediated signaling (13). Initial clinical data indicated that ZD1839 has good oral bioavailability, a long half-life, and was well tolerated at effective doses (14,15), with the most common toxicity being an acneiform skin rash, and diarrhea being a common dose-limiting toxicity on clinical trials. Daily dosing achieved a maximum concentration in the blood of 5 mM at a dose of 500 mg/day, and even concentrations in the 1- to 2-mM range produced complete or nearly complete inhibition of EGFR signaling in many cell lines. Results from several early clinical studies for noncentral nervous system solid tumors have demonstrated activity of ZD1839 as a single agent. However, large phase III studies in patients with advanced small cell lung cancer failed to demonstrate a convincing benefit of adding this agent to regimens including either gemcitabine/cisplatin or paclitaxel/carboplatin (16).

Response to ZD1839 is strongly influenced by tumor EGFR status, confirming that this agent may be an exquisitively selective inhibitor in appropriate tumors (17). Twenty-five of 275 patients treated with ZD1839 were noted to have objective therapeutic responses; eight of the nine who had tumor specimens available for mutational analysis were observed to have mutations within the EGFR gene, generally involving gain-of-function changes close to the adenosine triphosphate (ATP)–binding pocket of the tyrosine kinase domain (16). In contrast, none of the seven patients with no response to ZD1839, who were analyzed in parallel, had mutations. In two cases in which the functional effect of the mutation on ZD1839 sensitivity was examined, it was observed that this was increased 10-fold, with complete inhibition of protein activity at a concentration of 0.2 mM versus 2 mM with the wild-type receptor. These observations emphasize the importance of studies of tumor genotype and phenotype in considerations of both study design and response analysis.

It is likely that not only the presence, but also the type of such mutations may influence the effect of ZD1839. In contrast to the above results showing increased therapeutic efficacy with certain types of mutations, other groups have observed that the most common mutational phenotype in gliomas (EGFRvIII) may confer reduced sensitivity to ZD1839 in in vivo brain tumor models, because this receptor is active independent of ligand binding (17). The involvement of other key signaling pathways driving tumor proliferation may counteract the effects of ZD1839 (18). For example, PTEN mutations, which are common in these tumors, appear to counteract the effect of EGFR inhibitors, on downstream growth and survival signaling (19), necessitating the use of multiple signaling inhibitors in order to achieve a growth inhibitory effect. Given this, phase I/II studies of ZD1839 have been initiated within the NABTC (for adults with malignant glioma and meningioma) and the Pediatric Brain Tumor Consortium (for children with recurrent malignant glioma and newly diagnosed brain stem malignant glioma). These studies are including analyses of receptor expression and mutational status. In the NABTC study, patients who were not receiving enzyme-inducing antiepileptic drugs (EIAD) or corticosteroids received a daily dose of 500 mg and those receiving corticosteroids were escalated incrementally to a dose of 1000 mg/day. A phase I study was conducted in patients receiving EIAD that established a maximum tolerated dose of 1500 mg/day. Among 55 patients with malignant gliomas who were in the first two groups, a phase II evaluation of activity identified partial responses in seven, although the median times to progression in patients with glioblastoma and anaplastic glioma were not superior to historical controls (8 and 12 weeks, respectively) (20). Therefore, it needs to be determined whether a certain molecular signaling profile will help to distinguish responders from nonresponders. Because a study of ZD1839 in patients with newly diagnosed malignant gliomas failed to demonstrate a significant improvement in survival, or an association between EGFR amplification status as assessed by fluorescence in situ hybridization and outcome, a more detailed analysis of mutations and signaling pathway phenotype will be required to identify an appropriate subset of patients for treatment with this agent. A small trial has reported good tolerance of ZD1839 and rapamycin in heavily pretreated glioblastoma patients (21). Studies are also in progress to determine whether combinations of ZD1839 with conventional chemotherapeutic agents such as temozolomide, may enhance efficacy.

Erlotinib

OSI-774 (Erlotinib), another small molecule inhibitor of EGFR, exhibits reversible inhibition of EGFR, by competition with the ATP-binding site, similar to ZD1839, with a median inhibitory concentration in the low nanomolar range. This agent inhibits EGFR autophosphorylation at concentrations in the range of 20 nM, and in cell lines dependent on EGFR for proliferation, inhibition of cell growth was observed in a comparable range (22). Higher concentrations induced apoptosis. As with ZD1839, this agent induces cell cycle arrest at G1, with accumulation of p27Kip1. A recently completed trial in adults with malignant glioma has demonstrated some efficacy (23). In the phase II part of this study, patients were treated with 150 mg/day; only 1 of 45 patients had an objective response, with median time to progression for the cohort no better than historical controls (24). Although a higher rate of responses was observed in a single-institution study using the same dose (4 of 16 patients), these responses were not durable and median time to progression was not improved compared to historical controls. A trial combining OSI-774 with temozolomide in children with recurrent glioma has recently been opened. Two other selective, reversible EGFR inhibitors that are in early phase trials are GW2016 (Lapatinib) and PKI166, both of which have demonstrated preclinical activity at submicromolar concentrations (25,26). GW2016 has activity against ErbB2-expressing tumors and is planned to be tested in childhood medulloblastoma and ependymoma. Irreversible EGFR inhibitors that are active against other ErbB family members are also being tested clinically. These include CI-1033, Cetuximab, and EKB-569. CI-1033 is currently tested in combination with temsirolimus, a mammalian target of rapamycin (mTOR) inhibitor, in a phase I/II clinical trial in recurrent malignant glioma (27).

Vascular Endothelial Growth Factor/Vascular Endothelial Growth Factor Receptor

Numerous clinical studies have been initiated to test antiangiogenic strategies on various malignancies employing synthetic as well as naturally occurring antiangiogenic compounds. Over 80 antiangiogenic agents are currently evaluated in clinical trials having enrolled over 10,000 patients. Several of these trials recruit patients with brain tumors [at the time of writing this article, an internet search revealed 14 ongoing trials (3,28,29) targeting different pathways (30)]. Current reports from phase I and II clinical trials conclude that antiangiogenic agents are well tolerated. However, despite promising results obtained in experimental tumor models, none or only limited therapeutic effects have been reported from clinical trials. Differences in tumor vasculature in humans and animals as well as the use of tumor models established from cell lines which seldom resemble the molecular and morphological heterogenous composition of primary tumors may be reasons for this discrepancy. The use of transgenic tumor models may be one of the means to improve experimental testing of therapeutic approaches. Moreover, combination therapies with established conventional treatment regimens have been suggested to enhance therapeutic potential.

Bevacizumab

Bevacizumab is an anti-VEGF monoclonal antibody currently under investigation in combination with CPT-11 in the treatment of patients with relapsed malignant glioma. Bevacizumab is administered at 5 mg/kg body weight over 60 to 90 minutes every two weeks. Following bevacizumab, and continuing weekly for four weeks, CPT-11 at $125 \, mg/m^2$ is administered. Toxicities attributed to Bevacizumab are intracranial hemorrhage (1/29 patients), bowel perforation (1/29), wound healing abnormalities (2/29), and epistaxis (5/29). More than half of the patients show a radiographic response during the first treatment cycle (31).

SU5416

This VEGFR2 inhibitor has been effective in preclinical glioma paradigms and is currently being investigated in metastasized colorectal cancer and Kaposi sarcoma in AIDS patients (27).

Reactive Oxygen Species

Generation of reactive oxygen species (ROS) may make glioma cells more vulnerable to oxidative stress, i.e., damage involving oxidation–reduction reactions, inflicted by radiation or chemotherapy. Generation of ROS promotes apoptosis. Motexafin gadolinium is the first of an investigational class of drugs called "texaphyrins," which are designed small molecules that accumulate inside cells with high rates of metabolism, including anaerobic glycolysis. Because motexafin gadolinium is a paramagnetic compound, its presence is visible with magnetic resonance imaging (MRI). A current study looks at the tolerability and efficacy in combination with temozolomide in progressive and recurrent malignant gliomas (27).

Protein Kinase C-β

The protein kinase C (PKC) family of serine–threonine PKs has been implicated in the processes that control tumor cell growth, survival, and progression. Early observations that PKCs are activated by tumor-promoting phorbol esters suggested that PKC activation may be involved in tumor initiation and progression. Tumor-induced angiogenesis requires activation of PKCs, particularly PKC-β. PKC activation also contributes to tumor cell survival and proliferation and has been repeatedly implicated in the malignant progression of human cancers, notably B-cell lymphomas, malignant gliomas, and colorectal carcinomas (32). PKC expression is specifically increased in patients with fatal/refractory diffuse large B-cell lymphoma, linking increased PKC expression to patient survival. PKC activation can trigger signaling through the ras/extracellular signal–regulated kinase pathway, which may be involved in controlling cellular proliferation and apoptosis as well as the induction of intestinal cell invasiveness.

Enzastaurin

These data have prompted the development of novel anticancer therapeutics targeting PKC. Enzastaurin (LY317615.HCl) was developed as a selective PKC-β inhibitor. Enzastaurin decreased microvessel density and VEGF expression in human tumor xenografts. In addition, enzastaurin directly suppresses proliferation, induces apoptosis of tumor cells in culture, and suppresses phosphorylation of glycogen synthase kinase (GSK) 3β, ribosomal protein S6, and AKT. Oral dosing of enzastaurin to achieve plasma concentrations of drug comparable with those achieved in clinical trials significantly suppresses the growth of human colon and glioblastoma xenografts. As in cell culture, GSK3β phosphorylation was suppressed in these tumor tissues. Moreover, GSK3β phosphorylation was suppressed to a similar extent and with a similar time course in peripheral blood mononuclear cells from these xenograft-bearing mice (33). These data support the notion that enzastaurin elicits an antitumor effect by suppressing signaling through the AKT pathway, directly inducing tumor cell death and suppressing tumor cell proliferation. A large unicenter phase I/II study in progressive and recurrent malignant glioma, undertaken in patients with and without EIAD, with some efficacy parameters published to date (subjective responses in over 20% of more than 100 patients) (34), is prompting the design of a phase III randomized trial in recurrent glioblastoma and several phase I/II studies in newly diagnosed glioblastoma to be initiated in 2006.

TARGETS IN MOTILITY AND ANGIOGENESIS

Malignant progression correlates with increased migratory capacity of tumor cells involving a wide range of molecular mechanisms including metalloproteinolytic activity and integrin-dependent regulation of cell adhesion. Invasion of cells into the surrounding tissue is a multistep process that requires changes in cell–cell contacts, e.g., mediated by cadherins or the hyaluronic acid receptor CD44, cell substrate interactions, and degradation of the extracellular matrix by matrix metalloproteinases (MMP). Some cytokines such as EGF, hepatocyte growth factor, or transforming growth factor (TGF)-β_2 promote cell migration and invasion in a cell type– and context-dependent manner by triggering distinct intracellular signaling cascades. Accordingly, expression of TGF-β_2 correlates with glioma cell invasiveness, and inhibition of TFG-β by a neutralizing antibody or by a small molecule TGF-β receptor antagonist, SD-208, significantly reduced glioma cell migration (35).

Anti-Integrins

Cilengitide

Integrins are mediators of cell matrix interactions, which have important clinical consequences. Vitronectin, a glioma-derived extracellular matrix protein and $\alpha v\beta 3/5$ integrin ligand, protects tumor cells from apoptotic death, probably via upregulated genes including PI3-kinase. Targeting integrin signaling through the PI3kinase/AKT pathway by integrin-linked kinase (ILK) inhibitors effectively inhibits the ILK-AKT cascade, blocking both basal and EGF-induced phosphorylation of AKT downstream targets, including p70S6K and GSK3α/β. ILK inhibitors reduce growth and invasion in U87 glioma cells. The integrin antagonist EMD 121974 (Cilengitide) induces apoptosis in brain tumor cells growing on vitronectin and tenascin and shows efficacy in vivo using orthotopic glioma models (36). The agent is a cyclic pentapeptide, which binds to the RGD sequence of the integrin, interrupting ligand interaction and blocking downstream signaling including focal adhesion kinase–dependent cell survival pathways. New Approaches to Brain Tumor Therapy (NABTT) clinical trials with cilengitide have demonstrated some objective responses and some long-term disease stabilizations. In these trials, perfusion-sensitive MRI studies have been shown to serve as potential measures of treatment efficacy.

In summary, cilengitide is not highly cytotoxic and its effects in restoring sensitivity to proapoptotic stimuli require cotreatment for full effect. In breast cancer and also glioma xenografts, cilengitide targeting of $\alpha v\beta 3$ integrin receptor synergizes with radiotherapy and radioimmunotherapy. Current brain tumor clinical trials test concurrent cilengitide with the radio-chemotherapy applied in the EORTC 26981 study (2).

Inhibitors of Matricellular Proteins

Antitenascin Monoclonal Antibody

The only matricellular protein target taken to clinical trial is tenascin-C. After demonstrating that antitenascin monoclonal antibody 81C6 exhibited therapeutic potential in subcutaneous and intracranial human xenografts in athymic mice, a study demonstrated that the ^{131}I-labeled antibody demonstrated selective intracranial localization upon systemic administration (37). Currently, a clinical study assessing the efficacy and maximum tolerated dose of 81C6 by bolus injection or microinfusion is underway.

MMP Inhibitors

RO28-2653

MMP inhibition with RO-28-2653 that predominantly inhibits MMP-2/-9 was effective in vitro and by oral administration in vivo. In a paradigm of B-cell leukemia (Lymphoma-title like protein) BCL-X$_L$–induced glioma satellite formation in xenografted glioma in nude mice, MMP inhibition resulted in loss of gelatinolytic activity and prevention of tumor satellite formation (38).

Marimastat

Marimastat is a low-molecular-weight peptide mimetic inhibitor of MMP. In vitro studies of Marimastat demonstrated significant inhibition of invasion of glioma cell lines. Marimastat administered adjuvantly to patients with glioblastoma after radiotherapy did not show significant efficacy (unpublished data). In another trial, the combination of temozolomide and Marimastat appeared to result in some benefit (39). Therefore, anti-invasion therapy might preferentially be combined with proapoptotic therapies. Another MMP inhibitor, Col-3, has been used in a single-agent phase I/II study for a continuous oral schedule in patients with recurrent high-grade glioma with good safety, but limited efficacy (40). Cathepsin B and urokinase plasminogen activator and receptor inhibition have shown some efficacy in preclinical models, but no inhibitors have demonstrated the same in clinical use.

MEASURES TO ENHANCE THE APOPTOTIC MACHINERY IN GLIOMA CELLS

Dysregulation of Apoptotic Pathways

Human glioma cell lines express a variety of antiapoptotic and proapoptotic BCL-2 family proteins, and it has been shown that overexpression of BCL-2 and BCL-X$_L$ protects these cells from apoptosis induced by diverse stimuli. An upregulation of BCL-2 and BCL-X$_L$, but a downregulation of BCL-2-associated X-Protein (BAX), has been described in recurrent glioblastoma independent from treatment, suggesting therapy-independent pressures for the development of an apoptosis-resistant phenotype. In contrast, BCL-2 or BCL-X$_L$ expression has not consistently shown to be associated with increasing World Health Organization (WHO) grade. Overexpression of BCL-2 or BCL-X$_L$ induces complex changes of the glioma cell phenotype in that it not only protects glioma cells from various proapoptotic stimuli, but also enhances their motility via mechanisms independent from the prevention of apoptosis (38). p53 may be the most common target gene for mutational inactivation in human cancers. p53 mutations are rather common (65%) in secondary glioblastomas, thought to be derived through the malignant progression from grade II or III astrocytomas. In these patients, the same p53 mutations are already found in the less malignant precursor lesion in approximately 90%. In contrast, only 10% of primary glioblastomas exhibit p53 mutations. Interestingly, p53 mutations and amplification of the EGFR gene appear to be mutually exclusive. The molecular basis for this phenomenon remains to be identified.

In untransformed cells, the loss of p53 may enhance rather than decrease the vulnerability to apoptosis. However, within the process of neoplastic transformation, the loss of p53 probably allows the cell to accumulate random genetic and chromosomal aberrations without triggering the endogenous p53-controlled cell death pathway. In human malignant glioma cell lines, there is no apparent correlation between the sensitivity to cytotoxic therapy and genetic or functional p53 status or expression of p53-response genes (41).

Apoptosis Modulators

BCL-2

The neutralization of antiapoptotic BCL-2 family proteins by antisense technology or by overexpression of proapoptotic BCL-2 family proteins has remained an active area of apoptosis research for more than a decade. Natural born killer (NBK) is a prototype member of the proapoptotic BH-3–only BCL-2 family members which heterodimerizes with BCL-2 and BCL-X$_L$. Adenoviral transfer of NBK induces cell death independent of activation of caspases 3, 7, 8, 9, and 10. The most widely used and most experimentally advanced DNA therapeutic is the antisense oligonucleotide. These oligomers are predominantly used to inhibit mRNA expression. For cancer chemotherapy, the BCL-2 antisense oligonucleotide (oblimersen sodium, G3139, and genasense by Genta Inc., New Jersey, U.S.A.) is currently in multiple phase II and III clinical trials for myeloma, non-Hodgkin's lymphoma, colorectal cancer, and solid tumors in children except for brain tumors (42).

p53

A phase I study of adenoviral p53 gene therapy in patients with malignant glioma demonstrated that ectopic expression of p53 can induce apoptosis in vivo, but transduction efficiency was too low for clinically relevant impact of this strategy (43). The stabilization of mutant p53 proteins by small molecules that act in a chaperone-like fashion and promote wild-type p53 activity is another promising approach to cancer therapy. In human malignant glioma cells, the compound CP-31398 induces cell death in both p53 mutant and p53 wild-type cell lines, but not in the p53-null LN-308 cell line. Cell death in this paradigm had some features of apoptosis, namely phosphatidylserine exposure on the outside of the cell membrane, but was independent of BCL-X$_L$ and lacked caspase activation. The proximate cause of death thus remained obscure. In addition, p53-independent cytotoxic effects of CP-31398 may limit the usefulness of this specific compound. However, a number of related agents with supposedly more specificity are currently being developed (44).

Death Ligands

Death ligands are naturally occurring effector molecules of the tumor necrosis factor family, which serve as an endogenous pathway to eliminate dispensable or dangerous cells, e.g., virally infected or cancer cells. The presence of both agonistic and antagonistic (decoy) receptors for Apo2L/TRAIL may be of special importance because the differential distribution of these receptors in tumor cells and normal tissue has been proposed to underlie the selective activity of Apo2L/TRAIL against tumor cells. A preferential expression of agonistic Apo2L/TRAIL receptors is also seen in malignant glioma cells. Downstream effectors of death receptor–mediated apoptosis, the caspases, have been successfully employed to promote glioma cell death in vitro and in vivo, too. Yet, targeting potent intracellular mediators of apoptosis is only feasible clinically if major problems of therapeutic gene delivery will be solved, involving both efficacy and specificity. Thus, caspase 3 gene transfer will only kill cancer cells that are transduced. Caspase 3 is also a potent inducer of apoptosis in neurons, suggesting that neurotoxicity might become a problem in vivo.

In the field of death ligands and receptors, inducing cancer cell apoptosis via local or systemic application of Apo2L/TRAIL is one of the most promising strategies. The growth of intracranial human glioma xenografts in nude mice is inhibited by the locoregional administration of Apo2L/TRAIL (45). Convection-enhanced delivery of Apo2L/ TRAIL can also enhance the effect of systemic treatment of temozolomide in an intracranial glioma model. Differences in the intracellular actions of CD95L and Apo2L/TRAIL can account for selective sensitivity of glioma cell lines to either ligand, and combined treatment with adenovirally delivered Apo2L/TRAIL and CD95L may have synergistic effects in some cell lines. A potentially clinically applicable strategy to promote glioma cell apoptosis consists of the combination of peptides derived from the Smac protein with chemotherapy or Apo2L/TRAIL. Smac is a potent inhibitor of members of the inhibitor of apoptosis proteins (IAP) family of caspase inhibitors, and overexpression of Smac or the treatment with cell-permeable Smac peptides bypasses the BCL-2 block to apoptosis and greatly facilitates chemotherapy and Apo2L/TRAIL-mediated apoptosis in vitro. Even more impressive, intracranially grafted U87MG human malignant glioma cells were eradicated by local combination treatment with Smac peptides and Apo2L/TRAIL in a mouse model (46). While the application of Smac peptides is hampered by technical problems, nonpeptidyl small molecule drugs, which mimic the inhibitory action of Smac on IAPs, are already tested in preclinical studies.

Inactivation of X-inhibitor of apoptosis protein (XIAP) by an antisense construct is another strategy, and there is a phase I clinical study with the XIAP antisense molecule AEG35165 (47). For survivin, proapoptotic effects of either antisense oligonucleotide-mediated downregulation or functional suppression through transduction with a dominant negative mutant have been reported. A clinical trial with survivin antisense oligonucleotides has also been announced.

Targeting Nonclassical Players Involved in Apoptosis

In addition to the direct targeting of classical players involved in apoptosis, such as BCL-2, p53 or death receptors, there are some novel approaches to induce apoptosis in glioma cells which appear to be close to a clinical assessment. A report of antitumoral actions of cannabinoids, thought to act via the ceramide pathway, in a rat glioma model in vivo in the absence of neurotoxicity is provoking in this regard. However, lower levels of cannabinoids transactivate the EGFR and enhance tumor cell proliferation. Glioma cells with deregulated activity of the EGFR pathway may also display enhanced sensitivity for Ras inhibition by farnesyltransferase inhibitors. However, we have recently found that inhibition of EGFR signaling may also mimic a "starvation signal" and thus protect glioma cells from acute hypoxia by decreasing energy demand (48). While the importance of this phenomenon for the therapy of human tumors is not yet known, it may be prudent to consider ambiguous effects of therapies targeting the EGFR when pronounced hypoxia is present, e.g., concurrent treatment with angiogenesis inhibitors. An ongoing phase I/II study in recurrent and progressive glioblastoma uses the combination of the farnesyltransferase inhibitor tipifarnib and radiochemotherapy with temozolomide (2).

NF-kB is activated by chemotherapeutic agents and may mediate antiapoptotic transcriptional responses in malignant glioma cells. Expression of dominant negative I-kB inhibits the nuclear translocation of NF-kB and augments the cytotoxicity of carmustine, carboplatin, and SN-38. Exposure to sulfasalazine, a potent inhibitor of NF-kB, has differential effects on CD95L and Apo2L/TRAIL-mediated apoptosis—the former is inhibited while the latter is enhanced. Intriguingly, these effects appear to be independent from the inhibitory action on NF-kB, but require protein synthesis and possibly p21.

Histone deacetylase (HDAC) inhibitors have been identified as promising compounds for the treatment of various types of neoplasms. They induce differentiation, growth arrest, and apoptotic cell death. Acetylation and deacetylation of core histones represent regulatory mechanisms of gene expression. In general, histone acetylation opens the chromatin structure and thereby promotes gene transcription, whereas histone deacetylation induces an opposite effect mediated by chromatin condensation. In addition, normal cell differentiation and adjustment of metabolic activity require coordinated gene transcription and balanced activity of histone acetyltransferases (HAT) versus HDAC. Accordingly, deletions or inactivating mutations of HAT are associated with tumor progression in humans. Thus, HDAC inhibitors provide the intriguing opportunity to pharmacologically modulate gene activity by epigenetic regulation. FR901228 is the first novel HDAC inhibitor analyzed in a National Institute of Health (NIH) clinical trial (28).

Suicide Gene Therapy

Herpes Simplex Virus–Thymidine Kinase

In the classical paradigm of retroviral gene therapy, actively dividing cells are transduced by prodrug gene therapy with the herpes simplex virus (HSV) thymidine kinase (TK) gene and subsequently treated with the antiviral drug ganciclovir. The viral enzyme phosphorylates the prodrug into ganciclovir triphosphate, which acts as an inhibitor of DNA synthesis and leads to cell death. Prodrug/suicide gene therapies exhibit bystander effects leading to the killing of infected as well as nontransduced tumor cells by the cell-to-cell transfer of phosphorylated ganciclovir through gap junctions as well as an immune response. Phase I/II clinical trials demonstrated low toxicity and some tumor responses. In contrast, when efficacy was tested in newly diagnosed glioblastoma in a phase III randomized controlled trial of 240 patients, no significant advantage over standard therapy was found. This could be due to limitations of the ganciclovir thymidine-kinase (GCV/TK) system itself because ganciclovir poorly crosses the blood–brain barrier and the transduction efficacy of tumor cells was very low. Application of ganciclovir directly into the tumor or different prodrug/suicide gene systems, e.g., cyclophosphamide/cytochrome P450 2B1, in which the prodrug can cross the blood–brain barrier, is being developed (49).

Oncolytic Viruses

Oncolytic virotherapy uses viruses such as adenoviruses or HSVs with the natural ability to kill their host cells. An infected cell undergoes lysis and thereby thousands of new virus particles are released and new cells are infected and killed in successive rounds of infection and cytolysis. By the use of mutant/attenuated viruses that preferentially replicate in tumor cells or through engineered viruses in which genes that are essential for replication are placed under tumor-specific promoters, cell death is restricted to tumor cells. The dl1520 (ONYX-015) replication-competent adenovirus replicates preferentially in p53-deficient cells because it carries a mutation that renders those cells deficient in viral E1B-55K expression. Normally, E1B-55K protein binds and inactivates p53 thereby preventing p53-mediated induction of growth arrest or apoptosis in infected cells. The disadvantage is that E1B-55K wild-type viruses could replicate in nontumor as well as in tumor cells. In tumor cells that are deficient for p53 function, E1B-55K is dispensable for p53 inactivation and viral replication proceeds unimpaired. Phase I/II clinical trials showed safety and some signs of efficacy of dl1520. A NABTT trial of injection of dl1520 at 10^7 to 10^{10} plaque-forming units in 24 recurrent glioblastoma after surgical resection of tumor exhibited no maximum tolerated dose at 10^{10} plaque-forming units, and a median time to tumor progression of 67.5 days with a median survival time of 176.6 days (50). Dl1520 was safe but time to progression was short and only one patient showed a subjective partial response. This limited efficacy may be due to several factors: (i) This virus lacks E1B-55K functions. Hence, its cytolytic capacity is lower relative to wild-type adenovirus; (ii) viral infection rate was low because the glioma cells do not express the viral receptor; (iii) intratumoral spread was found to be insufficient; and (iv) reresections in two patients revealed that some antiviral immune responses might have limited its spread and efficacy. More promising results have been found in trials combining radiotherapy with dl1520.

IMMUNOTHERAPY: STRATEGIES TO OVERCOME THE DISEASE

Glial tumor therapy is hampered by extensive spread of tumor cells in the brain, a lack of effective immune responses to glial tumor cells that has been attributed to the blood–brain barrier, a lack of lymphatic vessels, and local release of immunosuppressive factors, as well as limitations or toxicities of other therapies. Therefore, immunotherapy is attractive as it is designed to specifically target tumor but not normal cells and to enable the host immune system to combat the disease. In general, the immune system can be divided into innate and adaptive components. The innate immune system uses microbial nonself, missing-self, and induced-self recognition. Missing-self recognition is due to absence of inhibitory markers of normal-self activating the immune system. This concept was introduced to explain the preferential attack of target cells that express few or no major histocompatibility complex (MHC) class I proteins by natural killer (NK) cells. The paradigm of induced self-recognition relies on the detection of markers that are induced upon infection or cellular transformation. These excessive cellular stressors promote the expression of molecules that highlight affected cells for attack preferentially by NK cells. These molecules interact with a recently described activating receptor, NKG2D. Why are glioma cells that express NKG2DL nonetheless not effectively targeted by NK cells? A recent paper provides evidence that NKG2DL expression in glioma cells might be outbalanced by MHC class I expression inhibiting NK cell–mediated killing. The immunosuppressive molecule TGF-β, produced by glioma cells, down-regulates NKG2D on NK and CD8+ T-cells. This limits the NKG2DL/NKG2D interactions. Further, TGF-β induces MMP that cleave NKG2DL and suppress NKG2D mRNA levels in glioma cells (51,52). A specific anti-tumor cytotoxicity depends on the identification of specific tumor antigens.

The adoptive component of the immune system involves T- and B-cells. Recent advances in genome-wide expression analyses and tools to predict immunogenic epitopes enhance the probability of identifying brain tumor–associated antigens. Continuous progress in the understanding of the molecular mediators of the immune response will also promote the incompletely understood immune escape mechanisms of brain tumors. Passive and vaccine-based (active) immunotherapies are discussed as principally different approaches.

Active Immunotherapy

Vaccination aims to augment the existing or to create a new antitumor immune response. Primarily cytokines such as interleukin (IL)-2, IL-4, IL-7, IL-12, granulomonocytic colony–stimulating factors (GM-CSF), macrophage colony–stimulating factor, and interferons have been used to augment antitumor immunity. In these experiments, the predominant role of antigen-presenting cells in the initiation of the immune response became evident. Professional antigen-presenting cells, such as dendritic cells, capture tumor antigens, process them, and present them on MHC molecules to T-cell receptors. T-cell activation requires a second stimulatory signal provided by costimulatory molecules, e.g., B7 on antigen-presenting cells engaging CD28 on T-cells. Once properly activated, these T-cells will launch a potent tumor-specific immune response. Because under normal conditions brain cells exhibit a low expression of MHC class I and II molecules, they are not recognized as a target by antigen-specific T-cells. Functionally intact neurons suppress the induction of immune molecules on surrounding glial cells, e.g., by expression of nerve growth factor. Recent approaches have attempted to prime dendritic cells with antigen in vitro and reinjecting these cells into the patient to activate a T-cell response. This peripheral subcutaneous immunization has been shown to elicit systemic and intratumoral immune responses in a phase I/II clinical trial for glioblastoma. However, the induction of systemic effector cells did not necessarily translate into objective clinical responses or increased survival, particularly for patients with actively progressing tumors or those with tumors expressing high levels of TGF-β$_2$. In reoperated patients, the magnitude of the tumor T-cell infiltration was inversely correlated with the expression levels of TGF-β (53). Experimental combination of intratumorally delivered interferon-α–transduced dendritic cells with subcutaneously administered IL-4 or GM-CSF expressing glioma cells enhanced the antitumor efficacy compared to peripheral vaccination alone. This was dependent on TRAIL/Apo2L-sensitive tumor-specific cytotoxic T-cells (54).

Passive Immunotherapy

Passive immunotherapy is defined as the transfer of molecules immuno-competent for a specific antigen into a host that is immunopassive for that antigen or the transfer of immune cells. These molecules can be antibodies, the cells are T-cells or lymphokine-activated killer cells, and activated tumor infiltrating lymphocytes (the latter is also called "adoptive transfer"). A number of antibodies coupled to radioisotopes or immunotoxins have been tested in clinical trials.

Neutralizing TGF-β

Antisense Strategies

Antisense oligonucleotides to TGF-β_2 have been used for almost 10 years to inhibit the synthesis of TGF-β and to thereby promote the immune-mediated lysis of glioma cells. A rat 9L glioma model was used to demonstrate that sub-cutaneous vaccination with TGF-β_1 antisense cDNA-transfected glioma cells inhibited intracranial tumor growth. Similarly, stable TGF-β_2 antisense-transfected C6 glioma cells, injected subcutaneously seven days after the implantation of an intracranial C6 glioma, led to smaller tumor sizes and prolonged survival of Wistar rats compared with animals treated with control-transfected C6 cells (55). More recently, RNA interference targeting TGF-β_1 and TGF-β_2 was shown to abrogate the subcutaneous and intracra-nial tumorigenicity of human glioma cells in nude mice (53) and also to greatly diminish the invasion of monolayer glioma cells through matrigel-coated membranes and of glioma cell spheroids into a collagen matrix.

Inhibition of TGF-β Processing

One would anticipate that the inhibition of TGF-β–processing furin-like proteases results in a depletion of TGF-β and a reversal of the local milieu of immunosuppression. Glioma cells express furin and possibly other related proprotein convertases, and furin inhibition by the synthetic antitrypsin analog α-antitrypsin portland (PDX) or synthetic pseudosubstrate inhibi-tors expectedly reduced TGF-β activity in the cell culture supernatant. Inter-estingly, furin inhibitor–treated glioma cells showed an accumulation of the 55 kD TGF-β precursor protein in the supernatant, not in the cellular lysate, consistent with the notion that these cells release furin-like proteases which then process TGF-β extracellularly. Pharmacological agents for clinical use would therefore probably not have to be cell-permeable molecules.

Inhibition of TGF-β Signaling

The desired prevention of biological effects of enhanced TGF-β activity could also be achieved by rendering the target cells, which include mostly host cells, but also the tumor cells, resistant to TGF-β. Small molecule inhibitors targeting TGF-βR1–associated kinase activity have recently become available. SD-208, a prototypic agent of this new class of agents, inhibits TGF-β signaling at an EC_{50} concentration of 30 nM. It abrogates autocrine TGF-β effects such as Smad2/3 phosphorylation and migration in glioma cells, prevents the inhibitory effects of glioma cell supernatants on immune cell function, and delays the growth of syngeneic SMA-560 gliomas in VM/Dk mice (35). The clinical evaluation of similar agents in recurrent malignant glioma should be the next step to determine whether this simple strategy should be further pursued as a part of changing the natural course of this disease.

Anti-TGF-β Strategies in the Clinic

Based on the experience derived from a small phase I/II evaluation that disclosed essentially no dose-limiting toxicity, an antisense oligonucleotide to TGF-$β_2$ referred to as AP-12009 is currently being assessed in a randomized phase II trial for recurrent malignant glioma in Germany, Austria, Israel, Russia, and India. AP-12009 is administered by convection-enhanced delivery through a continuous pump infusion following a one-week on/one-week off schedule for up to six months. The control arm is chemotherapy, that is, temozolomide for patients pretreated with nitrosoureas and vice versa, and either of these for patients who have had radiotherapy only as their first line treatment. The primary endpoint is progression-free survival at six months. Results from this trial will be available at the end of 2006.

Perspectives

TGF-β may be considered one of the most promising target molecules for biological treatment approaches to glioblastoma. A wide variety of small molecule inhibitors of TGF-β signaling are under development. This notion is supported by the profound inhibitory effects of TGF-β on the immune system as well as the phenotype of increased motility, invasiveness, and angiogenesis associated with elevated TGF-β activity. It is now necessary to evaluate the feasibility of these strategies in the clinic, with the option to combine these approaches or to use TGF-β antagonism in order to permit the success of more sophisticated immunotherapies based on vaccination strategies. Such concepts should not only result in a better therapeutic outcome for human glioma patients, but also may have broader relevance for other types of cancers associated with enhanced TGF-β activity.

FUTURE PROSPECTS

Neural Stem Cells and the Origin of Gliomas

Recent reports on the identification of glioma-initiating cells, which may lead to improved understanding of the cellular origin of gliomas and better therapeutic targeting, have raised a lot of enthusiasm in the field (56).

Basically, there are obvious similarities between glioma and neural stem cells: high motility, robust proliferative potential, association with blood vessels and white matter tracts, and immature expression profiles (expression of nestin, EGFR and PTEN), as well as activity of the hedgehog and Wnt pathways and telomerase activity. The next step would be to (i) develop an assay to detect these glioma subsets for clinical practice, (ii) investigate putative differential sensitivity between tumor-initiating (stem) cells and cells that do not exhibit these properties, (iii) identify molecular alterations in these cells that could predict therapeutic response, or (iv) help monitor tumor control with molecular imaging.

Cell-Based Therapy

Adult Stem Cells

A different aspect is the use of stem cells as a versatile vehicle for glioma therapy. An easily accessible autologous cellular vector that targets disseminated glioma cells and expresses a therapeutic transgene would represent a major step ahead in the experimental treatment of these tumors. Neural stem cells from the cortex of C57BL 6 mice have been used as vehicles to deliver IL-4 to C6 experimental rat gliomas in Sprague-Dawley rats and to GL261 mouse gliomas in C57BL6 mice. Animals treated with stem cells delivering IL-4 lived significantly longer than animals treated with fibroblast-derived packaging cells for in vivo transfer of IL-4. Further, LacZ-expressing cells derived from the immortalized murine neuronal precursor cell line C17.2, injected into either an experimental CNS-1 rat glioma, the tail vein, or nontumorous brain tissue, diffusely transmigrated the whole glioma diameter within three days (57).

Adult hematopoietic progenitor cells are a highly migratory cell population of the bone marrow. Primary nontransformed adult bone marrow–derived cells with neuronal properties efficiently migrate toward distant sites of brain tumor when injected intracranially (58). The molecular mechanisms underlying the phenomenon of a possible lesion- or tumor-directed migration of adult hematopoietic stem cells involve two TGF-β–dependent pathways, namely CXC chemokine ligand 12 (CXCL12) synthesis, and MMP-9–mediated cleavage of stem cell factor, facilitating the promigratory effect of CXCL12 (59). At present, it remains uncertain whether sufficient quantities of any of these stem cell populations can be generated and safely applied. Further, appropriate therapeutic molecules to be delivered by these carriers need to be identified, although in some paradigms the administration of autologous cells, e.g., neural stem cells to the tumor bed themselves conferred some therapeutic effect.

ACKNOWLEDGMENTS

The authors received support from the German Research Council, the German Cancer Council, and the Landesstiftung Baden-Württemberg.

REFERENCES

1. Krause DS, Van Etten RA. Tyrosine kinases as targets for cancer therapy. N Engl J Med 2005; 353(2):172–187.
2. Stupp R, Mason WP, Van den Bent MJ, et al. On behalf of the European Organization for Research and Treatment of Cancer (EORTC) Brain Tumor and Radiotherapy Groups and National Cancer Institute of Canada Clinical Trials Group (NCIC CTG). Radiotherapy plus concomitant and adjuvant temozolomide for patients with newly diagnosed glioblastoma. N Engl J Med 2005; 352(10):997–1003.
3. http://www.cancer.gov/clinicaltrials.
4. Druker BJ, Tamura S, Buchdunger E, et al. Effects of a selective inhibitor of the Abl tyrosine kinase on the growth of Bcr-Abl positive cells. Nat Med 1996; 2(5):561–566.
5. Druker BJ, Sawyers CL, Kantarjian H, et al. Activity of a specific inhibitor of the BCR-ABL tyrosine kinase in the blast crisis of chronic myeloid leukemia and acute lymphoblastic leukemia with the Philadelphia chromosome. N Engl J Med 2001; 344(14):1038–1042.
6. Druker BJ, Talpaz M, Resta DJ, et al. Efficacy and safety of a specific inhibitor of the BCR-ABL tyrosine kinase in chronic myeloid leukemia. N Engl J Med 2001b; 344(14):1031–1037.
7. Apperley JF, Gardembas M, Melo JV, et al. Response to imatinib mesylate in patients with chronic myeloproliferative diseases with rearrangements of the platelet-derived growth factor receptor beta. N Engl J Med 2002; 347(7):481–487.
8. Pietras K, Sjoblom T, Rubin K, et al. PDGF receptors as cancer drug targets. Cancer Cell 2003; 3(5):439–443.
9. Raymond E, Brandes A, Van Oosterom A, et al. Multicentre phase II study of imatinib mesylate in patients with recurrent glioblastoma: an EORTC:NDDG/BTG intergroup study. Proc ASCO 2004:107.
10. Katz A, Barrios CH, Abramoff R, et al. Imatinib (STI 571) is active in patients with high-grade gliomas progressing on standard therapy. Proc ASCO 2004:117.
11. Dresemann G. Imatinib (STI571) plus hydroxyurea: safety and efficacy in pretreated progressive glioblastoma multiforme patients. Proc ASCO 2004:119.
12. Wakeling AE, Guy SP, Woodburn JR, et al. ZD1839 (Iressa): an orally active inhibitor of epidermal growth factor signaling with potential for cancer therapy. Cancer Res 2002; 62(20):5749–5754.
13. Raymond E, Faivre S, Armand JP. Epidermal growth factor receptor tyrosine kinase as a target for anticancer therapy. Drugs 2000; 60(suppl 1):15–23.

14. Lorusso PM. Phase I studies of ZD1839 in patients with common solid tumors. Semin Oncol 2003; 30(suppl 1):21–29.
15. Herbst RS, Giaccone G, Schiller JH, et al. Gefinib in combination with paclitaxel and carboplatin in advanced non-small-cell lung cancer: a phase III trial—Intact 2. J Clin Oncol 2004; 22(5):785–794.
16. Lynch TJ, Bell DW, Sordella R, et al. Activating mutations in the epidermal growth factor receptor underlying responsiveness of non-small-cell lung cancer to gefitinib. N Engl J Med 2004; 350(21):2129–2139.
17. Heimberger AB, Hlatky R, Uki D, et al. Prognostic effects of epidermal growth factor receptor and EGFRvIII in glioblastoma multiforme patients. Clin Cancer Res 2005; 11(4):1462–1466.
18. Li B, Chang C-M, Yuan M, et al. Resistance to small molecule inhibitors of epidermal growth factor receptor in malignant gliomas. Cancer Res 2003; 63(21):7443–7450.
19. Bianco R, Shin I, Ritter CA, et al. Loss of PTEN/MMAC1/TEP in EGF receptor-expressing tumor cells counteracts the antitumor action of EGFR tyrosine kinase inhibitors. Oncogene 2003; 22(18):2812–2822.
20. Lieberman FS, Cloughesy T, Fine H, et al. NABTC phase I/II trial of ZD-1839 for recurrent malignant gliomas and unresectable meningiomas. Proc ASCO 2004:109.
21. Das A, Badruddoja D, Tryciecky D, et al. Phase I study of gefitinib and rapamycin in patients with recurrent or progressive glioblastoma (GBM). Proc ASCO 2005:1572.
22. Moyer JD, Barbacci EG, Iwata KK, et al. Induction of apoptosis and cell cycle arrest by CP 358–774, an inhibitor of epidermal growth factor receptor tyrosine kinase. Cancer Res 1997; 57(21):4838–4848.
23. Prados M, Chang S, Burton E, et al. Phase I study of OSI-774 alone or with temozolomide in patients with malignant glioma. Proc ASCO 2003:394.
24. Raizer JJ, Abrey LE, Wen P, et al. A phase II trial of erlotinib (OSI-774) in patients with recurrent malignant gliomas not on EIACDs. Proc ASCO 2004:107.
25. Vogelbaum MA, Peereboom D, Stevens G, et al. Phase II trial of the EGFR tyrosine kinase inhibitor erlotinib for single agent therapy of recurrent glioblastoma multiforme: interim results. Proc ASCO 2004:121.
26. Burris HA. Dual kinase inhibition in the treatment of breast cancer: initial experience with the EGFR/ErbB-2 inhibitor lapitinib. Oncologist 2004; 9(suppl 3):10–15.
27. http://www.nci.nih.gov.
28. http://www.clinicaltrials.gov.
29. http://www.virtualtrials.org/index.cfm.
30. van Meir E, Bellail A, Phuphanich S. Emerging molecular therapies for brain tumors. Semin Oncol 2004; 31(suppl 4):38–46.
31. http://virtualtrials.com.
32. Goekjian PG, Jirousek MR. Protein kinase C inhibitors as novel anticancer drugs. Exp Opin Invest Drugs 2001; 10(12):2117–2214.
33. Graff JR, McNulty AM, Hanna KR, et al. The protein kinase Cb-selective inhibitor, enzastaurin (LY317615.HCL), suppresses signaling through the AKT

pathway, induces apoptosis, and suppresses growth of human colon cancer and glioblastoma xenografts. Cancer Res 2005; 65(16):7462–7469.

34. Fine HA, Kim L, Royce C, et al. Results from phase II trial of enzastaurin (LY317615) in patients with recurrent high grade gliomas. Proc ASCO 2005:1504.

35. Uhl M, Aulwurm S, Wischhusen J, et al. SD-208, a novel TGF-b receptor I antagonist, inhibits growth and invasiveness and enhances immunogenicity of murine and human glioma cells in vitro and in vivo. Cancer Res 2004; 64(21):7954–7961.

36. MacDonald TJ, Taga T, Shimada H et al. Preferential susceptibility of brain tumors to the antiangiogenic effects of an av integrin antagonist. Neurosurgery 2001; 48(1):151–157.

37. Zalutsky MR, Moseley RP, Coakham HB, et al. Pharmacokinetics and tumor localization of 131I-labeled anti-tenascin monoclonal antibody 81C6 in patients with gliomas and other intracranial malignancies. Cancer Res 1989; 49(10): 2807–2813.

38. Weiler M, Bähr O, Hohlweg U, et al. BCL-x_L: time-dependent dissociation between modulation of apoptosis and invasiveness in human malignant glioma cells. Cell Death Differ. In press.

39. Groves MD, Puduvalli VK, Hess KR, et al. Phase II trial of temozolomide plus the matrix metalloproteinase inhibitor, marimastat, in recurrent and progressive glioblastoma multiforme. J Clin Oncol 2002; 20(5):1383–1388.

40. New P, Mikkelsen T, Phuphanich S, et al. A phase I/II study of col-3 administered on a continuous oral schedule in patients with recurrent high grade glioma: preliminary results of the NABTT 9809 clinical trial A237. Neurooncology 2002; 4:373.

41. Weller M, Rieger J, Grimmel C, et al. Predicting chemoresistance in human malignant glioma cells: the role of molecular genetic analyses. Int J Cancer 1998; 79(6):640–644.

42. Coppelli FM, Grandis JR. Oligonucleotides as anticancer agents: from the benchside to the clinic and beyond. Curr Pharm Des 2005; 11(22):2825–2840.

43. Lang FF, Bruner JM, Fuller GN, et al. Phase I trial of adenovirus–mediated p53 gene therapy for recurrent glioma: biological and clinical results. J Clin Oncol 2003; 21(13):2508–2518.

44. Bykov VJ, Issaeva N, Shilov A, et al. Restoration of the tumor suppressor function to mutant p53 by a low-molecular-weight compound. Nat Med 2002; 8(3):282–288.

45. Roth W, Isenmann S, Naumann U, et al. Locoregional Apo2L/TRAIL eradicates intracranial human malignant glioma xenografts in athymic mice in the absence of neurotoxicity. Biochem Biophys Res Commun 1999; 265(2):479–483.

46. Fulda S, Wick W, Weller M, et al. Smac agonists sensitize for Apo2L/TRAIL- or anticancer drug-induced apoptosis and induce regression of malignant glioma in vivo. Nat Med 2002; 8(8):808–815.

47. Schimmer AD. Inhibitor of apoptosis proteins: translating basic knowledge into clinical practice. Cancer Res 2004; 64(20):7183–7190.

48. Steinbach JP, Klumpp A, Wolburg H, et al. Inhibition of epidermal growth factor receptor signaling protects human malignant glioma cells from hypoxia-induced cell death. Cancer Res 2004; 64(5):1570–1574.

49. Rainov NG. A phase III clinical evaluation of herpes simplex virus type 1 thymidine kinase and ganciclovir gene therapy as an adjuvant to surgical resection and radiation in adults with previously untreated glioblastoma multiforme. Hum Gene Ther 2000; 11(17):2389–2401.

50. Chiocca EA, Abbed KM, Tatter S, et al. A phase I open-label, dose-escalation, multi-institutional trial of injection with an E1B-attenuated adenovirus, ONYX-015, into the peritumoral region of recurrent malignant gliomas, in the adjuvant setting. Mol Ther 2004; 10(5):958–966.

51. Friese MA, Platten M, Lutz SZ, et al. MICA/NKG2D-mediated immunogene therapy of experimental gliomas. Cancer Res 2003; 63(24):8996–9006.

52. Friese MA, Wischhusen J, Wick W, et al. RNA interference targeting transforming growth factor-beta enhances NKG2D-mediated antiglioma immune response, inhibits glioma cell migration and invasiveness, and abrogates tumorigenicity in vivo. Cancer Res 2004; 64(20):7596–7603.

53. Liau LM, Prins RM, Kiertscher SM, et al. Dendritic cell vaccination in glioblastoma patients induces systemic and intracranial T-cell responses modulated by the local central nervous system tumor microenvironment. Clin Cancer Res 2005; 11(15):5515–5525.

54. Kuwashima N, Nishimura F, Eguchi J, et al. Delivery of dendritic cells engineered to secrete IFN-a into central nervous system tumors enhances the efficacy of peripheral tumor cell vaccines: dependence on apoptotic pathways. J Immunol 2005; 175(4):2730–2740.

55. Wick W, Naumann U, Weller M. Transforming factor-b: a molecular target for the future therapy of glioblastoma. Curr Pharm Des. 2006; 12(3):341–349.

56. Sanai N, Alvarez-Buylla A, Berger MS. Neural stem cells and the origin of gliomas. N Engl J Med 2005; 353(8):811–822.

57. Aboody KS, Brown A, Rainov NG, et al. Neural stem cells display extensive tropism for pathology in adult brain: evidence from intracranial gliomas. Proc Natl Acad Sci USA 2000; 97(23):12,846–12,851.

58. Lee J, Elkahloun AG, Messina SA, et al. Cellular and genetic characterization of human adult bone marrow-derived neural stem-like cells: a potential anti-glioma vector. Cancer Res 2003; 63(24):8877–8889.

59. Tabatabai G, Bahr O, Mohle R, et al. Lessons from the bone marrow: how malignant glioma cells attract adult hematopoietic progenitor cells. Brain 2005; 128(Pt 9):2200–2211.

5

Imaging in Neurooncology

Wilhelm Küker

Department of Neuroradiology, The Radcliffe Infirmary, Oxford, U.K.

Thomas Nägele

Department of Neuroradiology, University Hospital Tuebingen, School of Medicine, Tuebingen, Germany

Imaging is indispensable for the management of neoplastic disorder affecting the brain. The first step in this process is the detection of a lesion causing the clinical symptoms of the patient. When an abnormality is found, the next task is to elucidate its pathologic significance and to decide whether it is the cause of the clinical symptoms. The next step is then the differential diagnosis of the brain lesion and its basic classification as neoplastic, inflammatory, vascular, or of developmental origin. If the lesion is thought to be a neoplasm, further differential diagnosis should place it into one of the relevant subgroups such as primary or metastatic, congenital or acquired, glial, neuronal, lymphomatous, or embryologic. Imaging should then supply an evaluation of the grade of malignancy and the prospective speed of proliferation. If all these tasks have been accomplished the role of imaging is far from over. The planning of any treatment requires the evaluation of tumor location and extension relative to eloquent brain areas. After any therapeutic procedure, imaging is required to monitor the extent of resection and the response to radio- and chemotherapy. Follow-up scans should detect tumor recurrence and indicate treatment side effects such as radionecrosis or leukoencephalopathy.

The imaging modality best suited to address most of these tasks is magnetic resonance imaging (MRI). In addition to traditional imaging with T2- and T1-weighted images, new methods of physiological imaging have become available, which significantly enhance the role of MRI for specific tasks in the evaluation of patients with neoplastic brain disease.

This chapter is intended to give an overview of the best diagnostic strategies to address the different tasks mentioned above, with a focus on MRI. This will also include the application of MRI techniques such as proton spectroscopy, diffusion- and diffusion-tensor–weighted imaging, or perfusion studies where appropriate. The description of individual imaging characteristics is given in the chapters outlining the diseases and is not incorporated into this overview.

DETECTING A LESION

Primary Brain Neoplasms

The initial clinical presentation of primary and secondary cerebral neoplasms is dominated by the occurrence of seizures. Fits are the most frequent first symptom of a cerebral neoplasm, and the onset of seizures should always induce a thorough imaging workup because the underlying tumor may be small at this stage.

The second most frequent clinical presentation of a cerebral neoplasm is a progressive neurological deficit such as a hemiparesis, aphasia, or sensory symptoms. Lesions causing these symptoms due to mass effect or tissue destruction are usually large and hence readily detected by cranial imaging.

Headaches and a decreased level of consciousness are initial symptoms of mass lesions in the posterior fossa or third ventricle. The clinical findings are due to the increased pressure in the posterior fossa or the ensuing hydrocephalus. Primary neoplasms of the posterior fossa are more frequent in children than in adults. Most lesions large enough to cause considerable direct mass effect are readily visible on cerebral imaging studies. However, small neoplasms obstructing the cerebrospinal fluid (CSF) flow in the cerebral aqueduct or at the foramen of the fourth ventricle may be difficult to see on an unenhanced computed tomography (CT) scan.

Whereas most cerebral neoplasms are found because they cause neurological symptoms, the increasing availability of scanning facilities has also caused the detection of more asymptomatic brain neoplasms, mainly of low malignancy.

The imaging modalities used and the imaging strategies employed depend to a large extent on the local health-care systems and the available resources. The most sensitive first line imaging method for the detection of symptomatic brain lesions is gadolinium-enhanced MRI.

MRI is also well suited for the differential diagnosis of brain lesions, if physiological imaging modalities are employed. However, contrast-enhanced

CT is still the mainstay of cranial imaging in many countries and has a high sensitivity for brain tumors of higher malignancy or larger extent. It is also very well suited for the detection of calcified neoplasms and has therefore a role in differential diagnosis. It is of clearly limited value for posterior fossa, brain stem, or temporal lobe pathology. Unenhanced CT is sometimes used as a screening tool in patients with limited treatment options for cerebral neoplasms, such as very old patients. Whereas a subdural fluid collection as a cause of a neurological deficit should be treated in all age groups, the value of an aggressive tumor treatment in these patients seems to be very limited. Furthermore, large neoplasms are visible on unenhanced CT scans due to mass effect and edema. It should be remembered that the application of contrast agent in old patients with an unknown past medical history carries a considerable risk of adverse effects and should therefore be well considered.

Extra-Axial Tumors

The most frequent extra-axial intracranial tumors are of benign histology, but may become life threatening due to location and growth pattern. Symptoms occur, if these meningeomas or schwannomas exert a mass effect. This may result in focal neurological deficits, seizures, or behavioral changes in frontal lesions. Meningeomas may cause considerable cerebral edema and vestibular schwannomas brain stem compression as well as hydrocephalus. Meningeomas may be densely calcified.

For many of these lesions, CT is an adequate initial imaging method because the neoplasms are either big or calcified or have a perifocal edema. However, for the detection of smaller lesions that exert a mass effect in a small confined space such as vestibular schwannomas or perioptic meningeomas, thin slice contrast-enhanced MRI may prove to be indispensable.

Metastases

Metastases are the most frequent neoplastic brain lesions. Frequent sources are primary neoplasms of the lung, breast, skin, kidneys, and the gastrointestinal tract. Whereas most metastases occur in patients with known primary malignancies, up to 30% represent the first manifestation of the disease. Clinical presentation is not different from a primary brain neoplasm of high malignancy in the same location. Because secondary deposits of body tissue inherently lack a blood–brain barrier, contrast enhancement is a constant feature of metastases. Furthermore, secondary deposits are frequently surrounded by edema. Imaging for metastases follows the same principles as for highly malignant primary brain neoplasms. Symptomatic lesions are mostly visible on contrast-enhanced CT scans, which are also widely used for surveillance imaging. Treatment planning, differential diagnosis, or the occurrence of neurological symptoms not explained by

CT may, however, require contrast-enhanced MRI, which has a very high sensitivity for metastases and may be preferred if readily available. As an exception to this general rule, we would always favor MRI to search for metastases of small-cell lung cancer because these often lack a perifocal edema and show minor contrast enhancement.

The imaging of leptomeningeal disease clearly requires the application of contrast-enhanced MRI. Neoplastic deposits are usually nodular or linear structures on the surface of the brain or medullary cord. They are frequently found on the surface of the pons and in the foliae of the superior vermis of the cerebellum in sagittal contrast-enhanced T1-weighted images. Other locations often involved are the internal auditory meatus and the infundibular recessus of the third ventricle. MRI of the complete spinal canal is mandatory because the most distal parts of the dural sack may also be affected.

DIFFERENTIAL DIAGNOSIS

The diagnostic task after the detection of an abnormality is its differential diagnosis. Conventional MRI including T2- and T1-weighted images and contrast-enhanced scans are the most important imaging modalities. However, it may have to be supplemented by CT, magnetic resonance spectroscopy (MRS), and perfusion- and diffusion-weighted imaging (DWI), as well as positron-emission tomography (PET). It should always be remembered, that no imaging modality is as accurate as histology and may fully replace a biopsy. For many clinical purposes, however, the reliability of imaging is sufficient to direct the subsequent patient care.

Differential diagnosis is usually based on conventional MRI performed to investigate the presenting clinical symptoms of the patients. These investigations usually include T1- and T2-weighted images, frequently also dark fluid T2-weighted sequences such as fluid-attenuated inversion recovery (FLAIR) imaging as well as spin-density sequences. Intravenous gadolinium-based contrast is also commonly used in these patients. The tumors most frequently encountered and therefore the main differential diagnoses differ significantly according to the patient's age and the lesion's location. Furthermore, underlying clinical disorders such as neoplasms and infections have to be appreciated.

In adults, the most frequent brain neoplasms are metastases and gliomas. Metastases enhance after contrast injection and are often multifocal. Diagnosis is easy if an underlying metastasizing neoplasm is known. However, if a brain metastasis is the first and single manifestation of a tumor, differential diagnosis against other pathologies such as gliomas or inflammatory lesions may be difficult without biopsy. DWI and spectroscopy have been reported to help differentiate between neoplastic and inflammatory necrosis, which will be discussed in more detail with the malignant gliomas. Metastases are mostly encountered in patients most at risk of developing a carcinoma or sarcoma. They also tend to occur in the cerebellum, a location very rarely affected by a primary malignant brain tumor in adults.

The most frequent glial brain tumor by far is glioblastoma multiforme. It usually appears as a contrast-enhancing cerebral lesion with perifocal edema and central necrosis. Most tumors occur in the sixth and seventh decade of life. At the time of presentation, most lesions are of considerable size and easily detected with MRI, also with CT. Glioblastomas grow rapidly (Fig. 1).

Relevant differential diagnoses are metastases and cerebral abscesses. Whereas it may be impossible to differentiate a single metastasis from a malignant glioma, diffusion-weighted MRI may be useful for the differential diagnosis of pus and tumor necrosis (1,2). Inflammatory necrosis tends to contain more cellular particles such as bacteria and leukocytes than those in necrotic tumor. Hence, cerebral abscesses are of high signal intensity in diffusion-weighted images, indicating restricted diffusion of protons. Areas of tumor necrosis do not show restricted diffusion due to the breakdown of cell membranes and are dark on diffusion images (Fig. 2).

(A)   **(B)**

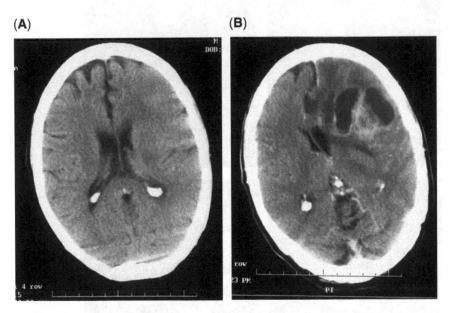

Figure 1   Development and natural course of glioblastoma in a 63-year-old man with new onset of seizures. (**A**) This initial unenhanced CT scan was performed in May 2004 for a new onset of seizures. An area of focal swelling in the left frontal lobe was not recognized at this stage. (**B**) This follow-up CT scan performed in November 2004 because of aphasia, hemiparesis, and drowsiness shows an extensive, ring-enhancing mass lesion in the left frontal lobe with massive compression of the ventricles and midline shift. Glioblastoma multiforme was found at biopsy.

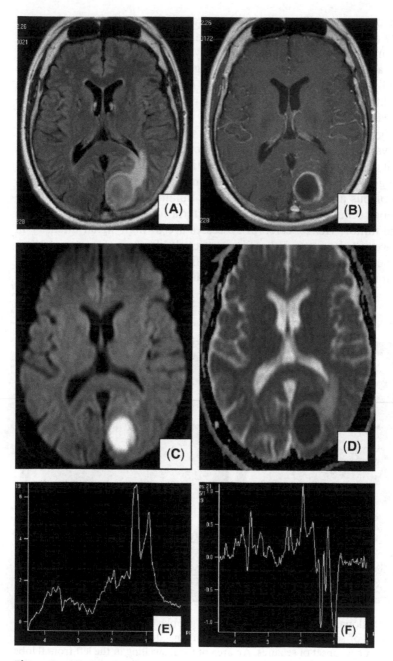

Figure 2 (*Caption on facing page*)

Proton MRS shows increased levels of lactate in inflammatory necrosis but not in necrotic neoplasms. This may also be used to differentiate both entities (3,4). However, it should be borne in mind that groups reporting on clinical studies undertaken in larger numbers of patients found exemptions to these rules (5). Therefore, in patients with equivocal MRI findings or a mismatch of clinical and imaging information, a rapid biopsy is still the procedure of choice to reach a definitive diagnosis.

Whereas high-grade gliomas are most prevalent in the elderly, glial tumors of lower malignancy are found in younger adults. These tumors of World Health Organization (WHO) grade II and III are mostly either astrocytomas or oligodendrogliomas or of a mixed oliogoastroglioma type. Ependymal tumors are comparatively rare. Although the prognosis does not significantly depend on timely diagnosis in glioblastoma patients, curative or long-term remissive surgery may be required in patients with low-grade gliomas. In these cases, the success of treatment does depend on the extension of the tumor at the time of detection and hence requires an early diagnosis.

Gliomas of WHO grade II do not enhance after contrast injection because the blood–brain barrier remains intact. The lesions are visible using MRI because the tissue water content is higher than in normally myelinated white matter due to increased cellularity. This causes increased signal intensity in T2-weighted images and decreased signal intensity in T1-weighted sequences. Differential diagnosis therefore needs to include all lesions of similar signal pattern. For various reasons, only few disorders are difficult to separate from a low-grade glioma. The application of new MRI techniques has significantly contributed to this differential diagnostics.

In all age groups, mostly in young patients, areas of acute demyelination may present as slightly expansive areas of high signal intensity in

---

Figure 2 (*Figure on facing page*) Value of diffusion-weighted imaging (DWI) and spectroscopy for the differential diagnosis of necrotic neoplasm and bacterial abscess in a 34-year-old man with headaches and new onset of seizures. (**A**) The T2-weighted fluid-attenuated inversion recovery (FLAIR) sequence shows a left occipital mass lesion. An area of perifocal high signal extends to the occipital horn of the lateral ventricle. (**B**) The T1-weighted sequence after contrast administration shows a left occipital rim-enhancing mass lesion, which appears sharply demarcated. Differential diagnoses include high-grade glioma, metastasis, and abscess. (**C**) DWI source image shows restricted diffusion of protons in the lesion. This finding is highly suggestive but not proof of a bacterial abscess. (**D**) The apparent diffusion coefficient (ADC) map confirms the finding of restricted proton diffusion. The center of the abscess appears dark on this image. (**E**) The single voxel proton spectroscopy (^{1}H-MRS) using a short echo time single-shot–stimulated echo acquisition mode (STEAM) sequence shows two high peaks in the right part of the spectrum. (**F**) Repetition of the spectroscopy at the same voxel position but with a long echo time STEAM sequence shows inversion of the two peaks, thereby proving the presence of lactate. This metabolite is frequently found in abscesses. An abscess was found at surgery.

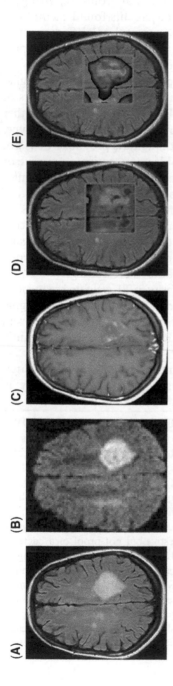

Figure 3 Value of diffusion-weighted imaging (DWI), chemical shift imaging (CSI), and single voxel proton magnetic resonance spectroscopy (^{1}H-MRS) with metabolite suppression for differential diagnosis of tumor mimicking demyelinating brain lesions in a 38-year-old man with rapid onset of left hemiparesis. (**A**) The T2-weighted fluid-attenuated inversion recovery (FLAIR) sequence shows a large left hemispheric hyperintense lesion in the white cerebral matter. The cortex is spared. Further, small lesions are seen in the callosal radiation on both sides. (**B**) DWI shows restricted diffusion of protons in the left hemispheric lesion. The small areas of T2-signal change are not affected. Diffusion abnormality was confirmed by calculation of apparent diffusion coefficient (ADC) values. (**C**) The T1-weighted sequence after contrast injection shows small areas of enhancement within the large lesion. Otherwise, the lesion is hypointense compared to normal brain parenchyma. (**D–G**) Chemical shift imaging. The concentrations of cerebral metabolites are overlying a T2-weighted FLAIR image. High concentrations are displayed by light gray, low concentrations by dark gray. (**D**) The map of N-acetyl-aspartate (NAA) concentrations shows a marked reduction in the left hemispheric lesion. The rest of the brain is not affected. (**E**) This map shows an increased concentration of lipids in the area of T2-signal abnormality. Increased lipid concentrations are encountered in acutely demyelinating lesions. (**F**) Single voxel proton spectroscopy using a short echo time and a stimulated echo acquisition mode sequence. The volume of interest is located in the center of the lesion. The proton spectrum shows increased concentration of choline and macromolecules. There is also a significant reduction of NAA. These findings are encountered in acutely demyelinating lesions. (**G**) This spectrum was acquired with the application of the metabolite suppression technique to expose the underlying macromolecules. The double peak displayed here is very characteristic of acute demyelination (7). The findings in this patient were regarded as reliable enough to avoid a biopsy. The diagnosis was confirmed by cerebrospinal fluid findings and the further clinical course.

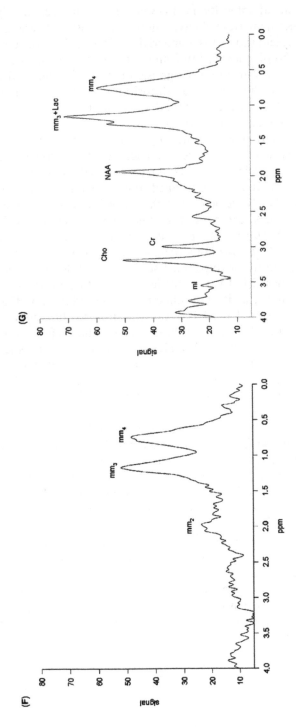

Figure 3 (*Continued*)

T2- and low signal intensity in T1-weighted sequences, mostly without contrast enhancement (tumefactive multiple sclerosis). These lesions may be the initial presentation of the underlying disease. Whereas conventional MRI may not be diagnostic, DWI and proton MRS have been shown to be of value for the differential diagnosis of demyelinating and neoplastic lesions. DWI may show restricted diffusion of protons in cases of acute demyelination (6), a feature not found in neoplasms (Fig. 3). Proton MRS has also been reported to contribute to a reliable differential diagnosis between demyelination and tumor by demonstration of elevated levels of macromolecules (7), which is not encountered in low-grade gliomas (Fig. 4A). Today, brain biopsy should be reserved for patients, in whom these modern imaging tools have failed to establish a reliable diagnosis.

It should also be remembered that a wait-and-see strategy may be applied in unclear cases, if invasive treatment may be delayed without detrimental effects. A 56-year-old patient developed a left hemiparesis over several days. The MRI was initially regarded as suggestive of a high-grade glioma, but revision prior to planned surgery raised doubts. Under steroid medication, a repeat MRI two weeks later showed resolution of the lesion, which was therefore classified as inflammatory pseudotumor (Fig. 5).

Diffusion-weighted MRI is a valuable tool to differentiate ischemic and neoplastic brain lesions, even in the same patient (Fig. 4). Low-grade gliomas and infarcts may display identical signal characteristics in MRI and the same density in CT. However, signal changes are due to intracellular edema in ischemic lesions in contrast to interstitial water collection in a tumor. Hence, DWI shows restricted diffusion in ischemic tissue but not in the brain neoplasm.

DWI may also facilitate the diagnosis of viral encephalitis, which may have to be separated from low-grade glioma. Herpes simplex encephalitis often presents with seizures and conventional MRI frequently shows an area of high signal intensity on T2-weighted (Fig. 6) images and of low signal on T1-weighted sequences, initially without contrast uptake. Differential diagnosis is facilitated by the demonstration of restricted proton diffusion in the limbic system and insula (8).

A further disease caused by viral infection and of differential diagnostic significance to glioma is progressive multifocal leukoencephalopathy. This demyelinating disorder is caused by Jamestown Canyon (JC) virus activation in the central nervous system and occurs in patients with impaired T-cell function. It is hence mostly encountered in AIDS patients or in patients with an established history of immunosuppressive treatment after organ transplantation. Occasionally, the lesions may occur as the first manifestation of a disease and cause neurological symptoms. MRS and especially DWI are of great diagnostic value in these patients as areas of active demyelination show restricted diffusion of protons (Fig. 7) (9). The diagnosis is further confirmed by spectroscopic findings of acute demyelination.

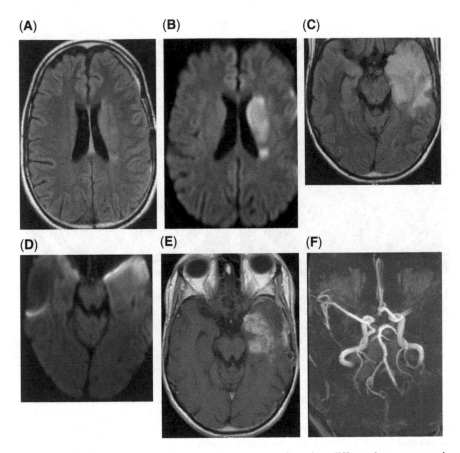

Figure 4 Diffusion-weighted magnetic resonance imaging differentiates vasogenic and cytotoxic edema in a 37-year-old man with anaplastic left temporal astrocytoma and sudden onset of aphasia and right-sided hemiparesis. (**A**) The T2-weighted fluid-attenuated inversion recovery (FLAIR) image through the cella media of the lateral ventricles shows subtle hyperintensity in the left caudate nucleus with narrowing of the lateral ventricle. (**B**) The diffusion-weighted imaging (DWI) sequence demonstrates restricted diffusion of protons in the left caudate nucleus and the adjacent white matter. This finding indicates cytotoxic edema and is commonly seen in stroke. (**C**) This T2-weighted FLAIR sequence shows a left temporal mass lesion of high signal intensity. (**D**) The DWI image in the same location as in (**C**) does not indicate restricted diffusion in most of the areas of high T2 signal. This indicates vasogenic edema as the probable cause of T2-signal change. There is, however, an area of restricted diffusion around the temporal pole. (**E**) The T1-weighted image after contrast injection demonstrates blood–brain barrier breakdown in the tumor, indicating anaplastic degeneration. The tumor is in broad contact with the left middle cerebral artery. (**F**) The magnetic resonance angiography using a time-of-flight sequence shows occlusion of the left middle cerebral artery. Tumor invasion of the vessel wall was found on surgery.

(A)   **(B)**

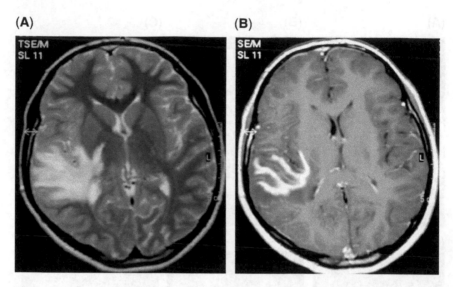

Figure 5 Inflammatory pseudo tumor mimicking high-grade glioma in a 56-year-old patient with rapidly progressive left hemiparesis and left hemianopia. **(A)** This T2-weighted image shows a mass lesion in the right temporal and parietal lobes, extending into the internal and external capsules. The optic radiation is heavily involved. The abnormalities predominately affects the white matter with only a very minor degree of cortical involvement. **(B)** This contrast-enhanced T1-weighted image shows massive enhancement in the subcortical regions around the Sylvian fissure, surrounded by edema. No necrosis is encountered. The appearance was found to be unusual for high-grade glioma or lymphoma and a repeat scan was performed after steroid treatment. Clinical symptoms and signal changes had disappeared after two weeks and no relapse has been encountered since.

Since the successful invention of PCV chemotherapy for oligodendro-gliomas and mixed gliomas, especially of the 1p19q subtype, the differential diagnosis between gliomas of the astrocytic and oligodendrocytic subtype has gained clinical significance. The most relevant imaging feature for this differential diagnosis is calcification, which is encountered in many oligodendrocytic tumors, but rarely in astrocytomas. Imaging of calcification is best performed with T2*-weighted gradient echo sequences in MRI or with plain CT.

Also of clinical importance for prognostic and therapeutic purposes is the discrimination of WHO grade II and III tumors (Figs. 8–10). Whereas the efficacy of any treatment for diffuse grade II gliomas is still highly controversial, the benefit of radiotherapy is established in grade III and IV gliomas. Whereas significant contrast enhancement reliably indicates a high-grade glioma, the lack of contrast uptake does not rule out a grade III lesion. Enhancement after contrast injection in conventional MRI corresponds to leaking of the blood–brain barrier, not necessarily to the overall

(A)　　　　　　　　　　　　　**(B)**

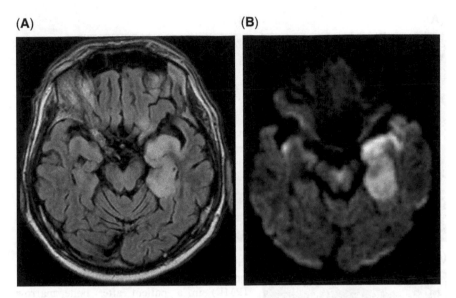

Figure 6　Herpes simplex encephalitis in a 68-year-old man with sudden onset of sei-zures. (**A**) The T2-weighted fluid-attenuated inversion recovery sequence shows an area of signal abnormality with moderate mass effect in the left temporal lobe, mainly involving the cortex. (**B**) The diffusion-weighted image clearly indicates restricted diffusion of protons in the involved area [verified by apparent diffusion coefficient (ADC) calculation]. This finding is not encountered in brain neoplasms, but in cerebral ischemia or encephalitis. There may also be an area of restricted diffusion on the right, not visible on the T2-weighted images. Herpes simplex encephalitis was verified by cerebrospinal fluid tests.

vascularity of a brain lesion. Perfusion-weighted MRI has overcome this problem because this dynamic method clearly visualizes areas of increased vascular density, a characteristic feature of high-grade gliomas. If dynamic MRI studies are not available, intra-arterial digital subtraction angiography may also be used to identify increased tumor vascularity in grade III glio-mas or pathological tumor vessels as in glioblastoma multiforme. This invasive procedure is now only rarely performed for the imaging of cerebral neoplasms.

Proton MRS and PET have been shown to differentiate metabolites characteristic for high- and low-grade tumors (10). The availability of PET is restricted and the accuracy of proton MRS is usually not regarded sufficient to replace brain biopsy (11). However, perfusion-weighted MRI (Fig. 9), proton MRS (Fig. 8), and PET (Fig. 10) may be helpful in selecting the best location for a biopsy because the overall tumor grade is determined by its most anaplastic component. This may be difficult in large, long-standing tumors, which eventually undergo focal anaplastic change.

(A) (B)

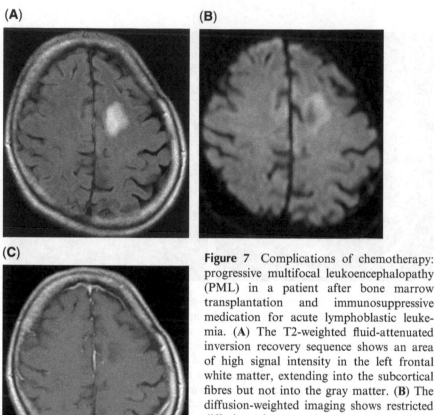

(C)

Figure 7 Complications of chemotherapy: progressive multifocal leukoencephalopathy (PML) in a patient after bone marrow transplantation and immunosuppressive medication for acute lymphoblastic leukemia. (**A**) The T2-weighted fluid-attenuated inversion recovery sequence shows an area of high signal intensity in the left frontal white matter, extending into the subcortical fibres but not into the gray matter. (**B**) The diffusion-weighted imaging shows restricted diffusion of protons in the periphery of the lesion, but not in its center. Areas of diffusional abnormality are currently undergoing demyelination and indicate disease progression. (**C**) The T1-weighted image shows the lesion to be hypointense compared to adjacent brain but lacking contrast enhancement. PML was verified by demonstration of Jamestown Canyon (JC) virus in the cerebrospinal fluid by polymerase chain reaction.

Perfusion-weighted MRI has also been shown to facilitate the differential diagnosis between gliomas and cerebral lymphomas (12).

TREATMENT PLANNING

The first step in the treatment of brain neoplasms usually involves surgery, either to remove the tumor or to obtain tissue for histological examination.

Surgical planning depends on precisely identifying the extent of the neoplasm and its position in relation to eloquent brain areas. Conventional MRI using T2- and T1-weighted scans supplemented by contrast-enhanced sequences are the mainstay of anatomic imaging. For an increased spatial resolution, three-dimensional (3-D) images may be required. However, it should always be borne in mind that the tumor border seen on imaging studies is not necessarily the histologic tumor margin. Recent scientific work on tumor biology has demonstrated the ability of neoplastic glia cells to migrate quickly through the brain. Hence, at the time of initial presentation, tumor cells have usually spread far beyond the visible tumor borders. Signal changes in MRI appear, if the cell density has increased beyond a certain threshold causing its visibility against adjacent or contralateral brain tissue. Although migration and proliferation are features of all malignant gliomas, the relative proportion of these features differs between neoplasms.

Some gliomas of low malignancy (WHO grade II) seem to be fairly circumscribed because the neoplastic cells show significant local proliferation but only very limited migration. In these patients, subtotal or even curative resection seems possible if no eloquent structures are involved. Otherwise, glioma surgery is always for biopsy, cytoreduction, and debulking, but not for cure. Given these biological restrictions, aggressive surgery at the expense of neurological function should be avoided.

Areas of functional significance, such as the speech areas or the motor strip, are identified by their location on the brain surface. If these areas are not affected by the neoplasm, the risk of a treatment-related functional deficit is low. If, however, the tumor does involve an eloquent brain area without neurological deficits, advanced imaging techniques are needed to establish the exact location of the functional brain parenchyma.

The imaging modality usually employed for this task is functional MRI. Most modern MRI scanners are capable of acquiring appropriate data sets, and postprocessing tools are widely available. In a clinical setting, functional testing for easy motor, optical, and language tasks can be established with limited efforts. The evaluation of higher cognitive function is usually restricted to dedicated research labs. PET imaging is only rarely performed for presurgical cortical mapping in a routine clinical setting (Fig. 11).

A matter of major concern to the neurological surgeon is the integrity of deep white matter tracts such as the pyramidal tract. Until recently, the localization of white matter tracts was difficult to evaluate in the depths of the cerebral hemispheres, where anatomical landmarks are scarce. Neuronavigation is particularly difficult if the normal anatomy is distorted by a mass lesion or edema.

Diffusion tensor imaging (DTI) identifies the direction of white matter fibers. By acquiring multiple slices from one anatomic landmark to a second, it is often possible to reconstruct the course of a tract and thereby avoid its surgical damage (Fig. 12).

The role of imaging to identify the most malignant part of a tumor and therefore the most appropriate biopsy site has been mentioned in detail on page 103.

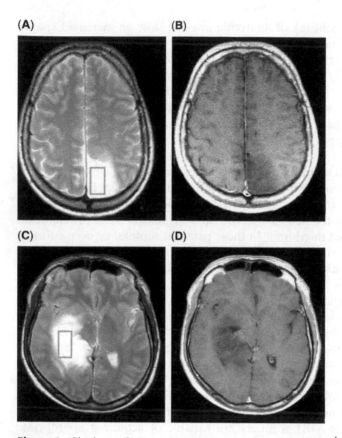

Figure 8 Single voxel proton magnetic resonance spectroscopy (^{1}H-MRS) with metabolite suppression for the grading of gliomas. T2- and T1-weighted images do not differentiate between World Health Organization (WHO) grade II and III gliomas. (**A**) The
T2-weighted image shows a hyperintense tumor in the left occipital lobe. The quadrangle
indicates the voxel of the proton spectroscopy. (**B**) The contrast-enhanced T1-weighted
scan does not indicate blood–brain barrier breakdown. The tumor is hypointense to normal brain parenchyma. The appearance is typical for a low-grade glioma. (**C**) This
T2-weighted image of a right temporal tumor, involving white matter and cerebral cortex,
is very similar to the tumor shown in (**A**). The voxel of spectroscopy is indicated by
a quadrangle. (**D**) The T1-weighted, contrast-enhanced image does not show tumor
enhancement. Although contrast uptake is seen in a considerable proportion of WHO
grade III gliomas, it is not encountered in all cases. Therefore, the absence of contrast
enhancement does not reliably differentiate between WHO grade II and III lesions.
(**E**) ^{1}H-MRS using a short echo time stimulated echo acquisition mode sequence shows
a reduction of N-acetyl-aspartate (NAA) and an elevation of choline. The underlying
dotted line is a spectrum applying the metabolite suppression technique (7). The concentration of lipids and macromolecules, which determine the course of the dotted line, is in
the range of normal. WHO grade II astrocytoma was found at surgery. (**F**) ^{1}H-MRS of the
second patient using the same technique as in the previous patient also shows a reduction
of NAA. (*Continued on facing page*)

(E)

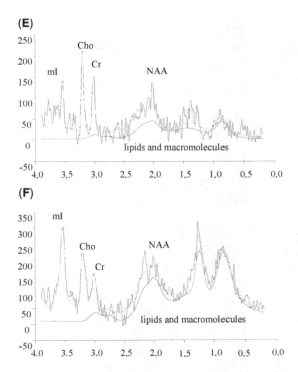

(F)

Figure 8 (*Continued from facing page*) In this patient, however, choline and creatine concentrations are also low with a less-severe choline reduction. Note the increase in myoinositol. The dotted line indicating the lipid and macromolecules shows an elevation of these substances. These concentrations were evaluated using the metabolite suppression technique as in (**E**). Elevated lipids and macromolecules are a hallmark of malignant neoplasms, even in the absence of contrast enhancement.

Intraoperative MRI or CT is used to facilitate the extent of surgery in patients suffering from a glioma. Up to now, high equipment costs, the delay in surgery, and the modest impact on patient survival have prevented a more widespread application.

Careful diagnostic evaluation using modern imaging techniques may be required in other patients. Although infrequent, seizures can cause cortical edema, which may be difficult to distinguish from cortical tumor infiltration. DWI may identify cortical edema due to repetitive seizures by demonstrating cytotoxic edema (13), not encountered in neoplasms (Fig. 13).

IMMEDIATE TREATMENT CONTROL

The evaluation of treatment success is an important imaging task in patients with neoplasms. It needs to be performed in individual patients as well as in treatment trial, the basis of all progress in tumor treatment.

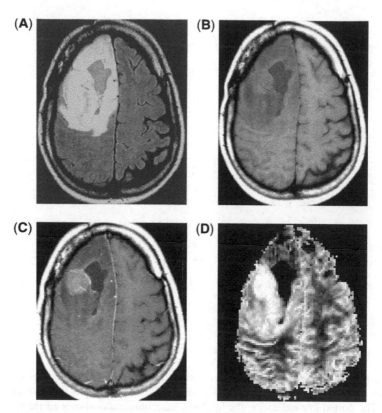

Figure 9 Perfusion magnetic resonance imaging identifies areas of anaplastic tumor degeneration in a 45-year-old woman 20 months after partial resection of right frontal astrocytoma World Health Organization (WHO) grade II. New onset of seizures. (**A**) The T2-weighted fluid attenuated inversion recovery sequence shows a right frontal tumor surrounding a cerebrospinal fluid–filled resection cavity. The neoplasm appears homogenously hyperintense to normal brain tissue on this image. (**B**) The T1-weighted image shows the tumor as hypointense mass lesion adjacent to the postsurgical defect. There is a nodular area of increased signal intensity protruding into the resection cavity. (**C**) The contrast-enhanced T1-weighted image shows enhancement of a nodular tumor component, which already appears slightly hyperintense on the unenhanced images. This tumor nodule represents a regrown neoplasm, extending into the resection defect. (**D**) This perfusion-weighted map shows areas of high perfusion hyperintense, although the source images were generated by dynamic contrast susceptibility imaging. The map indicates not only high perfusion of the contrast-enhancing nodule but also tumor areas with intact blood–brain barrier. Other parts of the tumor do not display increased perfusion. On surgery, areas of high perfusion were found to be astrocytoma of WHO grade III, whereas the rest of the tumor retained histologic features of a WHO grade II glioma. The neoplasm was reclassified according to its most malignant parts as WHO grade III lesion.

(A)

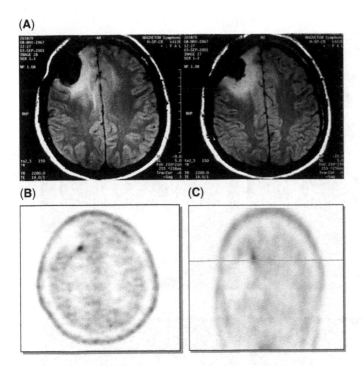

(B)　　　　　　　　　**(C)**

Figure 10 ^{11}C methionine positron-emission tomography (PET) identifies areas of focal anaplasia in a glioma in a 38-year-old patient with five-year history of right frontal fibrillary astrocytoma World Health Organization (WHO) grade II and previous partial resection, now experiencing increasing frequency of seizures. (**A**) The T2-weighted axial fluid attenuated inversion recovery images show a right frontal tumor with central defect after previous partial resection. The tumor margin is uniformly hyperintense. No focal abnormality or contrast enhancements were seen (no picture). (**B**) ^{11}C methionine PET. This axial scan shows a focal area of high tracer activity within the tumor, whereas in most regions of the neoplasm the activity does not differ from normal brain parenchyma. The postsurgical brain defect is clearly visible anterior and lateral to the lesion. (**C**) This coronal reformatted image of the PET scan shows the location of the anaplastic area in relation to the surgical brain defect. Focal tumor anaplasia (WHO grade III) was confirmed at surgery.

Because contrast-enhancing scar tissue develops soon after surgery, imaging studies to evaluate the extent of the resection should be performed within the first one or two days. Again, MRI has a higher sensitivity to identify residual tumor than has CT, with the exemption of highly calcified neoplasms.

After radio- and chemotherapy, treatment response is usually seen later, and imaging is therefore delayed depending on the neoplasm. Unless treatment-related adverse effects are suspected or the patient's condition deteriorates, treatment success is monitored after the end of radiotherapy

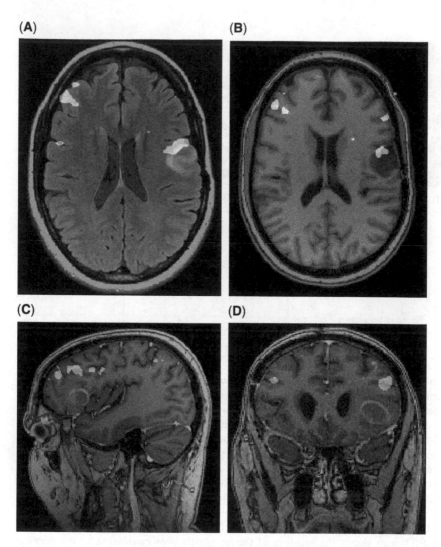

Figure 11 Functional magnetic resonance imaging (fMRI) for the presurgical location of eloquent brain areas in a 36-year-old patient with low grade left frontal glioma. (**A**) fMRI with task to locate motoric language area overlying T2-weighted fluid attenuated inversion recovery image. The activated area is clearly seen anteriorly to the lesion. (**B**) This image shows an overly of fMRI data on a T1-weighted image, which also shows the area of abnormality in the left frontal lobe. (**C**) 55-year-old female patient with high-grade glioma in the left frontal lobe. The overly of fMRI data of a language task on the T1-weighted, contrast-enhanced sagittal reconstruction shows displacement of Brocas area upwards. (**D**) This overly on a coronal reformatted 3-D data set also clearly shows the anatomical location of the eloquent brain areas in relation to the contrast-enhancing lesion. Surgery could, in both patients, be performed without neurological deficit.

(A)   **(B)**

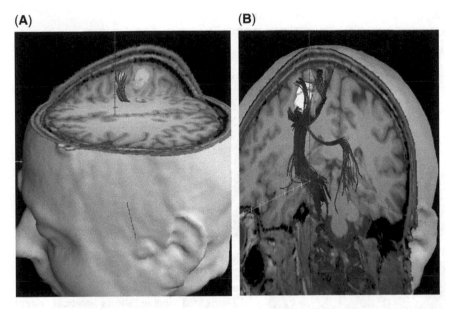

Figure 12 Diffusion tensor imaging (DTI) for the presurgical location of fiber tracts in a 44-year-old man with right parietal mass lesion. (**A**) This DTI sequence was used to identify fiber tracts. These were superimposed on a 3-D T1-weighted anatomical data set. The image presented here shows the lesion in the subcortical white matter of the right parietal lobe. The fibers of the pyramidal tract (dark gray) are displaced anteriorly. (**B**) For this image, a wedge-shaped section of the data set was removed. The overlay shows the pyramidal tract and crossing fibers in the corpus callosum (dark gray), both displaced by the mass. A cavernoma was found at surgery and could be removed without neurological deficit. *Source*: Courtesy of Dr. Gharibagi, Tuebingen, Germany.

or the initial chemotherapy; hence at a time, when, according to the initial response, the future treatment strategy has to be decided.

The evaluation of treatment response in neurooncology is usually performed according to guidelines proposed by MacDonald et al. (14) This scale is based on the evaluation of contrast-enhanced CT scans of high-grade glioma patients, but widely applied to other imaging modalities and neoplasms.

In this scale, the absence of contrast-enhancing tissue is regarded as complete response, a reduction of contrast-enhancing tissue by more than 50% but less than 100% is a partial remission, any change between 50% decrease and 25% increase in tumor volume is rated as stable disease, and any increase of more than 25% or the development of new enhancing lesions is regarded as progressive disease. Some modifications of these criteria have recently been proposed for cerebral lymphoma (Fig. 14) (15).

(A)   (B)

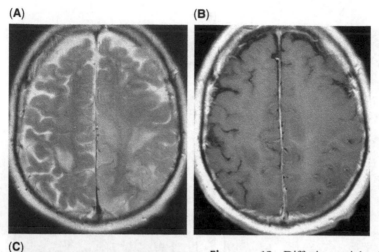

(C)

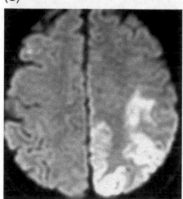

Figure 13 Diffusion-weighted imaging (DWI) abnormality in focal status epilepticus due to underlying low-grade glioma. **(A)** The T2-weighted image shows cortical signal changes in the left hemisphere and hyperintense white matter abnormalities on both sides. Direct cortical tumor infiltration was noted on previous scans. **(B)** The T1-weighted image after contrast injection does not show areas of enhancement suggesting anaplastic tumor degeneration or ischemia. **(C)** DWI shows restricted diffusion of protons in the left occipital and parietal cortex. These findings were reversible after the seizure was terminated. No residual defect was encountered. *Source*: Courtesy of Dr. Pretorius, Oxford, U.K.

Adverse treatment effects also have to be considered on posttreatment images. After surgery, cerebral hemorrhage and other surgical complications may prevent the patient's recovery. Radiosurgery may induce acute radionecrosis and cerebral edema. Chemotherapy with various cytotoxic agents may cause acute neurological deficits due to toxic demyelination (Fig. 15) (16). Other causes of treatment-related neurological deficits are arterial and venous infarcts as well as cerebral infections. The latter may be caused by surgery or can be due to immunological impairment. Frequent infectious agents are *Staphylococcus aureus* and other bacteria after surgery. Cellular parasites such as *Toxoplasma gondii* and viruses such as JC virus are encountered after chemotherapy. The identification of the infectious agents usually requires CSF sampling or even biopsy.

(A) (B)

(C) (D)

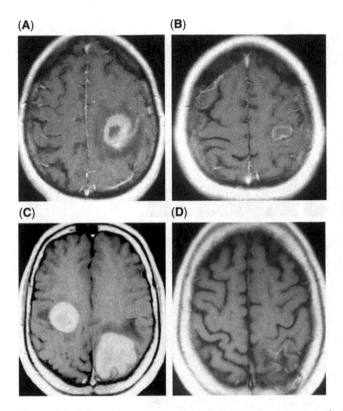

Figure 14 Magnetic resonance imaging–based response evaluation of primary lymphomas of the central nervous system. Residual areas of contrast uptake not indicating viable tumor tissue in two patients. (**A**) This T1-weighted image after contrast injection shows a lesion centered in the left precentral gyrus. There is an area without contrast enhancement in the center. Central necrosis is infrequent in cerebral lymphoma and mainly found in patients with AIDS. (**B**) The follow-up scan six months after biopsy and chemotherapy shows a residual ring lesion. This finding was regarded as scar tissue rather than viable tumor and further treatment was withheld. No local relapse has evolved over more than three years. (**C**) Two large areas of contrast uptake are seen in this patient with primary central nervous system lymphoma. Open biopsy was performed in the left parietal lobe, complicated by a small hemorrhage. (**D**) The T1-weighted image after contrast administration shows a contrast uptake at the edge of the postsurgical left parietal brain defect. No tumor growth was seen over more than two years.

FOLLOW-UP

Follow-up scans are performed to detect any tumor growth or regrowth. The time intervals between the surveillance scans depend on the rate of tumor proliferation and on the available treatment options. Imaging is either performed

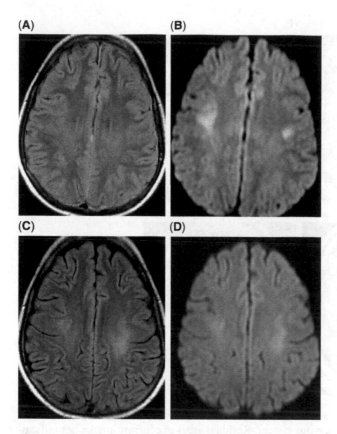

Figure 15 Diffusion-weighted imaging (DWI) shows early side effects of chemotherapy in a 16-year-old boy presenting with right sided hemiparesis seven days after intrathecal methotrexate (MTX) administration for relapse of acute lymphoblastic leukemia. (**A**) The T2-weighted fluid attenuated inversion recovery (FLAIR) sequence shows very subtle signal changes in the subcortical white matter on both sides. (**B**) DWI identifies areas of high signal intensity in both hemispheres, more pronounced on the right, but affecting the pyramidal tract on the left. (**C** and **D**) Follow-up scans two weeks after resolution of symptoms. (**C**) The T2-weighted FLAIR images now show areas of high signal intensity in both hemispheres. (**D**) In DWI, the affected areas are slightly hyperintense. These changes are caused by T2-shine-through, i.e., the T2 sensitivity of the DWI sequence. This was proven by calculation of an apparent diffusion coefficient (ADC) map. Restricted diffusion of protons in this patient was caused by acute demyelination, which has been reported as a rare early side effect of high-dose MTX treatment.

with CT or MRI, usually after contrast injection. Treatment response is evaluated according to the MacDonald criteria as described above.

While postsurgical complications are prevalent in the early phase after treatment, adverse effects of radio- and chemotherapy are mainly

(A) (B)

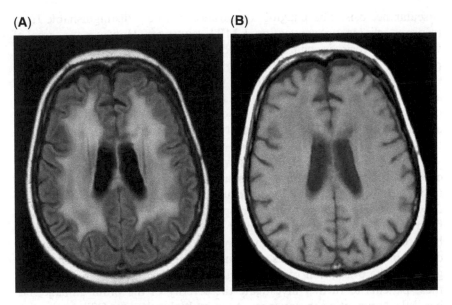

Figure 16 Chemotherapy-induced leukoencephalopathy after radiochemotherapy of primary central nervous system lymphoma and intrathecal methotrexate administration. (**A**) T2-weighted fluid attenuated inversion recovery image. There are bilateral, diffuse white matter signal changes, extending from the ventricular walls to the subcortical regions. (**B**) The T1-weighted image shows white matter signal loss, most pronounced in the frontal and parietal regions. T1-signal changes tend to correlate more with clinical defects than the more sensitive T2 abnormalities.

encountered after months to years. White matter damage is caused either by toxic demyelination or due to endothelial injury and hence microvascular damage. Due to its slowly progressive nature, these changes may proceed to outright necrosis with blood–brain barrier breakdown.

During this phase of imaging, the main task is the differentiation of adverse effects and scar tissue from progressive or recurrent tumor, which has to be expected in patients with glial tumors.

This differential diagnosis is facilitated by comparison with preceding examinations and relevant clinical data such as the radiotherapy fields and the details of the chemotherapy such as the route of application.

Contrast-enhancing scar tissue has to be encountered after open biopsy and resection, especially after postsurgical hemorrhage and infection. Direct comparison with postsurgical images is therefore extremely helpful. Further studies will have to determine the efficacy of PET to differentiate scar tissue and residual or recurrent cerebral neoplasms.

Radiation necrosis is a rare complication of cerebral radiotherapy due to the presently applied treatment protocols. However, necrosis may occur up to three years after the termination of the treatment due to delayed vascular necrosis. The imaging appearance can be indistinguishable from recurrent glioma on conventional MRI sequences. However, an area of vascular necrosis is characterized by reduced metabolic activity and perfusion. Hence, physiological imaging modalities are most appropriate to differentiate these entities. PET is well suited to evaluate the metabolic activity and the perfusion of brain tissue and is therefore regarded as the most specific imaging modality. However, due to its high cost and limited availability, MRI has become the most commonly used tool for this differential diagnosis by employing perfusion-weighted imaging and proton MRS.

Apart from outright necrosis with blood–brain barrier breakdown, chronic demyelination (Fig. 16) is a dreaded consequence of radiochemotherapy because it may be associated with severe cognitive decline. To fully appreciate the possible development of this leukoencephalopathy, follow-up scans should be performed after at least 12 months. It needs to be stressed that the association of white matter changes and cognitive deficits may not be as close as previously thought. Perfusion-weighted imaging and the evaluation of brain metabolic activity may be performed in these patients to further investigate the severity of the brain damage, but has little therapeutic consequences. As in multiple sclerosis, DTI can be used to further delineate the extent of white matter damage in normal appearing white matter and in homogenously affected brain tissue. Although further studies are required, the early detection and careful evaluation of white matter lesions during treatment may potentially have a significant impact on the further treatment of brain neoplasm.

REFERENCES

1. Guo AC, Provenzale JM, Cruz LC Jr., Petrella JR. Cerebral abscesses: investigation using apparent diffusion coefficient maps. Neuroradiology 2001; 43:370–374.
2. Nadal Desbarats L, Herlidou S, de Marco G, et al. Differential MRI diagnosis between brain abscesses and necrotic or cystic brain tumors using the apparent diffusion coefficient and normalized diffusion-weighted images. Magn Reson Imaging 2003; 21:645–650.
3. Garg M, Gupta RK, Husain M, et al. Brain abscesses: etiologic categorization with in vivo proton MR spectroscopy. Radiology 2004; 230:519–527.
4. Mishra AM, Gupta RK, Jaggi RS, et al. Role of diffusion-weighted imaging and in vivo proton magnetic resonance spectroscopy in the differential diagnosis of ring-enhancing intracranial cystic mass lesions. J Comput Assist Tomogr 2004; 28:540–547.
5. Hartmann M, Jansen O, Heiland S, Sommer C, Munkel K, Sartor K. Restricted diffusion within ring enhancement is not pathognomonic for brain abscess. AJNR Am J Neuroradiol 2001; 22:1738–1742.
6. Kuker W, Ruff J, Gaertner S, Mehnert F, Mader I, Nagele T. Modern MRI tools for the characterization of acute demyelinating lesions: value of chemical shift and diffusion-weighted imaging. Neuroradiology 2004; 46:421–426.

7. Mader I, Seeger U, Weissert R, et al. Proton MR spectroscopy with metabolite-nulling reveals elevated macromolecules in acute multiple sclerosis. Brain 2001; 124:953–961.
8. Kuker W, Nagele T, Schmidt F, Heckl S, Herrlinger U. Diffusion-weighted MRI in herpes simplex encephalitis: a report of three cases. Neuroradiology 2004; 46:122–125.
9. Mader I, Herrlinger U, Klose U, Schmidt F, Kuker W. Progressive multifocal leukoencephalopathy: analysis of lesion development with diffusion-weighted MRI. Neuroradiology 2003; 45:717–721.
10. Kaminogo M, Ishimaru H, Morikawa M, et al. Diagnostic potential of short echo time MR spectroscopy of gliomas with single-voxel and point-resolved spatially localized proton spectroscopy of brain. Neuroradiology 2001; 43:353–363.
11. Howe FA, Barton SJ, Cudlip SA, et al. Metabolic profiles of human brain tumors using quantitative in vivo IH magnetic resonance spectroscopy. Magn Reson Med 2003; 49:223–232.
12. Hartmann M, Heiland S, Halting I, et al. Distinguishing of primary cerebral lymphoma from high-grade glioma with perfusion-weighted magnetic resonance imaging. Neurosci Lett 2003; 338:119–122.
13. Senn P, Lovblad KO, Ziitter D, et al. Changes on diffusion-weighted MRI with focal motor status epilepticus: case report. Neuroradiology 2003; 45:246–249.
14. Macdonald DR, Cascino TL, Schold SC, Cairncross JG. Response criteria for phase II studies of supratentorial malignant glioma. J Clin Oncol 1990; 8:1277–1280.
15. Kuker W, Naegele T, Thiel E, Weller M, Herrlinger U. Primary central nervous system lymphomas (PCNSL): MRI response criteria revised. Neurology, 2005 In press.
16. Kuker W, Bader P, Herrlinger U, Heckl S, Nagele T. Transient encephalopathy after intrathekal methotrexate chemotherapy: diffusion-weighted MRI. J Neurooncol 2005; 73:47–49.

6

Neurooncological Syndromes

Joachim M. Baehring
Yale University School of Medicine,
New Haven, Connecticut, U.S.A.

INTRODUCTION

The clinical presentation of neoplasms of the nervous system is nonspecific and entirely location dependent. However, certain syndromes exist, recognition of which, in combination with neuroimaging data, laboratory evaluations, and histopathology is crucial in establishing a specific diagnosis and developing a treatment plan. This chapter does not intend to provide a full account of topical diagnoses in neurooncology, but rather focuses on peculiar presentations of cancer patients and points out similarities to and distinction from respective syndromes in noncancer patients.

SYNDROMES OF THE CENTRAL NEURAXIS

Syndromes of the Cerebral Hemispheres

Intracranial neoplasms typically come to medical attention when a new headache develops, a chronic headache changes its pattern, seizures ensue, or signs of increased intracranial pressure (ICP) arise. Gaze paresis to the side opposite the lesion indicates involvement of the frontal center for horizontal gaze. However, this is only observed with acute tumor manifestations such as intratumoral hemorrhage or a focal seizure. Posterior frontal masses cause contralateral hemiparesis and, when the dominant hemisphere is affected, expressive dysphasia. Bilateral prefrontal involvement, by either infiltrative or extra-axial neoplasms, is characterized by psychomotor slowing and loss of sphincter control. Hemianesthesia, apraxia, visuospatial disorientation, or complex neglect syndromes reflect parietal lobe pathology. Hemi- or quadrantanopsias, less congruent than with lesions of the primary visual cortex, are seen in temporal lobe disease. Furthermore, temporal lobe tumors can give rise to the whole spectrum of temporal lobe epilepsy with auditory, olfactory, gustatory, or visual hallucinations and anxiety attacks (Fig. 1A). Dominant hemispheric lesions give rise to receptive dysphasias. Profound short-term memory loss accompanies paraneoplastic limbic encephalitis or tumor infiltration of fornices and hippocampi. Occipital lobe disease causes visual field deficits. Time course of the neurological syndrome reflects the tumor's growth dynamics. Subtle personality changes such as social dysinhibition evolving over years have been described with giant meningiomas compressing the frontal lobes (olfactory groove meningioma); worsening of cognitive skills over weeks accompanies rapidly growing tumors such as malignant gliomas and lymphoma; a fulminant presentation soon followed by signs of increased ICP characterizes true gliomatosis ("neoplastic encephalitis"). Infiltration of the corpus callosum is the basis for disconnection syndromes such as alexia without agraphia (splenium) or transcortical dysphasias (genu or body). Personality disorders and psychoses can be a predominant feature at presentation or after tumor removal. Although locations in temporal and parietal lobe predominate, a definitive relationship between neuroanatomical location and syndrome is difficult to ascertain as neoplasms and psychiatric disorder may be coincidental.

Stroke-like presentations are common in cancer patients and can reflect a direct tumor effect (hemorrhage into a primary or metastatic tumor), dural sinus thrombosis, vascular compression as part of a herniation syndrome, a hypercoaguable state, marantic endocarditis, or an acute chemotherapy-related toxicity (methotrexate and ifosfamide; Fig. 1B).

Diencephalic Tumor Syndromes

Thalamic deficits are rarely complete, and even diffuse infiltration can remain asymptomatic in slow growing tumors. Unilateral tumors cause contralateral hypaesthesia and hemiataxia. Hemiparesis results from infiltration of the posterior limb of the internal capsule. Thalamic pain syndromes are characterized by contralateral hyperpathia and allodynia (Dejerine–Roussy syndrome). Language disturbances are complex and involve receptive and expressive functions. Bilateral involvement of nuclei of the reticular-activating system causes somnolence even in the absence of spinal fluid obstruction. Psychomotor slowing and profound memory impairment have been described, usually with bilateral lesions. Destruction of subthalamic and basal ganglionic structures elicits extrapyramidal syndromes. Infiltration of the hypothalamus disrupts the hypothalamopituitary hormonal axis and

(A)   (B)   (C)

(D)   (E)   (F)

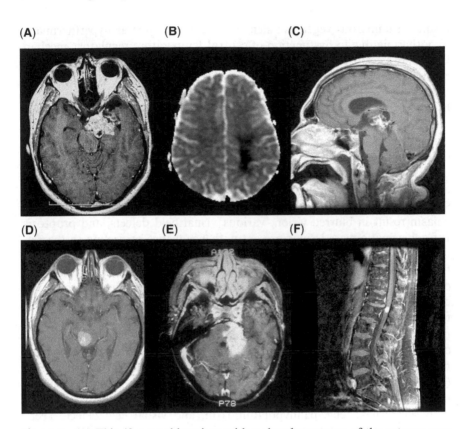

Figure 1 (**A**) This 42-year-old patient with a chondrosarcoma of the petrous apex presented with ictal episodes of extreme sadness and crying (dacrystic seizures). (**B**) A 17-year-old girl with acute lymphoblastic leukemia suddenly developed right hemiparesis and right hemibody numbness. She had received intrathecal methotrexate (12 mg) seven days prior for central nervous system prophylaxis. Apparent diffusion coefficient map showed an area of restricted proton diffusion consistent with cytotoxic edema. Her symptoms resolved as did the observed diffusion abnormality. (**C**) A 26-year-old man with a yolk sac tumor of the pineal region presented with severe headache, nausea, vomiting, lethargy, and confusion. He had a partial Parinaud syndrome with light-near dissociation of pupillary response and impaired upgaze. (**D**) This 55-year-old man with metastatic non–small cell cancer of the lung complained of a dull, relentless pain involving the left side of his body. (**E**) A 68-year-old woman developed sequential cranial neuropathies on the left side (V, VI, VII, VIII, and X; Garcin syndrome) and a right hemiparesis. (**F**) A 62-year-old man with metastatic papillary thyroid carcinoma complained of progressive weakness in his distal left lower extremity and difficulty initiating micturition. Magnetic resonance imaging (MRI) of the lumbosacral spine revealed an intramedullary metastasis within the conus medullaris. (**A, C, D,** and **E**) T1-weighted MRI with gadolinium; (**B**) Apparent diffusion coefficient map; (**F**) T1-weighted MRI with gadolinium and fat suppression.

results in numerous vegetative signs or symptoms such as hyperthermia or hypothermia due to dysfunction of central temperature regulatory mechanisms and electrolyte imbalances (central diabetes insipidus and syndrome of inappropriate adiuretin secretion). Hyperphagia has been linked to destruction of a satiety center located in the ventromedial nucleus of the hypothalamus. Emaciation due to destruction of a hypothalamic appetite center has not been clearly established in adults. In children, progressive emaciation despite normal food intake occurs with hypothalamic tumors. Other manifestations of hypothalamic neoplasms are hypersexuality or loss of sexual interest, pubertas praecox in children, disturbances of affect control (pathological laughter or crying, rage), amnestic syndromes, and somnolence or disturbance of sleep–wake cycles. Gliomas of the optic chiasm result in blurred vision, various visual field defects, and proptosis. Infrachiasmatic mass lesions present with headaches projecting to the center of the forehead. Pressure on the optic chiasm from below is the basis for a heteronymous bitemporal hemianopsia, the classical visual field defect from a pituitary adenoma. Partial field defects affecting the upper quadrants of the temporal visual fields may be an early sign. In addition to nonspecific, pressure-related effects, symptoms caused by pituitary tumors reflect their hormone-producing status. Non–hormone-producing pituitary adenomas, infrachiasmatic meningiomas, or metastases cause panhypopituitarism with lethargy, heat–cold intolerance, and lack of sexual interest (hypogonadotropic hypogonadism). Hemorrhage into a pituitary tumor—pituitary apoplexy—constitutes a neurosurgical emergency and presents with severe headache, panhypopituitarism, and visual field defect. Tectal syndromes are observed with pineal region tumors. Parinaud's syndrome with conjugate upgaze inhibition, light-near dissociation of pupillary contraction, pathologic lid retraction (Collier's sign) and retractory nystagmus is rarely complete, but partial variants are common.

Tumor Syndromes of the Brain Stem and Cranial Nerves

The clinical syndrome and its dynamics serve as important clues to the diagnosis of brain stem neoplasms. In this location, the clinician may be dependent on indirect diagnostic means because tissue acquisition is limited to stereotactic biopsy or not possible at all due to unacceptable morbidity associated with the procedure. It remains surprising how little symptoms an encapsulated neoplasm such as a metastasis can cause. Even in this anatomical "bottle neck" of the central neuraxis, neoplasms can grow in a compressive fashion without giving rise to symptoms. On the other side, infiltrative tumors such as lymphoma or malignant gliomas cause substantial morbidity early in their course (Fig. 2). Infiltrative tumors migrate along long white matter tracts such as corticospinal tract, spinothalamic tract, or fasciculus longitudinalis medialis. Invasion of the area postrema is the basis

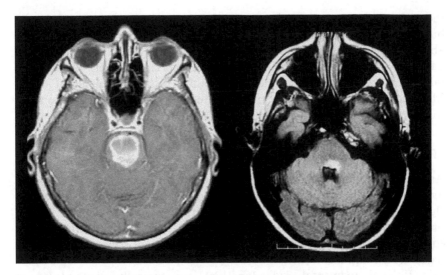

Figure 2 *Left*: A 52-year-old woman with ovarian cancer complained of a mild intermittent headache and left facial numbness. Magnetic resonance imaging revealed a large metastasis occupying the entire basis pontis (T1 with gadolinium). *Right*: A 43-year-old woman with primary central nervous system lymphoma complained of horizontal diplopia. Neurological examination revealed a Bell's palsy on the left and bilateral internuclear ophthalmoplegia with complete horizontal gaze paresis on the left (one-and-a-half syndrome; T1 with gadolinium).

for intractable nausea. Neuropathic pain affecting the same side of the patient's face or the opposite side of trunk and extremities arises from tumors affecting the trigeminal nerve or its root entry zone or the spinothalamic tract (Fig. 1D). Parenchymal invasion of the mesencephalon is the basis for nuclear third nerve palsies. A peculiar syndrome is associated with tumors growing along the craniocaudal axis of the brain stem while respecting the midline of the brain stem. This growth pattern gives rise to cranial nerve dysfunction restricted to one side (Garcin syndrome; Fig. 1E). The small size of the infratentorial compartment results in early signs of spinal fluid obstruction, upward or downward herniation. Appendicular ataxia characterizes cerebellar hemispheric lesions, whereas midline tumors predominantly affect stance and gait. A severe, rapidly evolving, and usually irreversible diffuse cortical cerebellar syndrome is seen with paraneoplastic cerebellar degeneration.

Myelopathies

Extrinsic pressure on the spinal cord invariably gives rise to a transverse myelopathy. Asymmetric cord syndromes can only result from cord infiltration by tumor. A classical Brown–Secquard syndrome with upper motor neuron signs and proprioceptive loss on the side of tumor infiltration and thermal anesthesia on the opposite side below the level of the lesion is rare but incomplete variants are not uncommon. Radicular pain is typically absent as opposed to epidural cord compression. However, neuropathic pain may complicate the clinical picture, especially when the cord is infiltrated by a tumor growing centripetally within a segmental nerve. Metastases or primary tumors of the conus medullaris cause saddle anesthesia and loss of sphincter tone (Fig. 1F).

PERIPHERAL SYNDROMES

Asymmetric multilevel radiculopathies and cranial neuropathies characterize meningeal carcinomatosis and lymphomatosis. The syndrome also includes signs of meningeal irritation (nausea, vomiting, headache, back pain, and photo- and phonophobia) and cognitive decline. Involvement of the cauda equina is recognized when patients complain of low back pain, perineal paresthesias, and incontinence.

Isolated segmental radiculopathies are typically encountered in patients with nerve sheath tumors or metastases encasing the intervertebral foramen. Brachial plexopathies are typically seen in patients with breast cancer or lung cancer involving the lung apex (Pancoast tumor), lumbosacral plexopathies in patients with intrapelvic neoplasms (prostate, colon, uterus, and bladder; Fig. 3A). These can indicate tumor infiltration or the effects of radiotherapy. Clinically and radiographically, a definitive diagnosis is difficult. The presence of myokymia is more consistent with radiation plexopathy. Peripheral neuropathies are amongst the most common neurological findings in cancer patients. The majority of cases reflect toxicity of systemic chemotherapy (vinca alkaloids, taxanes, platinum compounds, and bortezomib). Sensory deficits distributed in a fiber length–dependent fashion predominate. Autonomic neuropathies with orthostatic hypotension, abdominal cramps, constipation, urinary retention, and sexual dysfunction occur as a consequence of amyloid deposition or an autoimmune-mediated (paraneoplastic) process. Isolated neuropathies are observed in patients with nerve sheath tumors or lymphoma (Fig. 3B). Paraneoplastic disorders can affect the neuromuscular junction, either presynaptically (Lambert–Eaton syndrome) or postsynaptically (Myasthenia gravis), and muscle. Myopathies also arise from metastatic spread to muscle (Fig. 3C).

SYNDROMES ASSOCIATED WITH INCREASED ICP, DISTURBANCES OF SPINAL FLUID FLOW, AND CEREBRAL HERNIATION

Headache is the most common complaint of patients with increased ICP. In its classical form, it is severe, resistant to common analgesics, and reaches maximum intensity upon awakening in the morning. Decreased venous

(A) (B)

(C)

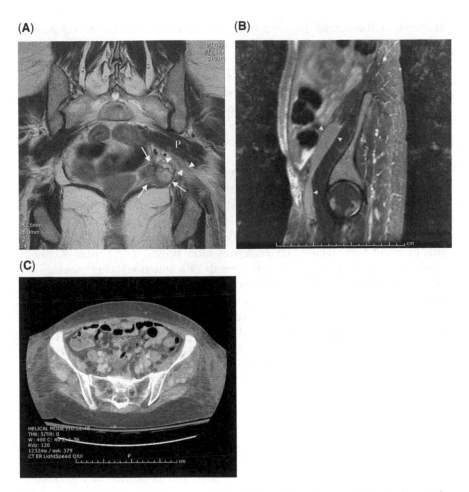

Figure 3 (A) A 54-year-old woman with a history of carcinoma of the uterine cervix nine years prior presented with severe pain in her left buttock radiating down the posterior aspect of her leg. Magnetic resonance imaging (MRI) of the lumbosacral plexus demonstrated a heterogeneous mass lesion (*arrows*) abutting the sciatic nerve (*arrow heads*) at its exit from the pelvis below the piriformis muscle (*P*) (T2-weighted MRI). (B) A 46-year-old woman with disseminated diffuse large B-cell lymphoma noticed weakness of knee extension and a dull pain on the anterior aspect of her left thigh. MRI showed enlargement and enhancement of the femoral nerve consistent with neurolymphomatosis (T1 with gadolinium). (C) A 60-year-old woman experienced progressive difficulty walking up the incline in her front yard to her mailbox. She had lost 30 lbs over the course of a few months. She was diagnosed with widely metastatic breast cancer. Computed tomography (CT) of the pelvis (with contrast) revealed multiple metastases in the gluteal and iliac muscles bilaterally.

drainage in the supine position likely accounts for this observation. Frequently patients report immediate relief from their headache by vomiting. However, the majority of patients have nonspecific tension-type or migraine-like headaches. If ICP continues to rise, nausea, vomiting, hiccoughing, and yawning ensue. Cognitive complaints such as slowness to respond and inattentiveness reflect frontal lobe dysfunction. The patient becomes increasingly somnolent and ultimately falls into a coma. In infants, prior to closure of the calvarial sutures, hydrocephalus is accompanied by enlargement of head circumference.

Chronic hydrocephalus can be recognized on plain radiographs of the skull as focal thinning of the tabula interna of the skull ("Lückenschädel"). Funduscopic examination reveals papilledema in about half of patients with increased ICP. Absence of venous pulsations within the center of the optic disc is an early finding, whereas papilledema with blurring of the disc margins or small hemorrhages characterizes later stages. The Foster Kennedy syndrome—optic nerve atrophy as a result of a sphenoid wing meningioma and contralateral papilledema from increased ICP—is rarely seen in the days of improved neuroimaging methods and earlier diagnosis. Paresis of extraocular muscles results from stretch injury of fourth or sixth nerve or uncal herniation with compression of the third nerve. However, the clinician must be aware of "false" localizing signs. Temporal lobe tumors can cause compression of the cerebral peduncle at the tentorial notch on the opposite side resulting in a hemiparesis on the same side as the mass lesion (Kernohan's syndrome).

In uncal herniation from temporal lobe masses or herpes encephalitis, ipsilateral compression of the third nerve leads to pupillary dilatation before extraocular dysmotility. With progression of shift of brain substance, a complete third nerve palsy ensues and signs of midbrain dysfunction appear. Patients develop contralateral hemiparesis from pressure on the cerebral peduncle and ultimately become stuporous. Increasing pressure from hemispheric or diencephalic mass lesions results in central (transtentorial) herniation. Central herniation leads to a progressive syndrome reflecting sequential damage to brain stem structures in a rostrocaudal fashion. At the early "diencephalic" stage, mild changes in the patient's alertness are accompanied by periodic breathing, yawning, or hiccoughing. Pupils are small but remain reactive to light. With further progression of central herniation, the patient becomes obtunded or stuporous. Roving eye movements reflect diffuse cortical dysfunction and preservation of lower brain stem gaze centers. Noxious stimuli elicit flexion of upper extremities and extension of lower extremities (decorticate posturing). Midsize pupils unresponsive to light indicate midbrain dysfunction. Damage to the mesencephalic reticular–activating system produces coma. Central neurogenic hyperventilation denotes a fast and regular breathing pattern. The triad of changes in breathing pattern, arterial hypertension, and bradycardia is known as the Kocher–Cushing reflex. Noxious stimulation elicits extension of all limbs (decerebrate posturing). Absence of oculocephalic reflex (doll's head maneuver) and horizontal eye movements to caloric stimulation of the vestibular system indicates damage to pontine structures. Breathing becomes apneustic. Further progression leads to herniation of the cerebellar tonsils through the foramen magnum. At the preterminal stage, breathing is ataxic and the blood pressure drops.

The syndrome of raised ICP and cerebral herniation can evolve slowly over days to weeks or acutely over hours. Rapid progression usually indicates hemorrhage. Subdural hematomas in patients with coagulopathies can evolve so rapidly that signs of cerebral herniation are present before an imaging study can be obtained. Hemorrhage into a metastatic focus is typically characterized by the sudden onset of focal neurological signs including seizures. Intraparenchymal hemorrhage as a result of coagulopathy leads to slowly progressive neurological deterioration.

A peculiar syndrome is associated with tumors causing a pressure valve effect such as a colloid cyst of the foramen of Monro. Patients, typically in their late childhood or early adulthood, report sudden onset of severe imbalance, headache, and nausea that is frequently brought on by positional changes (bending down) or Valsalva maneuvers. Sudden deaths have occurred.

Idiopathic intracranial hypertension (Pseudotumor cerebri) is mostly characterized by nocturnal or hypnopompic headaches aggravated by Valsalva maneuver. Nonspecific visual changes, diplopia due to sixth nerve palsy or transient visual obscuration are less frequent manifestations. On physical examination, papilledema is the most striking abnormality. The blind spot is enlarged. It is presumed that the disorder is due to decreased cerebrospinal fluid absorption.

Another characteristic clinical syndrome is recognized in patients with chronic disturbance of spinal fluid reabsorption (Fig. 4, right). These patients or, more likely, their family members report a combination of cognitive decline, precipitate micturition, and gait apraxia. Dementia is usually of the subcortical type. Precipitate micturition reflects dysfunction of the cortical center for bladder control (paracentral lobule). Minimal bladder filling results in the uncontrollable urge to urinate. The gait disturbance is characterized by difficulty initiating ambulation and postural instability with retropulsion. Strength is preserved.

MENINGEAL SYNDROMES

Meningeal spread of cancer is recognized as a complex syndrome comprising headache, nausea, vomiting, asymmetric cranial neuropathies, and painful radiculopathies affecting multiple levels of the neuraxis. However, signs of meningeal irritation may be entirely absent, and the disease can take a more subacute course mimicking a dementing illness.

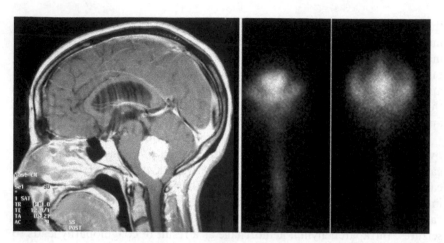

Figure 4 *Left*: A 37-year-old woman complained of progressive headache, nausea, and imbalance. Magnetic resonance imaging with gadolinium demonstrated a large enhancing mass lesion obstructing the fourth ventricle. The tumor was removed and found to be a choroid plexus papilloma. *Right*: A 58-year-old woman, in remission from Non-Hodgkin lymphoma after autologous stem cell transplantation, developed imbalance, cognitive decline, and urinary incontinence. Cerebrospinal fluid analysis confirmed leptomeningeal relapse. A cisternography showed early ventricular and late subarachnoid filling over the hemispheres suggestive of aresorptive hydrocephalus.

EXTRADURAL SYNDROMES OF CRANIUM, SKULL BASE, AND SPINAL CANAL

Intracranial Extra-Axial and Skull Base Syndromes

Dural mass lesions overlying the hemispheres can remain silent until the tumor has reached a considerable size. The rare rapidly growing neoplasms such as multiple myeloma, dural sarcomas, or lymphomas are detected as "soft spots" within the cranial vault, rapidly progressive headache or signs resulting from cerebral parenchymal infiltration. Infiltration or obstruction of dural venous sinuses leads to a syndrome reminiscent of pseudotumor cerebri. Tumors arising from the dura of the lesser wing of the sphenoid bone infiltrate the cavernous sinus resulting in ocular dysmotility due to compression of cranial nerve III, IV, VI, and facial paraesthesias. Cerebrovascular complications in the territory of encased blood vessels (such as the cavernous portion of the internal carotid artery) are surprisingly rare and more commonly reflect the effects of surgical intervention or radiation. Metastases or the rare primary tumors affecting the base of the skull give rise to complex syndromes (Fig. 5). Paragangliomas (glomus tympanicum and glomus jugulare tumors) grow through the jugular foramen into the parapharyngeal space resulting in dysfunction of cranial nerves IX, X

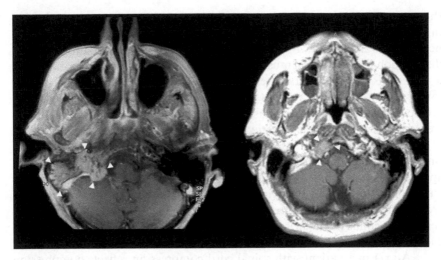

Figure 5 *Left*: A 72-year-old woman suffered from recurrent pneumonias. She was hoarse, and her right trapezius muscle was visibly atrophic (Vernet syndrome). Laryngoscopy showed a right vocal-cord paralysis. Otoscopic examination revealed a purplish mass in her middle ear. Tumor biopsy was consistent with Glomus tympanicum tumor (T1 with gadolinium). *Right*: A 62-year-old man with metastatic papillary thyroid carcinoma noticed difficulty maneuvering food with his tongue from the left to the right side and into the gullet. He started choking on his food and his speech became slurred. Magnetic resonance imaging (MRI) of the brain with gadolinium revealed a metastasis to the hypoglossal canal on the right side.

(hoarseness and dysphagia), XI (weakness of the trapezius muscle), and XII (homolateral tongue atrophy). Glomus tympanicum tumors are visible as purplish masses within the middle ear through inspection of external auditory canal.

Squamous cell carcinomas of the face, melanomas, adenoid cystic carcinomas, malignant tumors of paranasal sinuses, and skin appendages have a predilection for centripetal growth along peripheral nerves. Initial symptoms reflect involvement of terminal branches ("numb chin syndrome"). Once the cancer cells reach intracranial structures, more complex syndromes arise from invasion of the cavernous sinus or even the cerebral parenchyma.

Epidural Spinal Cord Compression

Epidural spinal cord compression is one of the most devastating neurological complications of systemic cancer. Metastases usually arise from the axial skeleton. Pain ensues when the richly innervated periosteum is involved. The vertebral body affected by metastatic spread is tender to percussion. The pain resulting from epidural mass effect is typically exacerbated by sneezing, coughing, or the Valsalva maneuver. As the recumbent position aggravates the pain, many patients experience maximum pain intensity upon awakening in the morning or even have to sleep in a sitting position. Compression of a nerve root is associated with excruciating pain in the corresponding radicular distribution. Paravertebral muscle spasm caused by nerve root irritation from a metastasis results in straightening of the physiologic cervical or lumbar lordosis. Straight leg raising (Lasegue maneuver) or, more specifically, crossed straight leg raising (passive elevation of the contralateral, pain-free leg), exacerbate a radiculopathy. Referred pain may mimic a radiculopathy.

Neurological symptoms typically evolve within weeks to months of the onset of back pain. Motor dysfunction (paraparesis or quadriparesis and spasticity) is the earliest sign and occurs before sensory disturbance. Typical early complaints are leg "heaviness," difficulty climbing stairs, or getting up from a chair. Epidural progression of metastases to the upper lumbar spine results in a conus medullaris syndrome with distal lower extremity weakness, saddle paraesthesias, and overflow leakage from bladder and bowel.

Ataxia in a patient with spinal cord compression reflects compression of spinocerebellar pathways. Tingling paresthesias radiating down the spine into the extremities upon brisk flexion of the neck (Lhermitte's sign) indicate an intrinsic or extrinsic spinal cord process. Alarming symptoms of bladder dysfunction are hesitancy and urinary retention.

Presence of a Horner's syndrome (the combination of miosis, ptosis, and enophthalmus) indicates transforaminal progression of tumors located at the level of the cervicothoracic junction and infiltration of the stellate ganglion.

7

Pathology and Classification of Tumors of the Nervous System

Serguei Bannykh

Department of Pathology and Laboratory Medicine, Yale University School of Medicine, New Haven, Connecticut, U.S.A.

The classification and grading of primary tumors of the nervous system have been in flux ever since the first system was introduced. The revised World Health Organization (WHO) Classification (Table 1) (1) may prove to be the most widely accepted classification, but, as it remains morphology based, will likely undergo further refinement. Interobserver variability continues to be a problem and the availability of more objective, prognostically meaningful markers would be desirable. This chapter provides an overview of the current classification system and summarizes the main histological and molecular features of nervous system tumors.

NEUROEPITHELIAL TUMORS

The category of neuroepithelial tumors comprises of gliomas as well as tumors with neuronal differentiation and embryonal neoplasms.

Infiltrative Gliomas

Astrocytoma and *oligodendroglioma* share variable expression of glial fibrillary acidic protein, and a fraction of tumors shows overlapping features. Origin and pathogenesis of gliomas are controversial and likely multifactorial. It is plausible to assume that the tumors are driven by growth-signaling

(Text continues on page 137)

Table 1 World Health Organization Classification of Tumors of the Nervous System

Tumors of neuroepithelial tissue	
Astrocytic tumors	
Diffuse astrocytoma	9400/3
Fibrillary astrocytoma	9420/3
Protoplasmic astrocytoma	9410/3
Gemistocytic astrocytoma	9411/3
Anaplastic astrocytoma	9401/3
Glioblastoma	9440/3
Giant cell glioblastoma	9441/3
Gliosarcoma	9442/3
Pilocytic astrocytoma	9421/1
Pleomorphic xanthoastrocytoma	9424/3
Subependymal giant cell astrocytoma	9384/1
Oligodendroglial tumors	
Oligodendroglioma	9450/3
Anaplastic oligodendroglioma	9451/3
Mixed gliomas	
Oligoastrocytoma	9382/3
Anaplastic oligoastrocytoma	9382/3
Ependymal tumors	
Ependymoma	9391/3
Cellular	9391/3
Papillary	9393/3
Clear cell	9391/3
Tanycytic	9391/3
Anaplastic ependymoma	9392/3
Myxopapillary ependymoma	9394/1
Subependymoma	9383/1
Choroid plexus tumors	
Choroid plexus papilloma	9390/0
Choroid plexus carcinoma	9390/3
Glial tumors of uncertain origin	
Astroblastoma	9430/3
Gliomatosis cerebri	9381/3
Chordoid glioma of the third ventricle	9444/1
Neuronal and mixed neuronal-glial tumors	
Gangliocytoma	9492/0
Dysplastic gangliocytoma of cerebellum (Lhermitte-Duclos)	9493/0
Desmoplastic infantile astrocytoma/ganglioglioma	9412/1
Dysembryoplastic neuroepithelial tumor	9413/0
Ganglioglioma	9505/1
Anaplastic ganglioglioma	9505/3

(*Continued*)

Table 1   World Health Organization Classification of Tumors of the Nervous System (*Continued*)

Central neurocytoma	9506/1
Cerebellar liponeurocytoma	9506/1
Paraganglioma of the filum terminale	8680/1
Neuroblastic tumors	
Olfactory neuroblastoma (Aesthesioneuroblastoma)	9522/3
Olfactory neuroepithelioma	9523/3
Neuroblastomas of the adrenal gland and sympathetic nervous system	9500/3
Pineal parenchymal tumors	
Pineocytoma	9361/1
Pineoblastoma	9362/3
Pineal parenchymal tumor of intermediate differentiation	9362/3
Embryonal tumors	
Medulloepithelioma	9501/3
Ependymoblastoma	9392/3
Medulloblastoma	9470/3
Desmoplastic medulloblastoma	9471/3
Large cell medulloblastoma	9474/3
Medullomyoblastoma	9472/3
Melanotic medulloblastoma	9470/3
Supratentorial primitive neuroectodermal tumor	9473/3
Neuroblastoma	9500/3
Ganglioneuroblastoma	9490/3
Atypical teratoid/rhabdoid tumor	9508/3
Tumors of peripheral nerves	
Schwannoma (neurilemmoma, neurinoma)	9560/0
Cellular	9560/0
Plexiform	9560/0
Melanotic	9560/0
Neurofibroma	9540/0
Plexiform	9550/0
Perineurioma	9571/0
Intraneural perineurioma	9571/0
Soft tissue perineurioma	9571/0
MPNST	
Epithelioid	9540/3
MPNST with divergent mesenchymal and/or epithelial differentiation	9540/3
Melanotic	9540/3
Melanotic psammomatous	9540/3
Tumors of the meninges	
Tumors of meningothelial cells	
Meningioma	9530/0

(*Continued*)

Table 1 World Health Organization Classification of Tumors of the Nervous System (*Continued*)

Meningothelial	9531/0
Fibrous (fibroblastic)	9532/0
Transitional (mixed)	9537/0
Psammomatous	9533/0
Angiomatous	9534/0
Microcystic	9530/0
Secretory	9530/0
Lymphoplasmacyte-rich	9530/0
Metaplastic	9530/0
Clear cell	9538/1
Chordoid	9538/1
Atypical	9539/1
Papillary	9538/3
Rhabdoid	9530/3
Anaplastic meningioma	9530/3
Mesenchymal, nonmeningothelial tumors	
Lipoma	8850/0
Angiolipoma	8861/0
Hibernoma	8880/0
Liposarcoma (intracranial)	8850/3
Solitary fibrous tumor	8815/0
Fibrosarcoma	8810/3
Malignant fibrous histiocytoma	8830/3
Leiomyoma	8890/0
Leiomyosarcoma	8890/3
Rhabdomyoma	8900/0
Rhabdomyosarcoma	8900/3
Chondroma	9220/0
Chondrosarcoma	9220/3
Osteoma	9180/0
Osteosarcoma	9180/3
Osteochondroma	9210/0
Hemangioma	9120/0
Epithelioid hemangioendothelioma	9133/1
Hemangiopericytoma	9150/1
Angiosarcoma	9120/3
Kaposi sarcoma	9140/3
Primary melanocytic lesions	
Diffuse melanocytosis	8728/0
Melanocytoma	8728/1
Malignant melanoma	8720/3
Meningeal melanomatosis	8728/3
Tumors of uncertain histogenesis	
Hemangioblastoma	9161/1

(*Continued*)

Table 1 World Health Organization Classification of Tumors of the Nervous System (*Continued*)

Lymphomas and hemopoietic neoplasms	
Malignant lymphomas	9590/3
Plasmacytoma	9731/3
Granulocytic sarcoma	9930/3
Germ cell tumors	
Germinoma	9064/3
Embryonal carcinoma	9070/3
Yolk sac tumor	9071/3
Choriocarcinoma	9100/3
Teratoma	9080/1
Mature	9080/0
Immature	9080/3
Teratoma with malignant transformation	9084/3
Mixed germ cell tumors	9085/3
Tumors of the sellar region	
Craniopharyngioma	9350/1
Adamantinomatous	9351/1
Papillary	9352/1
Granular cell tumor	9582/0
Metastatic tumors	

Note: Morphology code of the International Classification of Diseases for Oncology and the Systematized Nomenclature of Medicine. Behavior is coded /0 for benign tumors, /1 for low or uncertain malignant potential or borderline malignancy, /2 for in situ lesions, and /3 for malignant tumors.
Abbreviation: MPNST, malignant peripheral nerve sheath tumor.

abnormalities affecting a primitive cell with a limited range of possible differentiations. Exact nature of signaling pathways mediating growth of low-grade gliomas is largely unknown.

The incidence of gliomas changes with aging. The most common neoplasms of young adults are low-grade astrocytoma and oligodendroglioma, whereas in older patients, anaplastic tumors and glioblastoma multiforme (GBM) predominate. Both oligodendroglioma and diffuse astrocytoma are infiltrative tumors (Fig. 1A) and have an intrinsic tendency to slow progression and degeneration into anaplastic tumors and GBM. However, the majority of oligodendrogliomas with "classic" morphology and complete losses of chromosomal arms 1p and 19q tends to have much slower rate of progression. Only a fraction of diffuse astrocytomas behave in a similar indolent fashion (2).

A distinction between oligodendroglioma and astrocytoma is based on a set of morphologic and molecular criteria. Classic astrocytoma is composed of elongated cells with angulated hyperchromatic nuclei; Glial fibrillary acidic protein (GFAP) is strongly expressed (Fig. 1C). There are three somewhat overlapping morphological patterns of astrocytoma: protoplasmic, fibrillary, and gemistocytic. The protoplasmic variant is controversial because of inter-observer variability. It features mucoid background, low cellularity, and contains tumor cells with a few thin processes. The most predominant type is fibrillary astrocytoma, displaying dense GFAP-positive fibrillary background

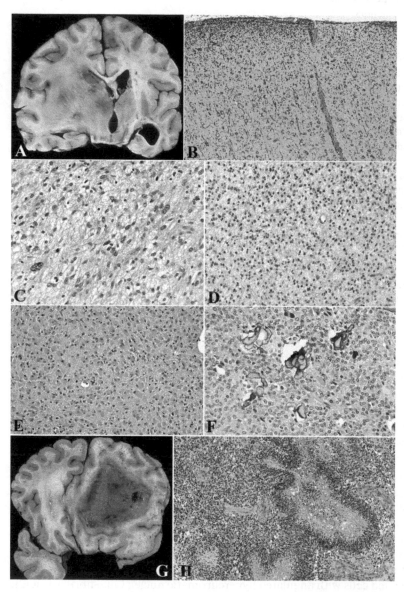

Figure 1   (*Caption on facing page*)

and typical angulated hyperchromatic nuclei. The gemistocytic type contains cells with expanded GFAP- and vimentin-positive cell bodies (Fig. 1E). Oligodendroglioma cells features round nuclei with open chromatin pattern and clear perinuclear halos, and are nurtured by delicate blood vessels of uniform thin diameter and regular branching giving rise to a "chicken-wire" pattern on get ridoff reticulin staining (Figs. 1D and F) (3). In our experience, the classic oligodendroglial and astrocytic morphology are rather rare and the majority of low-grade gliomas falls in the mixed category (4). Both tumors contain microcysts and calcification, although these features are more prominent in oligodendrogliomas. The infiltrative capacity of gliomas manifests in the formation of the so-called secondary structures of Scherer: clustering of migrating tumor cells around blood vessels, underneath the pia and ependyma, and around neurons (perineuronal satellitosis) (Fig. 1B). The secondary structures of Scherer are likely to reflect the capacity of tumor cells to interact dynamically with receptors on respective structures, which facilitates tumor migration and may prove to be a target for tumor therapy. Grading of gliomas relies on a common set of criteria, including presence of necrosis, endothelial proliferation, number of mitotic figures in 10 high-power fields (HPF), and nuclear atypia (5). Presence of nuclear atypia and mitoses defines WHO Grade III tumor (anaplastic astrocytoma), whereas tumors additionally displaying endothelial proliferation or necrosis are diagnosed as WHO Grade IV astrocytoma (GBM) (Figs. 1G and H). Grading of oligodendrogliomas is more controversial, which primarily reflects the ambiguity of morphologic diagnosis. Whereas a few mitotic figures in a tumor are sufficient for upgrading an astrocytic tumor to the anaplastic category, presence of at least 6 mitoses/10 HPF in combination with endothelial proliferation is needed to grade an oligodendroglioma as anaplastic (WHO Grade III). The mitotic count depends on cell density and therefore, more objective

---

Figure 1 (*Facing page*) (**A**) An infiltrative diffuse astrocytoma [World Health Organization (WHO) Grade III)] shows expansion and obscuration of the outlines of normal brain structures, with compression of lateral ventricle and midline shift. (**B**) Secondary structures of Scherer in WHO Grade II oligodendroglioma. Note the clustering of tumor nuclei underneath the pia (*top*), spread along blood vessels and accumulation around neurons (perineuronal satellitosis). (**C**) WHO Grade III astrocytoma features nuclear angulation, hyperchromasia, and pleomorphism on a dense fibrillary background. Mitoses are rare. (**D**) Oligodendroglioma, WHO Grade II. Uniform round nuclei with perinuclear halos. (**E**) Gemistocytic astrocytoma, WHO Grade II. Hyperchromatic nuclei are surrounded by abundant brightly eosinophilic cytoplasm with numerous cell processes. (**F**) Oligodendroglioma, WHO Grade II. Numerous calcifications. (**G**) Hyperemic rim surrounds a necrotic center in this glioblastoma multiforme. Note the transfalcian herniation. (**H**) High cell density, palisading necrosis, and florid endothelial proliferation in glioblastoma multiforme.

estimates of proliferative activity are gaining wide acceptance. In particular, a highly reproducible immunohistochemical stain with MIB-1 antibody, which visualizes Ki-67 antigen present in the nucleus during G1, S, G2, and M phases, allows for a precise count of the percentage of dividing cells. We routinely use MIB-1 on all gliomas, reporting a value obtained in the focus of the highest density of the immunoreactive nuclei. Ki-67 index has the most significance in poorly preserved specimens with compact nuclei and in tumors of the intermediate grade (Grade II/III). It has no predictive value for patients with GBM and the threshold has to be high enough to reveal aggressive tumors. We routinely use a value of 10% as an indicator of worrisome properties (6), but the marker is only used as an adjunct to the mitotic count and endothelial proliferation. Validation across institutions is pending.

Although the histologic diagnosis of GBM in most cases does not present any difficulties, a few examples of GBM are rather distinct. These include gliosarcoma (GS), giant cell GBM, GBM with metaplastic changes, such as formation of bone, cartilage, skeletal, and smooth muscle, advanced squamous differentiation, GBM with granular cell changes, epithelioid and rhabdoid GBM. All of these tumors display GFAP reactivity, infiltration, endothelial proliferation, and necrosis. Giant cell GBM is characterized by predilection for younger age (mean age approximately 40 years), demarcation on imaging, and distinct perilesional edema mimicking metastasis. Giant cell GBM contains bizarre multinucleated and aneuploid cells, which often deposit a reticulin network (7). GS is composed of alternating areas of GFAP-positive foci of typical GBM and GFAP negative, but reticulin-positive foci, reminiscent of a sarcoma. GBM with granular cell changes has a slightly more aggressive course (8) and more frequent chromosomal alterations (9). Predominant epithelioid and rhabdoid morphology in GBM are rare and these peculiar phenotypes are important to keep in mind while differentiating between metastases and primary gliomas. Gliomatosis cerebri (GC) is a distinct variant of glioma with a marked propensity for brain infiltration in dissociation from other features of high-grade glioma, such as endothelial proliferation or necrosis. Definition of GC requires involvement of more than two lobes but currently tends to disregard morphologic appearance and biological property of the tumor by lumping together extensively infiltrative lesions without a distinct nodule and infiltrative tumors associated with nodule. We opt to retain the designation of GC only to the former category. Constituent cells of GC typically show hyperchromatic and angulated nuclei, characteristic of astrocytes. However, oligodendroglial-like morphology in GC has also been reported. Cytogenetic studies of GC are limited. Chromosome 1p and 19q are intact but multiple deletions have been found elsewhere (10).

Classic oligodendroglioma and astrocytoma have very distinct molecular signatures and corresponding tests are now considered to be a standard of care in many institutions. The majority (60–80%) of oligodendrogliomas have combined loss of the entire short arm of chromosome 1 and the entire long arm of chromosome 19 (11). On the contrary, fibrillary astrocytomas have a low rate of 1p19q loss but a very high (40–90%) rate of mutations in *TP53* (11). *TP53* mutations are rare in pure oligodendrogliomas and seem mutually exclusive with 1p- and 19q loss. Testing for 1p19q loss can be performed by various techniques, including comparative genomic hybridization (12), polymerase chain reaction–based studies to evaluate loss of heterozygosity (LOH) of microsatellite DNA, or by fluorescence in situ hybridization (FISH) (13). Each technique has advantages and problems. FISH can visualize LOH in a minor fraction of tumor cells infiltrating normal tissue. This can be useful in the evaluation of small core biopsies of highly invasive tumors (14). However, it can theoretically miss some of the rare cases of interstitial deletions, since only a single probe is used to visualize each chromosomal arm. LOH studies generally require the predominance of tumor cells in the tissue sample and therefore can be of limited value to study invasive tumors of low cellularity.

Abnormalities of *TP53* are pivotal in the pathogenesis of low-grade astrocytomas (15). *TP53* interacts with *MDM2* and *p14^{ARF}*. Function of *TP53* can be altered either by mutations of the constituent genes of this complex or by promotor methylation of either *TP53* or *p14^{ARF}*. Mutations of *TP53* or promoter methylation of either *TP53* or *p14^{ARF}* are detected in 80% to 90% of both oligodendroglioma and astrocytoma (16). Techniques to assess alterations in the *TP53* pathway are laborious and not available for routine diagnostic use. Instead, an immunohistochemistry (IHC)-based technique is widely used to indirectly assess the *TP53* mutation status. Whereas normal *TP53* has a short half-life due to its binding to *MDM2* and subsequent degradation by a proteasome, mutant protein often is unable to enter the degradation pathway, accumulates in the nucleus and can thus be detected by IHC (17). Consequently, it has been demonstrated that IHC detection of *p53* in gliomas correlates with mutations of the protein and can be used as a diagnostic and prognostic marker (18), although *TP53*-immunoreactivity can occur in tumors with no mutations (19). Technically, a strong expression of *TP53* in the majority of nuclei is required to raise a suspicion of *TP53* mutations (20). An application of these tests allows a prognostically useful separation of anaplastic oligodendrogliomas into subcategories (21). Presence of the combined loss of 1p and 19q predicts response to therapy and overall long survival. Mutations in *TP53* were associated with a modest response to chemotherapy, but relatively long survival. Lack of 1p19q codeletion and *TP53* mutations correlated with loss of 10q, amplification of epidermal growth factor receptor (*EGFR*), alteration of phosphatase and tensin homology (*PTEN*), and deletion of *CDKN2A*, and were associated with poor chemotherapy response and short survival.

The majority of GBMs are primary tumors, which form de novo without evidence of preexisting low-grade tumor. In any GBM, there is derangement in two major signaling networks: *EGFR*/platelet-derived growth factor receptor/*PTEN*/*PI3 kinase*/*Akt* pathway and retinoblastoma *RB* (retinoblastoma) /*TP53* pathway. Secondary GBM, which form by degeneration of WHO Grade II tumors, only rarely show amplification of *EGFR* or *MDM2*. Anaplastic progression in some oligodendrogliomas is linked to deletions of *CDKN2A* gene and to amplification of proto-oncogenes.

Giant cell GBM is characterized by a high rate of mutations in *TP53* and *PTEN* (7). Genetic alterations of GS and GBM are similar, except for a lack of *EGFR* amplification in GS. Microdissection analysis confirms the monoclonal origin of both glial and sarcomatous components.

It is convenient to assume that infiltrative gliomas originate from precursor cells of glial lineage, and therefore already have a certain degree of morphologically obvious glial differentiation. Genetic events driving tumor growth work in the context of a preexisting differential repertoire and do not necessarily change phenotype. In this context, identical genetic events in oligodendroglial precursors will produce tumors with oligodendroglial morphology, whereas those affecting astrocytic or neuronal precursors will correspondingly give rise to astrocytomas and neuronal tumors. In this line of thought, the morphologic identification of lineage is not directly linked to the biology of genetic events and consequently to tumor growth and prognosis. The correlation between morphology and genetics can be alternatively explained by a predisposition of neuroectodermal precursors to specific genetic errors during their differentiation, analogous to events described in lymphomas. Very little is known about the signaling cascades driving the growth of gliomas, but there is no doubt that the therapeutic approaches in the future will specifically target the upregulated signaling to inhibit proliferation and migration, and activate apoptosis. These will require a molecular, rather than mere morphological, diagnosis. Advanced data mining of gene expression profiling might be useful to reveal the molecular signatures of altered signaling pathways.

Noninfiltrative Gliomas

Several neuro-ectodermal tumors show distinct glial differentiation but generally lack a tendency for infiltration. These include: pilocytic astrocytoma (PA), pleomorphic xanthoastrocytoma (PXA), ependymomas, and ganglion cell tumors.

Pilocytic Astrocytoma

PA is a low-grade, well circumscribed, slowly growing, and frequently cystic glioma of young age, with a characteristic biphasic histology of alternating loose and densely structured areas and degenerative cytoplasmic features: Rosenthal fibers (RF) and eosinophilic granular bodies (EGBs) (Figs. 2A and B). RF are produced by aggregation of GFAP enmeshed by heat shock protein 27 and αB-crystallin. EGBs represent endosomal compartment. A fraction of PA is infiltrative, e.g., some brain stem gliomas, but nonetheless retains a favorable prognosis (22). Some tumors involve leptomeninges, but usually do not disseminate. Ki-67 index is low, only rarely exceeding 4% (23). Interestingly, despite the higher Ki-67 index and a higher rate of recurrence in younger (<14 years) patients, survival is superior in this category (24). A very small fraction of PA can undergo anaplastic transformation, morphologically identified as brisk mitotic activity, true endothelial proliferation, and necrosis in a background of a tumor either previously identified as PA by biopsy or by

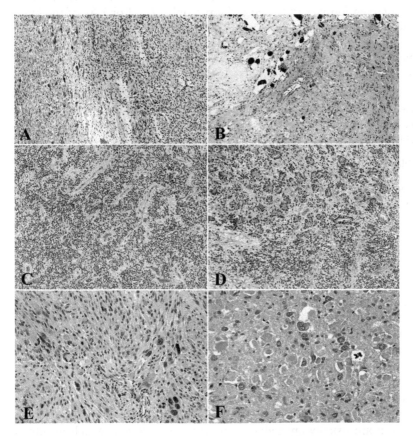

Figure 2 Morphology of noninfiltrative gliomas. (**A**) Pilocytic astrocytoma. Note a typical biphasic architecture with alternating loose (*right*) and dense fibrillary areas (*left*), containing numerous Rosenthal fibers. (**B**) Abundant calcifications and eosinophilic granular bodies (round inclusions on the right side) are also features of pilocytic astrocytoma. (**C**) Perivascular pseudorosettes of ependymoma. (**D**) True ependymal rosettes with lumina (*top*) and perivascular pseudorosettes. (**E**) Intersecting fascicles of pleomorphic cells with frequent eosinophilic granular bodies (EGBs) are characteristic of pleomorphic xanthoastrocytoma. (**F**) Ganglion cell tumor shows tightly packed abnormal neurons with binucleation, calcification, EGBs, and perivascular lymphoid infiltrates (not shown).

the presence of numerous RF and EGBs. PA is frequent in patients with neurofibromatosis type I; in this setting, the tumors are often infiltrative and involve optic pathways. Although they cause pressure atrophy of the involved structures, the majority of these tumors appears nonprogressive (25). Inactivation of NF1 gene plays a role in their origin, while no involvement of NF1 was detected in sporadic PA, suggesting they represent two distinct entities (26). Prognosis is excellent for resectable tumors. A 100% 10-year survival follows gross total and subtotal resection, but only 74% is achieved in cases where surgical intervention was restricted to biopsy only (27). For PAs of the brain stem, five-year survival was reported as 80% (22).

The recently identified *pilomyxoid astrocytoma* has a mixed morphology (28). On one hand, it is discrete, noninfiltrative, and contrast enhancing, like PA, while on the other hand it lacks biphasic architecture and most importantly, degenerative features such as RF or EGB. The tumor cells are dishesive and tend to disseminate along leptomeninges. A more aggressive biology is suggested by limited progression-free (26 months) and overall survival (63 months) (29).

Pleomorphic Xanthoastrocytoma

PXA is a rare, leptomeningeal-based, well-circumscribed, often cystic glioma composed of specialized astrocytes capable of depositing reticulin fibers. The tumors predominantly affect adolescents and young adults and are predominantly located in the temporal lobe. The typical clinical presentation—seizures of long duration—attests to their slow growth and noninfiltrative nature. They are contrast enhancing and can be associated with perilesional calcifications. Intersecting fascicles of spindle cells with entrapped large pleomorphic cells, xanthic cells, frequent EGBs, and perivascular lymphocytes are hallmarks of this distinct entity (Fig. 2E) (30). Constituent cells have a tendency for neuronal differentiation, variably evident in individual examples (31). Despite of highly pleomorphic appearance, suggesting a diagnosis of leptomeningeal-based sarcoma, PXAs have very low proliferative potential. About one-third of the tumors have no detectable mitoses and only 18% show more than 5 mitoses/10 HPF (32). This group has a tendency for early recurrence. The majority of PXA behave in a benign fashion and are usually amenable to gross total resection, which results in cure in 70% of the cases. Residual tumors recur and show morphologic evidence of progression: increased mitotic count and endothelial proliferation. Still, the overall prognosis of PXA is favorable with 81% overall survival at 5 years and 70% at 10 years (32).

Ependymoma

Ependymoma is a noninfiltrative tumor of children and young adults with a distinct ependymal differentiation associated with ventricular lining. Whereas infratentorial ependymomas are solid tumors predominantly affecting young children and often occluding the fourth ventricle, supratentorial tumors are frequently cystic and also seen in adults. All ependymomas are well-circumscribed, contrast enhancing, and induce little edema in adjacent brain. Intralesional hemorrhage and necrosis are common. Morphologically, ependymomas share with other gliomas a dense fibrillary background and strong GFAP reactivity. Other histologic features are unique to and diagnostic of ependymomas. These include formation of perivascular pseudorosettes, true ependymal rosettes, and ependymal canals (Figs. 2C and D). Perivascular pseudorosettes are formed (Figs. 2C and D) as a result of the capacity of these polarized elongated tumor cells to maintain a uniform distance between their nuclei and a blood vessel. Interestingly, immunoreactivity for GFAP is strongest around the blood vessel. Normal ependymal cells have a rectangular shape with apical surface lining the ventricles. The apical surface is studded with microvilli and cilia. It is separated from the basolateral plasma membrane by highly specialized adhesive junctions. Ependymomas recapitulate such differentiation and can form true ependymal rosettes or even canals. However, in the majority of cases, the lumina are abortive and often intracellular. They however retain delineation by adhesive junctions and apical cilia or microvilli. This feature is highly useful for electron microscopic confirmation of the ependymal nature of poorly differentiated tumors. Lumina can also be highlighted by immunohistochemical stain with epithelial membrane antigen (EMA). In addition to the typical, so-called *cellular* ependymomas, several other morphologic variants are discerned, including "oligodendroglial-like" *clear cell* ependymomas, *tanycytic* ependymoma, *myxopapillary* ependymoma, and tumors with metaplastic changes: osseous, cartilaginous, melanocytic, signet-ring, and also giant cell variant. A differentiation between WHO Grade II and III (anaplastic) ependymoma relies on the presence of endothelial proliferation and brisk mitotic activity (over 7 mitoses/10 HPF) (33). However, widely accepted criteria have not been established, since several studies failed to find a correlation between mitotic activity, endothelial proliferation, and even cerebrospinal fluid (CSF) dissemination at presentation and survival (34). Anaplastic ependymomas have a significantly higher proliferative index, with reported values of 2% for Grade II and 34% for Grade III tumors (35). An inverse relationship between proliferative index and prognosis has been reported (36). We use a Ki-67 labelling index of 10% as a threshold value to raise a level of suspicion for anaplastic biology, as done in other gliomas. Being a noninfiltrative tumor, ependymoma is amenable to surgical excision, and the extent of resection has a major impact on prognosis (37). Spillage of the poorly cohesive tumor cells and contamination of the resection cavity are to be avoided. Prognosis also depends on age. Children younger than three years old tend to have more aggressive ependymomas and poor prognosis (38). In some series, the five-year survival of adult patients with supratentorial ependymomas approached 100% (39).

Molecular abnormalities leading to the development of ependymomas are poorly understood. Tumors in patients with NF2 have a higher incidence of ependymomas, and a genetic linkage to chromosome 22q12 was detected. A recent study revealed multiple alterations in the 4.1 family of proteins, including merlin, in a wide range of ependymomas (40).

Myxopapillary ependymoma is a distinct variant most commonly originating from the filum terminale of the spinal cord. It is characterized histologically by a distinct papillary growth and layered architecture. Within the center of each papilla, one finds a hyalinized blood vessel, which is surrounded by hyaluronic acid-rich spaces, which are in turn collared by perivascular arrangements of a single layer of ependymal cells. The tumor carries an excellent prognosis, but relapses occur after incomplete resection.

Subependymoma is a highly fibrillary ependymoma, typically protruding into a ventricle. Morphologically, the tumor is characterized by clustering of small nuclei, abundant microcysts, and dense fibrillary matrix with occasional RF and calcifications. Tumors have very low proliferative potential, are often amenable to gross total resection, and recur only years after incomplete removal.

Astroblastoma is a well-circumscribed, generally noninfiltrative glioma with a generic relationship to ependymomas. The cellular processes directed toward blood vessels are shorter than in ependymomas, and the vessel walls are frequently hyalinized. Grading of astroblastomas is controversial but relies on the presence of brisk mitotic activity (over 5 mitoses/10 HPF), endothelial proliferation, and necrosis (41). The proliferative index in well-differentiated astroblastomas ranges from 1% to 8%, whereas Ki-67 in the group of "malignant" astroblastomas varies between 6% and 22%. Similar to ependymomas, survival appears to be related to both malignant morphology and the extent of surgical resection.

One more recently described tumor of periventricular location and ependymal differentiation is *chordoid glioma of the third ventricle* (42). This sharply delineated, contrast-enhancing tumor is located within the third ventricle. The morphology is characterized by clustered epithelioid cells, strongly positive for GFAP, embedded in mucinous stroma, and associated with lymphoplasmacytic infiltrates. Despite of the lack of mitotic activity, the tumor's location often precludes complete resection resulting in recurrences and death of disease in a significant number of cases (43).

Neuronal tumors are discussed in detail in Chapter 13.

Choroid Plexus Tumors

Choroid plexus tumors include papilloma and carcinoma. *Choroid plexus papilloma* (CPP) is a benign proliferation of the epithelial lining of the choroid plexus. The majority of CPPs are located within the lateral ventricles (50%) and the fourth ventricle (40%); only a minor fraction involves the third ventricle (5%). The vast majority of the tumors in lateral ventricles occurs during the first decade of life, whereas the age distribution of CPP in the fourth ventricle is more even. Clinical presentation is related to obstruction of CSF flow and overproduction of CSF by the tumor. Tumors are discrete and contrast enhancing, and can be calcified. Morphology discloses a cauliflower-like growth of papillary fronds, lined by cuboidal to columnar epithelium. The apical surfaces of the tumor cells lose the typical tombstone appearance of the normal choroid plexus and appear flattened. Various "metaplastic" changes such as foci of melanocytic, osseous, cartilaginous, or oncocytic differentiation can be seen. No mitoses, necrosis, or brain invasion are detected. The tumor cells express cytokeratin, GFAP, S100, and transthyretin. Ki-67 index averages approximately 2%. One-, five-, and 10-year survival rates for CPP are 90%, 81%, and 77%, respectively.

Choroid plexus carcinomas (CPC) are rare with a CPP:CPC ratio of 5:1 and tend to affect patients during the first three years of life. CPC show fusion of papillae and loss of normal architecture, obvious cytologic atypia, numerous mitoses, necrosis, and brain invasion. The proliferative index exceeds 10% and survival rates drop from 71% at 1 year to 41% at 5 and 35% at 10 years (44).

Pineal Parenchymal Tumors

Pineal region tumors represent a large variety of neoplasms including germ cell tumors, pineal parenchymal tumors, tumors of meninges, gliomas, ependymomas, and papillary neuroectodermal tumor of the pineal region.

Pineal parenchymal tumors are divided into pineoblastoma, pineocytoma, pineal parenchymal tumor of intermediate differentiation, and mixed pineoblastoma and pineocytoma. *Pineoblastoma* is a highly aggressive small blue cell tumor of children with a tendency to dissemination along CSF pathways and distal metastasis, and an association with the retinoblastoma cancer predisposition syndrome. Neuronal differentiation is recognized by formation of Homer-Wright rosettes. Flexner-Wintersteiner rosettes, fleurettes, and expression of retinal S-antigen indicate retinal differentiation. Five-year survival with modern treatment exceeds 50% (45). *Pineocytoma* is a slow-growing neuronal neoplasm in young adults. It presents with aqueductal obstruction and is contrast enhancing. Morphologic examination reveals a lobular pattern of mitotically inactive, synaptophysin-positive neurocytes forming large irregularly shaped zones of nuclei-free neuropil, called pineocytomatous rosettes. Prognosis is excellent. *Mixed pineal parenchymal tumors* contain foci of pineoblastoma and are more aggressive than *tumors of intermediate differentiation* (46).

A recently described entity of *papillary neuroectodermal tumor of the pineal region* is a rare neoplasm of adults with characteristic papillary morphology, expression pattern of cytokeratin, transthyretin, and neural cell adhesion molecule (NCAM). No GFAP staining is detected, but the tumor shows a distinct ependymal ultrastructure and is hypothesized to originate from the subcommissural organ (47).

Embryonal Tumors

Embryonal tumors include medulloblastoma (MB), ependymoblastoma, medulloepithelioma, supratentorial primitive neuroectodermal tumor (PNET), and atypical teratoid/rhabdoid tumor (AT/RT).

Medulloblastoma (MB) is the most common form of embryonal tumor and is by definition a tumor of the cerebellum. The peak incidence is seven years with male predominance. Clinical presentation is dominated by cerebellar signs and consequences of CSF flow obstruction. Pediatric tumors tend to involve the vermis, while tumors in young adults are hemispheric. Imaging shows a contrast-enhancing mass with frequent seeding of leptomeninges. Several variants are discerned, including "undifferentiated or classic," nodular or desmoplastic, MB with extensive nodularity and advanced neuronal differentiation and large cell MB. The classic variant is characterized by a patternless growth of small blue cells with no obvious neuronal differentiation. Desmoplastic MB shows pale islands of cells with neurocytic, slightly enlarged nuclei within a synaptophysin-positive neuropil, separated by reticulin-rich areas of densely packed small blue cells without differentiation. This pattern appears inverted in MB with extensive nodularity and advanced neuronal differentiation, a variant carrying a better prognosis (48). Rarely, MB shows glial and myoid differentiation. A recent attempt to grade MBs disclosed a prognostic significance of what was previously considered a large cell variant. The current approach is to identify anaplastic features such as nuclear enlargement (over twice that of red blood cells), hyperchromasia, wrapping, and numerous mitoses. About a quarter of MB demonstrates such features that carry an adverse prognosis (49).

Prognosis of MB is improving with current modalities of treatment. The pathogenesis of MB is uncertain. The most common cytogenetic abnormality is isochromosome 17q. There is an indication that the desmoplastic variant might have an origin from the external granular cell layer of the cerebellum, a transient structure, populated by migrating neuroblasts, whereas the classic variant is derived from neuroblasts of subependymal origin. On the molecular level, it is known that disruption of the *hedgenog/ patched* and *APC/Wnt* signaling pathways can result in medulloblastoma.

Medulloepithelioma is a rare embryonal neoplasm morphologically mimicking neural tube with a characteristic multilayered arrangement of tumor cells to form hollow tubes. Mitoses are predominantly seen within the luminal aspect. The outer surface is surrounded by a basal lamina. The tumors are bulky, rapidly growing, and aggressive.

Ependymoblastoma is an embryonal tumor of childhood, morphologically characterized by rosette-like arrangements of cells with ependymal differentiation. Lumina contain abortive cilia, and in contrast to medulloepithelioma, no deposition of basal lamina is seen. This tumor is also aggressive.

Supratentorial PNET is an embryonal neoplasm with divergent neuronal, ependymal, astrocytic, muscular, or melanotic differentiation. Its cytogenetic properties are distinct from MB and peripheral PNET.

AT/RT is a neoplasm, predominantly affecting newborns, usually involving the cerebellum and morphologically characterized by jumbled areas of nondescript small cell, epithelial, or mesenchymal morphology. Rhabdoid cells with large vesicular nuclei, prominent nucleoli, and brightly eosinophilic paranuclear round inclusion are best appreciated on frozen sections, but can be inconspicuous on permanent preparations. Coexpression of EMA and smooth muscle actin is typical to this neoplasm. The tumors are part of the rhabdoid predisposition syndrome and related to loss of both copies of INI1, a tumor suppressor gene on 22q11.2. FISH studies for LOH and immunohistochemical examination for loss of nuclear expression of the protein using BAF47 antibodies have become routine in the diagnosis. Prognosis of patients with AT/RT is dismal.

TUMORS OF THE MENINGES

Meningiomas represent the most common meningeal tumor. A multitude of other meningeal lesions is described, which includes hemangiopericytoma, solitary fibrous tumor (SFT), various sarcomas (chondrosarcoma, osteosarcoma, leiomyosarcoma, rhabdomyosarcoma, malignant fibrous histiocytoma, and angiosarcoma) and their benign counterparts, and epithelioid hemangioendothelioma, as well as primary melanocytic tumors of meninges (melanocytoma and melanoma).

Tumors of Meningothelial Cells

Meningiomas

Meningiomas are tumors of meningothelial differentiation, most commonly seen in middle-age adults with a predilection for women. They represent 15% to 25% of intracranial tumors and are associated with neurofibromatosis type II. Meningiomas have a tendency to send tongues of tissue into the meninges and appear multicentric. Recurrences are common. About 5% to 7% of meningiomas show atypical histology and about 2% of meningiomas are anaplastic. Clinical presentation relates to mass effect of the tumor on underlying brain or nerves. Imaging discloses contrast-enhancing mass with a characteristic "dural tail." Calcifications can be detected. Intraventricular location is not uncommon. Morphologic examination focuses on typical features of meningothelial cells: formation of whorls and psammoma bodies. These are virtually pathognomonic for meningiomas. Several histologic variants are discerned, some of which are of prognostic relevance. The majority of histologic variants typically follow a benign course. These include meningotheliomatous, fibrous, transitional, psammomatous, angiomatous, microcystic, lymphoplasmacyte-rich, secretory, oncocytic, and metaplastic variants. Rhabdoid and papillary morphologies are uncommon and herald WHO Grade III anaplastic tumors. Clear cells and chordoid morphologies indicate WHO Grade II biology. Several histologic features have an independent association with more aggressive behavior. Combination of these permits identification of atypical WHO Grade II and anaplastic WHO Grade III tumors. Atypical meningiomas show more than 4 mitoses/10 HPF and also three or more of the following features: prominent nucleoli, increased cellularity with nuclear sheeting, small cells with high nuclear/cytoplasmic ratio, and foci of necrosis. Anaplastic tumors display severe cytologic atypia and over 20 mitoses/10 HPF (50). Brain invasion, defined by an infiltration of narrow irregular tongues of tumors cell directly into the brain parenchyma and eliciting reactive gliosis, indicates a high likelihood of early recurrence. Ki-67 index corresponds to tumor grade averaging 3.8% for WHO Grade I, 7.2% for WHO Grade II, and 14.7% for WHO Grade III tumors (51). Immunohistochemically, the vast majority of tumors are at least focally positive for EMA and may show S100 staining. Pathogenesis of meningiomas is multifactorial (52,53) and involves abnormalities in merlin, the related protein *DAL-1*, chromosomal losses on 1p, 9p, 10q, and 14q and amplification of 17q. A history of irradiation predisposes to development of meningiomas with a latency of 20 to 40 years for children and shorter periods for adults.

Mesenchymal, Nonmeningothelial Tumors

Hemangiopericytoma is an aggressive meningeal neoplasm, predominantly involving middle-aged men. Clinical presentation, imaging, and gross appearance resemble that of meningioma. Morphologic features include dense cellularity, chaotic orientation of small angulated nuclei, "staghorn-like" vasculature, and scattered mitoses. Tumor cells are enmeshed by reticulin fibers and are variably positive for CD34. The tumor is considered to be a low-grade sarcoma with 5-, 10-, and 15-year survival rates of 67%, 40%, and 23%, respectively (54).

SFT of meninges is a recently defined entity, which has to be differentiated from hemangiopericytoma. Clinical presentation and imaging of SFT is similar to meningiomas. Morphology is rather nondescript and is characterized by intersecting fascicles of predominantly elongated cells often depositing prominent bundles of collagen. Immunohistochemical stains for CD34 and EMA are useful in the differential diagnosis (55). Biology of the tumor is poorly defined, but appears to be more favorable than that of hemangiopericytoma.

Primary Melanocytic Lesions

Leptomeningeal melanocytes give rise to primary *melanocytoma* and *melanoma* of the CNS. The tumors are predominantly found in the posterior fossa and spinal canal, and affect all ages with a predilection for males. Imaging discloses T1-hyperintense and T2-hypointense, enhancing lesion. Typical morphology is characterized by nested or spindle cell arrangements of focally pigmented cells, strongly expressing S100 and other melanocytic markers such as MelanA and HMB45. Presence of prominent nucleoli, numerous mitoses, and necrosis indicate malignant properties (primary melanoma). Ki-67 index ranges from 0% to 2% for melanocytoma and 2% to 15% for melanoma (56).

Tumors of Uncertain Histogenesis

Hemangioblastomas are richly vascularized tumors of unknown histogenesis intimately associated with leptomeninges. They are frequently seen in the patients with von Hippel-Lindau syndrome. One of the favorite locations is the cerebellar hemisphere, with clinical presentation related to CSF flow occlusion and cerebellar dysfunction. Tumor cells secrete erythropoietin. Imaging shows a cystic mass with an enhancing mural nodule. The tumor is composed of irregular clusters of foamy stromal cells embedded in a network of ectatic vessels. Stromal cells are the only tumor cell population and their histogenesis is uncertain. They contain neutral lipid, which can be visualized on frozen sections with Oil-Red-O stain. A large fraction of tumors are strongly positive with neuron-specific enolase inhibin. The tumors are benign, but can be multifocal.

TUMORS OF THE SELLAR REGION

Craniopharyngioma is a benign epithelial tumor of the suprasellar region, presumably derived from the lining of Rathke's pouch. Two distinct varieties are discerned: adamantinomatous and papillary. Adamantinomatous craniopharyngioma (AC) is a tumor of childhood, with a peak incidence between 5 and 15 years, accounting for 10% of pediatric and 3% of all intracranial tumors (57). The lesions are often bulky, cystic, and frequently calcified and are detected by pituitary deficiencies and visual problems. Magnetic resonance imaging (MRI) shows contrast-enhancing lesions with cystic component, relatively smooth contour, and minimal perilesional edema. Intraoperatively, the cysts contain brown, machine oil–like content with discernable cholesterol flakes. Microscopy is of interconnected lichen-like growths of epithelial islands lined by a picket-fence palisading arrangement of tall columnar cells encircling looser areas, referred to as stellate reticulum, with incrustations of anuclear mulberry-like morules of "wet" keratin. Calcification and ossification of the keratin nodules can be seen, reminiscent of pilomatrixoma, a benign skin tumor with similar molecular pathogenesis. The epithelial cells of stellate areas are dishesive, conferring an edematous appearance on such foci. True cysts with necrotic debris, cholesterol crystal clefts, and foreign body giant cells are frequent. The tumor is intimately associated with brain and elicits intense reactive gliosis, rich in RF. Papillary craniopharyngioma (PC) is a tumor of adults, which is histologically characterized by a solid growth of poorly polarized squamous epithelium, supported by fibrovascular stroma. No cholesterol-rich cystic fluid is present. Peripheral palisading, stellate reticulum, and wet keratin nodules are not seen. These two variants of craniopharyngioma also have very distinct molecular pathogenesis. AC almost invariably harbor mutations in β-catenin gene, which renders the protein inaccessible to phosphorylation-dependent degradation, induces accumulation of the protein, its translocation from the plasma membrane to the nucleus followed by the activation of the Wnt pathway (58). Much less is currently known about the molecular events leading to PC, but no abnormalities in the Wnt pathway have been detected to date.

GERM CELL TUMORS

Germ cell neoplasms are rare, except for Far East countries. Their location is equally split between the pineal gland and suprasellar area. The germ cell tumors of the pineal region have a distinct male predilection of 9:1, which is in contrast to approximately equal sex distribution in the suprasellar region. Most tumors manifest during the second decade of life. Several histologic variants are discerned including germinoma, choriocarcinoma, yolk sac tumor, embryonal carcinoma, mature, and immature teratoma. Germinoma is composed of lobules of large cells with centrally located vesicular nuclei and prominent nucleoli, surrounded by fragile glycogen-rich cytoplasm. Lymphocytic infiltrates are conspicuous. Occasional granulomas or syncytiotrophoblastic giant cells are seen. The tumors are positive for placental alkaline phosphatase. Yolk sac tumor has a characteristic loose myxoid background with embedded ribbons of germ cells. α-fetoprotein–positive hyaline globules are conspicuous and Schiller-Duval bodies can be found. Embryonal carcinoma is composed of larger clusters of CD30-positive germ cells. Choriocarcinoma features syncytiotrophoblast and cytotrophoblast and is immunoreactive for human chorionic gonadotrophin (β-HCG). α-fetoprotein and β-HCG are useful markers of tumor recurrence. Mature teratoma contains fully differentiated elements, whereas immature teratoma contains components resembling fetal tissue, such as neural tube. Teratoma with malignant transformation shows foci of aggressive malignancy within its teratomatous background. These include sarcomas, squamous, and adenocarcinomas.

Association of germ cell tumors with Klinefelter syndrome prompted molecular analysis for genetic status of X chromosome, which indeed revealed an extra copy of hypomethylated X chromosome in the vast majority of cases (59). In contrast, isochromosome 12p, which is a common finding in gonadal germ cell tumors, was relatively rare. The majority of germinomas express c-kit and up to 25% of them show c-kit mutations (60). Rising titers of the shed ligand–binding domain of c-kit in the CSF indicate recurrence (61). Prognosis of germ cell neoplasms has markedly improved in recent years due to aggressive chemo- and radiotherapy. Germinomas and mature teratomas can be cured while most patients with nongerminomatous germ cell tumors including malignant teratomas succumb to their disease (62).

TUMORS OF THE HEMATOPOIETIC AND LYMPHOID SYSTEM

Primary CNS lymphoma (PCNSL) is defined as involvement by the tumor of the CNS with no history of lymphoma outside of the nervous system. Typical PCNSL involves white matter, whereas the metastatic lymphoma presents as leptomeningeal disease (leptomeningeal lymphomatosis). However, PCNSL can also expand to leptomeninges.

PCNSL predominantly involves immunocompromised patients, in particular, AIDS patients, but can also affect the immunocompetent population, particularly the elderly. Posttransplant lymphoproliferative disorder involving CNS eventually progresses to full-blown lymphoma, which is generally similar to that seen in AIDS patients (63). The disease is usually multifocal with the larger lesions in the supratentorial white matter. Up to a quarter of the patients shows ocular disease. MRI reveals T1-hyper- or isodense lesions with or without enhancement and tends to underestimate the extent of the involvement (64). Lesions in AIDS patients are often necrotizing and rim enhancing. Butterfly-like involvement of the corpus callosum and subependymal spread are characteristic. Peritumoral edema is modest and disproportional to the size of the lesion. At the extreme of the spectrum of PCNSL is a widely infiltrative disease with no distinct tumor mass, which can present as a white matter dementia and is named lymphomatosis cerebri (65). Extension of the tumor to either leptomeninges or ventricles provides for detection of malignant cells in CSF. The vast majority of PCNSL cases represents diffuse large B-cell lymphoma (DLBCL), although other variants are also described. Molecular studies of tumor cells in CSF therefore include studies of immunoglobulin heavy chain gene rearrangement to detect clonality (66). Morphologic analysis of brain biopsy shows characteristic multifocal angiocentric accumulation of pleomorphic large cells with vesicular nuclei and prominent nucleoli. The tumor cells invade and expand blood vessels, but also spill over to neuropil. A variably prominent accompaniment of small reactive T-lymphocytes and macrophages is also seen. Tumor cells of DLBCL are positive for B-cell markers CD20 and CD19. Their clonality can also be confirmed by detection of λ- or κ-light chain restriction. Pathogenesis of PCNSL is unknown and appears to differ between immunocompromised and immunocompetent patients. Virtually all AIDS-related PCNSL show incorporation of genetic material from Epstein-Barr virus (67), whereas this is rare in immunocompetent hosts (68). Continuous antigenic stimulation by an as yet unknown pathogen is speculated to be involved in the pathogenesis of PCNSL. *Toxoplasma gondii* is a common parasite with a high prevalence of persistence of the pathogen in CNS. Isolated reports detected DNA of *T. gondii* or of JC virus in tumor cells of immunocompetent hosts, but their causative role remains undetermined (69,70). T-cell lymphomas constitute only a small fraction of PCNSL ranging from 2.4% to 8.5%. Diagnosis of T-cell lymphomas relies on cytologic atypia of the constituent cells, presence of which helps to differentiate lymphoma from CNS vasculitis (71). Molecular studies, in particular T cell receptor rearrangements are becoming indispensable diagnostic tools (72). A systemic disease, an *intravascular (angiotropic) lymphoma* clinically manifests as CNS dysfunction in 30% of the patients and is related to occlusion of small blood vessels by the tumor cells resulting in ischemia and infarction (73).

Acute myeloid leukemia rarely involves the CNS. However, occasionally dura-based mass lesions (*granulocytic sarcoma* or chloroma) are formed in the setting of or prior to manifestation of systemic leukemia. The name "chloroma" stems from a green tinge of freshly cut tumor related to myeloperoxidase of tumor cells. The deposits have a predilection for subperiosteum, in particular of sinuses and orbit. Three morphologic variants are described: blastic, immature, and differentiated. Presence of mature eosinophils, neutrophils, and immunoreactivity for CD45, CD68, and myeloperoxidase helps to differentiate them from lymphomas or other malignancies.

REFERENCES

1. Kleihues P, Louis DN, Scheithauer BW, et al. The WHO classification of tumors of the nervous system. J Neuropathol Exp Neurol 2002; 61:215–225.
2. Schramm J, Luyken C, Urbach H, Fimmers R, Blumcke I. Evidence for a clinically distinct new subtype of grade II astrocytomas in patients with long-term epilepsy. Neurosurgery 2004; 55:340–347.
3. Coons SW, Johnson PC, Scheithauer BW, Yates AJ, Pearl DK. Improving diagnostic accuracy and interobserver concordance in the classification and grading of primary gliomas. Cancer 1997; 79:1381–1393.
4. Bannykh SI, Stolt CC, Kim J, Perry A, Wegner M. Oligodendroglial-specific transcriptional factor SOX10 is ubiquitously expressed in human gliomas. J Neurooncol 2006; 76(2):115–127.
5. Daumas-Duport C, Scheithauer B, O'Fallon J, Kelly P. Grading of astrocytomas. A simple and reproducible method. Cancer 1988; 62:2152–2165.
6. Ho DM, Wong TT, Hsu CY, Ting LT, Chiang H. MIB-1 labeling index in nonpilocytic astrocytoma of childhood: a study of 101 cases. Cancer 1998; 82:2459–2466.

7. Peraud A, Watanabe K, Schwechheimer K, Yonekawa Y, Kleihues P, Ohgaki H. Genetic profile of the giant cell glioblastoma. Lab Invest 1999; 79:123–129.
8. Brat DJ, Scheithauer BW, Medina-Flores R, Rosenblum MK, Burger PC. Infiltrative astrocytomas with granular cell features (granular cell astrocytomas): a study of histopathologic features, grading, and outcome. Am J Surg Pathol 2002; 26:750–757.
9. Castellano-Sanchez AA, Ohgaki H, Yokoo H, et al. Granular cell astrocytomas show a high frequency of allelic loss but are not a genetically defined subset. Brain Pathol 2003; 13:185–194.
10. Hecht BK, Turc-Carel C, Chatel M, et al. Chromosomes in gliomatosis cerebri. Genes Chromosomes Cancer 1995; 14:149–153.
11. Okamoto Y, Di Patre PL, Burkhard C, et al. Population-based study on incidence, survival rates, and genetic alterations of low-grade diffuse astrocytomas and oligodendrogliomas. Acta Neuropathol (Berl) 2004; 108:49–56.
12. Cowell JK, Barnett GH, Nowak NJ. Characterization of the 1p/19q chromosomal loss in oligodendrogliomas using comparative genomic hybridization arrays (CGHa). J Neuropathol Exp Neurol 2004; 63:151–158.
13. Kelley TW, Tubbs RR, Prayson RA. Molecular diagnostic techniques for the clinical evaluation of gliomas. Diagn Mol Pathol 2005; 14:1–8.
14. Perry A, Fuller CE, Banerjee R, Brat DJ, Scheithauer BW. Ancillary FISH analysis for 1p and 19q status: preliminary observations in 287 gliomas and oligodendroglioma mimics. Front Biosci 2003; 8:a1–a9.
15. Kleihues P, Cavenee WK. Pathology and genetics of tumours of the nervous system. Lyon: IARC Press, 2000:314.
16. Amatya VJ, Naumann U, Weller M, Ohgaki H. TP53 promoter methylation in human gliomas. Acta Neuropathol (Berl) 2005; 110:178–184.
17. Finlay CA, Hinds PW, Tan TH, Eliyahu D, Oren M, Levine AJ. Activating mutations for transformation by p53 produce a gene product that forms an hsc70-p53 complex with an altered half-life. Mol Cell Biol 1988; 8:531–539.
18. Pollack IF, Finkelstein SD, Woods J, et al. Expression of p53 and prognosis in children with malignant gliomas. N Engl J Med 2002; 346:420–427.
19. Lang FF, Miller DC, Pisharody S, Koslow M, Newcomb EW. High frequency of p53 protein accumulation without p53 gene mutation in human juvenile pilocytic, low grade and anaplastic astrocytomas. Oncogene 1994; 9:949–954.
20. Burger PC, Minn AY, Smith JS, et al. Losses of chromosomal arms 1p and 19q in the diagnosis of oligodendroglioma. A study of paraffin-embedded sections. Mod Pathol 2001; 14:842–853.
21. Ino Y, Betensky RA, Zlatescu MC, et al. Molecular subtypes of anaplastic oligodendroglioma: implications for patient management at diagnosis. Clin Cancer Res 2001; 7:839–845.
22. Fisher PG, Breiter SN, Carson BS, et al. A clinicopathologic reappraisal of brain stem tumor classification. Identification of pilocystic astrocytoma and fibrillary astrocytoma as distinct entities. Cancer 2000; 89:1569–1576.
23. Giannini C, Scheithauer BW, Burger PC, et al. Cellular proliferation in pilocytic and diffuse astrocytomas. J Neuropathol Exp Neurol 1999; 58:46–53.

24. Haapasalo H, Sallinen S, Sallinen P, et al. Clinicopathological correlation of cell proliferation, apoptosis and p53 in cerebellar pilocytic astrocytomas. Neuropathol Appl Neurobiol 1999; 25:134–142.
25. Listernick R, Louis DN, Packer RJ, Gutmann DH. Optic pathway gliomas in children with neurofibromatosis 1: consensus statement from the NF1 Optic Pathway Glioma Task Force. Ann Neurol 1997; 41:143–149.
26. Wimmer K, Eckart M, Meyer-Puttlitz B, Fonatsch C, Pietsch T. Mutational and expression analysis of the NF1 gene argues against a role as tumor suppressor in sporadic pilocytic astrocytomas. J Neuropathol Exp Neurol 2002; 61:896–902.
27. Abdollahzadeh M, Hoffman HJ, Blazer SI, et al. Benign cerebellar astrocytoma in childhood: experience at the Hospital for Sick Children 1980–1992. Childs Nerv Syst 1994; 10:380–383.
28. Tihan T, Fisher PG, Kepner JL, et al. Pediatric astrocytomas with monomorphous pilomyxoid features and a less favorable outcome. J Neuropathol Exp Neurol 1999; 58:1061–1068.
29. Komotar RJ, Burger PC, Carson BS, et al. Pilocytic and pilomyxoid hypothalamic/chiasmatic astrocytomas. Neurosurgery 2004; 54:72–79; discussion 79–80.
30. Kepes JJ, Rubinstein LJ, Eng LF. Pleomorphic xanthoastrocytoma: a distinctive meningocerebral glioma of young subjects with relatively favorable prognosis. A study of 12 cases. Cancer 1979; 44:1839–1852.
31. Powell SZ, Yachnis AT, Rorke LB, Rojiani AM, Eskin TA. Divergent differentiation in pleomorphic xanthoastrocytoma. Evidence for a neuronal element and possible relationship to ganglion cell tumors. Am J Surg Pathol 1996; 20:80–85.
32. Giannini C, Scheithauer BW, Burger PC, et al. Pleomorphic xanthoastrocytoma: what do we really know about it? Cancer 1999; 85:2033–2045.
33. Zamecnik J, Snuderl M, Eckschlager T, et al. Pediatric intracranial ependymomas: prognostic relevance of histological, immunohistochemical, and flow cytometric factors. Mod Pathol 2003; 16:980–991.
34. Hamilton RL, Pollack IF. The molecular biology of ependymomas. Brain Pathol 1997; 7:807–822.
35. Rushing EJ, Brown DF, Hladik CL, Risser RC, Mickey BE, White CL III. Correlation of bcl-2, p53, and MIB-1 expression with ependymoma grade and subtype. Mod Pathol 1998; 11:464–470.
36. Rickert CH, Paulus W. Prognosis-related histomorphological and immunohistochemical markers in central nervous system tumors of childhood and adolescence. Acta Neuropathol (Berl) 2005; 109:69–92.
37. Pollack IF, Gerszten PC, Martinez AJ, et al. Intracranial ependymomas of childhood: long-term outcome and prognostic factors. Neurosurgery 1995; 37:655–666.
38. Horn B, Heideman R, Geyer R, et al. A multi-institutional retrospective study of intracranial ependymoma in children: identification of risk factors. J Pediatr Hematol Oncol 1999; 21:203–211.
39. Schwartz TH, Kim S, Glick RS, et al. Supratentorial ependymomas in adult patients. Neurosurgery 1999; 44:721–731.
40. Rajaram V, Gutmann DH, Prasad SK, Mansur DB, Perry A. Alterations of protein 4.1 family members in ependymomas: a study of 84 cases. Mod Pathol 2005; 18:991–997.

41. Brat DJ, Hirose Y, Cohen KJ, Feuerstein BG, Burger PC. Astroblastoma: clinicopathologic features and chromosomal abnormalities defined by comparative genomic hybridization. Brain Pathol 2000; 10:342–352.
42. Brat DJ, Scheithauer BW, Staugaitis SM, Cortez SC, Brecher K, Burger PC. Third ventricular chordoid glioma: a distinct clinicopathologic entity. J Neuropathol Exp Neurol 1998; 57:283–290.
43. Pasquier B, Peoc'h M, Morrison AL, et al. Chordoid glioma of the third ventricle: a report of two new cases, with further evidence supporting an ependymal differentiation, and review of the literature. Am J Surg Pathol 2002; 26:1330–1342.
44. Vajtai I, Varga Z, Aguzzi A. MIB-1 immunoreactivity reveals different labelling in low-grade and in malignant epithelial neoplasms of the choroid plexus. Histopathology 1996; 29:147–151.
45. Schild SE, Scheithauer BW, Schomberg PJ, et al. Pineal parenchymal tumors. Clinical, pathologic, and therapeutic aspects. Cancer 1993; 72:870–880.
46. Jouvet A, Saint-Pierre G, Fauchon F, et al. Pineal parenchymal tumors: a correlation of histological features with prognosis in 66 cases. Brain Pathol 2000; 10:49–60.
47. Jouvet A, Fauchon F, Liberski P, et al. Papillary tumor of the pineal region. Am J Surg Pathol 2003; 27:505–512.
48. Giangaspero F, Perilongo G, Fondelli MP, et al. Medulloblastoma with extensive nodularity: a variant with favorable prognosis. J Neurosurg 1999; 91:971–977.
49. Eberhart CG, Kepner JL, Goldthwaite PT, et al. Histopathologic grading of medulloblastomas: a Pediatric Oncology Group study. Cancer 2002; 94: 552–560.
50. Perry A, Scheithauer BW, Stafford SL, Lohse CM, Wollan PC. "Malignancy" in meningiomas: a clinicopathologic study of 116 patients, with grading implications. Cancer 1999; 85:2046–2056.
51. Maier H, Wanschitz J, Sedivy R, Rossler K, Ofner D, Budka H. Proliferation and DNA fragmentation in meningioma subtypes. Neuropathol Appl Neurobiol 1997; 23:496–506.
52. Lamszus K. Meningioma pathology, genetics, and biology. J Neuropathol Exp Neurol 2004; 63:275–286.
53. Perry A, Gutmann DH, Reifenberger G. Molecular pathogenesis of meningiomas. J Neurooncol 2004; 70:183–202.
54. Guthrie BL, Ebersold MJ, Scheithauer BW, Shaw EG. Meningeal hemangiopericytoma: histopathological features, treatment, and long-term follow-up of 44 cases. Neurosurgery 1989; 25:514–522.
55. Perry A, Scheithauer BW, Nascimento AG. The immunophenotypic spectrum of meningeal hemangiopericytoma: a comparison with fibrous meningioma and solitary fibrous tumor of meninges. Am J Surg Pathol 1997; 21:1354–1360.
56. Brat DJ, Giannini C, Scheithauer BW, Burger PC. Primary melanocytic neoplasms of the central nervous systems. Am J Surg Pathol 1999; 23:745–754.
57. Adamson TE, Wiestler OD, Kleihues P, Yasargil MG. Correlation of clinical and pathological features in surgically treated craniopharyngiomas. J Neurosurg 1990; 73:12–17.
58. Sekine S, Shibata T, Kokubu A, et al. Craniopharyngiomas of adamantinomatous type harbor beta-catenin gene mutations. Am J Pathol 2002; 161:1997–2001.

59. Okada Y, Nishikawa R, Matsutani M, Louis DN. Hypomethylated X chromosome gain and rare isochromosome 12p in diverse intracranial germ cell tumors. J Neuropathol Exp Neurol 2002; 61:531–538.

60. Sakuma Y, Sakurai S, Oguni S, Satoh M, Hironaka M, Saito K. c-kit gene mutations in intracranial germinomas. Cancer Sci 2004; 95:716–720.

61. Miyanohara O, Takeshima H, Kaji M, et al. Diagnostic significance of soluble c-kit in the cerebrospinal fluid of patients with germ cell tumors. J Neurosurg 2002; 97:177–183.

62. Dearnaley DP, A'Hern RP, Whittaker S, Bloom HJ. Pineal and CNS germ cell tumors: Royal Marsden Hospital experience 1962–1987. Int J Radiat Oncol Biol Phys 1990; 18:773–781.

63. Castellano-Sanchez AA, Li S, Qian J, Lagoo A, Weir E, Brat DJ. Primary central nervous system posttransplant lymphoproliferative disorders. Am J Clin Pathol 2004; 121:246–253.

64. Lai R, Rosenblum MK, DeAngelis LM. Primary CNS lymphoma: a whole-brain disease? Neurology 2002; 59:1557–1562.

65. Bakshi R, Mazziotta JC, Mischel PS, Jahan R, Seligson DB, Vinters HV. Lymphomatosis cerebri presenting as a rapidly progressive dementia: clinical, neuroimaging and pathologic findings. Dement Geriatr Cogn Disord 1999; 10:152–157.

66. Baehring JM, Hochberg FH, Betensky RA, Longtine J, Sklar J. Immunoglobulin gene rearrangement analysis in cerebrospinal fluid of patients with lymphoproliferative processes. J Neurol Sci 2006; EPub Jun 7.

67. MacMahon EM, Glass JD, Hayward SD, et al. Epstein-Barr virus in AIDS-related primary central nervous system lymphoma. Lancet 1991; 338:969–973.

68. Bashir R, Luka J, Cheloha K, Chamberlain M, Hochberg F. Expression of Epstein-Barr virus proteins in primary CNS lymphoma in AIDS patients. Neurology 1993; 43:2358–2362.

69. Tuaillon N, Chan CC. Molecular analysis of primary central nervous system and primary intraocular lymphomas. Curr Mol Med 2001; 1:259–272.

70. Del Valle L, Pina-Oviedo S. HIV disorders of the brain: pathology and pathogenesis. Front Biosci 2006; 11:718–732.

71. Gijtenbeek JM, Rosenblum MK, DeAngelis LM. Primary central nervous system T-cell lymphoma. Neurology 2001; 57:716–718.

72. Assaf C, Hummel M, Dippel E, et al. High detection rate of T-cell receptor beta chain rearrangements in T-cell lymphoproliferations by family specific polymerase chain reaction in combination with the GeneScan technique and DNA sequencing. Blood 2000; 96:640–646.

73. Glass J, Hochberg FH, Miller DC. Intravascular lymphomatosis. A systemic disease with neurologic manifestations. Cancer 1993; 71(10):3156–3164.

8

Astrocytic Tumors

Martin J. van den Bent

Neuro-Oncologie Unit, Daniel den Hoed Cancer Center/Erasmus University Medical Center, Rotterdam, The Netherlands

INTRODUCTION

Gliomas account for 70% of all primary brain tumors, the vast majority (about 80%) of which are of astrocytic origin. Most astrocytic tumors are so-called diffuse astrocytomas, because of their infiltration of adjacent and distant brain structures, regardless of grade. Diffuse astrocytoma represents a continuum, with a grading dependent on the presence or absence of anaplastic features. According to the World Health Organization (WHO) classification (1), low grade astrocytoma (grade II) is defined as an astrocytic neoplasm, with a high degree of cellular differentiation, slow growth, and diffuse infiltration of neighboring brain. The tumor is considered an anaplastic astrocytoma (or grade III) if focal or dispersed anaplasia is present, with increased cellularity, distinct nuclear atypia and marked mitotic activity. The presence of endothelial proliferation and necrosis is the hallmark of the glioblastoma multiforme (GBM) (grade IV). This tumor, with its median survival of 9 to 12 months makes up 60% to 80% of the diffuse astrocytic tumors.

The current chapter considers the clinical features and treatment of diffuse tumors of astrocytic origin. In addition, it describes pilocytic astrocytoma, pleomorphic xanthoastrocytoma and subependymal giant cell astrocytoma (SEGA) that, although more well circumscribed, are also counted amongst the astrocytic tumors. Gliomatosis cerebri is by definition a diffuse glial tumor infiltrating the brain extensively so as to involve more than two lobes, and often bilaterally or extending infratentorially or into the spinal cord (2). This is basically a neuroimaging diagnosis; histologically these tumors may be either low-grade or high-grade, and either of astrocytic or of oligodendroglial lineage.

General Remarks

The clinical presentation of all brain tumors depends on the localization of the tumor and the rate of growth. Many of the low-grade astrocytoma patients present with seizures only, which may be related to their lower growth rate. In contrast, more malignant astrocytoma often present with focal deficits, cognitive disturbances and increased intracranial pressure. Within the group of diffuse astrocytoma, there is a strong association between tumor grade and age at presentation. Astrocytomas have a peak incidence at the age of 30 to 40 years. Glioblastoma affects primarily an older age category; the median age at presentation is between 50 and 60 years and in one-third of patients it is over 65 to 70 years of age. The peak incidence of anaplastic astrocytoma lies in between that of low-grade astrocytoma patients and that of glioblastoma patients.

Etiology of Astrocytomas

Little is known about the cause of astrocytomas. Most cases of astrocytoma are sporadic, although familial predispositions exist. In some well-described familial cancer syndromes, brain tumors occur, including astrocytic tumors: Li-Fraumeni syndrome (*TP53* germ line mutations), neurofibromatosis type 1 and 2, and Turcot syndrome (*APC* and *hMLH1/hPSM2* germ line mutations). NF1 is in particular related to optic nerve pilocytic astrocytomas, but other astrocytomas may also arise. In NF2 in particular spinal cord ependymomas are observed, but other gliomas do occur as well. Radiotherapy (RT) to the brain in particular at young age, is the only environmental factor unequivocally associated with an increased risk of developing brain tumors including astrocytic tumors (3). SEGA is almost exclusively observed in the tuberous sclerosis syndrome.

Prognosis: General Remarks

The prognosis of astrocytoma is mainly determined by tumor grade. With a median survival of 5 to 10 years, low-grade astrocytoma has the best outcome (4). Large studies reported a median survival in anaplastic astrocytoma or grade III astrocytoma of two to four years, although in some series outcome was much worse (5–7). With a median survival of 9 to 12 months, the outcome of GBM is grim, although recent trials show that for some subsets of patients, outcome may be improved by combined modality treatment (8).

For all glial tumors, age and clinical condition of the patient (as measured by the ECOG performance status or Karnofsky index) are independent prognostic factors. Some of the differences in outcome between the astrocytoma tumor grades are also related to the difference in age, at which these tumors generally arise. For both low-grade astrocytoma and glioblastoma astrocytoma a short bedside evaluation of the mental status of patients, the mini mental status examination (MMSE) has been found to be an independent predictor of survival (9,10).

DIFFUSE ASTROCYTOMA (WHO GRADE II)

Most textbooks on primary brain tumors lump grade II astrocytoma together with the oligoastrocytoma and oligodendroglioma in one chapter on low-grade glioma. The rationale for this is that these tumors pose similar clinical problems [young adults presenting with seizures only, and an unenhancing lesion on magnetic resonance imaging (MRI)], share a better prognosis as compared to their anaplastic counterparts and, perhaps most importantly, guidelines on the treatment of these tumors must be obtained from studies that included all three histologies. Furthermore, the large interobserver variation with respect to the histological diagnosis of these tumors hampers the clinical distinction between them. It is now clear that at least oligodendroglial tumors with combined 1p/19q loss have a markedly better outcome than astrocytoma. Also, most mixed oligoastrocytoma carry either typical oligodendroglial genetic lesions (1p/19q loss) or *TP53* mutations suggestive of an astrocytic lineage. Thus, there is compelling evidence mixed oligoastrocytoma are not true mixed tumors but are either of astrocytic or of oligodendroglial lineage (11). Most likely, in the near future the diagnosis of these tumors will be based on molecular analysis, but this is not yet the case. At present, most new cooperative group trials on low-grade glioma include all three histologies albeit after stratification for 1p and 19q loss. Despite their being named "benign glioma," earlier on low-grade astrocytoma are by no means benign tumors. With two- and five-year survival rates of 80% to 85% and 50% to 55% in large prospective trials, most patients die of recurrent disease, at which time 65% of tumors are transformed into a high-grade tumor (4,10).

Histology

Three histological subtypes of grade II astrocytoma are recognized: fibrillary astrocytoma, gemistocytic astrocytoma, and the rare protoplasmic astrocytoma. This distinction has little clinical relevance, although it is generally assumed that gemistocytic astrocytomas have a more aggressive course than the more common fibrillary astrocytomas (12).

Molecular Biology

Trisomy or polysomy 7 (or 7 q) is frequent in grade II astrocytomas; this is found in up to 50% to 65% of cases and has been correlated with poor survival (13). About 60% of cases have *TP53* mutations, although this figure may be even higher in gemistocytic astrocytoma. The simultaneous overexpression of platelet-derived growth factor receptor (PDGFR) and its ligand PDGF is also frequent, suggestive of the presence of an autocrine loop, in which the tumor cells are expressing both the receptor and its ligand (and the cells are stimulating themselves) (14).

Neuroimaging

On computed tomography (CT) scan, low-grade astrocytomas present as low density lesions with or without mass effect. These lesions can easily be mistaken for ischemic vascular lesions. The lesions are hypointense on T1- and hyperintense on T2-weighted images (Fig. 1). The margins on T2 may be either sharp or somewhat diffuse. Although the area with signal intensity appears rather homogeneous, this is not invariably the case. Most astrocytomas arise supratentorially and do not show enhancement, but exceptions do occur. Nevertheless, if histological examination of an enhancing tumor suggests a grade II astrocytoma, the diagnosis should be doubted. Many clinicians tend to treat these patients as bearing a high-grade tumor especially if the diagnosis was obtained by biopsy and sampling error is likely. The differential diagnosis of the neuroimaging findings includes ischemic lesions and white matter diseases.

(A)   **(B)**   **(C)**

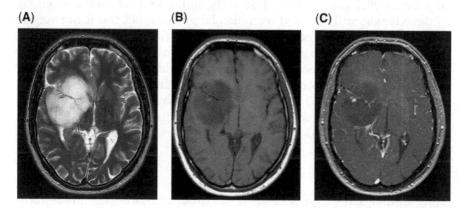

Figure 1   Magnetic resonance imaging of a right temporal low-grade astrocytoma: high signal intensity on T2 imaging (**A**), low signal intensity on T1-weighted imaging (**B**) but no enhancement on T1-weighted imaging after intravenous contrast administration (**C**). The tumor is relatively well demarcated on both T1- and T2-weighted images.

Prognosis

Two large phase III European Organization for Research and Treatment of Cancer (EORTC) studies identified five independent poor prognostic factors in low-grade glioma: astrocytic histology (vs. oligodendroglial or mixed), greater than 6-cm tumor diameter, midline involvement, neurological deficits and age more than 40 years (4). In the presence of three or more factors survival decreased to three to four years while survival was more than seven years in patients with less than three factors present (Table 1 and Fig. 2). A phase III Radiation Therapy Oncology Group (RTOG) study confirmed the prognostic significance of histology, tumor size, and age (10). These factors basically outweigh the influence of treatment on survival in low-grade glioma (15). The usefulness of these factors in current practice is limited, because these studies included oligodendroglial tumors, and the size and extension of tumors were assessed with CT scanning. Their significance should be reassessed using MRI in trials on astrocytic tumors only (or preferably on a set of tumors without 1 p/19 q loss). As for glioblastoma and brain metastases, the MMSE has been identified as a prognostic variable. Enhancement of tumors and extent of resection was identified in some retrospective series as an independent factor, but not in all series (16). A first analysis of a RTOG study on 111 patients under 40 years of age with a low-grade astrocytoma that had undergone a gross total resection failed to find a relation between the time to progression and enhancement (17).

Treatment of Diffuse Astrocytoma

General Remarks

The optimal treatment of low-grade astrocytoma is controversial. First of all, there is a debate on the best treatment in the good-prognosis subset of patients: young patients presenting with seizures only. As such patients may do well for a prolonged period of time without any treatment and many physicians defer diagnostic procedures and treatment as long as possible, whereas others advocate early treatment consisting of an extensive resection with or without adjuvant radiation therapy (18,19). Arguments against early treatment are derived from the observation that many patients remain asymptomatic (apart from the seizures) for a prolonged period of time, and may deteriorate following treatment. Arguments for early treatment are uncertainty as to the diagnosis and potentially improved survival after early treatment. Moreover, even so-called stable untreated low-grade gliomas show a constant tendency to grow over time (on average 4.1 mm per year) (20). This implies that in patients followed with a wait-and-see policy, once treatment is initiated, the tumor will be larger than at the time of initial presentation. RTOG study 9802 has an observation-only arm on the subgroup of young patients (under 40 years of age) who have undergone a

Table 1 Median Survival by Risk-Group Based on the Prognostic Score of EORTC Study 22844 and 22845

Risk group	Score	EORTC 22844, Construction set (N = 281)			EORTC 22845, Validation set (N = 253)		
		O/N	Median survival years (95% CI)	HR (95% CI)	O/N	Median survival years (95% CI)	HR (95% CI)
Low risk	0–2	90/200	7.72 (6.55–9.25)	1	72/195	7.80 (6.77–8.90)	1
High risk	3–5	61/81	3.20 (2.95–3.99)	1.62 (1.38–1.92)	39/58	3.67 (2.89–4.69)	1.83 (1.48–2.26)

Abbreviations: O/N, observed endpoints/total number of patients; HR, hazard ratio; EORTC, European Organization for Research and Treatment of Cancer.
Source: From Ref. 4.

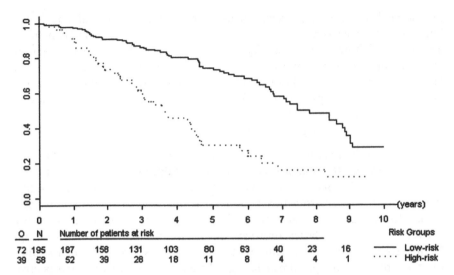

Figure 2 Survival in low-grade glioma depending on three or more ("high risk") versus less than three ("low risk") poor prognostic factors (see also Table 1). *Source*: Adapted from Ref. 4.

gross total resection (17). At first analysis both tumor diameter over 4 cm and astrocytic histology proved to be poor prognostic factors for progression. After two and five years of follow-up 67% and 34% of patients with an astrocytoma larger than 4 cm in diameter were still free from progression, in contrast to 93% and 78% for patients with an oligodendroglioma with a diameter of less than 4 cm. The presence of residual disease following surgery was strongly associated with progression during follow-up. More detailed data are needed for a full interpretation of these results, but they are in line with the observation that many "stable" astrocytomas tend to grow during follow-up.

Apart from this issue, the impact on survival of patients on whom of more extensive resections and of early radiation therapy are matters of debate, and the role of chemotherapy is not defined. With respect to clinical decision making two situations must be distinguished: (i) patients presenting with a presumed LGG, and (ii) patients with histologically proven astrocytoma. For an optimal management of these patients several questions must be considered:

What Is the Reliability of the Neuroradiological Diagnosis "Presumable LGG"? Several series on consecutive patients with unenhancing intra-axial lesions have shown, that 30% to 45% of these patients carry a high-grade glioma—usually an anaplastic astrocytoma (19,21,22). Vice versa, 31% of anaplastic astrocytoma and 4% of GBM were nonenhancing on contrast-enhanced CT scan (23). Proponents of an early intervention in presumed low-grade glioma patients see this as an argument to obtain early histological verification; however the assumption that an early diagnosis will improve outcome has never been proven in clinical trials (19). Timely neuroradiological follow-up will identify those patients with progressive lesions requiring histological diagnosis and treatment. It should be clear though that lack of enhancement couldn't be taken as proof of the low-grade nature of a glioma. Especially in patients over 40 years of age, the histology of the lesion may still be anaplastic. If a wait and see policy is chosen, careful follow-up is required to detect early progression.

What Is the Evidence Available to Decide on the Moment, At Which the Diagnosis Should Be Obtained and Treatment Initiated?   To give at least a clue as to the value of early diagnosis and treatment in low-grade glioma-like lesions, studies addressing this issue should include all patients with presumed low-grade glioma and not be limited to patients with histologically proven tumors as the latter approach does not consider patients with long-lasting stable lesions or patients with anaplastic lesions (24). Such studies on both proven and presumed low-grade glioma are scarce, retrospective and are of small size. One retrospective study compared 26 patients with presumed low-grade glioma patients having presented with seizures only and in whom treatment was deferred to a non-matched group of 20 patients that underwent early surgery. No differences were found between both groups with regard to time to malignant transformation and to overall survival (18). Another study investigated quality of life and cognitive function in 24 patients with suspected low-grade glioma and compared this to 24 matched patients with proven but not irradiated low-grade glioma (25). All patients had presented with seizures and were without focal neurological deficits at the time of testing. Patients with biopsied or resected tumors were found to have a worse quality of life and cognitive status in comparison to patients with suspected LGG. In contrast to these early data, a recent large study on cognitive deficits in low-grade glioma patients using several nonglioma control groups did not find an association between prior RT and cognitive deficits, provided the RT was given in fractions of 2 Gy or less (26). Cognitive deficits were in particular found in patients that had been treated with RT fraction size exceeding 2.0 Gy and in patients on antiepileptic drugs. Whether the latter observation is due to the presence of uncontrolled seizures or due to the use of antiepileptic drugs remains to be established. A randomized trial has shown that early RT improves progression free survival, without affecting overall survival (27). This suggests that with respect to survival, delaying RT does not adversely affect outcome.

Can We Select Patients on Whom Early Diagnosis and Treatment Is Indicated?   It has been assumed that the presence of poor prognostic factors can be used to identify patients that require treatment, especially in older patients or after a limited resection. This assumption has never been validated in prospective series. Given the worse prognosis, the higher risk of malignant transformation, and the possible higher risk of high grade tumors presenting as unenhancing lesions in elderly patients, a more prudent approach in patients over 45 to 50 years of age with presumed or proven LGG is indicated (22,28). However, no strict cut-off level with regard to age can be distilled from the presently available literature.

In contrast, the need to immediately treat patients with focal deficits or raised intracranial pressure is undisputed. The presence of a lesion exerting mass effect or progressing on imaging studies during follow-up also provides an indication for treatment, as this heralds focal deficits or a rise in intracranial pressure. Intractable seizures may also constitute an indication for treatment, as treatment may improve seizure control (27,29–31).

In young patients, with an unenhancing intracerebral lesion, suspected to be a low-grade astrocytoma, without mass effect and without symptoms other than well-controlled seizures, a wait-and-see policy can be followed, provided the patient is carefully monitored. A first follow-up scan should then be obtained within two to three months of the first scan to detect early progression of a high-grade tumor. In those cases that are being followed, histological confirmation can be postponed until the time start of treatment is clinically indicated (e.g., in case of radiological progression, clinical deterioration, uncontrolled seizures).

Options for Diffuse Astrocytoma Treatment

Surgery: There are four theoretical reasons to perform surgery in astrocytoma:

1. Histological confirmation of the nature of the lesion,
2. Improvement of the neurological condition of the patient,
3. To minimize the risk of tumor progression, and
4. To prevent malignant transformation.

The first of these is an obvious one. Small retrospective series suggest that surgery may improve the neurological condition and the control of seizures (24,32). There are no randomized trials though on the significance of the extent of resection in LGG with regard to the survival of the patient. Several large retrospective series identified the extent of resection in multivariate analysis as an important prognostic factor but others were unable to confirm this (4,16,33). Most of these studies however did not evaluate the extent of resection by direct postoperative CT or MR scan. Several studies that quantitated the extent of resection with neuroimaging observed an association between the extent of resection and survival (34,35). The first analysis of the RTOG study 9802 on low-grade glioma confirms this: subtotally resected patients with a residual lesion of more than 2 cm had a higher risk of radiological progression than those with a smaller residual lesion (17). However, at multivariate analysis only preoperative tumor size and histology were significant. Indeed, survival in low-grade glioma is better in smaller tumors, not crossing the midline—a subset of patients who are much more likely to undergo extensive surgery (4,36,37). Thus, one might argue that the improved outcome of more extensively operated tumors is due to patient selection. Nevertheless, in view of the observed improved outcome in some series, it is advisable that once surgery is considered, the resection should be as extensive as safely possible. To obtain this goal, specialized procedures such as craniotomy with the patient kept awake, functional neuroimaging (Fig. 3) and intraoperative MRI evaluation of extent of resection should be considered in patients with tumors in eloquent areas (35,38).

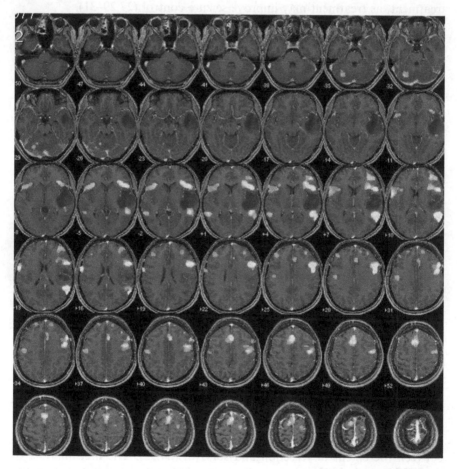

Figure 3 Functional magnetic resonance imaging in a young patient with a presumed low-grade glioma in the left temporal region scheduled for an awake resection. The patient was given verbal tasks. Motor and sensory speech centers are seen as colored areas just frontal and posterior of the tumor. The absence of eloquent areas within the tumor allowed for nearly complete resection.

Radiation Therapy: The efficacy of radiation therapy in low-grade glioma has been demonstrated by a large randomized trial that showed an increase in time to progression after early radiation therapy in comparison to observation (and radiation therapy at the time of progression) (27). Early RT (to a dose of 54 Gy in fractions of 1.8 Gy) improved the median progression-free survival from 3.4 years (95% CI: 2.9, 4.4) to 5.3 years (95% CI: 4.6, 6.3; 1 log rank < 0.0001). However, early radiation therapy did not improve overall survival. As most patients in the observational arm however received RT at the time of recurrence, this points to the effectiveness of salvage RT at progression. The overall picture that emerges from this trial is that the timing of RT is less relevant as long as it is given. The trial did not provide data on "time to neurological deterioration," but at one year, seizures were better controlled in the RT arm. Another prospective trial observed a clear radiological response to radiation therapy in almost one third of patients, and small retrospective surveys have suggested improvement of neurological function or improved seizure control after radiation (10,31,39). Because even after involved field irradiation virtually all recurrences of LGG after radiation therapy occur within the irradiated volume, one might have expected a better local control after a higher dose of irradiation. However, two large randomized multicenter trials totaling 590 patients failed to detect an improved outcome survival after 59, 4 to 64, and 8 Gy as compared to 45 to 50, 4 Gy, using involved fields radiation therapy (10,40). In the high-dose radiation therapy groups, slightly more toxicity was observed and lower levels of quality of life were reported (10,41). Currently it is advised to treat these tumors to a dose of 50 to 54 Gy in fractions of 1.8 Gy.

Chemotherapy: There is only one small ($n = 60$) and prematurely closed phase III trial on adjuvant chemotherapy (with lomustine) after radiation therapy in low-grade glioma (42). The small sample size precludes a meaningful analysis. The results of an RTOG study on adjuvant chemotherapy with procarbazine, lomustine, and vincristine (PCV) after RT are pending. In recent small phase II trials, favorable response rates to temozolomide were also obtained in astrocytic tumors, either at the first diagnosis or at the recurrence (30,43,44). The role of chemotherapy in newly diagnosed low-grade astrocytoma needs further prospective phase III studies; in fact, several trials are ongoing. Until results of these trials are available, chemotherapy in newly diagnosed astrocytoma must be considered experimental. For progressive astrocytoma after RT, chemotherapy is often the only remaining treatment option. Trials have shown a 30% to 60% response rate to temozolomide. This compound would appear to be the drug of choice as other compounds have either not been systematically evaluated or were proved to be inactive.

HIGH-GRADE ASTROCYTOMAS

In any patient in whom a high-grade glioma is presumed, treatment should be initiated without delay. Given the usually aggressive behavior of these tumors, any deferral of the therapy will put the patient at risk of rapid neurological deterioration. In general, on MR or CT scanning, histologically proven diffuse astrocytoma with enhancing lesions should be treated as high-grade glioma. If histology fails to provide evidence for a high-grade lesion, the possibility of a sampling error should be considered, especially in patients who underwent stereotactic biopsy. Many treatment guidelines are based on trials that included grade IV tumors and anaplastic glioma. Table 2 summarizes median one- and two-years survival, as reported in different randomized clinical trials on high-grade gliomas. Currently, most trials address specific subtypes of gliomas.

Anaplastic Astrocytoma

Histology

Similar to the histological diagnosis of other glial tumors, the diagnosis of anaplastic astrocytoma is troublesome. With respect to grading, anaplastic astrocytomas fall in between diffuse astrocytoma and GBM. Pure astrocytic tumors have to be distinguished from oligoastrocytoma, which by definition are tumors containing elements of both oligodendroglioma and astrocytoma.

Table 2 Median, 1- and 2-Year Survival in High-Grade Glioma After Various Postoperative Adjuvant Treatments

References	Postsurgical treatment	Median survival (mo)	1-year survival (%)	2-year survival (%)
Walker	Supportive care	3	3	0
et al. (45)	BCNU	4	12	0
	RT	8	24	1
	RT + BCNU	7.5	32	5
Bleehen and	RT: 20×2.25 Gy	9	29	8
Stenning (46)	RT: 30×2 Gy	12	39	12
Souhami	RT + BCNU	14.1	NS	22
et al. (47)	RT + BCNU + SRS	13.7	NS	16
Westphal	RT	11.6	49.6	NS
et al. (48)	RT + BCNU wafer	13.9	59.2	NS
Stupp	RT	12.1	50.6	10.4
et al. (8)	RT plus temozolomide	14.6	61.1	26.5

Abbreviations: RT, radiotherapy; SRS, stereotactic radiosurgery; BCNU, carmustine; NS, not stated.

In the absence of objective grading criteria and established tumors markers, this classification remains very subjective, and is subject to the significant interobserver variability (49). In addition, particularly in incompletely resected or stereotactically biopsied cases, the sample may simply not be representative of the entire tumor. Furthermore, at progression most low-grade and anaplastic astrocytomas have transformed into glioblastoma, which adds to the blurred distinction between these tumor grades. Nevertheless, from a clinical perspective the diagnosis of anaplastic astrocytoma makes sense. Patients with newly diagnosed anaplastic astrocytoma have a much better prognosis than patients with glioblastoma, and anaplastic astrocytomas were shown to be much more sensitive to temozolomide chemotherapy at recurrence than glioblastoma.

Over the past decade, anaplastic astrocytomas appear to have been decreased in frequency. Two factors are responsible for this development. Firstly, the histological definition of anaplastic astrocytoma has changed over the past years. In studies before the 1990s, the diagnosis anaplastic astrocytoma allowed the presence of endothelial proliferation. This is no longer the case since the introduction of the most recent WHO classification of brain tumors (1). Although this change has been questioned, older studies have shown that the presence of endothelial proliferation has indeed a great impact on the survival of patients, shortening the median existence from 5.5 to 3.5 years (50). Vice versa, GBM with only endothelial proliferation were shown to have a better outcome than GBM with necrosis: a two-year survival of 27% versus 13% for patients with necrosis (51). The difference is only modest however, and the overall outcome of glioblastoma patients without endothelial proliferation fits better with that of GBM with necrosis than with the typical three- to four-year survival of anaplastic astrocytoma patients. Secondly, the criteria for oligodendroglial tumors have been changing, resulting in a wider definition and increasing the number of mixed oligoastrocytomas (52). This process is now being reversed, because trials on anaplastic oligodendrogliomas have shown that the prognosis of anaplastic oligodendroglial tumors or mixed gliomas without combined 1p/19q loss is two to three years, very similar to the expected survival in anaplastic astrocytoma and much worse than those with combined 1p/19q loss (53). New trials are now considering to combine all anaplastic gliomas, provided they do not have 1p/19q loss.

Molecular Biology

Gain of chromosome 7 and TP53 mutations are similarly frequent in anaplastic astrocytoma as in grade II astrocytomas (14). In contrast to glioblastoma, in which the of loss of heterozygosity for chromosome 10, EGFRvIII mutations, PTEN mutations, and mutations of the Rb pathway are *not* of prognostic significance, these alterations become of prognostic significance once diagnosed in an anaplastic astrocytoma (54). If present in anaplastic astrocytoma (55,56), the clinical outcome is more consistent with that of

GBM. Gain of chromosome 7p has also been associated with older age, which may account for the prognostic significance of age in anaplastic astrocytoma (57). Again, these data and the 1p/19q data suggest that molecular markers are more predictive for the outcome of anaplastic glioma patients than a subjective morphologic classification, but it will take some years before molecular markers are of use for the daily management of anaplastic glioma.

Neuroimaging

Also with respect to neuroimaging, anaplastic astrocytoma shares features of both diffuse astrocytoma and glioblastoma. Although most anaplastic astrocytoma are enhancing, in one study 31% of anaplastic astrocytoma were nonenhancing, on contrast-enhanced CT scan (Fig. 4) (23). Most tumors show some mass effect. Ring enhancement with a necrotic center on MRI scanning is more suggestive of a glioblastoma.

Treatment

Most guidelines on the treatment of anaplastic astrocytoma are derived from studies on high-grade glioma that included all histologies, provided anaplastic characteristics were present. As a consequence, most patients

(A)   **(B)**

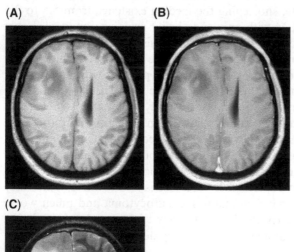

(C)

Figure 4 Magnetic resonance imaging of an anaplastic astrocytoma in a young patient presenting with seizures. T1 and T2 (**A**) signal intensities reflect the abnormalities observed in low-grade astrocytoma, except for some increased signal intensity within the T1-weighted images (**B**). Note the absence of contrast enhancement (**C**). The presence of mass effect initiated treatment in this patient. Histology revealed a anaplastic astrocytoma.

with an anaplastic astrocytoma are treated similarly to patients with glioblastoma, with surgery followed by RT to a dosage of 60 to 65 Gy and with or without chemotherapy. Only recently it became commonplace to develop separate trials for GBM, and we are now facing the question whether clinical data derived from glioblastoma trials can be extrapolated to patients with anaplastic astrocytoma. There is no answer to this question, in particular in view of the molecular differences between these tumor grades.

In the past it has been assumed that standard adjuvant chemotherapy with PCV offered a better outcome than carmustine (BCNU) in anaplastic astrocytoma, but a meta-analysis of several studies, which took prognostic factors into account could not find any evidence for this assumption (5). Patients with recurrent astrocytoma following RT show a much higher response rate to temozolomide chemotherapy than glioblastoma, with 35% of anaplastic astrocytoma patients responding and 45% of patients free from progression at six months (58). In contrast to the reported 40% to 50% response rates of newly diagnosed glioblastoma to temozolomide if given prior to irradiation, trials on preirradiation chemotherapy in anaplastic glioma provide disappointing response rates, with 17% to 30% of patients responding (59,60). Whatever the explanation, the currently available data fail to provide any evidence that the increased chemosensitivity of recurrent anaplastic astrocytoma as compared to glioblastoma is reflected in a higher response rate to neoadjuvant chemotherapy (61). A currently ongoing trial investigates if classical adjuvant temozolomide provides a superior result as compared to adjuvant BCNU chemotherapy.

With the improved outcome after treatment with adjuvant and concomitant temozolomide in glioblastoma (see the section on glioblastoma), the question is whether this treatment should also be applied to anaplastic astrocytoma (8). In view of the superior outcome of combined modality treatment this seems logical, but it is at present unknown if combined modality treatment may cause an increased delayed neurotoxicity in patients with a longer survival. Reviews of old RTOG/ECOG studies suggested a decreased survival in more aggressively treated anaplastic astrocytoma patients (62). These data should be viewed with caution, as they were not the result of a randomized prospective study. However, they may serve as a reminder that treatments showing a superior outcome in glioblastoma may not necessarily provide a superior outcome in anaplastic astrocytoma. A pragmatic approach may be to treat patients with poor clinical or molecular prognostic factors (and more indicative of a glioblastoma) with combined modality treatment. The others could be treated with RT only, while reserving chemotherapy for the time of progression.

Glioblastoma Multiforme

GBM, the most malignant astrocytic tumor, is histologically characterized by necrosis and/or endothelial proliferation. The entity GBM has been separated into so-called de novo and secondary glioblastoma, the latter having developed from a less malignant precursor lesion (either from a low-grade astrocytoma or an anaplastic astrocytoma). The latter occur in younger patients, and are characterized by *TP53* mutations and LOH of chromosome 10 q, which occur during progression (63). De novo GBM arise in older patients and are characterized by EGFR amplification/mutations, *PTEN* mutations, p16 deletions, or MDM2 overexpression (64). The MIB proliferation index was reported to be higher in elderly glioblastoma patients (65).

Although at the molecular level clear differences may be observed between de novo and secondary GBM, at the clinical level the prognosis seems similar once a lower grade tumor has transformed into an anaplastic tumor (66). Whether the distinction between de novo and secondary glioblastoma holds for all patients, is questionable; for instance *TP53* mutations have also been described in de novo glioblastoma, and were associated with a better survival (67). It is important to realize that the histological diagnosis GBM is a wastebasket diagnosis, in which different lesions with different molecular lesions are collected because of morphological similarities. However, the currently available molecular sub classifications are similarly artificial. One might expect that a better understanding of the molecular lesions of glioblastoma will allow for a better classification system—and hopefully a better and more tailored treatment.

Histological Subtypes

Giant cell glioblastoma is a histological variant of GBM, which may have a somewhat better outcome. Perhaps this is due to younger age at presentation and frequent *TP53* mutations. Gliosarcomas are bimorphic tumors containing elements of malignant gliomas and sarcomas. At the molecular level these tumors appear similar to glioblastoma, with similar genetic lesions in both morphological parts of the tumor (68). This suggests that both histological elements arise from the same precursor cells, with only a different phenotype in the various parts of the tumor. At the clinical level, the outcome of gliosarcoma patients is similar to GBM patients (69). Thus, in all respects these tumors can be considered as glioblastoma. Apart from these histological subtypes, some patients suffer from so-called multifocal glioma, with seemingly separate areas of tumor. Presumably these tumors represent a brain diffusely infiltrated by tumor cells, with only limited neuro-radiological abnormalities.

Prognosis

A large recursive partitioning analysis of three prospective trials on high-grade glioma showed that GBM patients below 50 years of age and in good clinical condition had a median survival of 17 months, whereas patients over 50 years of age with cognitive deficits and with a poor performance status had a median survival of only 4.6 months (70). In virtually all trials on high-grade glioma, age and performance status are very strong prognostic factors. These nontreatment-related factors have such a large impact on the overall outcome that they should be considered while planning treatment in individual patients. With the novel combined modality treatment, in which glioblastoma patients are treated with temozolomide in combination with RT, the methylation status of the *MGMT* promoter gene appears to be the most significant prognostic factor of glioblastoma patients (71). Similar to low-grade astrocytoma, the MMSE is an important prognostic factor in glioblastoma.

Neuroimaging

As a rule, glioblastoma presents as an enhancing tumor, often with mass effect and more irregularly shaped and less well defined borders than brain metastases (Fig. 5). Most lesions are rather large, but smaller lesions may mimic brain metastases. There may be extensive involvement of the corpus callosum and tumor growth into the other hemisphere ("butterfly glioma"). Necrotic areas and cysts are common. Occasionally, enhancing areas are seen at relatively large distances- the so-called multifocal glioblastoma. Brain metastases, lymphoma, and infectious lesions are the most important differential diagnostic considerations for single enhancing and space occupying lesions.

(A) **(B)**

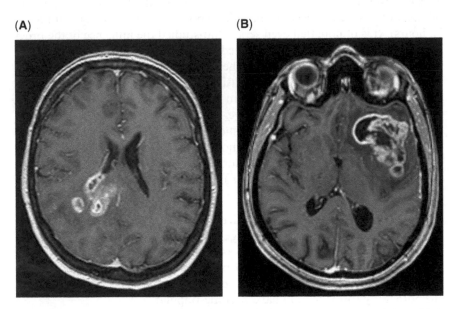

Figure 5 Magnetic resonance imaging of glioblastoma multiforme: (**A**) multiple enhancing lesions with central necrosis, extending into the corpus callosum; (**B**) left temporal glioblastoma with irregular enhancement and necrotic areas.

Treatment

Surgery: In malignant glioma, surgery serves three major objectives: obtaining tissue for diagnosis, reducing increased intracranial pressure and focal deficits by removal of a space occupying lesion, and improving the prognosis by reducing the tumor load. The first goal can be achieved by a biopsy. In general, biopsy is considered to be a safe procedure, with about 4% serious morbidity and 1% mortality (72,73). The need to reduce an intracranial space-occupying lesion to ameliorate clinical signs and symptoms is obvious. Whether a gross total resection improves the prognosis of patients with high-grade glioma, is controversial. Many uncontrolled studies and retrospective analyses have suggested that a more extensive resection improves the outcome of a patient. However, the crucial question is whether it is the extent of resection or the localization and size of the tumor (and thereby the chances for an extensive resection) that determines the prognosis. In other words, "Is the prognosis of a patient with a deep seated lesion in the basal ganglia poor, because a resection is not possible or because this localization gives rise to severe signs and symptoms at an earlier stage than a superficial and small lesion?" As an example, one retrospective study found a negative impact on survival of involvement of the corpus callosum (74). Many of the studies on the influence of an extensive resection have been based on the neurosurgeons estimate during the operation of the extent of resection. This is however not a reliable measure; the only good estimate of the amount of resection can be obtained by immediate postoperative imaging (within 24–72 hours). It is of note that even series that studied the influence of the prognosis of clearly different surgical procedures (biopsy vs. gross total resection) showed conflicting results (75,76). Other studies though, have suggested that the prognosis improves if postoperative imaging shows that virtually all tumors have been removed (77,78). In view of the many studies suggesting a better outcome after more extensive resections, it is generally agreed that the goal of the surgical intervention should be to remove as many tumor as safely possible. The morbidity and mortality of a neurosurgical procedure appears mainly dependant on the localization of the tumor and on the patient (age, condition, etc.) and not on the type of procedure (biopsy vs. resection) (79).

Radiation Therapy: Randomized controlled clinical trials have demonstrated that RT with a dosage of 60 Gy improves the survival of high-grade glioma patient (Table 2) (45,80,81). Furthermore, RT with or without chemotherapy was found to be more effective than chemotherapy alone (45,82,83). This is important to realize, now that trials on neoadjuvant chemotherapy (prior to RT) have become popular.

The issue of the required target volume of the radiation therapy has only been studied retrospectively; no study ever compared whole-brain RT with a dose level of 60 Gy to involved fields (equal to tumor area on

CT/MRI scan with a margin of 2–3 cm). Although high-grade gliomas often give the impression to be a localized disease on CT or MRI, histological examination may reveal tumor cells well outside the area that shows enhancement or edema on CT or MRI (84). The question is, therefore, whether a glioma should be seen as a focal disease or as a diffuse disease involving large areas of the brain. However, retrospective studies of focal brain RT demonstrate that the large majority of recurrences arise within the irradiated volume (85,86). Treatment of larger areas of the brain with radiation therapy also increases the risk of leukoencephalopathy and late cognitive side effects of the treatment. These considerations have resulted from the mid-eighties onward in treatment of glioma patients with involved field irradiation. The only trial that explored the reduction of the RT field compared whole-brain RT with a dosage of 60.2 to 43 Gy whole brain RT followed by a boost of 17.2 Gy to the tumor area (87). No survival difference was found. At present, it is widely recognized that involved field RT is sufficient, which is defined by the area with abnormalities on the T2-weighted MRI scan. However, studies on the correlation between CT and pathology or comparing metabolic imaging with MRI show, that the actual delineation of the RT field is not as straightforward as one would hope (84,88). Still, there is no need for whole brain RT except for some cases with gliomatosis cerebri or multifocal GBM. Also, in general there is no need to use 2- to 3-cm zones around the visible tumor, which inevitably results in very large RT fields.

Radiation therapy of the involved field with a dosage of 60 Gy in fractions of 2 Gy was found superior to 45 Gy in fractions of 2.25 Gy (Table 2) (46). No further improvement was observed if after 60 Gy involved field RT, a boost of 10 Gy was given to the tumor bed (89). Randomized controlled trials with hyperfractionation, (1.2 or 1.6 Gy twice daily) with a dosage of 70 to 81.6 Gy did not show a better survival as compared to conventional schedules with a dose level of 60 Gy, in once daily fractions (90,91). Similarly, dose-intensified RT after conventional 60 Gy external standard radiation, delivered either by interstitial brachytherapy implanted radioactive pellets or by a single 15 to 24 Gy stereotactic boost failed to improve outcome (Table 2) (47,92,93). One trial showed an improved outcome if 60 Gy external RT was followed by a boost given by interstitial RT combined with hyperthermia; the control arm received the interstitial brachytherapy boost without hyperthermia (94). Because of the many selection criteria, only a few patients were eligible for the interstitial part of the treatment. To conclude, for most patients 60 to 64 Gy RT in fractions of 1.8 Gy provides the optimum RT results, which takes some six weeks of daily treatment.

Chemotherapy: A recent EORTC/NCI-C study on 570 glioblastoma patients has identified combined 60 Gy RT with daily temozolomide at a dosage of 75 mg/m^2, followed by 150 to 200 mg/m^2 adjuvant temozolomide in the classical day 1 to 5 every four weeks as the standard of care for GBM patients (8). With this combined modality treatment, two-year survival increased from 11% to 26%. Subgroup analyses suggested that patients of all age groups (patients up to the age of 70 years were allowed) and those who were independent of prior tumor resection benefited from this treatment, the only exception being patients in a modest clinical condition (WHO performance status 2). Overall, the combined treatment was well tolerated, the main reason for early discontinuation being disease progression. The trial also identified the methylation of the promotor gene of alkyltransferase, *MGMT*, as the major factor that determines outcome (9). This DNA repair enzyme is a major resistance mechanism against alkylating and methylating chemotherapy, which is often epigenetically silenced in tumors through methylation of promoter regions. A subgroup analysis of the study strongly suggests that the *MGMT* methylation status is a predictive marker for benefit from temozolomide chemotherapy. For patients treated with temozolomide, the two-year survival rate was 46% when their tumor presented a methylated *MGMT* status in contrast to only 14% in patients with an unmethylated *MGMT* gene promoter (Table 3). Thus, in this molecularly defined subgroup temozolomide was more effective, while patients with an unmethylated *MGMT* gene promoter had little if any benefit from concurrent and adjuvant temozolomide.

This is the first trial that showed a clinically significant benefit from adjuvant chemotherapy in GBM. Most of the earlier randomized trials on adjuvant chemotherapy failed to show a difference in survival or revealed only a small and statistically insignificant increase in survival following adjuvant chemotherapy (Table 2) (45,82,95). These trials investigated mostly

Table 3 Median Survival and 2-Year Survival in European Organization for Research and Treatment of Cancer Study 26981 in Relation to the Methylation Status of the *MGMT* Promoter

	Median survival (mo)		2-year survival (%)	
	Radiotherapy[a]	Radiotherapy plus temozolomide	Radiotherapy[a]	Radiotherapy plus temozolomide
Unmethylated *MGMT* promotor	11.8	12.7	< 2	13.8
Methylated *MGMT* promotor	15.3	21.7	22.7	46

[a]72% of the patients in the radiotherapy-arm received alkylating chemotherapy at recurrence.
Source: From Ref. 9.

adjuvant treatment with nitrosoureas, which cannot be combined on a daily basis with RT. This suggests that it is the combined part of the temozolomide treatment that actually made the difference between the recent EORTC trials and the many historical trials on adjuvant chemotherapy. Still, it is the combination of concurrent and adjuvant temozolomide that provided the survival difference, and at present all other viewpoints are speculative.

Other Routes of Chemotherapy Administration: In line with these findings are the results of a study on post surgery intratumoral BCNU chemotherapy administered through BCNU loaded wafers (Table 2) (48). This resulted in a two-month increase of the median survival in a study on anaplastic glioma, without a clear difference in long term survival. Moreover, the survival difference was statistically not significant in the subset of glioblastoma patients. Currently, the combination of BCNU wafers treatment followed by combined modality treatment with temozolomide and RT is being advocated, but clinical data are not available. Clinical trials on adjuvant intra-arterial chemotherapy did not improve outcome as compared to intravenous chemotherapy (96,97). Early uncontrolled studies on high dose chemotherapy with autologous bone marrow transplantation reported favorable results, but these were most probably the result of the selection of good prognosis patients for this treatment. The only randomized study of this treatment comparing high dose BCNU to standard dose BCNU was prematurely closed after including 69 patients for excessive toxicity in the high dose chemotherapy arm; survival analysis failed to show any benefit of the high dose regimen (98). No randomized controlled clinical trials exist for the concept of chemotherapy of brain tumors after blood–brain barrier modification with intra-arterial mannitol.

Treatment of Elderly and Poor Prognosis Patients: Several investigators have tried to shorten the treatment period for poor prognosis patients (usually defined as patients in poor clinical condition, or with an age over 65–70 years) by giving hypofractionated RT. The validity of this approach was recently shown in a Canadian trial in elderly patients, which did not show a difference in survival between standard 60 Gy RT and a shortened course of RT (40 Gy in 15 fractions) (99). The advantage of this shortened schedule in elderly patients is of course the much shorter treatment duration. In many institutions the value of RT in elderly patients is doubted. A French study compared 50 Gy in 28 fractions to best palliative care in patients over 70 years of age (100). RT increased progression free survival from 7 weeks to 14 weeks and median survival from 17 to 28 weeks. Although RT clearly increases survival, the prognosis in this age category is very limited, with at best a modest increase after RT. One may consider treating elderly patients only if they are in exceptionally good condition, in which case a short course of RT may be considered.

Treatment of Recurrent High-Grade Glial Tumors: Once a high-grade glioma recurs, the further treatment strategy should depend on the condition of the patient, the type of the tumor, the time between the first treatment and the recurrence, and the localization of the recurrence. At the time of recurrence the performance status is the most important predictor for survival, irrespective of treatment.

Second Surgery. In selected cases, a reresection can contribute to the preservation or even improvement of the quality of life. Most patients undergoing reresection also receive other treatments; for that reason it is often difficult to determine the role of reresection for the overall outcome. In two series, the median survival after reresection was 36 weeks; and patients were in a good clinical condition during 18 to 26 weeks (101,102). A second resection offers the best possibility for rapid tumor reduction and symptom control, but appears of little value if only a modest part of the tumor can be removed.

Reirradiation. It is generally felt that if a glioma recurs within the radiation field following 50 to 60 Gy RT, the surrounding normal brain tissue will not tolerate reirradiation. Nonetheless, in several small phase II studies with various irradiation techniques (conventional fractionated RT, interstitial brachytherapy, and stereotactic radiosurgery) an acceptable treatment result was reported. Median survival after reirradiation was between 8 and 11 months (103). The modest survival in this patient category will limit the hazard of delayed neurotoxicity to the normal brain. There are no data as to whether there is a minimum interval between first RT and the recurrence, after which reirradiation may be beneficial.

Chemotherapy. For many patients with recurrent high-grade tumors, medical treatment is the only remaining treatment option. Second surgery is frequently precluded, or medical treatment is given following reresection. At present, temozolomide is the only drug that has been well investigated in recurrent anaplastic astrocytoma, with one third of patients responding and about 45% of patients still free from progression at six months (58). In recurrent glioblastoma, responses are reported in 5% to 8% of patients, with about 20% of patients still free from progression at six months (104,105). Today, many patients at first relapse will have already received temozolomide as part of the initial treatment. It is unknown if temozolomide is a useful treatment for progressive tumors after this combined modality treatment. It is, of course not logical to retreat patients relapsing during or shortly after temozolomide treatment with the same agent. Other recently investigated drugs include CPT-11 alone or in combination with BCNU, cyclophosphamide, and paclitaxel. None of these drugs provide satisfactory responses in recurrent glioblastoma; this situation is clearly an unmet clinical need. "Old-fashioned" combinations such as procarbazine and lomustine may still be considered (106). Whatever regimen is chosen, toxicity of the used regimen should be a major consideration in view of the modest efficacy. The use of many drugs is hampered because of induction of the cytochrome CYP3A4 by some of the anti-epileptic agents (in particular phenytoin, carbamazepine, and phenobarbital). This results in increased metabolism of many cytotoxic and cytostatic agents (107).

A randomized study of the effect of intratumoral BCNU following second surgery using a BCNU loaded polymer showed a small but statistically significant increase in survival (108). The median survival increased from 23 weeks to 31 weeks, the six-months survival from 47% to 60%. The high cost of the wafer in combination with the small improvement of outcome has hampered the widespread use of the BCNU-wafer.

Experimental Treatments. Recent studies are investigating biologically "targeted therapies," in which specific cell proteins are inhibited. Theoretically, interesting targets for this approach are cell surface receptors that are involved in the abnormal cell signaling of gliomas (e.g., EGFR amplification or PTEN mutations), or proteins that are involved in the growth of gliomas (e.g., VEGF signaling, PDGF autocrine loops). In a number of trials, small molecule inhibitors of these receptors and of components of the Ras/Raf and PI3K/AKT pathways have been investigated (e.g., inhibition of the mammalian target of rapamycine (mTOR) by CCI-779; inhibition of the EGFR receptor by gefitinib or erlotinib; inhibition of the PDGFR by STI571; inhibition of the vascular endothelial growth factor by PTK787/ZK22584 and SU5416). In a few of these trials some activity has been observed, but so far none of these drugs has been the long awaited "magic bullet."

A theoretically attractive approach is the use of genetically engineered fusion proteins comprised of toxins (e.g., pseudomonas toxin, diphtheria toxin) linked to ligands of cell surface receptors selectively expressed by glioma cells but not normal neurons or glia (e.g., IL-13, IL-4, transferring). These compounds are locally administered through convection-enhanced delivery. Several trials are ongoing. The interest in gene therapy has subsided with the negative results of the phase III study on the herpes virus construct. Problems that must be solved are the limited penetration of the viruses into the tumor.

NON-INFILTRATIVE ASTROCYTIC TUMORS

Pilocytic Astrocytoma

Pilocytic astrocytomas are circumscribed tumors occurring predominantly in children. They arise mostly in the cerebellum (especially in children) and in the temporal lobe, but also in other supratentorial regions such as the optic pathways and the thalamic region. Pilocytic astrocytoma constitutes about 5% of all gliomas, but it is the most common glioma in children. Median age at presentation in one study was 19 years, with 40% of patients being younger than 15 years (109). Although rare, these tumors may also arise in young adults (20 to 50 years). These tumors differ from the diffuse astrocytoma by the absence of infiltration of adjacent brain; if completely resected most patients are cured. Pilocytic astrocytoma is considered a WHO grade I tumor. In particular, optic nerve pilocytic astrocytoma is associated with neurofibromatosis type I. Pilomyxoid astrocytoma is a histological variant of the pilocytic astrocytoma.

Neuroimaging

Typically, patients present with circumscribed and enhancing lesions (despite their benign nature). Often they present with a cystic lesion with an enhancing mural nodule (Fig. 6). Mass effect and edema is common (110). Pilocytic tumors in the chiasmatic region are solid, with areas of necrosis. Brain stem pilocytic tumors frequently have an exophytic component, and involve the floor of the fourth ventricle.

Treatment

Complete resection is the treatment of choice if safely feasible (110,111). After subtotal resection, five-year progression-free survival decreases to 50% to

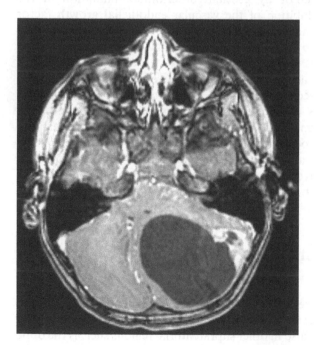

Figure 6 Magnetic resonance imaging of a pilocytic astrocytoma in a young patient with signs of increased intracranial pressure. Note the enhancing nodule on the left side of the cyst.

70%. However, even incompletely resected pilocytic astrocytoma may remain stable for prolonged periods of time. Incompletely resected tumors requiring further therapy can be controlled with RT. Several series reported excellent local control of unresectable tumors with stereotactic RT (112). Especially in younger patients with unresectable tumors and in whom one wants to avoid RT local control can be achieved with chemotherapy (113).

Prognosis

The prognosis is excellent if complete resection is achieved. Most series report 10-year survival rates exceeding 80% to 95% and up to 100% survival in completely resected patients, even in adults (109,111). Several trials found some association between the proliferation marker MIB-1 and outcome, but usually of borderline significance (110,114). MIB-1 labeling has not been validated across institutions. Nonetheless, long lasting stabilization or even regression has been observed after incomplete resections (115). In progressive cases multicentric spread may occur, perhaps more so in hypothalamic pilocytic tumors.

Pleiomorphic Xanthoastrocytoma

Pleiomorphic xantroastrocytoma is a rare tumor considered to be of astrocytic origin accounting for less than 1% of astrocytic tumors. They are usually found in a superficial supratentorial location and leptomeningeal invasion is common. On imaging studies a cyst is distinguished from a uniformly enhancing solid component (116). They typically occur in young patients, present with seizures and have ominous histological characteristics (marked cellular pleomorphism, nuclear atypia, and bizarre giant cells). Despite this histology, the prognosis is favorable after complete resection but in 15% to 40% of patients the tumor recurs, at which time it may show anaplastic transformation. TP53 mutations and other genetic aberrations found in diffuse glioma are rare, which implies different pathogenetic mechanisms (117,118). Clinical series have identified extent of resection, mitotic index, and presence of necrosis as indocators of a favorable prognosis (116,119). However, recurrence may occur even years after a complete resection.

Subependymal Giant Cell Astrocytoma

SEGA is a rare astrocytic tumor that may arise sporadically but occurs mainly in the context of tuberous sclerosis. Tuberous sclerosis is an autosomal dominant neurocutaneous syndrome, characterized by facial angiofibromas, mental retardation, seizures, and a variety of tumors. Various central nervous system lesions may occur: tubers, subependymal nodules, and SEGA, the latter complicating 5% to 14% of tuberous sclerosis cases. On CT scan these are usually calcified tumors. On MRI they are characterized by homogeneous enhancement (120). These tumors develop usually at the inferolateral wall of the lateral ventricles, often bilateral and in the region of the foramen of Monro. It is unclear if SEGA represent transformed subependymal nodules, as nodules distant from the Monro zone appear to remain stable (121). Subependymal nodules that are less than 5 mm in diameter, completely calcified, and incompletely enhancing are less likely to show growth during follow-up (122). Because of the relation of SEGA to the foramen of Monro they may give rise to hydrocephalus, which is major cause of mortality in tuber sclerosis. A surveillance program is therefore advised for tuberous sclerosis patients. The tumors are well circumscribed, and can be completely resected with excellent outcome (121,123). The presence of cytological atypia, mitotic activity, vascular proliferation, and necrosis do not have prognostic significance (121,123). As a rule, adjuvant treatment after surgery is not required, but tumors may recur.

ACKNOWLEDGMENT

The critical review and comments of Ms J.E.C. Bromberg, MD PhD are gratefully acknowledged.

REFERENCES

1. World Health Classification of tumours. In: Pathology and Genetics of Tumours of the Nervous System. Lyon: International Agency for the Research on Cancer, 2000.
2. Lantos PL, Bruner JM. Gliomatosis cerebri. In: Kleihues P, Cavenee WK, eds. Pathology and Genetics of Tumours of the Nervous System. Lyon: IARC, 2000:92–93.
3. Ohgaki H, Kleihues P. Epidemiology and etiology of gliomas. Acta Neuropathol 2005; 109:93–108.
4. Pignatti F, van den Bent MJ, Curran D, et al. Prognostic factors for survival in adult patients with cerebral low-grade glioma. J Clin Oncol 2002; 20:2076–2084.
5. Prados MD, Scott C, Curran WJ, et al. Procarbazine, lomustine, and vincristine (PCV) chemotherapy for anaplastic astrocytoma: a retrospective review of radiation oncology group protocols comparing survival with carmustine or PCV adjuvant chemotherapy. J Clin Oncol 1999; 17:3389–3395.
6. Prados MD, Seiferheld W, Sandler HM, et al. Phase III randomized study of radiotherapy plus procarbazine, lomustine, and vincristine with or without BUdR for treatment of anaplastic astrocytoma: final report of RTOG 9404. Int J Radiat Oncol Biol Phys 2004; 58:1147–1152.
7. Buckner JC, Schomberg PJ, McGinnis WL, et al. A phase III study of radiation therapy plus carmustine with or without recombinant interferon-alpha in the treatment of patients with newly diagnosed high-grade glioma. Cancer 2001; 92:420–433.
8. Stupp R, Mason WP, van den Bent MJ, et al. Radiotherapy plus concomitant and adjuvant temozolomide for glioblastoma. N Engl J Med 2005; 352:987–996.

9. Hegi ME, Diserens A-C, Gorlia T, et al. MGMT gene silencing and benefit from temozolomide in glioblastoma. N Engl J Med 2005; 352:997–1003.
10. Shaw E, Arusell RM, Scheithauer B, et al. A prospective randomized trial of low versus high dose radiation in adults with a supratentorial low grade glioma: initial report of a NCCTG-RTOG-ECOG study. J Clin Oncol 2002; 20: 2267–2276.
11. Maintz D, Fiedler K, Koopmann J, et al. Molecular genetic evidence for sub-types of oligoastrocytomas. J Neuropathol Exp Neurol 1997; 56:1098–1104.
12. Krouwer HGJ, Davis RL, Silver P, Prados MD. Gemistocytic astrocytomas: a reappraisal. J Neurosurg 1991; 74:399–406.
13. Wessels PH, Twijnstra A, Ummelen MIJ, et al. Gain of chromosome 7 as detected by in situ hybridization correlates with shorter survival in strocytoma grade II. Genes Chromosom Cancer 2002; 33:279–284.
14. Reifenberger G, Collins VP. Pathology and molecular genetics of astrocytic gliomas. J Mol Med 2004; 82:656–670.
15. Bauman G, Lote K, Larson D, et al. Pretreatment factors predict overall sur-vival for patients with low grade glioma: a recursive partitioning analysis. Int J Radiation Oncol Biol Phys 1999; 45:923–929.
16. Leighton C, Fisher B, Bauman G, et al. Supratentorial low-grade glioma in adults: an analysis of prognostic factors and the timing of radiation. J Clin Oncol 1997; 15:1294–1301.
17. Shaw E, Won M, Brachman DG, et al. Preliminary results of RTOG protocol 9802: a phase Ii study of observation in completely resected adult low grade glioma [abstr 7]. Neuro-Oncology 2005; 7:284.
18. Recht LD, Lew R, Smith TW. Suspected low-grade glioma: is deferring treat-ment safe? Ann Neurol 1992; 31:431–436.
19. Kondziolka D, Lunsford LD, Martinez AJ. Unreliability of contemporary neu-rodiagnostic imaging in evaluating suspected adult supratentorial (low-grade) astrocytoma. J Neurosurg 1993; 79:533–536.
20. Mandonnet E, Delattre JY, Tanguy ML, et al. Continuous growth of mean tumor diameter in a subset of grade II gliomas. Ann Neurol 2003; 53: 524–528.
21. Ginsberg LE, Fuller GN, Hashmi M, Leeds NE, Schomer DF. The significance of lack of MR contrast enhancement of supratentorial brain tumors in adults: histopathological evaluation of a series. Surg Neurol 1998; 49:436–440.
22. Barker FG, Chang CH, Huhn SL, et al. Age and the risk of anaplasia in mag-netic resonance-nonenhancing supratentorial cerebral tumors. Cancer 1997; 80:936–941.
23. Chamberlain MC, Murovic JA, Levin VA. Absence of contrast enhancement on CT brain scans of patients with supratentorial malignant gliomas. Neurol-ogy 1988; 38:1371–1374.
24. van Veelen MLC, Avezaat CJJ, Kros JM, van Putten WL, Vecht CJ. Supraten-torial low grade astrocytoma: prognostic factors, dedifferentiation, and the issue of early versus late surgery. J Neurol Neurosurg Psych 1998; 64:581–587.
25. Reijneveld JC, Sitskoorn MM, Klein M, Nuyen J, Taphoorn MJB. Cognitive status and quality of life in suspected versus proven low-grade gliomas. Neurol-ogy 2001; 56:618–623.

26. Klein M, Heimans JJ, Aaronson NK, et al. Effect of radiotherapy and other treatment-related factors on mid-term to long-term cognitive sequelae in low grade gliomas: a comparative study. Lancet 2002; 360:1361–1368.
27. van den Bent MJ, Afra D, De Witte O, et al. Long term results of EORTC study 22845: a randomized trial on the efficacy of early versus delayed radiation therapy of low-grade astrocytoma and oligodendroglioma in the adult. Lancet 2005. In Press.
28. Shafqat S, Hedley-Whyte ET, Henson JW. Age-dependant rate of anaplastic transformation in low grade astrocytoma. Neurology 2001; 52:867–869.
29. Soffietti R, Borgogne M, Ducati A, et al. Efficacy of radiation therapy on seizures in low-grade astrocytomas [abstr 422]. Neuro-Oncology 2005; 7:389.
30. Brada M, Viviers L, Abson C, et al. Phase II study of primary temozolomide chemotherapy in patients with WHO grade II gliomas. Ann Oncol 2003; 14:1715–1721.
31. Rogers LR, Morris HH, Lupica K. Effect on cranial irradiation on seizure frequency in adults with low-grade astrocytoma and medically intractable epilepsy. Neurology 1993; 43:1599–1601.
32. Britton JW, Cascino GD, Sharbrough FW, Kelly PJ. Low-grade glial neoplasms and intractable partial epilepsy: efficacy of surgical treatment. Epilepsia 1994; 35:1130–1135.
33. Shaw EG, Daumas-Duport C, Scheithauer B, et al. Radiation therapy in the management of low grade supratentorial astrocytomas. J Neurosurg 1989; 70:853–861.
34. Berger MS, Deliganis AV, Dobbins J, Keles GE. The effect of extent of resection on recurrence in patients with low grade cerebral hemisphere gliomas. Cancer 1994; 74:1784–1791.
35. Duffau H, Lopes M, Arthuis F, et al. Contribution of intraoperative electrical stimulations in surgery of low grade gliomas: a comparative study between two series without (1985–1996) and with (1996–2003) functional mapping in the same institution. J Neurol Neurosurg Psych 2005; 76:845–851.
36. Scerrati M, Roselli R, Iacoangeli M, Pompucci A, Rossi GF. Prognostic factors in low grade (WHO II) gliomas of the cerebral hemispheres: the role of surgery. J Neurol Neurosurg Psych 1996; 61:291–296.
37. Touboul E, Schlienger M, Buffat L, et al. Radiation therapy with or without surgery in the management of low-grade brain astrocytomas. A retrospective study of 120 patients. Bull Cancer/Radiother 1995; 82:388–395.
38. Claus E, Horlacher A, Hsu L, et al. Survival rates in patients with low-grade glioma after intraoperative magnetic resonance image guidance. Cancer 2005; 103:1227–1233.
39. Bauman G, Pahapill P, Macdonald D, et al. Low grade glioma: measuring radiographic response to radiotherapy. Can J Neurol Sci 1999; 26:18–22.
40. Karim ABMF, Maat B, Hatlevoll R, et al. A randomized trial on dose-response in radiation therapy of low grade cerebral glioma: European Organization for Research and Treatment of Cancer (EORTC) study 2284. Int J Radiation Oncol Biol Phys 1996; 36:549–556.
41. Kiebert GM, Curran W, Aaronson NK, et al. Quality of life after radiation therapy of cerebral low-grade gliomas of the adult: results of a randomised phase III trial on dose response (EORTC trial 22844). Eur J Cancer 1998; 34:1902–1909.

42. Eyre HJ, Quagliana JM, Eltringham JR, et al. Randomised comparison of radiotherapy and CCNU versus radiotherapy, CCNU plus procarbazine for the treatment of malignant gliomas following surgery. J Neuro-Oncol 1993; 1:171–177.
43. Pace A, Vidiri A, Galie E, et al. Temozolomide chemotherapy for progressive low grade glioma: clinical benefits and radiological response. Ann Oncol 2003; 14:1722–1726.
44. Quinn JA, Reardon DA, Friedman AH, et al. Phase II trial of temozolomide in patients with progressive low-grade glioma. J Clin Oncol 2003; 21:646–651.
45. Walker MD, Alexander E, Hunt WE, et al. Evaluation of BCNU and/or radiotherapy in the treatment of anaplastic gliomas. A cooperative clinical trial. J Neurosurg 1978; 49:333–343.
46. Bleehen NM, Stenning SP. A medical research council trial of two radiotherapy doses in the treatment of grades 3 and 4 astrocytoma. Br J Cancer 1991; 64:769–774.
47. Souhami L, Seiferheld W, Brachman D, et al. Randomized comparison of stereotactic radiosurgery followed by conventional radiotherapy with carmustine to conventional radiotherapy with carmustine for patients with glioblastoma multiforme: report of radiation therapy oncology group 93–05 protocol. Int J Radiation Oncol Biol Phys 2004; 60:853–860.
48. Westphal M, Hilt DC, Bortey E, et al. A phase 3 trial of local chemotherapy with biodegradable carmustine (BCNU) wafers (Gliadel wafers) in patients with primary malignant glioma. Neuro-Oncology 2003; 5:79–88.
49. Scott CB, Nelson JS, Farnan NC, et al. Central pathology review in clinical trials for patients with malignant glioma. Cancer 1995; 76:307–313.
50. Fulling KH, Garcia DM. Anaplastic astrocytoma of the adult cerebrum. Prognostic value of histologic features. Cancer 1985; 55:928–931.
51. Barker FG, Davis RL, Chang SM, Prados MD. Necrosis as prognostic factor in glioblastoma multiforme. Cancer 1996; 77:1161–1166.
52. Coons SW, Johnson PC, Scheithauer BW, Yates AJ, Pearl DK. Improving diagnostic accuracy and interobserver concordance in the classification and grading of primary gliomas. Cancer 1997; 79:1381–1391.
53. van den Bent MJ, Delattre J-Y, Brandes AA, et al. First analysis of EORTC trial 26951, a randomized phase III study of adjuvant PCV chemotherapy in patients with highly anaplastic oligodendroglioma [abstr 1503]. Proc Am Soc Clin Oncol 2005; 23:114s.
54. Balesaria S, Brock C, Bower M, et al. Loss of chromosome 10 is an independent prognostic factor in high-grade gliomas. Br J Cancer 1999; 81:1371–1377.
55. Backlund LM, Nilsson BR, Liu L, Ichimura K, Collins VP. Mutations in Rb1 pathway-related genes are associated with a poor prognosis in anaplastic astrocytomas. Br J Cancer 2005; 93:124–130.
56. Aldape KD, Ballman K, Furth A, et al. Immunohistochemical detection of EGFRvIII in high malignancy grade astrocytomas and evaluation of prognostic significance. J Neuropathol Exp Neurol 2004; 63:700–707.
57. Kunwar S, Mohapatra G, Bollen A, et al. Genetic subgroup of anaplastic astrocytomas correlate with patient age and survival. Cancer Res 2001; 61:7683–7688.
58. Yung WK, Prados M, Yaya-Tur R, et al. Multicenter phase II trial of temozolomide in patients with anaplastic astrocytoma or anaplastic oligoastrocytoma at first relapse. J Clin Oncol 1999; 17:2762–2771.

59. Chang SM, Prados MD, Yung WK, et al. Phase II study of neoadjuvant 1, 3-bis (2-chloroethyl)-1-nitrosourea and temozolomide for newly diagnosed anaplastic glioma: a North American Brain Tumor Consortium Trial. Cancer 2004; 100:1712–1716.

60. Rao RD, Krishnan S, Fitch TR, et al. Phase II trial of carmustine, cisplatin, and oral etoposide chemotherapy before radiotherapy for grade 3 astrocytoma (anaplastic astrocytoma): results of North Central Cancer Treatment Group trial 98-72-51. Int J Radiat Oncol Biol Phys 2005; 61:380–386.

61. Brada M, Ashley S, Dowe A, et al. Neoadjuvant phase II multicentre study of new agents in patients with malignant glioma after minimal surgery. Report of a cohort of 187 patients treated with temozolomide. Ann Oncol 2005; 16:949.

62. Fischbach AJ, Martz KL, Nelson JS, et al. Long-term survival in treated anapalstic astrocytomas. A report of combined RTOG/ECOG studies. Am J Clin Oncol 1991; 14:365–370.

63. Fujisawa H, Kurrer M, Reis RM, et al. Acquisition of the glioblastoma phenotype during astrocytoma progression is associated with loss of heterozygosity on 10q25-qter. Am J Pathol 1999; 155:387–394.

64. Tohma Y, Gratas C, Biernat W, et al. PTEN (MMAC1) mutations are frequent in primary glioblastoma 9de novo) but not in secondary glioblastomas. J Neuropathol Exp Neurol 1998; 57:684–689.

65. McKeever PE, Junck L, Strawderman MS, et al. Proliferation index is related to patient age in glioblastoma. Neurology 2001; 56:1216–1218.

66. Dropcho EJ, Soong S. The prognostic impact of prior low grade histology in patients with anaplastic gliomas. Neurology 1996; 47:684–690.

67. Schmidt MC, Antweiler S, Urban S, et al. Impact of genotype and morphology on the prognosis of glioblastoma. J Neuropathol Exp Neurol 2002; 61: 321–328.

68. Boerman RH, Anderl K, Herath J, et al. The glial and mesenchymal elements of gliosarcoma share similar genetic alterations. J Neuropathol Exp Neurol 1996; 55:973–981.

69. Galanis E, Buckner JC, Dinapoli RP, et al. Clinical outcome of gliosarcoma compared with glioblastoma multiforme: North Central Cancer Treatment Group results. J Neurosurg 1998; 89:425–430.

70. Curran WJ, Scott CB, Horton J, et al. Recursive partitioning analysis of prognostic factors in three radiation therapy oncology group malignant glioma trials. J Natl Canc Inst 1993; 85:704–710.

71. Hegi ME, Diserens A-C, Godard S, et al. Clinical trial substantiates the predictive value of O-6-methylguanine-DNA methyltransferase promoter methylation in glioblastoma patients treated with temozolomide. Clin Canc Res 2004; 15:1871–1874.

72. Jackson RJ, Fuller GN, Abi-Said D, et al. Limitations of stereotactic biopsy in the initial management of gliomas. Neuro-Oncology 2001; 3:193–200.

73. Hall WA. The safety and efficacy of stereotactic biopsy for intracranial lesions. Cancer 1998; 82:1749–1755.

74. Stelzer KJ, Sauvé KI, Spence AM, Griffin TW, Berger MS. Corpus callosum involvement as a prognostic factor for patients with high-grade astrocytoma. Int J Radiat Oncol Biol Phys 1997; 38:27–30.

75. Nijjar TS, Simpson WJ, Gadalla T, McCartney M. Oligodendroglioma. The Princess Margaret Hospital Experience (1958–1984). Cancer 1993; 71:4002–4006.
76. Kreth FW, Berlis A, Spiropoulou V, et al. The role of tumor resection in the treatment of glioblastoma multiforme in adults. Cancer 1999; 86:2117–2123.
77. Lacroix M, Abi-Said D, Fourney DR, et al. A multivariate analysis of 416 patients with glioblastoma multiforme: prognosis, extent of resection, and survival. J Neurosurg 2001; 95:190–198.
78. Wood JR, Green SB, Shapiro WR. The prognostic importance of tumor size in malignant gliomas: a computed tomographic scan study by the brain tumor cooperative group. J Clin Oncol 1988; 6:338–343.
79. Fadul C, Wood J, Thaler H, et al. Morbidity and mortality of craniotomy for excision of supratentorial gliomas. Neurology 1988; 38:1374–1379.
80. Kristiansen K, Hagen S, Kolleveld T, et al. Combined modality therapy of operated astrocytomas grade III and IV. Confirmation of the value of postoperative irradiation and lack of potentiation of bleiomyycin on survival time. Cancer 1981; 47:649–652.
81. Andersen AP. Postoperative irradiation of glioblastomas. Acta Radiol Oncol 1978; 17:475–484.
82. Walker MD, Green SB, Byar DP, et al. Randomized comparisons of radiotherapy and nitrosoureas for the treatment of malignant glioma after surgery. N Engl J Med 1980; 303:1323–1329.
83. Sandberg-Wollheim M, Malmström P, Strömblad LG, et al. A randomized study of chemotherapy with procarbazine, vincristine and lomustine with and without radiation therapy for astrocytoma grades 3 and/or 4. Cancer 1991; 68:22–29.
84. Halperin EC, Bentel G, Heinz ER, Burger PC. Radiation therapy treatment planning in supratentorial glioblastoma multiforme: an analysis based on post mortem topographic anatomy with CT correlations. Int J Radiation Oncol Biol Phys 1989; 17:1347–1350.
85. Aydin H, Sillenberg I, von Lieven H. Patterns of failure following CT-based 3-D irradiation for malignant glioma. Strahlenther Onkol 2001; 8:424–431.
86. Garden AS, Maor M, Yung WKA, et al. Outcome and patterns of failure following limited -volume irradiation for malignant astrocytomas. Radioth Oncol 1991; 20:99–110.
87. Shapiro WR, Green SB, Burger PC, et al. Randomized trial of three chemotherapy regimens and two radiotherapy regimens in postoperative treatment of malignant glioma. J Neurosurg 1989; 71:1–9.
88. Miwa K, Shinoda J, Yano H, et al. Discrepancy between lesion distributions on methionine PET and MR images in patients with glioblastoma multiforme: insight from a PET and MR fusion image study. J Neurol Neurosurg Psychiatry 2004; 75:1457–1462.
89. Chang CH, Horton J, Schoenfeld D, et al. Comparison of postoperative radiotherapy and combined postoperative radiotherapy and chemotherapy in the multidisciplinary management of malignant gliomas. Cancer 1983; 52:997–1007.
90. Werner-Wasik M, Scott CB, Nelson DF, et al. Final report of a phase I/II trial of hyperfractionated and accelerated hyperfractionated radiation therapy with carmustine for adults with supratentorial malignant gliomas. Cancer 1996; 77:1535–1543.

91. Prados MD, Wara WM, Sneed PK, et al. Phase III trial of accelerated hyperfractionation with or without difluromethylornitine (DFMO) versus standard fractionated radiotherapy with or without DFMO for newly diagnosed patients with glioblastoma multiforme. Int J Radiation Oncol Biol Phys 2001; 49:71–77.

92. Selker RG, Shapiro WR, Burger P, et al. The brain tumor cooperative group NIH trial 87/01± a randomized comparison of surgery, external radiotherapy, and carmustine versus surgery, interstitial radiotherapy boost, external radiation therapy, and carmustine. Neurosurgery 2002; 51:343–357.

93. Laperriere NJ, Leung PKM, McKenzie S, et al. Randomized study of brachytherapy in the initial management of patients with malignant astrocytoma. Int J Radiation Oncol Biol Phys 1998; 41:1005–1011.

94. Sneed PK, Stauffer PR, McDermott MW, et al. Survival benefit of hyperthermia in a prospective randomized trial of brachytherapy boost $+/-$ hyperthermia for glioblastoma multiforme. Int J Radiation Oncol Biol Phys 1998; 40:287–295.

95. Glioma Meta-Analysis Group. Chemotherapy in adult high-grade glioma: a systematic review and meta-analysis of individual patient data from 12 randomised trials. Lancet 2002; 359:1011–1018.

96. Hiesiger EM, Green SB, Shapiro WR, et al. Results of a randomized trial comparing intra-arterial cisplatin and intravenous PCNU for the treatment of primary brain tumors in adults: Brain Tumor Cooperative Group trial 8420A. J Neuro-Oncol 1995; 25:143–154.

97. Shapiro WR, Green SB, Burger PC, et al. A randomized comparison of intra-arterial versus intravenous BCNU, with or without intravenous 5-fluorouracil for newly diagnosed patients with malignant glioma. J Neurosurg 1992; 76:772–781.

98. Liassier C, Ben Hassel M, Figarrella-Brancher D, et al. Phase III study comparing high dose BCNU with autologous blood stem cell support versus standard dose BCNU, in combination with radiotherapy after gross total resection in patients with supratentorial glioblastoma. Proc Am Soc Clin Oncol 2003; 22:100.

99. Roa W, Brasher PM, Bauman G, et al. Abbreviated course of radiation therapy in older patients with glioblastoma multiforme: a prospective randomized clinical trial. J Clin Oncol 2004; 22:1583–1588.

100. Keime-Guibert F, Chinot O-L, Taillandier L, et al. Phase 3 study comparing radiotherapy with supportive care in older patients with newly diagnosed anaplastic astrocytomas (AA) or glioblastoma multiforme (GBM): an ANOCEF group trial [abstr 260]. Neuro-Oncology 2005; 7:349.

101. Barker FG, Chang SM, Gutin PH, et al. Survival and functional status after resection of recurrent glioblastoma multiforme. Neurosurgery 1998; 42:709–723.

102. Ammirati M, Galicich JH, Arbit E, Liao Y. Reoperation in the treatment of recurrent intracranial malignant gliomas. Neurosurgery 1987; 21:607–614.

103. Veninga T, Langendijk HA, Slotman BJ, et al. Reirradiation of primary brain tumors: survival, clinical response and prognostic factors. Radioth Oncol 2001; 59:127–137.

104. Yung WK, Albright RE, Olson J, et al. A phase II study of temozolomide vs. procarbazine in patients with glioblastoma multiforme at first relapse. Br J Cancer 2000; 83:588–593.

105. Brada M, Hoang-Xuan K, Rampling R, et al. Multicenter phase II trial of temozolomide in patients with glioblastoma multiforme at first relapse. Ann Oncol 2000; 12:259–266.
106. Kappele AC, Postma TJ, Taphoorn MJ, et al. PCV chemotherapy for recurrent glioblastoma multiforme. Neurology 2001; 56:118–120.
107. Chang SM, Kuhn JG, Rizzo J, et al. Phase I study of paclitaxel in patients with recurrent malignant glioma: a north american brain tumor consortium report. J Clin Oncol 1998; 16:2188–2194.
108. Brem H, Piantadosi S, Burger PC, et al. Placebo-controlled trial of safety and efficacy of intraoperative controlled delivery by biodegradable polymers of chemotherapy for recurrent gliomas. Lancet 1995; 345:1008–1012.
109. Burkhard C, Di Patre P-L, Schüler D, et al. A population-based study of the incidence and survival rates in patients with pilocytic astrocytoma. J Neurosurg 2003; 98:1170–1174.
110. Fernandez C, Figarrella-Brancher D, Girard N, et al. Pilocytic astrocytomas in children: prognostic factors-a retrospective study of 80 cases. Neurosurgery 2003; 53:544–555.
111. Brown PD, Buckner JC, O'Fallon JR, et al. Adult patients with supratentorial pilocytic astrocytomas: a prospective multicenter clinical trial. Int J Radiat Oncol Biol Phys 2004; 58:1153–1160.
112. Boethius J, Ulfarsson E, Rähn T, Lippitz B. Gamma knife radiosurgery for pilocytic astrocytomas. J Neurosurg 2002; 97(suppl 5):677–680.
113. Brown T, Friedman HS, Oakes J, et al. Chemotherapy for pilocytic astrocytomas. Cancer 1993; 71:3165–3172.
114. Dirven CMF, Koudstaal J, Mooij JJ, Molenaar WM. The proliferative potential of the pilocytic astrocytoma: the relation between MIB-1 labeling and clinical and neuro-radiological follow-up. J Neuro-Oncol 1998; 37:9–16.
115. Palma L, Mariottini A. Long-term follow-up of childhood cerebellar astrocytomas after incomplete resection with particular reference to arrested growth or spontaneous tumor regression. Acta Neurochir (Wien) 2004; 146:581–588.
116. Fouladi M, Jenkins J, Burger P, et al. Pleiomorphic xanthoastrocytoma: favorable outcome after complete surgical resection. Neuro-Oncology 2001; 3:184–192.
117. Giannini C, Hebrink D, Scheithauer BW, Dei Tos AP, James CD. Analysis of p53 mutations and expression in pleiomorphic xanthoastrocytoma. Neurogenetics 2001; 3:159–162.
118. Klaulich K, Blaschke B, Numann A, et al. Genetic alterations commonly found in diffusely infiltrating cerebral gliomas are rare or absent in pleiomorphic xantroastrocytomas. J Neuropathol Exp Neurol 2002; 61:1092–1099.
119. Giannini C, Scheithauer BW, Burger PC, et al. Pleiomorphic xantroastrocytoma. What do we really know about it? Cancer 1999; 85:2033–2045.
120. Nishio S, Morioka T, Suzuki S, et al. Subependymal giant cell astrocytoma: clinical and neuro-imaging features of four cases. J Clin Neurosc 2001; 8:31–34.
121. Cuccia V, Zuccaro G, Sosa F, et al. Subependymal giant cell astrocytoma in children with tuberous sclerosis. Childs Nerv Syst 2003; 19:232–243.

122. Nabbout R, Santos M, Rollnad Y, et al. Early diagnosis of subependymal giant cell astrocytoma in children with tuberous sclerosis. J Neurol Neurosurg Psych 1999; 66:370–375.
123. Kim S-I, Wang K-C, Cho B-K, et al. Biological behaviour and tumorigenesis of subependymal giant cell astrocytomas. J Neuro-Oncol 2001; 52:217–225.

9

Oligodendroglioma and Mixed Tumors

Ravi D. Rao and Jan C. Buckner

Department of Oncology, Mayo Clinic College of Medicine,
Rochester, Minnesota, U.S.A.

Robert Jenkins

Department of Laboratory Medicine, Mayo Clinic College of Medicine,
Rochester, Minnesota, U.S.A.

INTRODUCTION

Oligodendrogliomas are a subset of primary brain tumors with characteristic pathological, genetic, and clinical features. Histologically, the tumor cells in oligodendrogliomas resemble normal oligodendroglial cells, hence the nomenclature. Tumors that have a combination of oligodendroglial and astrocytic elements are termed as "mixed" tumors or oligoastrocytomas. Because there are no objective diagnostic criteria established for these tumors, the determination that a tumor (or a portion of any given tumor) is an oligodendroglioma has been based to a large extent on a subjective decision on the part of the pathologist.

The defining clinical characteristic of oligodendroglial tumors is that they are significantly more responsive to chemotherapy and are associated with much better outcomes when compared to other gliomas. Genetically, these tumors are characterized by the common occurrence of deletions of 1p and/or 19q. This "genetic signature" appears to correlate with pathology (i.e., tumors with these deletions have a more classical morphology), clinical behavior (responsiveness to chemotherapy and duration of response), and perhaps with even certain imaging characteristics. Genetic testing for

193

detection of the 1p and 19q deletions has now become commercially available. The widespread use of these tests has resulted in a better understanding of the relationship between the morphology, genetics, and clinical behavior of these tumors. These developments have led to a more diligent effort by pathologists at identifying oligodendroglial tumors. As a result of these efforts, the proportion of primary gliomas that are identified as having an oligodendroglial component has increased from 5% in the past to approximately 15% in some recent studies.

Several effective chemotherapeutic regimens have been identified to treat these tumors. Ongoing research efforts are focused on obtaining a better understanding of the genetics of this disease (as it relates to pathogenesis and responsiveness to therapy), and to identify better treatment strategies.

EPIDEMIOLOGY AND ETIOLOGY

There are no data regarding the epidemiology of oligodendrogliomas as a distinct entity. These tumors are grouped together with other gliomas in most cancer epidemiological studies. Moreover, because there is no single defining characteristic of these tumors, the diagnosis is observer dependent. For these reasons, it is difficult to determine the exact population incidence of these tumors.

As with most other primary brain tumors, the etiology of oligodendrogliomas is not known. Most of these tumors occur sporadically. There are some anecdotal case reports of familial occurrences of oligodendrogliomas. However, for the vast majority of patients with these tumors, there is no evidence of any hereditary predisposition.

PATHOLOGY AND MOLECULAR PATHOGENESIS

Oligodendrogliomas are characterized by the presence of uniformly round-oval cells with round nuclei and bland chromatin. Another typical characteristic is the presence of a background of a network of delicate capillary proliferation, termed as "chicken wire vasculature." The tumor cells are often described as having a "fried egg appearance" due to the presence of a perinuclear halo (which is actually an artifact of fixation). The diagnosis of oligodendroglioma is made predominantly using these morphological characteristics; there are no distinguishing immunohistochemical staining patterns. "Pure" oligodendrogliomas are tumors that have cells of this description as the sole cell type. However, approximately one in three of these tumors has an admixture of cells that are morphologically astrocytic; these tumors are termed as "mixed" oligoastrocytoma. The percentage of each component needed to classify a tumor as mixed is not clearly defined. Therefore, the diagnosis is often subject to interobserver variation. Most studies and clinical trials of oligodendrogliomas include patients with both pure and mixed lineage. Oligodendrogliomas can be classified as either low-grade (grade 2) or high-grade (grade 3 or anaplastic) tumors based on morphological features such as necrosis, mitoses, and cellular atypical and endothelial proliferation. Approximately half of all oligodendroglial tumors are low-grade tumors (1). A majority of these low-grade oligodendroglial tumors eventually progress into higher grade tumors (1). The World Health Organization classification of primary brain tumors classifies all high-grade oligodendroglial tumors as anaplastic (analogous to grade 3 or anaplastic astrocytomas). However, there does appear to be distinct a subset of high-grade oligodendroglial tumors with morphological features that are typical for grade 4 astrocytoma, i.e., glioblastoma multiforme (2). Patients with tumors with these features have a prognosis that is similar to (though somewhat better than) that of those with pure grade 4 astrocytoma patients (i.e., glioblastoma multiforme).

The characteristic genetic lesions seen in oligodendroglial tumors are the deletions of the short arm of chromosome 1 (1p) and long arm of chromosome 19 (19q) (3). These deletions are independently associated with responsiveness to chemotherapy, with duration of response to chemotherapy, and with better overall survival (independent of therapy received) (4,5). The exact etiological role of the genes deleted at these sites in the causation of these tumors is not known. Observations regarding the correlation between these mutations and histology, chemotherapy sensitivity, and survival provide insights into the function of the genes at these locations. It is postulated that a tumor suppressor gene as well as other gene(s) associated with chemotherapy resistance is located at these sites. One pertinent observation has been the correlation between these deletions and the inactivation of the DNA repair enzyme O6-methylguanine DNA methyltransferase, which has been associated with sensitivity to alkylating chemotherapy agents in gliomas (6).

Deletions at either locus (1p or 19q) occur in 75% of all low-grade (i.e., grade 2) oligodendroglial tumors (3,7). Simultaneous deletions of both loci occur in approximately two-thirds of all low-grade oligodendroglioma. Because the diagnostic criteria for these tumors are variable, the proportions of patients found to have tumors carrying these mutations vary between different reports. High-grade oligodendroglioma are also characterized by a similar incidence of 1p and 19q deletions. Additionally, high-grade tumors have been found to have several nonrandom mutations; these include loss of 9p, 10q, and the CDKN2A gene (8), mutations that are typically found in high-grade astrocytomas. The occurrence of these additional genetic abnormalities has been correlated with the presence of tumor necrosis and microvascular proliferation—morphological characteristics that define high-grade histology. These additional mutations, as a rule, do not occur in low-grade oligodendrogliomas, suggesting that they may be involved in tumor dedifferentiation. The presence of deletions of 1p and 19q are closely associated with the typical morphological appearance of pure oligodendroglioma, and occur less often in tumors with atypical or mixed histology.

In contrast to pure oligodendrogliomas, tumors with a mixed histology have a less-specific genetic signature. Deletions of 1p and 19q occur less frequently (~20–40% of these tumors), and are accompanied by several other genetic mutations. Interestingly, when these mutations occur in mixed oligodendrogliomas (or in pure astrocytomas, where they occur in ~5% of cases), they appear to portend a more favorable prognosis (9).

Much attention has been focused on the association between deletions of 1p/19q and a good prognosis. While the presence of 1p/19q deletions is associated with an unusual degree of sensitivity to chemotherapy, the absence of these deletions does not imply chemotherapy resistance–a large proportion of tumors with intact 1p/19q chromosomes are chemotherapy sensitive. Therefore, the mutational states of 1p and 19q should not be used to make clinical decisions. This issue will be highlighted later in the text. Because the 1p/19q status is a very powerful prognostic factor, testing for these mutations has become an important tool for physicians and patients.

CLINICAL PRESENTATION AND DIAGNOSIS

Low-grade oligodendroglial tumors occur in young patients: median age of these patients is in their late 30s or early 40s (1). Higher grade tumors seem to occur in somewhat older patients (in their 50s). There appears to be a slight male predominance among patients enrolled in clinical trials, suggesting a gender difference. Patients with oligodendroglioma are almost always detected when they develop symptoms from their brain tumor. In a vast majority (>70%) of patients with these tumors, the onset of seizures prompts the diagnosis (1). Other common symptoms include headaches and cognitive and focal neurological deficits. The most common location is the frontal lobe. Low-grade tumors uncommonly (≤10%) demonstrate enhancement with intravenous contrast on computed tomography or magnetic resonance imaging, while high-grade tumors typically (>80%) do so. Around half of oligodendroglial tumors demonstrate calcification on imaging studies, a radiological feature that may help distinguish them from other primary brain tumors.

PROGNOSIS

Several clinical, radiological, pathological, and genetic factors have been noted to be of prognostic value in these patients. In a variety of prospective and retrospective studies, the following features have been noted to be associated with better outcomes: younger age, presentation with seizures, better performance score, absence of neurological deficits at diagnosis, lack of cognitive deficits (at diagnosis), lack of enhancement with contrast use on imaging studies, lower grade of tumor, pure histology (as opposed to tumors with a mixed histology), low mitotic index, larger extent of resection, deletions of 1p or 19q or the combination, and lack of additional genetic mutations (e.g., loss of 10p, epidermal growth factor receptor (EGFR) amplification, CDKN2A deletion). Because many of these factors are known to be associated with a better prognosis in diffuse glial tumors in general, the finding of these associations in patients with oligodendroglial tumors is not necessarily unexpected. Not surprisingly, factors that portend a favorable (or poor) prognosis are strongly correlated with each other, e.g., younger patients more often present with low-grade tumors, which do not have contrast enhancement. The best validated *independent* favorable prognostic factors are young age, good performance score, low grade, and loss of 1p and 19q (5).

Younger patients with oligodendrogliomas have consistently been shown to have better outcomes than older patients. Similarly, patients with low-grade tumors have a better prognosis than those with high-grade tumors. Patients with low-grade oligodendrogliomas have a median survival of 7 to 10 years (1), while patients who are initially diagnosed as having an anaplastic (i.e., grade 3) oligodendroglioma have a median survival of three to five years (5,10). Patients with grade 4 oligodendrogliomas have a survival that is relatively poor, with a median of one to two years.

Much attention has recently been drawn to the association between the loss of 1p and 19q and good prognosis in these patients. This association in anaplastic oligodendroglioma was first noted by Cairncross et al. in Canada (4), and subsequently has been confirmed in many prospective and retrospective studies of these tumors (5,10,11). The association between 1p and 19q deletions and prognosis also holds true for low-grade tumors (12). To summarize the findings so far (i) combined loss of 1p and 19q is the most powerful good prognostic factor predicting better overall survival in patients in oligodendroglioma, and is more powerful than histology (i.e., grade of tumor) in this regard, (ii) loss of 1p (either as the sole abnormality or in combination with other abnormalities) has a strong association with sensitivity to alkylating chemotherapeutic agents, and with the duration of such a response, (iii) patients whose tumors have intact 1p and 19q have shorter progression-free durations and overall survival when compared to those with these deletions, (iv) differences in outcomes between the 1p/19q deletion and 1p/19q intact groups persist even after the use of optimal chemotherapy and radiation therapy, (v) even though patients with 1p/19q deletions are chemotherapy sensitive, using chemotherapy in the up-front therapy of these patients has so far not demonstrated improved survival (when compared to a strategy of delaying chemotherapy use till disease progression), and (vi) subsets of oligodendroglioma that have mutations more characteristic of high-grade astrocytomas (e.g., EGFR, p53 mutations) have a prognosis that is worse than that of patients without these mutations. Indeed, the data available regarding this issue suggests that there may be several clinically relevant groups of oligodendrogliomas based on genetic typing (13). This last observation has not been confirmed in prospective clinical trials.

THERAPY

Therapy of oligodendroglioma patients needs a multidisciplinary approach. The medical team needs to consist of neurosurgeons, neurologists, and medical and radiation oncologists. Additional help from several ancillary specialists (e.g., psychology and physical therapy) and diagnostic specialties (neuroradiology, neuropathology, and laboratory-based genetic diagnostics) may be invaluable. The care of these patients is perhaps best done at (or at least coordinated by) tertiary-care medical centers, where such specialists are available. This approach also has the additional advantage of allowing patients to have access to the most current clinical trials.

Typically, therapy of primary brain tumors requires a combination of surgery, radiation, and chemotherapy. Our understanding of the relative roles of radiation and chemotherapy in the up-front therapy of oligodendroglioma patients is currently in a state of flux, as is our understanding of the interaction between 1p and 19q deletions, responses to therapy, and outcomes.

SURGERY

Surgical therapy of oligodendroglioma and mixed tumors follows the same principles as those of other gliomas. Surgical resection is indicated for the following reasons: (i) to obtain a tissue diagnosis, (ii) to obtain a reduction of symptoms (especially seizures), and (iii) to reduce morbidity due to mass effect. The degree of resection that a neurosurgeon can perform depends upon several factors, including the location of the tumor, size, and the technical expertise of the sureon. Surgery undoubtedly has a beneficial effect on cancer-related outcomes, though the degree of correlation between the completeness of resection and the improvement in outcomes is unclear. Patients who have a more extensive resection appear to have better outcomes, though it is unclear if this relationship is actually due to the beneficial effect of extensive debulking or merely due to the correlation between tumor location and surgical resectability. Many of these questions regarding relationship between the extent of resection and prognosis cannot be practically answered by a randomized clinical trial. Hence a reasonable approach to surgery would be to perform the most extensive resection possible without causing excessive neurological damage.

RADIATION

High-Grade Oligodendroglioma

Several clinical trials have conclusively demonstrated that in newly diagnosed high-grade glioma patients, treatment with radiation after surgical resection clearly improves progression-free survival, overall survival, and quality of life. Most of these trials enrolled patients with high-grade gliomas of all subtypes, including many patients with oligodendroglial tumors; hence the conclusions are readily applicable to this subgroup. Attempts to improve outcomes by modifying radiation protocols (e.g., increasing doses and changing fractionation schedules) have been attempted, and not found to improve outcomes. The current standard is to use 60 Gy in 30 fractions to treat the tumor along with a 2-cm margin.

The use of chemotherapy early in the therapy of these patients is currently under investigation. The rationale behind these investigations is that the use of effective chemotherapy in conjunction with radiation would result in improvements in cancer-related outcomes with less neurologic toxicity. This approach will be discussed later in the chapter.

Low-Grade Oligodendroglioma

There is some divergence of opinion regarding the optimal management of patients with low-grade tumors, mainly related to the timing of radiation therapy. A logical argument can be made for observing relatively asymptomatic patients without active anticancer therapy and to intervene only when required to do so by tumor progression. The main arguments in favor of this approach is that (i) low-grade oligodendroglioma are relatively slow growing tumors, and if left untreated after diagnosis, become symptomatic only after a long interval of many years, (ii) all therapeutic modalities are associated with toxicities that impact on quality of life, and most importantly, (iii) none of the therapy options available are definitively curative [though prolonged (e.g., >15 years) survival without recurrence has been known to occur after therapy]. Thus, early decrements in quality of life caused by therapy need to be considered in the context that the therapy is not curative and does not prolong survival. Retrospective data suggests that patients who have radiologically suspected low-grade gliomas, but are observed without active therapy, have outcomes that are similar to those who underwent immediate therapy (14). This approach would avoid the adverse effects of therapy (especially decreases in cognitive function) in this young patient population. An alternate approach would be to treat with radiation at the time of diagnosis, with the expectation that this would delay the onset of tumor-related symptoms.

An attempt was made to answer this debate with the conduct of a randomized clinical trial by European investigators, which compared the strategies of using early versus delayed radiation therapy (15). Patients with low-grade gliomas with a good performance status and few or no neurological symptoms were randomized to receive therapy according to each strategy. This trial found that early radiation resulted in an improvement in progression-free survival, but did not impact on overall survival. There were no significant decrements in quality of life with the early-treatment approach. The result of this important clinical trial can be interpreted that either approach is equivalent from an oncological standpoint. Therefore, treatment decisions can be individualized based on patient and physician preferences. Although this study included low-grade gliomas of all histologies, a significant proportion (one-third) of all patients enrolled in this study had an oligodendroglial component, thus the results are readily applicable to these patients.

The impact of radiation on cognition in patients with low-grade tumors remains under investigation. Cognitive changes that occur in these patients have often been attributed to radiation. However, retrospective data is confounded by the use of different overall doses, fraction sizes, and the presence of other comorbid conditions. Radiation-induced cognitive deficits appear to be associated with the use of larger fraction sizes (>2 Gy) and are uncommon with the currently used fractionation schemes (16). An under-recognized confounding factor is the concomitant common use of anticonvulsant medications in this population, which may be associated with significant impairment of cognition. Data from some prospective studies in this patient population suggests that the cognitive deficits are mostly attributable to the tumor (at baseline) and to growth of the tumor, rather than to therapy (17). Most patients who have stability of their tumor do not have significant changes in their cognitive status (18). Thus, when these factors are accounted for, the use of standard fractionated radiation may not be associated with excessive neurotoxicity.

Another controversial issue in the past was regarding the optimal dose of radiation to be used to treat these patients. This issue was tested in two trials where patients were randomized to receive high- and low-dose schedules of radiation. Radiation dose escalation did not translate into an improved outcomes and was associated with significant toxicity and deterioration in quality of life measures (19,20).

CHEMOTHERAPY

High-Grade Oligodendroglioma

High-grade oligodendrogliomas are chemotherapy-sensitive tumors. This observation was made by investigators in the late 1980s and early 1990s (21). These observations resulted in the conduct of a prospective North American trial led by the National Cancer Institute, Canada, to test the utility of treating patients with anaplastic oligodendroglioma with procarbazine, CCNU, and vincristine (PCV) chemotherapy (22). Chemotherapy administration resulted in response rates of 75%, which is a remarkable degree of chemosensitivity for a high-grade primary brain tumor. Subsequent studies have demonstrated that the sensitivity is not limited merely to PCV, but that some of these tumors respond to a variety of alkylating chemotherapy agents, including temozolomide (TMZ) and carmustine (BCNU) (10,21,23). Most recent investigations have focused on temozolomide, a drug that is less toxic than the PCV combination.

On average, the response rates for these chemotherapy regimens when used in the first line setting are 60% to 70% (22,24), with a median progression-free survival of one to two years. Whether chemotherapy changes the natural history of this disease is not known, because no trials comparing them to best supportive care have been performed.

A strategy under intense investigation is to use chemotherapy early (in an adjuvant manner after initial surgery), either before, during, or immediately after radiation. The benefits of such an approach would be to delay tumor progression, reduce potential radiation-induced toxicity (as the tumor size may be reduced), and possibly to improve survival by the combined use of the most effective therapies early in the course of the disease. Several studies are currently in progress to clarify these questions.

The first of these studies to be reported was RTOG 94–02. Patients with anaplastic pure or mixed oligodendroglioma were randomized to receive immediate radiation therapy (59.4 Gy), or four cycles of PCV followed by radiation. Most patients in the radiation-alone arm received PCV therapy when they eventually progressed. The preliminary results of this study were reported in June 2004. Only a small fraction (20%) of patients progressed during the chemotherapy phase. PCV use was associated with significant toxicity, with a substantial proportion (one-fourth) of patients not being able to complete the stipulated therapy due to (mainly hematological) toxicity. Progression-free survival was longer in the combination therapy arm (median of 2.5 years), when compared to those treated with radiation alone (median 1.9 years) ($p = 0.053$). However, this benefit did not translate into an improvement in overall survival (median of 4.9 years in the combined therapy arm and 4.7 years in the radiation-alone arm) in the combined modality arm. Upon subset analysis, the prolongation in the progression free survival in the chemotherapy arm was present in those with intact 1p/19q (though the benefit was somewhat less than that seen in patients with 1p/19q deletion). In spite of the benefit noted from chemotherapy in the 1p/19q deletion subset, this group did not demonstrate a survival benefit over those not treated with chemotherapy. Overall, the median survival in all patients with combined loss of 1p/19q is more than 6 years, and 2.8 years in those without (5). These preliminary data suggest that adjuvant PCV delivered prior to radiation may be an appropriate choice for patients with anaplastic oligodendroglial tumors (5). This large prospective trial confirms the impressive prognostic value of 1p/19q deletional status of tumors. The results of this trial also argue against using the 1p/19q status to make clinical decisions regarding chemotherapy use.

More recently, early results of a related European study, EORTC 26591, were presented (10). This study investigated the possibility that the use of adjuvant PCV *after* completion of radiation would improve outcomes. Patients who completed radiation (33 Gy) were randomized to receiving six cycles of PCV, or to an observation arm. Only 25% were able to complete the entire course of six cycles of therapy, with the most common reason for therapy discontinuation being hematological toxicity from PCV. The progression-free survival was significantly improved (median increased from 12 to 23 months), while the overall survival demonstrated a minor, statistically nonsignificant improvement in those treated with PCV. Most patients who progressed (on either arm) were treated with additional chemotherapy (either PCV or TMZ), a factor that may have masked a potential survival benefit. This study can be interpreted as a comparison between early and late chemotherapy strategies, and suggests that both seem to be appropriate choices. The benefits of chemotherapy (in terms of effect on progression-free survival) were not limited to the 1p/19q deletion group, as even those without these mutations benefited (again arguing against using this factor to make clinical decisions). Similar to RTOG 94-02, this study found that when adjusted for 1p/19q deletion status, the overall survival was not dependent upon the therapy received. Again, similar to the findings in RTOG 94-02, the chemotherapy-related improvements in response rates in the 1p/19q deletion subset did not translate into prolongation of survival.

Another relevant study in this regard that explored the use of TMZ in this disease setting is RTOG 0131 (11). This is a single-arm phase II study that evaluated the role of TMZ in the adjuvant phase, before the use of radiation (with a strategy similar to that tested in RTOG 94-02). Patients with anaplastic oligodendroglioma were treated with six months of TMZ before undergoing radiation. Almost all patients had either a response or stable disease when treated with TMZ. Early results are encouraging; only 10% of patients progressed before completion of the stipulated course of TMZ (which compares favorably with data from RTOG 94-02). Data on correlations between genotype and responses are not currently available and would be important in interpreting the results of this study when available. Because TMZ is less toxic than PCV and appears to be at least as effective as PCV, TMZ may be the drug of choice in future trials. With this emerging data about the benefits of using chemotherapy up front in the therapy of these patients, an interesting research (and practice) question will be to determine if concurrent radiation and chemotherapy result in improvements in survival in this patient population when compared to radiation alone. This strategy seems promising as it has been shown to improve survival in grade 4 astrocytoma patients, a disease that is inherently more therapy resistant than does oligodendroglioma (25). When this strategy is adopted, TMZ will likely prove to be the drug of choice, as the safety of combining it with radiation has been established (25).

Because oligodendrogliomas are responsive to chemotherapy, the idea of dose escalation, in conjunction with an autologous stem cell transplant, has also been investigated in refractory or recurrent anaplastic oligodendroglioma. In one study, 40% of those enrolled had long lasting responses after high-dose chemotherapy (thiotepa) and stem cell rescue (26). Of all patients enrolled, a significant proportion (43%) was unable to undergo a transplant for a variety of reasons (mainly disease progression). Not surprisingly, patients who had residual tumor enhancement toward the completion of high-dose therapy (i.e., presumably had chemotherapy resistant tumors) had the highest risk of relapse after the transplant. Currently, this approach should be considered experimental and should not be used outside of a clinical trial setting.

Low-Grade Oligodendroglioma

Low-grade oligodendroglioma are also chemotherapy-sensitive tumors (27). However, the use of systemic chemotherapy at the time of initial diagnosis may not be appropriate for these tumors without comparing this to other therapy modalities (e.g., radiation, observation with delayed therapy). Because these patients are often asymptomatic, the use of potentially toxic, and noncurative, therapy is not justifiable in the absence of data suggesting that early chemotherapy has some long-term benefits. The use of such a strategy in high-risk patients (who are most likely to progress) remains the subject of ongoing investigation.

Relationship Between Genetic Abnormalities and Chemotherapy Response

Tumors that have deletions of 1p are unusually sensitive to chemotherapy; almost all patients harboring such tumors respond to alkylating agents (4). Similarly, loss of 19q is associated with a high response rate to chemotherapy. However, the latter correlation does not persist once adjustments are made for the 1p status. Absence of these deletions, however, does not imply chemotherapy resistance: up to one-third of those patients in this category can still respond to chemotherapy (13). Data from prospective studies suggests that patients with intact 1p/19q also benefit from the use of chemotherapy (as indicated by prolongations in progression-free survival), though to lesser extent than those with these mutations (5,10). Therefore, based on these data, the currently available data do not support limiting chemotherapy use only to those with 1p/19q deletions.

Progressive Oligodendroglioma

In spite of this tumor being sensitive to therapy, all patients with oligodendroglioma eventually progress and become symptomatic. Radiation therapy–naïve patients with progressive oligodendroglioma have the option of being treated with radiation. Surgery may be considered if the tumor is associated with mass effect and can be safely debulked. The use of PCV or single-agent TMZ appears to lead to responses in large proportions of patients with progressive high-grade oligodendroglial tumors (28,29). The rates of response and disease stabilization as high as 70% have been reported in some of these trials. For those patients who achieve a response, the response lasts typically for one to two years. Response to therapy may not be different in those who received prior radiation when compared to radiation-naïve patients (22), though it remains to be seen if patients who have previously received up-front chemotherapy at the time of diagnosis (as in RTOG 94-02 or EORTC 26591) remain as chemotherapy sensitive when treated at relapse many years later. Currently available data demonstrates that when tumors progress while on chemotherapy, they continue to maintain responsiveness to other second- and third-line chemotherapy agents (28,30). One caveat in interpreting these study results is that biopsies were not obtained at time of progression; therefore, the exact pathological status of the tumor at the time of radiological progression was unknown. The implications of a response to either of these regimens on overall neurological status, long-term disease-free survival, or overall survival remain to be evaluated.

REFERENCES

1. Shaw EG et al. Oligodendrogliomas: the Mayo Clinic experience. J Neurosurg 1992; 76(3):428–434.
2. Kraus JA et al. Molecular genetic alterations in glioblastomas with oligodendroglial component. Acta Neuropathol (Berl) 2001; 101(4):311–320.
3. Reifenberger J et al. Molecular genetic analysis of oligodendroglial tumors shows preferential allelic deletions on 19q and 1p. Am J Pathol 1994; 145(5): 1175–1190.
4. Cairncross JG et al. Specific genetic predictors of chemotherapeutic response and survival in patients with anaplastic oligodendrogliomas. J Natl Cancer Inst 1998; 90(19):1473–1479.
5. Cairncross G et al. An intergroup randomized controlled clinical trial (RCT) of chemotherapy plus radiation (RT) versus RT alone for pure and mixed anaplastic oligodendrogliomas: initial report of RTOG 94–02. Abstract No: 1500. J Clin Oncol 2004; 22:14S.
6. Mollemann M et al. Frequent promoter hypermethylation and low expression of the MGMT gene in oligodendroglial tumors. Int J Cancer 2005; 113(3):379–385.
7. Smith JS et al. Localization of common deletion regions on 1p and 19q in human gliomas and their association with histological subtype. Oncogene 1999; 18(28):4144–4152.
8. Bigner SH et al. Molecular genetic aspects of oligodendrogliomas including analysis by comparative genomic hybridization. Am J Pathol 1999; 155(2):375–386.
9. Ino Y et al. Long survival and therapeutic responses in patients with histologically disparate high-grade gliomas demonstrating chromosome 1p loss. J Neurosurg 2000; 92(6):983–990.
10. van den Bent M et al. First analysis of EORTC trial 26951, a randomized phase III study of adjuvant PCV chemotherapy in patients with highly anaplastic oligodendroglioma. Abstract No: 1503. J Clin Oncol 2005; 23:16S.

11. Vogelbaum M et al. RTOG 0131: phase II trial of pre-irradiation and concurrent temozolomide in patients with newly diagnosed anaplastic oligodendrogliomas and mixed anaplastic oligodendrogliomas. Abstract No: 1520. J Clin Oncol 2005; 23:16S.

12. Buckner J et al. Diagnostic and prognostic significance of 1p and 19q deletions in patients with low-grade oligodendroglioma and astrocytoma: NCCTG 94–72–53. Abstract No: 1502. J Clin Oncol 2005; 23:16S.

13. Ino Y et al. Molecular subtypes of anaplastic oligodendroglioma: implications for patient management at diagnosis. Clin Cancer Res 2001; 7(4):839–845.

14. Recht LD, Lew R, Smith TW. Suspected low-grade glioma: is deferring treatment safe? Ann Neurol 1992; 31(4):431–436.

15. Karim AB et al. Randomized trial on the efficacy of radiotherapy for cerebral low-grade glioma in the adult: European organization for research and treatment of cancer study 22845 with the medical research council study BRO4: an interim analysis. Int J Radiat Oncol Biol Phys 2002; 52(2):316–324.

16. Taphoorn MJ. Neurocognitive sequelae in the treatment of low-grade gliomas. Semin Oncol 2003; 30(6 suppl 19):45–48.

17. Brown PD et al. Effects of radiotherapy on cognitive function in patients with low-grade glioma measured by the folstein mini-mental state examination. J Clin Oncol 2003; 21(13):2519–2524.

18. Laack NN et al. Cognitive function after radiotherapy for supratentorial low-grade glioma: a north central cancer treatment group prospective study. Int J Radiat Oncol Biol Phys 2005; 63(4):1175–1183.

19. Karim AB et al. A randomized trial on dose-response in radiation therapy of low-grade cerebral glioma: European Organization for Research and Treatment of Cancer (EORTC) Study 22844. Int J Radiat Oncol Biol Phys 1996; 36(3): 549–556.

20. Shaw E et al. Prospective randomized trial of low- versus high-dose radiation therapy in adults with supratentorial low-grade glioma: initial report of a north central cancer treatment group/radiation therapy oncology group/eastern cooperative oncology group study. J Clin Oncol 2002; 20(9):2267–2276.

21. Cairncross JG, Macdonald DR. Successful chemotherapy for recurrent malignant oligodendroglioma. Ann Neurol 1988; 23(4):360–364.

22. Cairncross G et al. Chemotherapy for anaplastic oligodendroglioma. National Cancer Institute of Canada Clinical Trials group. J Clin Oncol 1994; 12(10): 2013–2021.

23. Peterson N et al. Salvage chemotherapy for recurrent malignant oligodendrogliomas. Abstract No: 294. Proc Annu Meet Am Soc of Clin Oncol 1995.

24. van den Bent MJ et al. Phase II study of first-line chemotherapy with temozolomide in recurrent oligodendroglial tumors: the European organization for research and treatment of cancer brain tumor group study 26971. J Clin Oncol 2003; 21(13):2525–2528.

25. Stupp R et al. Radiotherapy plus concomitant and adjuvant temozolomide for glioblastoma. N Engl J Med 2005; 352(10):987–996.

26. Abrey LE et al. High-dose chemotherapy with stem cell rescue as initial therapy for anaplastic oligodendroglioma. J Neurooncol 2003; 65(2):127–134.

27. Brada M et al. Phase II study of primary temozolomide chemotherapy in patients with WHO grade II gliomas. Ann Oncol 2003; 14(12):1715–1721.

28. van den Bent MJ et al. Second-line chemotherapy with temozolomide in recurrent oligodendroglioma after PCV (procarbazine, lomustine and vincristine) chemotherapy: EORTC brain tumor group phase II study 26972. Ann Oncol 2003; 14(4):599–602.

29. Brandes AA et al. Efficacy and feasibility of standard procarbazine, lomustine, and vincristine chemotherapy in anaplastic oligodendroglioma and oligoastrocytoma recurrent after radiotherapy. A phase II study. Cancer 2004; 101(9): 2079–2085.

30. Triebels VH et al. Salvage PCV chemotherapy for temozolomide-resistant oligodendrogliomas. Neurology 2004; 63(5):904–906.

10

Ependymal Tumors

Mark Dannenbaum and Raymond Sawaya

Department of Neurosurgery, Baylor College of Medicine, and Department of Neurosurgery, The University of Texas M.D. Anderson Cancer Center, Houston, Texas, U.S.A.

INTRODUCTION

Ependymal tumors represent a diverse collection of brain neoplasms with a multitude of clinical presentations. This chapter will analyze the salient clinical features necessary for the clinician to successfully diagnose and manage ependymoma and anaplastic ependymoma, intramedullary ependymoma, myxopapillary ependymoma, and subependymoma. These neoplasms are of neuroectodermal origin and arise from the neuroepithelial lining of the ventricles, central canal of the spinal cord, choroid plexus, white matter adjacent to a ventricular surface, and filum terminale. They are classified by the World Health Organization (WHO) as subependymoma (grade I), ependymoma (grade II), anaplastic ependymoma (grade III), and myxopapillary ependymoma (grade I). The focus of this review will be on epidemiology, specific clinical features, therapy, and prognosis, as detailed reviews of pathology and radiology are addressed elsewhere. The unifying theme among the ependymal tumors is that they all require surgical resection as the exclusive therapy or as part of it.

EPENDYMOMA

Epidemiology

Intracerebral ependymoma is a rare tumor with an incidence of 0.3 per 100,000 patient-years (at risk) in adults and children (1). These tumors primarily affect young children and constitute the third most common histologic type of brain tumor in children, after primitive neuroectodermal tumors (PNET) and astrocytomas. They account for approximately 5% to 10% of all childhood primary brain tumors and roughly 1% to 5% of adult intracranial tumors. The mean age of diagnosis is between 3 and 6, with a male to female ratio of 1.4 to 1 (1). Patients with neurofibromatosis type II (NF-2) develop ependymoma with a greater frequency than is seen in the general population. Although ependymoma has no clear-cut environmental cause, there is some epidemiologic evidence linking it to the oncogenic DNA virus—simian virus 40 (SV40) (2). Ependymomas frequently originate from the floor of the fourth ventricle, with 75% occurring below the tentorium (3). Posterior fossa ependymomas are more common in children less than three years old, whereas supratentorial lesions tend to be more common in children over age 3 (4). Supratentorial ependymomas arise more often in the lateral ventricle or, when intraparenchymal, they are in proximity to a surface lined by ependyma. When located supratentorially, they are frequently considered more readily resectable but are more often of high grade (5).

Clinical Presentation

Ependymomas frequently produce nonspecific symptoms of increased intracranial pressure (ICP) as a result of their propensity to cause hydrocephalus. Patients commonly present with headache, nausea, vomiting, and lethargy. Often patients will experience a headache in the morning that improves throughout the day and becomes more persistent as the disease progresses. If the cerebellar tonsils herniate into the cervical canal, a head tilt (mimicking torticollis) may occur. Patients may experience nausea without other symptoms of increased ICP, if the tumor arises in the area postrema or obex. A somewhat distinctive feature of ependymoma is its tendency to grow into the cerebellopontine (CP) angle via the foramen of Luschka and produce facial weakness, hearing loss, and dysphagia.

Preoperative Workup

Most patients will undergo magnetic resonance imaging (MRI) and computed tomography (CT) scanning of the brain, with and without contrast enhancement. These studies not only assist in surgical planning but also help guide the judgment of the treatment team, based on the presence of preoperative disseminated disease. In such cases, the surgical resection will usually be less aggressive when gross-total resection is not possible and risks of

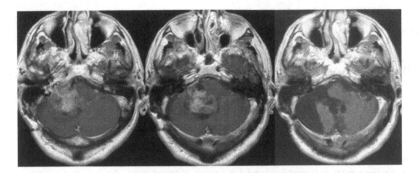

Figure 1 Magnetic resonance images (MRIs), of a patient with ependymoma. Preoperative T1-weighted contrast-enhanced MRI showing an axial view of a large fourth ventricle ependymoma extending through the right foramen of Luschka and attaching to the dura of the cerebellopontine angle (*left* and *center*). Postoperative axial T1-weighted contrast-enhanced MRI showing gross-total resection of the tumor (*right*).

neurologic morbidity cannot be justified. CT scans in most cases reveal a heterogeneous mass, associated with calcifications, that squeezes through the fourth ventricular outlet foramina into the CP-angle cistern and cisterna magna. MRI (Fig. 1) reveals heterogeneous signals on both T1 and T2 images, with variable contrast enhancement.

As mentioned earlier, patients commonly have significant hydrocephalus preoperatively. No consensus exists regarding the optimum management of this situation. Some advocate steroid administration and early tumor resection, whereas others believe that performing a preoperative ventriculostomy or placing a ventriculoperitoneal shunt prior to tumor removal is more advantageous. A review by McLaurin points out that the risks and benefits of these approaches balance each other (6). More recently, Saint-Rose et al. proposed the use of a preoperative endoscopic third ventriculostomy prior to definitive surgery in patients with posterior fossa masses (7).

Diagnosis and Differential Diagnosis

In children, PNET, cerebellar pilocytic astrocytoma, and atypical rhabdoid/teratoid tumor need to be considered in the differential diagnosis of ependymoma. In adults, the differential is more location dependent but will include choroid plexus papilloma, subependymoma, oligodendroglioma, and glioblastoma multiforme. Microscopically, these tumors display perivascular pseudorosettes and, less often, will have accompanying true ependymal rosettes. They show positive immunohistochemical staining for S100, glial fibrillary acidic protein, and vimentin. Ependymoma is considered a WHO grade II neoplasm, whereas its counterpart, the anaplastic ependymoma, is considered WHO grade III. The significance of histologic grade will be addressed in the section on prognosis.

Therapy

As previously mentioned, the primary treatment for ependymoma is surgical resection. Aggressive attempts should be made to achieve gross-total resection of the tumor (Fig. 1) to relieve the mass effect and to reestablish the cerebrospinal fluid flow. Prognostic factors will be addressed in another section, but the extent of the surgical resection is the unifying element across series regarding patient survival and outcome in terms of time to progression. The quality and extent of the ependymoma resection is affected most often by a tumor that is located in an area difficult to access surgically, such as the third ventricle or CP angle. Moreover, Figarella-Branger et al. reported that high quality resections were less likely to be achieved in patients four years old and younger (8). Few studies have addressed the treatment of postoperative residual tumor with a second resection (9,10). Furthermore, there is disagreement among neurooncologists regarding the use of interval chemotherapy between resections. Chemotherapy in this context may render the tumor more amenable to surgical resection and may also prevent tumor progression in the interval between resections.

As the pattern of recurrence in ependymoma is primarily local, most neurooncologists advocate local postoperative radiotherapy. Although the optimal dose remains controversial, data from the University of Pennsylvania and Princess Margaret Hospital indicate an overall survival improvement with doses of 4500 cGy or more (11,12). The University of Texas M. D. Anderson Cancer Center study on ependymomas in children showed a survival advantage with doses greater than 5000 cGy (13). It should be noted that the optimal radiation therapy dose is uncertain, because the evaluation of a dose–response relationship for a specific tumor type requires prospective evaluation. Craniospinal irradiation is reserved for the small percentage of patients with neuraxis dissemination and has limited benefit owing to the lower total dose administered to the tumor in the neuraxis (14). Conformal radiation therapy (CRT) limits the highest dose to the primary tumor site and decreases the doses received by the surrounding tissues. The best and most recent data on CRT are from a phase II trial at St. Jude Children's Research Hospital from 1997–2003 (14). They were able to limit the dose of radiation to a 10-mm anatomically defined clinical target volume, with patients receiving radiation therapy doses of 54 to 59.4 Gy, without affecting disease control rates in localized ependymoma (15).

Ependymomas are considered relatively chemoresistant. Although many agents have been used for adjuvant therapy with ependymoma, no clear impact on outcomes has been demonstrated. Evans et al. showed no difference in survival rates among children who underwent craniospinal radiation therapy and were randomized to receive adjuvant lomustine, vincristine or, prednisone (16). The German prospective trials HIT 88/89 and HIT 91, which combined postoperative irradiation and chemotherapy, failed to show a treatment advantage regardless of the mode of chemotherapy used (17). The platinum-based regimens seem to be the most effective against ependymoma. Gornet et al. demonstrated an improved radiographic response with platinum-based therapeutic agents relative to nitrosourea-based agents (18). The standard chemotherapy consists of six 12-week cycles of cisplatin, cyclophosphamide, etoposide, and vincristine, whereas the dose-intensive chemotherapy regimen consists of eight 9-week cycles of the same agents, with differences in the relative intensities. As mentioned previously, the most promising application of chemotherapy in the treatment of intracranial ependymoma is the role it plays in the interval prior to repeat resection and the role it plays in making tumor resection more facile in hopes of a complete repeat resection.

Prognostic Factors

The extent of the surgical resection is the most universally accepted prognostic factor in the literature regarding treatment of intracranial ependymoma. Healy et al. demonstrated that the presence of residual disease, as visualized radiographically on postoperative MRI or CT images, was the most important prognostic factor for patients with intracranial ependymoma (19). Robertson et al. observed that the predictors of the duration of progression-free survival included an estimate of the extent of the resection at surgery as well as the amount of residual tumor seen on postoperative imaging studies (20).

Age is a prognostic factor examined in many series. It is generally agreed that children less than three years old have a worse prognosis than older children. The reasons for this are unclear but possibly relate to tumor biology and the hesitation to use radiation therapy in young patients. The Pediatric Oncology Group examined the effect on patients of delaying irradiation and showed significant differences in outcome based on age (21). They found a 63% five-year survival rate for children 24 to 35 months old in whom radiation therapy was delayed for one year and a 26% five-year survival rate for children 0 to 23 months old in whom it was delayed for two years. Pollack et al. reviewed age as a prognostic factor and found the five-year survival rate to be 75% in patients at least three years old and 22% in the patients less than three years old (22); of note, no patient younger than two years old survived longer than 39 months after surgery.

The use of tumor grade and histology as prognostic factors has generated considerable controversy in the literature. Numerous retrospective studies with small numbers of patients, spanning very long periods of time, have cited anaplastic tumor histology as a negative prognostic factor.

However, several better-designed studies, including those of the Children's Cancer Group (prospective randomized trial) and the Pediatric Oncology Group (prospective cohort study), found histologic grade to be of no prognostic significance. Recently, Korshunov et al. analyzed a series of 258 patients with intracranial ependymoma, including 115 children and 143 adults (23). They found increasing grade of malignancy to be associated strongly and independently with worse clinical outcomes in terms of both survival time without tumor recurrence and overall survival time. Likewise, they found that the effect of radiotherapy was related to histologic grade of the tumor and that it was more likely to benefit patients who had the anaplastic tumor variety and had undergone complete tumor removal.

There is some evidence to support consideration of tumor location as a prognostic variable. In pediatric patients, posterior fossa masses not showing lateral extension into the CP angle are associated with a better prognosis (24).

INTRAMEDULLARY EPENDYMOMA

Epidemiology

Ependymomas are the most common spinal cord tumors in adult patients, representing roughly 60% of all intramedullary tumors. Although they may occur at any age, they are noted to occur most frequently in middle-aged patients, and they have no particular gender predilection. There is an association between intramedullary ependymomas and NF-2. Likewise, most sporadic ependymomas also show mutations in the NF-2 gene (25). The full spectrum of ependymoma is encountered in the spinal cord—cellular, tanycytic, malignant, mixed, and myxopapillary ependymoma, as well as subependymoma. Most often, the myxopapillary ependymoma is found in the filum terminale or cauda equina and therefore is considered an extramedullary tumor. Most spinal ependymomas are histologically benign, rarely show infiltrative growth, and do not form tumor capsules; however, the interface between the tumor mass and the surrounding normal cord tissue is relatively well defined (26).

Clinical Presentation

Symptoms are nonspecific, develop over several years, and are attributed to chronic cord compression causing myelopathy. The differential diagnosis includes other intramedullary tumors such as astrocytomas and hemangioblastomas as well as nonneoplastic processes, such as demyelinating diseases and cervical spondylotic myelopathy. Dysesthesias caused by spinothalamic tract compression are the most common initial symptoms in numerous series (27,28). The MRI characteristics of intramedullary ependymoma, although nonspecific, classically reveal a low signal on T1-weighted images, high signal on T2-weighted ones, marked but heterogeneous contrast enhancement, and a well-demarcated tumor margin. A tumor-related syrinx occurs in approximately 50% of intramedullary ependymomas. In their series of 100 intramedullary spinal cord tumors, Samii and Klekamp reported that the more proximally the tumor mass was located, the more frequently a syrinx developed (29).

Therapy

In most instances, the tumor pathology is low grade, and therefore the primary treatment objective is to achieve a gross-total resection without inflicting additional neurological morbidity. The most important factor in determining the surgical objective is the plane between the tumor and the spinal cord (30). This interface can be accurately assessed via an adequate myelotomy that extends over the entire rostral caudal extent of the tumor. It is important to review the pathology from the initial biopsy prior to continuing with gross-total resection. If a malignant component is identified, the procedure should be stopped, as gross-total resection is of no benefit for malignant intramedullary neoplasms.

The use of adjuvant therapy in the treatment of intramedullary ependymoma is controversial. There is a general consensus that radiation is not required if gross-total resection is achieved. However, after subtotal resection, the recurrence rate for these tumors is unacceptably high. Unfortunately, the data favoring the use of radiation after subtotal tumor removal are not easily interpreted, as they are based on small patient populations with limited follow-up, and they lack matched controls treated without radiation.

Despite insufficient data, most clinicians advocate radiation therapy after subtotal resections. The proper dose to use, however, is in a quandary. Some series have reported tumor recurrence rates of up to 90% with treatment doses of less than 40 Gy. Likewise, local tumor control failures have been reported with doses as high as 55 Gy, where the risk of radiation myelopathy becomes considerable (31).

MYXOPAPILLARY EPENDYMOMA

Epidemiology

This rare tumor occurs mainly in middle-aged adults and only rarely in children. Of all intraspinal ependymomas, 50% are of the intramedullary form, and the remaining 50% occur in association with the terminal filum, cauda equina, and conus as intradural, extramedullary masses. Among lumbosacral masses, ependymomas account for 90% of intradural tumors (32). In the lumbosacral region, the majority of ependymomas arise from the intradural terminal filum. These are characteristically well-encapsulated, sausage-shaped tumors with the nerve roots of the cauda equina draped

over the surface of the lesion or enveloped by it (33). Extradural ependymomas are rare and occur in the extradural canal in association with the dural
part of the terminal filum, the bone substance of the sacrum, the pelvic cavity anterior to the sacrum, and the subcutaneous tissue dorsal to the sacrum.
These intraspinal extradural sacral ependymomas arise from ependymal cell
remnants in the extradural part of the terminal filum, whereas the other
extradural ependymomas probably arise from ependymal rests that are present at the time of birth.

Clinical Presentation

With tumors arising from the terminal filum, the most common symptoms
are back and radicular pain. With lesions involving the cauda equina, motor
and sensory symptoms, as well as bladder dysfunction, are frequently
encountered. The presentation of the extraspinal ependymomas is variable
and can range from radicular symptoms to a palpable sacral mass.

All patients with these symptoms should undergo contrast-enhanced
MRI to localize the lesion and to assist in operative planning if the patient
is a surgical candidate. Generally, MRI reveals a hyperintense mass on
T2-weighted sequences, as well as contrast enhancement. For extraspinal
ependymoma with pelvic mass effect, a CT scan should be performed
to evaluate bony erosion. Fasset and Schmidt recommend evaluation of
all presacral tumors preoperatively by an abdominal/pelvic surgical
specialist (33).

Therapy

Myxopapillary ependymoma is best treated surgically. Gross-total resection
should be attempted when possible, as it is associated with lower tumor recurrence rates than subtotal resection. Unfortunately, gross-total resection rates
for myxopapillary ependymoma are lower than for spinal ependymoma, most
likely because of their intimate involvement with the cauda equina roots and
propensity to disseminate in the neuraxis at the time of diagnosis (34).

There is no consensus for the use of radiation in the treatment of myxopapillary ependymoma. This is because only a few patients present with this
condition, and no prospective randomized trials have been conducted to
assess the benefit of radiotherapy. However, there is general clinical agreement that progress in patients who have undergone gross-total resection
may be followed using serial imaging, whereas those who have undergone
subtotal resection might benefit from radiotherapy. In general, a dose of
45 to 55 Gy to the tumor bed is recommended (35).

Prognosis

The prognosis for myxopapillary ependymoma is largely determined by the
surgical resection. These low-grade lesions carry a favorable prognosis when

gross-total resection can be achieved. Clover et al. note that many long-term survivors live with persistent or recurrent disease (36). Fourney et al. reviewed these multiple recurrences and found that they put patients at great risk for spinal instability, often necessitating thoracolumbopelvic stabilization (37).

SUBEPENDYMOMA

Epidemiology

Subependymomas are rare, benign, noninvasive, and slow-growing tumors. They are most often located in the fourth ventricle, with the next most common sites being the septum pellucidum and lateral ventricles. These tumors occur more frequently in males than females and usually present between the fourth and sixth decades of life, with symptoms related to increased ICP (38).

Clinical Presentation

These lesions are asymptomatic in many patients, and they are discovered incidentally at autopsy. When subependymomas become large enough to cause obstructive ventriculomegaly, they may result in nonspecific symptoms such as headache, nausea, and vomiting secondary to increased ICP. The presence of symptoms has been shown to correlate directly with tumor size, with lesions measuring 3 to 5 cm or more in maximum diameter generally producing symptoms (38). Ataxia is frequently encountered in patients with fourth ventricular ependymomas, whereas lesions centered around the septum pellucidum may produce personality changes and also cause impaired recent and remote memory.

Diagnosis and Differential Diagnosis

The differential diagnosis for a lateral ventricular mass includes central neurocytoma, choroid plexus papilloma, subependymal giant cell astrocytoma, meningioma, metastasis, subependymoma, and ependymoma. Subependymomas located in the lateral ventricles are noted to have poor contrast enhancement on MRI and lack calcification, whereas those located in the fourth ventricle are more likely to show calcification and contrast enhancement. Younger age and the observation of hyperdensity on images lacking contrast enhancement favor a diagnosis of ependymoma rather than subependymoma. Owing to the variable imaging features of subependymoma, its reliable preoperative diagnosis cannot be firmly assured (39).

The pathological diagnosis is established by observing a hypocellular lesion with tumor cells arranged in nests separated by glial processes. Malignant features such as nuclear pleomorphism and mitoses are generally absent, and there is a low to absent MIB-1 labeling index. This bland pathological appearance has led some investigators to believe that subependymoma represents a hamartoma rather than a true neoplasm (40).

Therapy and Prognosis

These lesions are cured by complete surgical resection. For lateral ventricular and septum pellucidum lesions, the transcallosal or transcortical, transventricular approach may be utilized, depending on the exact location of the tumor. Because these tumors are avascular, they can be removed with a clean, bloodless resection. Fourth ventricular subependymomas are approached via standard suboccipital craniectomy, with splitting of the vermis. If the tumor is attached to the floor of the fourth ventricle, a complete resection may not be possible.

The prognosis for these lesions is usually very good except for those that are situated in the floor of the fourth ventricle and those with a mixed ependymoma/subependymoma histology. In the absence of these features, recurrences are rare after complete resection, and postoperative radiation therapy is not warranted.

ACKNOWLEDGMENT

The authors thank David M. Wildrick, Ph.D. for editorial assistance with the manuscript.

REFERENCES

1. Comprehensive Brain Tumor Registry of the United States. First Annual Report, 1995.
2. Carbone M, Rizzo P, Pass H. Simian virus 40, poliovaccines and human tumors: a review of recent developments. Oncogene 1997; 15:1877–1888.
3. Agaoglu F, Ayan I, Dizdar Y, et al. Ependymal tumors in childhood. Pediatr Blood Cancer 2005; 45(3):298–303.
4. Smyth M, Horn B, Russo C, et al. Intracranial ependymomas of childhood: current management strategies. Pediatr Neurosurg 2000; 33:138–150.
5. Vinchon M, Soto-Ares G, Riffaud L, et al. Supratentorial ependymomas in children. Pediatr Neurosurg 2001; 34:77–87.
6. McLaurin R. On the use of precraniotomy shunting in the management of posterior fossa tumors in children: a cooperative study. In: Chapman P, ed. Concepts in Pediatric Neurosurgery. Vol. 6. Basel: Karger, 1985:1–5.
7. Saint-Rose C, Cinalli G, Roux F, et al. Management of hydrocephalus in pediatric patients with posterior fossa tumors: the role of endoscopic third ventriculostomy. J Neurosurg 2001; 95:791–797.
8. Figarella-Branger D, Civatte M, Bouvier-Labit C, et al. Prognostic factors in intracranial ependymoma in children. J Neurosurg 2000; 93:605–613.

9. Foreman N, Love S, Gill S, et al. Second look surgery for incompletely resected fourth ventricular ependymomas: technical case report. Neurosurgery 1997; 40:856–860.

10. Sanford R, Kun L, Heideman R, et al. Cerebellar pontine angle ependymoma in infants. Pediatr Neurosurg 1998; 28:135–142.

11. Garrett P, Simpson W. Ependymomas: results of radiation treatment. Int J Radiat Oncol Biol Phys 1983; 9:1121–1124.

12. Goldwein JW, Leahy JM, Packer RJ, et al. Intracranial ependymomas in children. Int J Radiat Oncol Biol Phys 1990; 19(6):1497–1502.

13. Chiu JK, Woo SY, Ater J, et al. Intracranial ependymoma in children: analysis of prognostic factors. J Neurooncol 1992; 13(2):283–290.

14. Merchant T, Sanford R. Ependymoma. In: Berger MS, Prados MD, eds. Textbook of Neuro-Oncology. Philadelphia: W. B. Saunders (Elsevier), 2004: 656–665.

15. Merchant TE, Mulhern RK, Krasin MJ, et al. Preliminary results from a phase II trial of conformal radiation therapy and evaluation of radiation-related CNS effects for pediatric patients with localized ependymoma. J Clin Oncol 2004; 22(15):3156–3162.

16. Evans AE, Anderson JR, Lefkowitz-Boudreaux IB, et al. Adjuvant chemotherapy of childhood posterior fossa ependymoma: craniospinal irradiation with or without adjuvant CCNU, vincristine, and prednisone: a children's cancer group study. Med Pediatr Oncol 1996; 27:8–14.

17. Timmerman B, Kortman R, Kuhl J, et al. Combined postoperative irradiation and chemotherapy for anaplastic ependymoma in childhood: results of the German prospective trials HIT 88/89 and 91. Int J Radiat Oncol Biol Phys 2000; 46:287–295.

18. Gornet M, Buckner J, Marks R, et al. Chemotherapy for advanced CNS ependymoma. J Neurooncol 1999; 45:61–67.

19. Healy E, Barnes P, Kupsky W, et al. The prognostic significance of postoperative residual tumor in ependymoma. Neurosurgery 1991; 28(5):666–671.

20. Robertson P, Zeltzer P, Boyett J, et al. Survival and prognostic factors following radiation therapy and chemotherapy for ependymoma in children: a report of the Children's Cancer Group. J Neurosurg 1998; 88:695–703.

21. Duffner P, Krischer J, Sanford R, et al. Prognostic factors in infants and very young children with intracranial ependymomas. Pediatr Neurosurg 1998; 28:215–222.

22. Pollack I, Gerszten P, Martinez A, et al. Intracranial ependymomas of childhood: long-term outcome and prognostic factors. Neurosurgery 1995; 37:655–666.

23. Korshunov A, Golanov A, Sycheva R, et al. The histologic grade is the main prognostic factor for patients with intracranial ependymoma treated in the microneurosurgical era. Cancer 2004; 100(6):1230–1237.

24. Merchant T, Haida T, Wang M, et al. Anaplastic ependymoma: treatment of pediatric patients with or without craniospinal radiation therapy. J Neurosurg 1997; 86:943–949.

25. Birch BD, Johnson JP, Parsa A, et al. Frequent type 2 neurofibromatosis gene transcript mutations in sporadic intramedullary spinal cord ependymomas. Neurosurgery 1996; 39:135–140.

26. Chang U, Choe W, Chung S, et al. Surgical outcome and prognostic factors of spinal intramedullary ependymomas in adults. J Neurooncol 2002; 57:133–139.
27. Shrivastava RK, Epstein FJ, Perin NI, et al. Intramedullary spinal cord tumors in patients older than 50 years of age: management and outcome analysis. J Neurosurg Spine 2005; 2(3):249–255.
28. Epstein F, Farmer J, Freed D. Adult intramedullary spinal cord ependymomas: the result of surgery in 38 patients. J Neurosurg 1993; 79:204–209.
29. Samii M, Klekamp J. Surgical results of 100 intramedullary tumors in relation to accompanying syringomyelia. Neurosurgery 1994; 35:865–873.
30. Schwartz T, Parsa A, McCormick P. Intramedullary ependymoma. In: Berger MS, Prados MD, eds. Textbook of Neuro-Oncology. Philadelphia: W. B. Saunders (Elsevier), 2004:497–500.
31. Linstadt D, Wara W, Leibel S, et al. Postoperative radiotherapy of primary spinal cord tumors. Int J Radiat Oncol Biol Phys 1989; 16:1397–1403.
32. Fourney DR, Fuller GN, Gokaslan ZL. Intraspinal extradural myxopapillary ependymoma of the sacrum arising from the filum terminale externa. Case report. J Neurosurg 2000; 93(suppl 2):322–326.
33. Fasset D, Schmidt M. Lumbosacral ependymomas: a review of the management of intradural and extradural tumors. Neurosurg Focus 2003; 15(5):Article 13.
34. Parney I, Parsa A. Myxopapillary ependymomas. In: Berger MS, Prados MD, eds. Textbook of Neuro-Oncology. Philadelphia: W. B. Saunders (Elsevier), 2004:493–495.
35. Schild S, Nisi K, Scheithauer B, et al. The results of radiotherapy for ependymomas: The Mayo Clinic experience. Int J Radiat Oncol Biol Phys 1998; 42: 953–958.
36. Clover L, Hazuka M, Kinzie J. Spinal cord ependymomas treated with surgery and radiation therapy. A review of 11 cases. Am J Clin Oncol 1993; 16:350–353.
37. Fourney DR, Prabhu SS, Cohen ZR, et al. Thoracolumbopelvic stabilization for the treatment of instability caused by recurrent myxopapillary ependymoma. J Spinal Disord Tech 2003; 16:108–111.
38. Scheithauer B. Symptomatic subependymoma: report of 21 cases with review of the literature. J Neurosurg 1978; 49:689–696.
39. Rath T, Sundgren P, Brahma B, et al. Massive symptomatic subependymoma of the lateral ventricles: case report and review of the literature. Neuroradiology 2005; 47(3):183–188.
40. Prayson R, Suh J. Subependymomas: clinicopathologic study of 14 tumors, including comparative MIB-1 immunohistochemical analysis with other ependymal neoplasms. Arch Pathol Lab Med 1999; 123:306–309.

11

Tumors of the Choroid Plexus

Adrienne C. Weeks and James T. Rutka

Division of Neurosurgery, The Hospital for Sick Children, The University of Toronto, Toronto, Ontario, Canada

HISTORY AND EPIDEMIOLOGY

Choroid plexus (CP) tumors are rare primary brain tumors arising from CP epithelium, which derives from specialized ventricular ependymal cells around certain segments of the neural tube. These neoplasms were first described in 1833 by Guerard and the first resective operation was preformed in 1906 by Bielschowsy.

Choroid plexus neoplasms represent 0.4% to 0.8% of all primary neoplasms of the brain. Although these tumors can occur in all age groups, the preponderance occurs in childhood with 70% being diagnosed before the age of two. Studies have suggested a skewed distribution in favor of the male gender 1 to 1.3:1 (1–3). The malignant counterpart to the CP papilloma (CPP), the CP carcinoma (CPC) represents 29% to 39% of all CP tumors and, again, occurs more frequently in infancy (1–4).

Anatomically, choroid plexus neoplasms occur most frequently in the lateral (50%), fourth (40%), and third (5%) ventricles. They have also occurred in the cerebellopontine angle (CPA) and in biventricular locations (5%) (1). However, the anatomical distribution differs markedly with relation to age. The vast of choroid tumors present in the lateral ventricles in children, while fourth ventricular and CPA tumors increase in frequency with the age of the individual (2). Primary extraventricular locations are the rarest sites, but tumors have been described in children in the suprasellar cistern, foramen magnum, and spinal arachnoid space (2,3). Metastatic disease from CPC has been documented; anywhere along the neural axis including leptomeninges, tibia, lung, and abdomen, at least one case. There is report of abdominal metastasis occurring in the setting of a ventriculoperitoneal shunt (1–3,5).

ETIOLOGY AND CYTOGENETICS

The exact mechanisms by which CPPs and CPCs arise remain to be elucidated. However, strides have been made in regard to the cytogenetics, virology, and molecular markers that could aid in a better understanding of the etiology of these tumors.

Choroid plexus tumors have been diagnosed on antenatal ultrasound suggesting a possible congenital etiology for this condition. As well, certain genetic syndromes predispose to the formation of CPP and CPC, such as Li–Fraumeni syndrome (an aberration in P53), neurofibromatosis type II, Aicardi's syndrome, Down's syndrome, and von Hippel-Lindau's disease (1). Germline mutations in TP53 and hSNF5/INI1 have been found in familial cases of choroid tumors, and similar mutations have been found in tumors of some sporadic cases of CPC and CPP (6,7).

No unequivocal chromosomal link has yet been identified, however multiple genetic chromosomal aberrations have been associated with CPP and CPC. Most notably, hyperdiploidy with gains on chromosomes 5, 7, 8, 9, 12, and 18 and losses on 10 and 22 are found in CPPs. CPCs have shown gains on 1, 4, 8, 10, 12, 14, and 20 and losses on 9, 11, 15 and 18; the loss of 9p and 10q may be linked to enhanced survival in CPCs (1,8).

DNA sequences of the simian virus SV40 have been postulated to play a role in the evolution of CPP and CPC. Newborn rodents inoculated with SV40 and transgenic mice expressing an SV40 large T-antigen develop CPC and CPP (1,3). Previous studies have shown that this large T-antigen is capable of inactivating factors of cell-cycle regulation (TP53, RB1, and p107). However, millions of humans accidentally infected with SV40 given concomitantly with polio vaccination in the 1950s failed to increase the incidence of CPP or CPCs (1). To date, there is no evidence to suggest that SV40 is more than a neutral bystander in the pathogenesis of CPP and CPC.

CLINICAL FEATURES

There are no distinguishing clinical signs to aid in the delineation of a malignant carcinoma of the CP from a benign papillary tumor. Both present as a constellation of four overlapping signs and symptoms: increased intracranial pressure (tense fontanelle, splayed sutures, vomiting, lethargy, irritability, and papilledema), seizures, hemorrhage, and focal neurological deficits. The mean time of duration of symptoms until diagnosis is two to six months (1–3). The majority of patients come to medical attention for investigation of hydrocephalus and/or macrocephaly.

Hydrocephalus is the cardinal feature of both CPPs and CPCs. The cause of the hydrocephalus is thought to be obstruction of the normal flow of cerebrospinal fluid (CSF) or overproduction of CSF. Overproduction of CSF by these tumors has attracted much interest and been the subject of numerous reports (1,3). An increased rate of CSF production has been unequivocally demonstrated with choroid plexus neoplasms, albeit proven in only a few patients (1,3). It has been suggested that although overproduction of CSF can cause hydrocephalus, a complex combination of CSF overproduction and limited outflow may be the cause in many patients. Elevation of CSF protein is found in the majority of patients, and xanthochromia in the CSF is common; frank hemorrhage is less common (1,3). The obstruction of CSF absorptive pathways may also explain why despite a gross total excision of tumor the hydrocephalus may persist. Approximately one-third to one-half of patients with choroid plexus neoplasms require permanent CSF diversion postoperatively even when the tumor is completely removed. An interesting, but well-documented phenomenon of "shunt resistant hydrocephalus" has been described in the literature due to the CSF-producing ability of these neoplasms. In fact, abdominal ascites has been described after placement of ventriculoperitoneal shunts prior to surgical excision (1,3).

IMAGING

The neuroimaging features on computed tomography and magnetic resonance imaging (MRI) are depicted in Table 1 (9). Imaging characteristics are neither specific nor sensitive in distinguishing CPP from CPC, as both show similar signal and enhancement characteristics and can show areas of focal parenchymal invasion (Figs. 1 and 2). Nevertheless, extensive parenchymal invasion, increased heterogeneity, and high peritumoral vasogenic edema are indicative of a CPC (9).

Angiographically, there may be a tumor blush due to the high vascularity of choroid plexus tumors (Fig. 2D). Tumors situated in the lateral or third ventricles receive blood supply from the anterior and posterior lateral choroidal arteries. These masses tend to displace the basal vein of Rosenthal and internal occipital artery inferiorly. Fourth ventricular tumors tend to be supplied from medullary or vermian branches of the posterior cerebral artery. Although conventional angiography does not play a role in diagnosis, it can be used as an adjunct to surgery as embolization can be employed to reduce vascularity.

Table 1 Imaging Characteristics of Choroid Plexus Neoplasms

CT	CT + contrast	MRI T1	MRI T2	MRI + gadolinium	MRI spectroscopy
Isodense to hyperdense	Intense and slightly heterogeneous	Isointense to grey matter	Heterogeneous hyperintensity	Marked enhancement	Prominent choline peak
25% Calcification		Hypointense at areas of calcification and vascularity			Absence of *N*-acetyl aspartate

Note: Imaging is neither sensitive nor specific in distinguishing choroid plexus papilloma from choroid plexus carcinoma (CPC). These imaging patterns are similar on CT and MRI, however increased heterogeneity, prominent peritumoral edema and diffuse parenchymal invasion are suggestive of CPC.
Abbreviations: CT, computed tomography; MRI, magnetic resonance imaging.

(A)   (B)

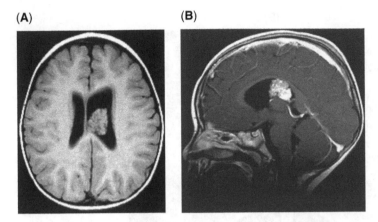

Figure 1 Choroid plexus papilloma in a three-year-old female presenting with hydrocephalus. Axial T1-weighted magnetic resonance imaging (MRI) without contrast (**A**) and sagittal T1-weighted MRI with gadolinium show a papillary homogeneously enhancing tumor within the left lateral ventricle (**B**).

The differential diagnosis of lesions in a similar area to CPP and CPC includes villous hypertrophy, metastasis (carcinoma metastasis in adult population), lymphoma, granulocytic sarcoma, atypical teratoid/rhabdoid tumors, and meningioma (3,9).

PATHOLOGY AND MOLECULAR MARKERS

Choroid Plexus Papillomas

CPP are considered World Health Organization (WHO) grade I lesions. Grossly, they are pink-gray, pedunculated soft neoplasms with the exception of the occasional foci of calcification. They are highly vascular with a "cauliflower" appearing surface, and less often they may have hemorrhagic or cystic components. Choroid plexus neoplasms tend to expand the ventricle locally, when in the lateral ventricle, and are attached to the normal CP at the confluence of the posterior and inferior horns. Histologically, CPPs are similar to normal CP; they show many papillae covered by simple columnar or cuboidal epithelium, eosinophilic cytoplasm, round to oval nuclei situated basally, and papillary fronds consisting of vascular connective stroma (1,3,5). This vascular connective stroma is the key to differentiation from papillary ependymoma. These neoplasms can take on acinar, tubular, adenomatous, xanthomatous, oncocytic, and pigmented patterns on occasion. CPP can seed throughout the neural axis but this is a rare phenomenon and a much more common occurrence in CPC (5). CPPs typically do not invade the surrounding brain parenchyma. However, consideration should be given to a lesion with otherwise benign cellular appearance except with

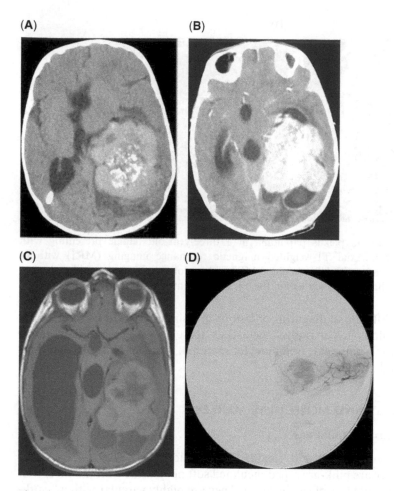

Figure 2 A two-year-old presenting with macrocephaly and hydrocephalus. Computed tomography with and without contrast dye (**A**, **B**). Note the placement of a ventriculoperitoneal shunt in (**B**). T1-weighted magnetic resonance imaging without gadolinium (**C**). Selective middle cerebral angiogram demonstrates a tumor blush (**D**).

stromal invasion and loss of normal villous architecture at this site alone, because these lesions may have a course more similar to CPP than CPC (10).

Atypical CPP

There is a subset of patients initially diagnosed with CPC that have a more benign course when compared to CPC. On histopathology, the distinction between CPP and CPC is not always clear-cut and a spectrum may exist. A subset of tumors may be classified as atypical CPP and exhibits one or only a few histological features of malignancy (1). This tumor subset, although recognized clinically, has yet to be well defined and therefore is not included in the current WHO classification.

Choroid Plexus Carcinoma

CPCs are designated WHO grade III and, as stated above, the vast majority occur in young children. As in other high-grade malignancy, CPC can show marked cytological atypia, nuclear pleomorphism, loss of polarity, high cellular density, frequent mitosis, necrosis, vascular proliferation, hemorrhage, and brain infiltration (5). Grossly, they are pinkish-yellow, soft, lobulated, invasive tumors typified by geographic foci of necrosis and hemorrhage. Although focally maintaining normal villous architecture, papillae of unorganized polygonal cells exhibiting irregular size and shape with high mitotic activity and lobulated nuclei are characteristic. Thus, the major pathological distinguishing features of CPC as compared to CPP are as follows: the degree of cytological atypia, evidence of brain invasion, and loss of normal papillary architecture (Fig. 2). Other features that can be seen are foamy macrophages, hemosiderin staining, cholesterol clefts, melanin, and psammoma bodies (5). CPC can metastasize along CSF pathways (Fig. 3) throughout the neural axis in addition to extraneural locations such as abdomen, lungs, tibia, and clavicle (1,3,5,11). In the report by Pencalet et al., 3 of 13 carcinoma patients had metastasis (11).

Immunohistochemical staining can aid in the delineation of CP neoplasms from normal choroid epithelium, and has some utility in differentiating

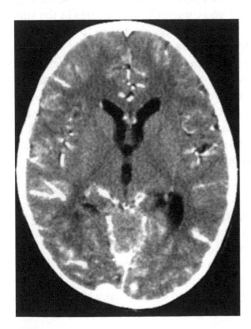

Figure 3 A four-year-old child with choroid plexus papilloma was treated with complete resection and chemotherapy. The child returned one year later with persistent headache. Contrast-enhanced computed tomography of the head demonstrates communicating hydrocephalus and meningeal enhancement consistent with leptomeningeal spread.

CPP from CPC. Normal choroid plexus epithelium and its associated tumors are immunohistochemically positive for vimentin, cytokeratins, transthyretin, and S-100 protein. CPP/CPC may express focal areas of glial fibrillary acidic protien (GFAP) positivity, whereas normal choroid plexus will not. It should be emphasized that there are no definitive antigenic profiles to delineate CPP from CPC. However, CPCs tend to express less S-100 and transthyretin and may express carcinogenic embryonic antigen (CEA). Ependymomas can be distinguished by widespread GFAP, reduced cytokeratin expression, and lack of a basement membrane (5). Metastatic carcinoma is GFAP negative and exhibits high CEA positivity.

TREATMENT

There is a general consensus in the literature that gross total resection (GTR) is curative in CPP and is the major prognosticator for survival in CPC (1,3). The role of adjunctive therapy such as chemotherapy and radiation in the treatment of CPC is still debated in the literature.

Surgical Considerations

Hydrocephalus is usually present at the time of diagnosis and may require treatment in the form of a CSF shunt. Third ventriculostomies frequently fail reflecting overproduction of CSF or communicating hydrocephalus.

The surgical approach is determined by the tumor's relationship to eloquent brain matter and location of the main vascular supply. The feeding arteries may be deep to the tumor bed and difficult to ligate early in the surgical procedure. An operative corridor providing early access to the feeding vessels facilitates removal of these highly vascularized tumors that not uncommonly results in loss of 1 to 1.5 times a child's blood volume. Mortality from intraoperative blood loss and cardiac arrest are not uncommon and severe hemorrhage is one of the main predictors of incompleteness of resection. Even biopsy of these tumors can result in catastrophic blood loss. At our institution, preoperative embolization is entertained for CPCs if the calibers of the child's vessels are large enough to make this presurgical adjunct useful in diminishing intraoperative hemorrhage.

Chemotherapy/Radiation

For CPP, no adjunctive therapy is required as GTR is curative. Chemotherapy for CPC has become a common treatment modality, but its true efficacy has been difficult to establish. There are a few case reports in the literature of response to various chemotherapeutic regimens either controlling disease or resulting in long-term survival after subtotal resection (2,11–14). The use of chemotherapy as an adjunctive therapy to GTR is even more difficult to interpret (15). The rarity of this tumor precludes the ability to perform a randomized trial, and a centralized registry, which tracks all cases, will be difficult to establish.

Chemotherapy may have a role in the neoadjuvant setting. There are numerous case reports of CPC patients receiving chemotherapy after biopsy or subtotal resection; during a second operation for more complete removal of residual tumor, blood loss was markedly reduced (3,4,11). The Hospital for Sick Children in Toronto showed a mean blood loss of 138% of blood volume for the first surgery and 15% of blood volume after a course of chemotherapy (4). Pathology showed fibrosis, hyalinization, and collagen in vessel adventitia after chemotherapy exposure.

The effectiveness of radiation is even more difficult to assess. Given the significant sequelae of radiation on the developing brain and the young age at which most patients are diagnosed, irradiation is probably best avoided especially in the young child. In children older than three years of age treated with radiotherapy, stable disease or long-term survival has been reported both in the presence and in the absence of chemotherapy (2,3,12–14). A meta-analysis suggested a survival benefit from radiation therapy. However, results of this study may have been confounded by the young age of patients who did not receive radiation (2,16).

PROGNOSIS

The majority of patients with CPP can expect an excellent outcome and long-term survival. A meta-analysis of the literature in 2002 revealed 1-, 5-, and 10-year survival rates for CPP of 90%, 81%, and 77%, respectively (2). If a GTR was achieved, 10-year survival increased to 85% as opposed to 56% without GTR and a one-year survival rate of 50% if biopsy was the only intervention performed (2). The GTR rate for CPP in the literature ranges from 80% to 96% (3). Despite its benign character, operative mortality has been reported to be 8% to 9.5%; this is in part due to the high vascularity of these lesions (3).

CPC runs a much more aggressive course and this is reflected in the long-term survival. One-, five-, and ten-year survival rates are 71%, 41%, and 35%, respectively (2). The literature agrees that the most important prognostic feature in CPC is the completeness of resection (2–4,11,12). The two-year survival rate for GTR was 72% as compared to 34% with subtotal resection (2). However, GTR was only accomplished in approximately 50% to 60% of CPC cases. This is in part due to the technical difficulty of removing these highly vascular, invasive lesions (2,4,11).

CONCLUSION

Choroid plexus tumors are rare tumors of childhood causing hydrocephalus, macrocephaly, and/or signs and symptoms of raised ICP. Surgical excision is recommended for both the benign CPP and the malignant CPC. While surgery is curative in CPP, it remains the best indicator for survival in CPC when resection can be complete. Chemotherapy and radiation have yet to prove survival benefit in CPC, but long-term survivors are identifiable. At the very least, preresection chemotherapy for CPCs may make the operative resection of these vascular tumors safer and easier to accomplish. Careful preoperative planning is essential in order to minimize the risks of surgery.

REFERENCES

1. Rickert CH, Paulus W. Tumours of the choroids plexus. Microsc Res Tech 2001; 52(1):104–111.
2. Wolff JE, Sajedi M, Brant R, et al. Choroid plexus tumours. Br J Cancer 2002; 87(10):1086–1091.
3. Gupta N. Choroid plexus tumours in children. Neurosurg Clin N Am 2003; 14(4):621–631.
4. St Clair SK, Humphreys RP, Pillay PK, et al. Current management of choroid plexus carcinoma in children. Pediatr Neurosurg 1991; 17(5):225–233.
5. Gaudio RM, Tacconi L, Rossi ML. Pathology of choroid plexus papillomas: A review. Clin Neurol Neurosurg 1998; 100(3):165–186.
6. Zakrzewska M, Wojcik I, Zakrzewski K, et al. Mutational analysis of *hSNF5/INI1* and TP53. Cancer Genet Cytogenet 2005; 156(2):179–182.
7. Taylor MD, Gokgoz N, Andrulis IL, et al. Familial posterior fossa brain tumours of infancy secondary to germline mutations. Am J Hum Genet 2000; 66(4):1403–1406.
8. Rickert CH, Wiestler OD, Paulus W. Chromosomal imbalances in choroid plexus tumours. Am J Pathol 2002; 160(3):1105–1113.
9. Guermazi A, De Kerviler E, Zagdanski AM, et al. Diagnostic imaging of choroid plexus disease. Clin Radiol 2000; 55(7):503–516.
10. Levy ML, Goldfarb A, Hyder DJ, et al. Choroid plexus tumours in children: Significance of stromal invasion. Neurosurgery 2001; 48(2):303–309.
11. Pencalet P, Sainte-Rose C, Lellouch-Tubiana A, et al. Papillomas and carcinomas of the choroid plexus in children. J Neurosurg 1998; 88(3):521–528.
12. Greenberg ML. Chemotheraphy of choroid plexus carcinoma. Childs Nerv Syst 1999; 15(10):571–577.
13. Berger C, Thiesse P, Lellouch-Tubiana A, et al. Choroid plexus carcinomas in childhood: clinical features and prognostic factors. Neurosurgery 1998; 42(3): 470–475.
14. Duffner PK, Kun LE, Burger PC, et al. Post-operative chemotherapy and delayed radiation in infants and very young children with choroid plexus carcinoma. Pediatr Neurosurg 1995; 22(4):189–196.
15. Fitzpatrick LK, Aronson LJ, Cohen KJ. Is there requirement for adjunctive therapy for choroid plexus carcinoma that has been completely resected. J Neurooncol 2002; 57(2):123–126.
16. Wolff JE, Sajedi M, Coppes MJ, et al. Radiation therapy and survival in choroid plexus carcinoma. Lancet 1999; 353(9170):2126.

12

Neuroepithelial Tumors of Unknown Origin

Jeffrey J. Raizer and Ed Olson
Department of Neurology, Feinberg School of Medicine, Northwestern University, Chicago, Illinois, U.S.A.

GLIOMATOSIS CEREBRI

Nevin first coined the term "gliomatosis cerebri" (GC) in 1938; he described a diffuse and infiltrative tumor-causing enlargement of cerebral structures without distortion of underlying tissue (1). The first ante mortem diagnosis was made in 1987 (2). The neuronal architecture is preserved in GC and it differs from multifocal gliomas by the lack of detectable connection between the tumors, lack of necrosis, lack of edema with mass effect, and differing enhancement patterns (3). The World Health Organization (WHO) classifies GC as a highly infiltrative neoplasm of the brain (WHO grade III), involving at least two lobes (often bilaterally), by astrocytes, oligodendroglial cells, or a mixture of both (4). GC can be divided into primary and secondary. Two types of GC are distinguished: diffuse infiltration without (type I) or with an associated mass (type II). Secondary GC denotes the remote and contiguous infiltration of tumor cells in a patient with a previously diagnosed glioma (5).

The peak incidence of GC occurs during the fifth decade, but the disease has been observed in neonates and the elderly (3,5). There is a slight male preponderance; women may present earlier. Most patients experience insidiously evolving symptoms over several months; however, symptom duration may range from a few days to as many as 23 years (5–7). Symptoms include cognitive or personality changes, seizures, aphasia, weakness and sensory complaints, and increased intracranial pressure (5–11).

Imaging

In general, computed tomography (CT) scans of the brain poorly visualizes GC because of the subtle infiltration of white matter, lack of clear margins, and absence of contrast enhancement in about half of the tumors (6–12). Prior to magnetic resonance imaging (MRI), the diagnosis of GC was generally established at autopsy or in rare patients undergoing several brain biopsies. MR sequences using fluid attenuated inversion recovery (FLAIR) or T2-weighted images provide the most information about the extent of disease (6,8,10,11,13). GC almost invariably involves the cerebral hemispheres and extends into the diencephalon and basal ganglia (Fig. 1); the brain stem is affected in about one-third of cases, and cerebellum or spinal cord is rarely involved. The primary area of involvement is the white matter (5,8,10,11,14). Nodules of contrast enhancement may be present, usually small nodules, but this does not appear to correlate with grade or outcome; some tumors may develop enhancement over time (6,8,10,11,13). Mass effect is noted in half of the cases and hydrocephalus in 10%.

Recent investigations with MR spectroscopy (MRS) have aimed at distinguishing GC from less-infiltrative gliomas and non-neoplastic processes (13). MRS demonstrates that both GC and low-grade gliomas are

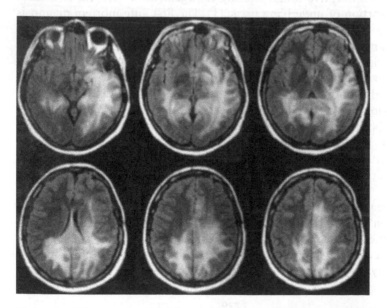

Figure 1 Gliomatosis cerebri low-grade oligodendroglioma (axial FLAIR).

characterized by elevated concentrations of choline (Cho), and reduced levels of *N*-acetyl aspartate (NAA). However, Cho levels are more elevated and NAA levels more reduced in low-grade gliomas than in GC. Levels of creatine (Cr) are elevated in GC but may be reduced in low-grade gliomas. GC also shows a greater elevation of myoinositol (MI) than low-grade gliomas. These spectroscopic differences suggest that glial proliferation may replace or destroy neurons in low-grade gliomas, whereas in GC there is relative preservation of normal brain or simply a lower density of tumor cells. Correlation between MRS and tumor grade was noted in a small series of patients (6). Mineura et al., using positron-emission tomography imaging with C-11 Methionine, found the total volume of tumor on MRI to be underestimated (15).

Cerebrospinal fluid analysis is unlikely to aid in the diagnosis, but protein may be elevated (16); fewer than five white blood cells/mm^3 may be seen and cytology is almost always negative (5,8,17).

Pathology

Histologic examination determines cell type—astrocytic, oligodendroglial, or mixed—and distinguishes GC from non-neoplastic processes. The cell of origin from which GC is derived is a matter of debate, hence its description as a "neuroepithelial tumor of unknown origin." Sanson et al. (9), however, were able to classify the underlying cell type in 94% of cases of GC as astrocytic, oligodendroglial, or mixed. GC is composed of elongated glial cells that often resemble astrocytes, with oval or fusiform nuclei (3). The cells form parallel rows among the nerve fibers when there is infiltration of myelinated tracts. There is variable glial fibrillary acid protein (GFAP) staining and mitotic activity, with an absence of vascular hyperplasia. Although by definition GC constitutes a grade III tumor (WHO classification), morphology ranges from benign to frank anaplastic.

Immunohistochemistry studies suggest that GC resembles astrocytic tumors. There is expression of GFAP, p53, MDM2, pRB, p16, and INK4A but lack of amplification of epidermal growth factor receptor (EGFR), expression of CDK4, or deletion of CDKN2A. Somatic mutations of TP53 and occasionally PTEN mutation are found (8). Alterations in other proteins controlling cell-cycle progression have been identified in accordance with findings in astrocytomas (18,19). Albeit a monoclonal disease at onset, GC progression is associated with successive somatic mutations leading to malignant transformation (4,18).

The invasive nature of GC remains unknown but several studies have documented possible mechanisms. In GC, there is an absence of genetic aberrations in the cell-cycle regulatory genes CDKN2 and CDK4 and a strong expression of p16[INK4a] and pRb; this suggests that the pRb cell-cycle checkpoint is commonly intact (8). In vitro studies of gliomas have suggested that a dichotomy exists in which actively migrating cells do not proliferate and proliferating cells do not migrate (20). There is speculation that upregulation of p16^{INK4a} is one mechanism leading to inhibition of proliferation of the highly migratory and invasive cells of GC (8). Tenascin-C and MMP-9, both of which aid in tumor migration, have no role in GC invasion but CD44 does appear to be involved (19).

Treatment

The optimal treatment of GC remains unclear, with modest results irrespective of therapy. About 50% of patients will die within 12 months of diagnosis, 63% by 24 months, and 73% by 36 months (5). The pathologic spectrum of GC may account for this variability; interestingly, response to treatment does not necessarily correlate with grade or cell type. An increased Ki-67 labeling index has a negative impact on survival; there does not appear to be a correlation between Ki-67 and enhancement on MRI (6).

The diffuse and extensive infiltration of GC leaves little role for surgery beyond a biopsy for diagnostic purposes. Once a tissue diagnosis is obtained, most patients are treated with radiation therapy (RT), chemotherapy, or both. Despite lack of a defined standard of treatment, radiographic and clinical responses are seen with both modalities and survival is increased over observation (6–11,21).

Radiation doses between 45 and 61.2 Gy have been used resulting in median overall survival not exceeding one year (7). While whole brain RT can stabilize or improve neurologic function, delayed neurotoxicity may be a complication in long-term survivors or those older than 60 years of age (22).

Two prospective studies have examined chemotherapy as the initial treatment of GC. Levin et al. (21) measured response in 11 patients treated with temozolomide (TMZ); six of which were changed from PCV (procarbazine, CCNU, vincristine) for clinical progression or toxicity. Seven patients had oligodendrogliomas (six grade II and one grade III), three astrocytomas (two grade II and one grade III), and one oligoastrocytoma (grade II). A median of 10 cycles of TMZ was administered (range 5–19). An objective response was observed in 45% of patients; median time to tumor progression was 13 months with a 12-month progression-free survival of 55%. The median overall survival was not reached at the time of publication. A larger study of 63 consecutive patients with GC compared the efficacy of TMZ with PCV (9). Patients were divided into either primary or secondary GC, the latter initially having a circumscribed glioma and later developed brain infiltration. Secondary GC occurred from 1 to 21 years (median 5.2 years) after the initial glioma was diagnosed. In the 49 patients with primary GC, 33 had oligodendrogliomas, 6 oligoastrocytomas, and 7 astrocytomas; 3 tumors were not classifiable. Ten of the 14 secondary GCs occurred in lesions that were initially grade II (six oligodendrogliomas and four astrocytomas) or grade III oligodendrogliomas (four patients). Patients with secondary GC all received prior RT. Seventeen patients were treated with PCV (median cycles 5, range 1–6) and 46 with TMZ (median courses 13, range 2–24). Progression-free survival was 16 months, and overall survival was 29 months for all patients. There was no significant difference in progression-free or overall survival between the two groups but greater toxicity in the PCV group. There was also no difference in outcome between primary and secondary GC, and prior RT did not affect response to chemotherapy. Patients with oligodendroglial GC had a significantly longer survival and overall survival than those with astrocytic or oligoastrocytic GC; a finding not seen by Peretti-Viton et al. (10). It is of interest to note that the maximal response seen in patients occurred between 6 and 18 months. The inherent sensitivity of oligodendroglial tumors has recently been show to have molecular correlate with 1p and/or 19q chromosomal loss (23). The pathogenetic relevance of 1p or 19q loss remains to be determined, but it may aid in the treatment decision-making process. Patients with loss of 1p or 19q might be offered initial treatment with chemotherapy whereas those without the deletion might be treated with RT. This approach needs to be validated in prospective studies, as does the determination of the optimal treatment.

ASTROBLASTOMA

Astroblastoma is a rare and controversial glial neoplasm first described by Bailey and Bucy in 1930 (24). The term "astroblastoma" is a misnomer as these tumors are not frankly astrocytic, nor do they have blastic features (25). The existence of this tumor as a distinct entity is controversial, however, there is a growing literature of well-demarcated tumors with pure, or almost pure, astroblastomatous architecture. As such, it remains a distinct entity in the WHO classification of central nervous system (CNS) tumors but without designation of grade (26).

Astroblastomas occur most frequently in young adults and less often in children, infants, and middle-to-older–aged individuals. Patients range between 1 and 58 years of age, with a slight female predominance (25,27–30). Most patients experience a relatively brief (one to six months) duration of symptoms before diagnosis; signs include increased intracranial pressure, focal neurologic deficits, and seizures (25,28–30). Astroblastomas are primarily supratentorial tumors, most often involving the frontal or parietal lobes (30). Involvement of the corpus callosum, cerebellum, optic nerve, brain stem, and cauda equina is reported (25,30–32). Astroblastomas are rarely noted in the ventricular system, in contradistinction to ependymomas with which they are often compared (26,28,30).

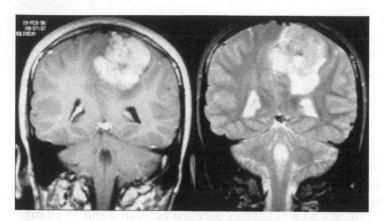

Figure 2   Astroblastoma (axial and coronal T1 postgadolinium and coronal T2).

Imaging

On MRI (Fig. 2), astroblastomas are well-circumscribed lobulated masses with a mixture of cystic and solid components (25,27,28). On T2, the solid component often has a "bubbly" appearance. Hemispheric tumors are generally peripheral with subcortical involvement and some extension into the cortex. The frontal, temporal, and parietal lobes are most commonly involved, with the tumors often encompassing more than one lobe. Enhancement is heterogeneous in the solid component and rim enhancing in the cystic component. Peritumoral edema can be present, but is minimal in most cases, especially given the size of many of the lesions (25,27). On CT scans of the brain, punctate calcifications may be seen (27).

Pathology

Grossly, tumors are well circumscribed and often lobulated, ranging in size from a few millimeters to more than 8 cm in diameter (30). These tumors are structurally homogeneous glial neoplasms characterized by a perivascular pseudorosette pattern of GFAP-positive cells with broad, nontapering processes radiating toward a central blood vessel. To be classified as an astroblastoma, these tumors should have the above findings throughout the tumor and lack of foci of conventional, infiltrative, fibrillary or gemistocytic astrocytoma, or ependymoma (26). The vascular architecture is the most striking feature of these tumors, often resulting in a papillary pattern. In about 60% of cases, a moderate to marked degree of collagen deposition and hyalinization is seen in the vessel walls; this sclerosis can be intense enough to cause luminal occlusions (30).

Astroblastoma can be subtyped into low or high grade (26,29,30). Low-grade tumors show a uniform perivascular arrangement of pseudorosettes (retaining a papillary appearance), low-to-moderate numbers of mitotic figures, little cellular atypia, minimal or no proliferation of the vascular endothelium, and often-prominent sclerosis of the vascular walls. High-grade tumors have increased cellularity with multiple cell layers piled upon the vascular walls, high mitotic rate, and cellular atypia, as well as hypertrophy and hyperplasia of the vascular endothelium without significant hyalinization of vascular walls. Necrosis may be seen in either grade of tumor (24,29); the labeling index is higher in anaplastic tumors (25). The proportion of low- and high-grade tumors is roughly even (25,27–30).

On immunohistochemical evaluation, astroblastomas exhibit GFAP, vimentin, S100, and epithelial membrane antigen (EMA) positivity (25,26,28,29).

The cell of origin of astroblastoma is unknown; but it may be derived from the tanycyte, a glial precursor cell normally found scattered along the ependymal lining of the embryonal and neonatal mammalian brain, but which is distinct from epithelial ependymocytes (33). Such an origin would account for many of the histologic findings as well as the structural features intermediate between ependymal and astrocytic cells. Additionally, the rarity of the astroblastoma could be explained by the short life span of the tanycyte during central neuroepithelial ontogeny (33).

Comparative genomic hybridization studies of seven tumors have revealed alterations dissimilar to those commonly seen in ependymomas and astrocytomas. The most frequent findings are gains of chromosome 19 and 20q; these gains are noted in both low- and high-grade tumors. Less commonly seen are loss on 9q, 10p and X (25).

Treatment

The peripheral location and well-circumscribed nature of astroblastomas often allows gross total resection by the surgeon (25,27–30). In most cases, low-grade tumors that are completely resected require no further therapy, except observation (25,27,29). Some patients have been treated with radiation and/or chemotherapy, but its impact on outcome is unclear as untreated patients do well (25,28–30).

High-grade tumors have a very different outcome, with most patients dying of progressive disease despite treatment with radiation or chemotherapy (28–30). Patients with high-grade tumors generally receive postoperative radiation with doses ranging from 38 to 72 Gy (25–30). The efficacy of radiation and the optimal field size remain unclear because in some cases there is distant CNS spread (28–30). The role of chemotherapy and optimal agent(s) selection is also unsolved; some chemotherapy regimens used include carboplatin and vincristine, paclitaxel and PCV, topotecan, and intensive chemotherapy followed by autologous stem-cell transplantation (28,29). Development of new treatment protocols is necessary, particularly in high-grade astroblastomas, but the rarity of this tumor will likely preclude large studies.

CHORDOID GLIOMA

Chordoid Glioma is a rare, low-grade primary brain tumor. It is located in the suprasellar region, arising from the third ventricular-hypothalamic area. Brat et al. first described this unique entity in 1998 (34), since then over 30 cases have been described, which have aided in our understanding of this rare lesion. Chordoid glioma primarily affects adults (median age, 45 years; range 12–70 years) with a female predominance (approximately 65%) (35). Presenting symptoms include the following: headache, nausea, and vomiting due to hydrocephalus; visual field deficits due to optic tract compression; endocrine abnormalities due to hypothalamic or pituitary compression; and personality changes including memory loss and psychosis due to affects on the lamina terminalis and trigone (36,37).

Imaging

Chordoid gliomas have stereotypic imaging features and must be considered in the differential diagnosis of suprasellar lesions (Fig. 3). They are solid, ovoid tumors, which occasionally have a central cystic or necrotic area (38). On CT, tumors are hyperdense to gray matter and homogeneously enhancing. MRI reveals a well-circumscribed mass, which is isointense to hyperintense on T1- and T2-weighted images (37); vasogenic edema has been seen extending into the optic tracts, and symmetrically into the basal ganglia and posterior limbs of the internal capsules (39). An MR perfusion study showed that the maximum cerebral blood volume ratio is significantly lower in chordoid gliomas than that observed in meningiomas or malignant gliomas, which may aid in diagnosis (37).

The radiologic differential diagnosis includes meningioma, craniopharyngioma, metastases, optic or hypothalamic pilocytic astrocytoma, giant

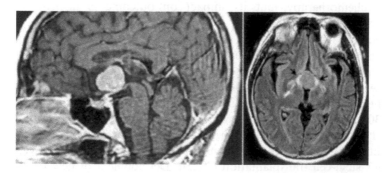

Figure 3 Chordoid glioma (sagittal T1 postgadolinium and axial FLAIR). *Source*: From Ref. 36.

aneurysm, lymphoma, and granulomatous disease. Tumors common to the third ventricle include ependymoma, choroid plexus papilloma/carcinoma, colloid cyst, and central neurocytoma (37,38). Pituitary adenoma is a consideration, but chordoid gliomas are usually clearly distinct from the pituitary gland and stalk; chordoid gliomas differ from Rathke cleft cysts and tuber cinereum hamartomas by displacing the infundibulum posteriorly rather than anteriorly (36).

Pathology

Histologic features of chordoid gliomas are consistent among all reports, and include cords and nests of epithelioid cells with abundant eosinophilic cytoplasm embedded in a mucinous matrix. Tumors exhibit prominent lymphoblastic infiltrates with Russell bodies. Nuclear features of anaplasia are not seen, and mitoses are rare (36). Proliferative activity as assessed by MIB-1 immunolabeling is uniformly low (34). Adjacent parenchyma exhibits chronic inflammation and piloid astrogliosis with Rosenthal fibers (36).

Immunohistochemical results commonly include diffuse GFAP, vimentin, and CD34 positivity (35). Some tumors contain cells that are reactive for S-100 protein and cytokeratins; EMA reactivity is inconsistent. All samples exhibit expression of EGFR and schwannomin/merlin (40). Tumors are negative for neuronal or neuroendocrine markers, desmin, estrogen or progesterone receptors, and p53, p21 (Waf-1), or Mdm2 proteins (36,40).

Molecular genetic analyses are limited, but can differentiate chordoid glioma from meningioma (no chromosome 22q deletions) and diffuse astrocytomas of adulthood (lack of amplification of EGFR, CKD4, or MDM2, and absence of mutations of TP53 and CDKN2A) (41). While chordoid gliomas appear to be of glial origin, their histogenesis remains unsettled (36). Ultrastructural studies have shown similarities to ependymomas, and, in particular, to specialized ependymal cells found in the subcommissural organ (SCO) (41). The SCO is a prominent circumventricular organ located in the dorsocaudal region of the third ventricle (42). However, given that tanycytes have an ependymal origin and arise from the anterior part of the third ventricle, as do chordoid gliomas, some authors have suggested that they may arise from embryonic tanycytes (43).

Treatment

Chordoid gliomas are relatively indolent tumors in almost all cases reported. Gross total resection is the treatment of choice, and no recurrences have been reported following total extirpation (36). However, complete resection is often impossible due to the proximity and adherence to critical structures (35,36). The role of RT remains unclear as results have been inconsistent (34,36). There are no reports using chemotherapy.

REFERENCES

1. Nevin S. Gliomatosis cerebri. Brain 1938; 61:170–191.
2. Troost D, Kuiper H, Valk J, Fleury P. Gliomatosis cerebri, report of a clinically diagnosed and histologically confirmed case. Clin Neurol Neurosurg 1987; 89: 43–47.
3. Lantos PL, Bruner JM. Gliomatosis cerebri. In: Kleihues P, Cavenee WK, eds. World Health Organization Classification of Tumours. Pathology and Genetics of Tumours of the Central Nervous System. IARC Press, 2000:92–93.
4. Kros JM, Zheng P, Dinjens WN, Alers JC. Genetic aberrations in gliomatosis cerebri support monoclonal tumorigenesis. J Neuropathol Exp Neurol 2002; 61: 806–814.
5. Jennings MT, Frenchman M, Shehab T, et al. Gliomatosis cerebri presenting as intractable epilepsy during early childhood. J Child Neurol 1995; 10:37–45.
6. Kim DG, Yang HJ, Park IA, et al. Gliomatosis cerebri: clinical features, treatment, and prognosis. Acta Neurochir (Wien) 1998; 140:755–762.
7. Elshaikh MA, Stevens GH, Peereboom DM, et al. Gliomatosis cerebri: treatment results with radiotherapy alone. Cancer 2002; 95:2027–2031.
8. Herrlinger U, Felsberg J, Kuker W, et al. Gliomatosis cerebri: molecular pathology and clinical course. Ann Neurol 2002; 52:390–399.
9. Sanson M, Cartalat-Carel S, Taillibert S, et al. Initial chemotherapy in gliomatosis cerebri. Neurology 2004; 63:270–275.
10. Peretti-Viton P, Brunel H, Chinot O, et al. Histological and MR correlations in gliomatosis cerebri. J Neurooncol 2002; 59:249–259.
11. Vates GE, Chang S, Lamborn KR, Prados M, Berger MS. Gliomatosis cerebri: a review of 22 cases. Neurosurgery 2003; 53:261–271.
12. Chamberlain MC. Gliomatosis cerebri: better definition, better treatment. Neurology 2004; 63:204–205.
13. Galanaud D, Chinot O, Nicoli F, et al. Use of proton magnetic resonance spectroscopy of the brain to differentiate gliomatosis cerebri from low-grade glioma. J Neurosurg 2003; 98:269–276.
14. Filley CM, Kleinschmidt-DeMasters BK, Lillehei KO, Damek DM, Harris JG. Gliomatosis cerebri: neurobehavioral and neuropathological observations. Cogn Behav Neurol 2003; 16:149–159.
15. Mineura K, Sasajima T, Kowada M, Uesaka Y, Shishido F. Innovative approach in the diagnosis of gliomatosis cerebri using carbon-11-L-methionine positron emission tomography. J Nucl Med 1991; 32:726–728.
16. Artigas J, Cervos-Navarro J, Iglesias JR, Ebhardt G. Gliomatosis cerebri: clinical and histological findings. Clin Neuropathol 1985; 4:135–148.
17. Miller RR, Lin F, Mallonee MM. Cytologic diagnosis of gliomatosis cerebri. Acta Cytol 1981; 25:37–39.
18. Mawrin C, Kirches E, Schneider-Stock R, et al. Alterations of cell cycle regulators in gliomatosis cerebri. J Neurooncol 2005; 72:115–122.
19. Mawrin C, Schneider T, Firsching R, et al. Assessment of tumor cell invasion factors in gliomatosis cerebri. J Neurooncol 2005; 73:109–115.
20. Giese A, Bjerkvig R, Berens ME, Westphal M. Cost of migration: invasion of malignant gliomas and implications for treatment. J Clin Oncol 2003; 21: 1624–1636.

21. Levin N, Gomori JM, Siegal T. Chemotherapy as initial treatment in gliomatosis cerebri: results with temozolomide. Neurology 2004; 63:354–356.
22. Abrey LE, DeAngelis LM, Yahalom J. Long-term survival in primary CNS lymphoma. J Clin Oncol 1998; 16:859–863.
23. Cairncross JG, Ueki K, Zlatescu MC, et al. Specific genetic predictors of chemotherapeutic response and survival in patients with anaplastic oligodendrogliomas. J Natl Cancer Inst 1998; 90:1473–1479.
24. Bailey P, Bucy PC. Astroblastomas of the brain. Acta Psychiatr Neurol 1930; 5:439–461.
25. Brat DJ, Hirose Y, Cohen KJ, Feuerstein BG, Burger PC. Astroblastoma: clinicopathologic features and chromosomal abnormalities defined by comparative genomic hybridization. Brain Pathol 2000; 10:342–352.
26. Lantos PL, Rosenblum MK. Astroblastoma. In: Kleihues P, Cavenee WK, eds. World Health Organization Classification of Tumours. Pathology and Genetics of Tumours of the Central Nervous System. IARC Press, 2000:88–89.
27. Port JD, Brat DJ, Burger PC, Pomper MG. Astroblastoma: radiologic-pathologic correlation and distinction from ependymoma. Am J Neuroradiol 2002; 23: 243–247.
28. Navarro R, Reitman AJ, de Leon GA, Goldman S, Marymont M, Tomita T. Astroblastoma in childhood: pathological and clinical analysis. Childs Nerv Syst 2005; 21:211–220.
29. Thiessen B, Finlay J, Kulkarni R, Rosenblum MK. Astroblastoma: does histology predict biologic behavior? J Neurooncol 1998; 40:59–65.
30. Bonnin JM, Rubinstein LJ. Astroblastomas: a pathological study of 23 tumors, with a postoperative follow-up in 13 patients. Neurosurgery 1989; 25:6–13.
31. Kim BS, Kothbauer K, Jallo G. Brainstem astroblastoma. Pediatr Neurosurg 2004; 40:145–146.
32. Russel DS , Rubinstein LJ. Pathology of Tumors of the Nervous System. 5th ed. Edward Arnold, London, 1989.
33. Rubinstein LJ, Herman MM. The astroblastoma and its possible cytogenic relationship to the tanycyte. An electron microscopic, immunohistochemical, tissue- and organ-culture study. Acta Neuropathol (Berl) 1989; 78:472–483.
34. Brat DJ, Scheithauer BW, Staugaitis SM, Cortez SC, Brecher K, Burger PC. Third ventricular chordoid glioma: a distinct clinicopathologic entity. J Neuropathol Exp Neurol 1998; 57:283–290.
35. Buccoliero AM, Caldarella A, Gallina P, Di LN, Taddei A, Taddei GL. Chordoid glioma: clinicopathologic profile and differential diagnosis of an uncommon tumor. Arch Pathol Lab Med 2004; 128:e141–e145.
36. Raizer JJ, Shetty T, Gutin PH, et al. Chordoid glioma: report of a case with unusual histologic features, ultrastructural study and review of the literature. J Neurooncol 2003; 63:39–47.
37. Grand S, Pasquier B, Gay E, Kremer S, Remy C, Le Bas JF. Chordoid glioma of the third ventricle: CT and MRI, including perfusion data. Neuroradiology 2002; 44:842–846.
38. Pomper MG, Passe TJ, Burger PC, Scheithauer BW, Brat DJ. Chordoid glioma: a neoplasm unique to the hypothalamus and anterior third ventricle. Am J Neuroradiol 2001; 22:464–469.

39. Pasquier B, Peoc'h M, Morrison AL, et al. Chordoid glioma of the third ventricle: a report of two new cases, with further evidence supporting an ependymal differentiation, and review of the literature. Am J Surg Pathol 2002; 26:1330–1342.
40. Reifenberger G, Weber T, Weber RG, et al. Chordoid glioma of the third ventricle: immunohistochemical and molecular genetic characterization of a novel tumor entity. Brain Pathol 1999; 9:617–626.
41. Cenacchi G, Roncaroli F, Cerasoli S, Ficarra G, Merli GA, Giangaspero F. Chordoid glioma of the third ventricle: an ultrastructural study of three cases with a histogenetic hypothesis. Am J Surg Pathol 2001; 25:401–405.
42. Rodriguez EM, Rodriguez S, Hein S. The subcommissural organ. Microsc Res Tech 1998; 41:98–123.
43. Sato K, Kubota T, Ishida M, Yoshida K, Takeuchi H, Handa Y. Immunohistochemical and ultrastructural study of chordoid glioma of the third ventricle: its tanycytic differentiation. Acta Neuropathol (Berl) 2003; 106:176–180.

13

Neuronal and Glioneuronal Neoplasms of the Central Nervous System

Tarik Tihan

Neuropathology Unit, UCSF School of Medicine, San Francisco, California, U.S.A.

James Waldron

*Department of Neurological Surgery, UCSF School of Medicine,
San Francisco, California, U.S.A.*

INTRODUCTION

Neuronal and glioneuronal tumors of the central nervous system (CNS) constitute a diverse group of lesions that includes hamartoma-like tumors as well as highly cellular and locally aggressive neoplasms. Poorly differentiated neuroblastic tumors are considered distinct from this group, and within the embryonal tumor category. Some suggest that glioneuronal hamartomas and neoplasms have common precursors that undergo abnormal divergence and differentiation (1). This suggestion is further supported by an increasing number of reported tumors with coexisting patterns, blurring the boundary between hamartoma and neoplasm.

The overwhelming majority of glioneuronal tumors shares three common features: (i) they occur in children and young adults, (ii) they are less aggressive than infiltrating astrocytomas, and (iii) they have at least two phenotypically distinct cell populations readily identified using neuronal and glial markers. Correct identification of glioneuronal tumors is critical in order to distinguish them from infiltrating high-grade gliomas, and avoid aggressive overtreatment.

Neurooncologists and neurosurgeons are confronted with an ever-increasing list of names within the glioneuronal tumor category that may not always correspond to clinically and radiologically distinct entities. Some of these names are not found in the 2000 World Health Organization (WHO) classification (2), and they do not have well-recognized treatment options or prognoses. These tumor names may reflect individual variations of an existing entity, or may be unique lesions for which molecular, genetic, and clinical characteristics can be defined.

GANGLIOCYTOMA AND GANGLIOGLIOMA

This group of indolent and well-circumscribed tumors is the most common glioneuronal tumors. Gangliocytoma is composed entirely of mature neuronal cells, and ganglioglioma is a combination of neoplastic glial and neuronal cells. Both neoplasms are considered within a single spectrum, hence the term, ganglion cell tumor (GaCT). Gangliocytomas are WHO grade I neoplasms, while gangliogliomas can be either grade I or grade II. A rare ganglioglioma with a malignant component is classified as anaplastic ganglioglioma, a WHO grade III neoplasm. There may be a common precursor to GaCTs and cortical dysplasia, since both lesions have similar clinicopathological and radiographic features.

Clinical Characteristics

Series of GaCTs report a frequency of up to 9% of all brain tumors (3). GaCTs occur equally in both sexes, and the median age at presentation between the second and the third decade of life. GaCTs are most common in the temporal lobe, but can occur throughout the neuraxis including cerebellum, optic chiasm, hypothalamus, brain stem, and the spinal cord. An unusual "gangliocytoma" can occur within the sella turcica. The most common presenting symptom for supratentorial GaCTs is seizures, followed by focal neurological deficits and headaches, but some GaCTs remain subclinical for many decades. Seizures may also antedate surgical intervention by many years. A study of gangliogliomas associated with partial complex seizures report a mean period of 11.5 years between the onset of seizures and radiological diagnosis (4).

Radiological Characteristics

Computerized tomography (CT) of GaCTs reveals a well-circumscribed, hypodense lesion with occasional isodense regions, calcifications, and variable contrast enhancement. On magnetic resonance imaging (MRI), the tumors are hypointense on T1 and iso- or hyperintense on T2-weighted sequences. Some GaCTs show partial enhancement after gadolinium injection (Fig. 1A). Cystic tumors are more common in children than older patients. Typically, there is no mass effect or surrounding edema, but peritumoral edema is rarely seen. Although GaCTs can be either cystic or solid, the

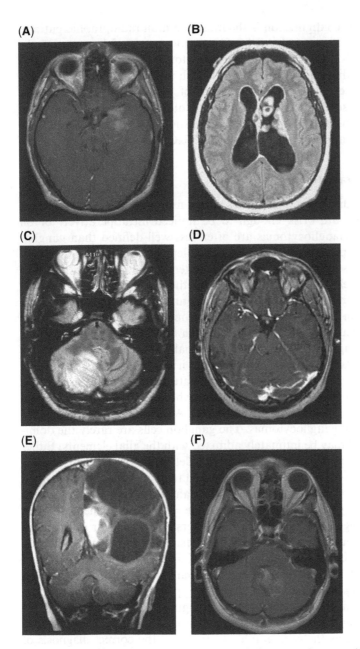

Figure 1   Typical radiographic appearance of glioneuronal tumors: (**A**) ganglioglioma—axial contrast-enhanced T1, (**B**) central neurocytoma—axial FLAIR, (**C**) Lhermitte-Duclos disease—axial T2, (**D**) dysembryoplastic neuroepithelial tumor—axial contrast-enhanced T1, (**E**) desmoplastic infantile ganglioglioma—coronal contrast-enhanced T1, and (**F**) rosette-forming glioneuronal tumor—axial contrast-enhanced T1.

cyst/mural nodule configuration is the most common radiographic pattern. Positron-emission tomography (PET) can show areas of hypermetabolic activity in GaCTs. Distinguishing gangliocytoma from ganglioglioma is challenging on radiographic grounds, although multicystic appearance and a leptomeningeal extension is more typical of ganglioglioma. GaCTs are slow-growing masses and can cause scalloping of the inner table of the skull. Due to the variability of imaging characteristics, both CT and MRI are recommended for appropriate evaluation of GaCT.

Pathological Characteristics

Most GaCTs are discrete, cystic lesions with a mural nodule. Rarely, superficial calcifications are brisk enough to be noticed intraoperatively or on gross inspection. Gangliocytomas are often less well defined than gangliogliomas. Most superficial GaCT may have leptomeningeal involvement, and the tumor cells in the subarachnoid space tend to be more spindled. The principal cellular elements of the GaCTs are the large and small neuronal cells. Gangliocytoma appears as an architecturally disorganized mixture of large neurons in a fine neuropil-like background composed of tumor cell processes. The cellularity is slightly higher than that of normal gray matter. The neoplastic ganglion cells are often abnormally clustered, have binucleation, and have vacuolated cytoplasm with irregularly distributed Nissl substance. A second component is the small mature neuronal cells accompanying the ganglion cells. Eosinophilic granular bodies (EGBs) are helpful in the diagnosis of GaCTs, and can be numerous. As a rule, gangliogliomas are more complex than gangliocytomas. The ganglion cells are rarely the dominant cell type, and may be intimately admixed with the glial elements. Either component can be small enough to avoid detection on frozen sections. Microcysts are common in gangliogliomas and may underlie the aggregated neoplastic ganglion cells, neuropil-rich lobules, and a collagen-rich internodular stroma. Some gangliogliomas demonstrate a glial component with an angiocentric arrangement (Fig. 2A), while others exhibit a clear cell pattern. The glial component is sometimes indistinguishable from a typical pilocytic astrocytoma. It is critical to distinguish GaCT from an infiltrating astrocytoma that invades the gray matter and trap ganglion cells. The distinction may be challenging in stereotactic biopsies. Trapped ganglia in an infiltrating astrocytoma may mislead the pathologist to diagnose a GaCT, only to be disappointed by an aggressive clinical outcome. It is important to consider the sample size as well as the radiographic features for the correct diagnosis of GaCT. This can be facilitated by a direct communication between the neurosurgeon and the neuropathologist, especially during frozen sections.

In GaCT, calcifications can be in the form of psammoma bodies or dystrophic clusters, and may involve vascular walls. Perivascular lymphocytic infiltrates are a frequent feature of GaCTs, and do not appear to have a

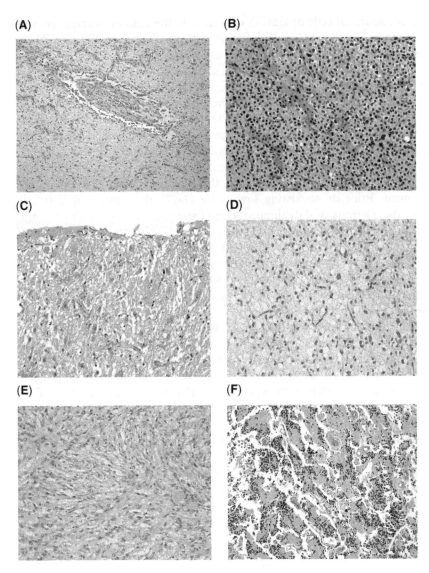

Figure 2   Typical histological patterns of glioneuronal tumors: (**A**) ganglioglioma (x100), (**B**) central neurocytoma (x200), (**C**) Lhermitte-Duclos disease (x200), (**D**) dysembryoplastic neuroepithelial tumor (x200), (**E**) desmoplastic infantile ganglioglioma (x200), and (**F**) rosette-forming glioneuronal tumor (x100).

particular prognostic significance. Pigmented cells found in GaCT can be lipofuscin, hemosiderin, or rarely melanin.

Neurofibrillary change and/or granulovacuolar degeneration, indistinguishable from those seen in neurodegenerative conditions, can be seen within the neuronal cells of GaCTs as well as in the adjacent cortex. Neuro-degenerative changes occur more often in patients older than 30 years. These changes are of no particular diagnostic significance.

One interesting feature of GaCTs is the presence of mixed lesions showing diverse histological patterns. Combination of GaCT and neurocytoma, GaCT and dysembryoplastic neuroepithelial tumor (DNT), and GaCT and PXA further challenge the definition of each entity. It has been suggested that such mixed lesions provide circumstantial evidence for a common precursor element for the glioneuronal tumors.

Anaplastic gangliogliomas are rare, but well recognized. The anaplastic features are expressed mostly within the glial, and rarely in the neuronal component. Prior or coexisting low-grade GaCT is required to correctly identify these lesions, and distinguish them from malignant gliomas or primitive neuroectodermal tumors with focal divergent differentiation identified on immunohistochemistry. In our experience, anaplastic gangliogliomas behave like malignant infiltrating gliomas of comparable grade.

The main utility of immunohistochemistry is the confirmation of the two components in GaCTs. Synaptophysin is the most commonly employed neuronal marker, followed by Neu-N, Anti-Hu, neurofilament protein, alpha-synuclein, and chromogranin. Interpretation of synaptophysin can be difficult and should be done with caution, and staining with neurofilament protein and Neu-N are often only focally positive. Chromogranin stains neuronal cells in exceptional tumors. The glial component of gangliogliomas is immunoreactive for vimentin, S-100 protein, and glial fibrillary acidic protein (GFAP). Typically, the latter stain inversely correlates with the neuronal stains. GaCTs can show immunohistochemical positivity for peptide hormones such as somatostatin, corticotropin-releasing hormone, beta-endorphin, or calcitonin.

Rarely, an ultrastructural examination is justifiable for the diagnosis of GaCTs. One can recognize multiple dense-core granules within neuronal cells, and since they are not found in large numbers within normal neurons, this is convincing of a neuronal neoplasm. In addition to dense-core granules, processes resembling Herring bodies and synaptic junctions are among the ultrastructural features of GaCTs.

Treatment and Prognosis

Surgery is the principal treatment of GaCTs, and the overall prognosis is good even in the case of partial resection, since the residual tissue will grow slowly, if at all. Some studies indicate that a prompt diagnosis, relatively soon after seizure onset, followed by gross total resection provides the best chance for curing epilepsy as well as the tumor (5). Even though recurrences may be related to high proliferative activity, this parameter is far from being a simple or reliable measure.

Patients with spinal cord gangliogliomas have a long term of progression-free survival. The majority of these tumors have an indolent course without the need for radiotherapy (6). Some reports of aggressive spinal cord gangliogliomas raise the suspicion of an infiltrating component or associated high-grade neoplasm in such examples. Temporal lobe tumors seem to have better long-term prognosis (7). Gangliogliomas involving the optic tract may cause visual loss, and the prognosis in this region may be less predictable (8). Supratentorial gangliogliomas that are higher grade (WHO grades II and III) tend to recur, but extent of resection is still the critical factor. It has also been suggested that the surgical approach and careful preoperative planning improve outcome and overall prognosis (9). The prognosis is more dependent on gross total resection and location rather than on the proliferative capacity. Anaplastic ganglioglioma or subsequent malignant transformation may require further treatment, and adjuvant therapy becomes important for such patients. Behavior of anaplastic gangliogliomas is akin to malignant gliomas of comparable histologic grade (10).

CENTRAL NEUROCYTOMA

The term "central neurocytoma" (CN) was initially coined by Hassoun et al. (11) in a report defining ultrastructural characteristics of two such neoplasms. This and subsequent studies define CN as a well-circumscribed intraventricular neoplasm, typically near the foramen of Monro. The neoplasm is considered grade II in the 2000 WHO system. It is probable that most, if not all, neoplasms previously reported as "intraventricular oligodendroglioma" can be reclassified as CN. Similar to the recommendations of the original authors, we suggest that the diagnosis of CN not be expanded to neoplasms that are purely intraparenchymal, have atypical histological features, or harbor significant percentage of blastic or glial components.

Clinical Characteristics

CNs are rare, intraventricular, primary CNS tumors, and comprise less than 1% of all brain tumors. They are equally distributed among sexes, and most patients are young adults. The median age at presentation is between the second and the third decades (12). Most patients present with signs or symptoms of cerebrospinal fluid outflow obstruction. Most common symptom is headache, followed by nausea and vomiting, visual disturbances, paresthesias, or weakness. Acute presentations can be attributed to intratumoral hemorrhage and/or occlusion of the foramen of Monro. Exceptional cases are incidental. The symptoms are usually present for a few weeks to months prior to diagnosis. There are rare examples of CNs involving the spinal cord or the cerebellum.

Radiological Characteristics

The tumors are well circumscribed, partly calcified masses within the lateral ventricle (Fig. 1B). They involve one or both of the lateral ventricles, or less commonly, arise from the third ventricle (12). Most tumors are associated with significant ventricular enlargement. CT scans typically demonstrate an iso- or hyperdense mass adjacent to the foramen of Monro or the septum pellucidum, and show conspicuous calcifications. On MRI, T1-weighted images are often isointense to gray matter or hypointense, and tumors variable intensity on T2-weighted images. Contrast enhancement is variable and can be brisk and homogenous in some tumors. Tumor margins are relatively well defined with a smooth contour and occasionally show cystic component or hemorrhage.

Pathological Characteristics

Intraoperatively, tumors are well circumscribed but are focally attached to septum pellucidum and/or ventricular walls, and rarely appear to infiltrate the parenchyma. Tumor fragments are often soft, fleshy in color, similar to gray matter, and may contain cysts.

CNs are cytologically and architecturally monomorphous with fried-egg cells and the so-called chicken-wire vascular network, that show a remarkable histological similarity to oligodendrogliomas (Fig. 2B). CN may also display nodules or clusters of tumor cells interspaced by a neuropil-like background. The tumor nuclei possess a finely distributed chromatin network, the so-called "salt and pepper" chromatin pattern. The perivascular fibrillary zones can give the impression of ependymal pseudorosettes. Some regions exhibit striking neurocytic differentiation with streaming cells similar to classic medulloblastomas. Rare tumors may contain lipofuscin or neuromelanin pigment. Tumors resembling CNs with foci of ganglion cells have been referred as "ganglioneurocytoma." The exact relationship of such lesions to CNs is unclear. Typical CN does not exhibit significant pleomorphism, vascular proliferation, or necrosis. Mitotic figures are rare, but may be numerous in unusual cases. Such neoplasms are considered "atypical" neurocytomas, and have a reportedly elevated incidence of local recurrence (13).

CNs are highlighted by a number of neuronal stains. Almost all tumors are positive with class-III b-tubulin, MAP-2, synaptophysin, and neuron-specific enolase, and generally lack reactivity for chromogranin. Most are focally positive for neurofilament proteins. Anti-Hu and Neu-N stain almost all the neoplastic nuclei in CNs. Some tumors may have a subpopulation of GFAP-positive neoplastic cells. Ki-67 staining can be useful to determine tumors with a higher likelihood of recurrence, and tumors with > 2% Ki-67 index are considered atypical (13). The ultrastructural features of CN include microtubules, terminations, clear vesicles, dense-core granules, and intercellular junctions. Well-formed synapses are rare. Alterations in chromosomes 2p,

7, 10q, 17, and 18q have been encountered in CNs. However, none of these putative changes have been reproducibly demonstrated as a distinguishing feature of CN. One pertinent negative finding is the absence of chromosomal alterations that are typically seen in oligodendroglial neoplasms.

Treatment and Prognosis

The principal treatment for CNs is gross total resection, which confers an excellent outcome (12,14). Craniospinal dissemination of CN is extremely rare. Gross total resection is not always possible due to attachment to surrounding ventricular surfaces, and, sometimes, inaccessible location within the ventricles. Following gross total resection, radiotherapy does not appear to provide additional benefit. In cases of incomplete resection or recurrence, either radiation or chemotherapy may be used as adjuvant therapy. Overall, the prognosis of CN is excellent; with about reported rate of 81% five-year survival (12). Atypical CNs with > 2% Ki-67 index tend to recur more often (13).

DYSPLASTIC GANGLIOCYTOMA OF CEREBELLUM (LHERMITTE-DUCLOS DISEASE)

Clinical Characteristics

Dysplastic gangliocytoma of cerebellum or Lhermitte-Duclos disease (LDD) is a tumoral but non-neoplastic developmental abnormality of the cerebellar cortex due to massive enlargement of neurons in the internal granule cell layer. The lesion arises sporadically or in the setting of Cowden syndrome. LDD, either within the spectrum of Cowden syndrome or in an isolated form, is extremely rare. Typically, the disease presents in adults at a mean age of 35 years (15). LDD has an equal gender distribution. The prevalence of Cowden disease is in the range of 1 in 250,000 in some populations with a low mutation frequency (16). Patients present in the second or third decades with headaches, nausea/vomiting, and vertigo, or macrocephaly (15). Less-common symptoms include seizures, orthostatic hypotension, or subarachnoid hemorrhage. Cowden syndrome patients with LDD also exhibit other lesions of the syndrome, which include thyroid disease, meningiomas, multiple tricholemmomas, oral papillomatosis and cutaneous keratoses, gastrointestinal polyps, and hamartomatous soft-tissue lesions. Breast cancer affects approximately one-third of women with Cowden syndrome. Patients with LDD should be comprehensively screened for all features of Cowden syndrome.

Radiological Characteristics

LDD is characterized as a slowly growing mass in the posterior fossa. CT scans suggest the diagnosis by showing a posterior fossa lesion, iso- and hypodense, partially calcified, and without contrast enhancement. The distinctive "tiger-striped" cerebellar mass that is hyperintense on T2-weighted, and hypointense on T1-weighted images is virtually pathognomonic (Fig. 1C). LDD rarely shows gadolinium enhancement, and may have restricted diffusion in diffusion-weighted images. Spectroscopic features of LDD demonstrate reduced N-acetyl aspartate/choline and N-acetyl aspartate/creatine, and normal choline/creatine. Peaks attributable to lactate can be seen.

Pathological Characteristics

Intraoperatively, distortion of the cerebellar hemispheric folia and displacement of cerebellar tonsils are helpful features. Macroscopically, the thickened folia produce a sizable increase in the volume of the affected hemisphere. Microscopically, there is replacement of internal granular cell layer by "hypertrophic" or bizarre ganglion cells (Fig. 2C), abnormal myelination of the molecular layer, and partial or complete loss of Purkinje cells. The extent of these changes varies markedly from case to case, and even within the same lesion. Typically, both the molecular layer and the internal granular layer exhibit increased cellularity. Microscopic calcifications, especially along the abnormal internal granular layer can be seen. While most of the abnormal neurons appear to be derived from granule cells, Purkinje cell–specific antibodies may be positive in hypertrophic neurons, which are also reactive with neurofilament antibodies. The neurofilament-staining pattern of hypertrophic cells is similar to normal cerebellar neurons suggesting a hamartomatous rather than neoplastic character. Electron-microscopic investigations highlighted the neuronal character of the hypertrophic granular cell neurons, excess of myelination of axons in the molecular layer, and degenerative changes within the remaining Purkinje cells.

Recent genetic advances in the studies of LDD have found germline PTEN mutations as the major genetic aberration in LDD with and without Cowden syndrome (16). This gene, located at chromosome 10q23–3, is a tumor suppressor gene that encodes a protein with phosphatase activity. PTEN mutations may not be readily demonstrable in some patients with LDD, and the genetic basis in such cases is unclear.

Treatment and Prognosis

LDD is a benign process, and surgical excision is the only satisfactory treatment for symptomatic patients. We have observed rare cases that have "recurred" after subtotal resection following a long quiescent period (15). This "recurrent" lesion is best treated with a subsequent resection rather than radiation or chemotherapy. When the diagnosis of LDD is established, it is imperative to search for lesions that occur in Cowden disease. Finally, a long-term follow-up of the patient is required and a thorough familial screening is necessary.

DYSEMBRYOPLASTIC NEUROEPITHELIAL TUMOR

Clinical Characteristics

DNT was originally described by Daumas-Duport et al. (17) as an intracortical multinodular mass, predominantly composed of oligodendrocyte-like cells. The neoplasm is considered a grade I lesion in the 2000 WHO system, and is classified within the neuronal or mixed glioneuronal tumors category, but its origin is not clear. DNT is typically seen within the first two decades, and the majority of patients are less than 15 years at the onset of their symptoms (17). The most common presentation is partial complex seizures, which last many years before the patients undergo surgery. Most DNTs are supratentorial, and temporal lobe is the most common site. DNT constitutes approximately 3% of cases among patients surgically treated for temporal lobe epilepsy. There has been little association of DNT with dysgenetic syndromes or familial seizure disorders, but a rare familial occurrence can be observed. DNTs have also been reported within the caudate nucleus, floor of the third ventricle, brain stem, and cerebellum. Rare tumors can be multifocal.

Radiological Characteristics

On CT, DNTs are cortically based, moderately hypodense lesions on non-contrast images, and some may show high-attenuation foci compatible with calcifications. The hypodense, cystic nature of the tumor can be better visualized, following contrast administration, which may show enhancing foci. Erosion of the inner table is common in DNTs that are juxtaposed to the skull. MRI demonstrates a well defined, T1-hypointense, T2-hyperintense lesion with intracortical nodular appearance (Fig. 1D). Typically, there is no associated edema or mass effect. Cortical localization may not be evident in the bulky masses. Gadolinium injection usually shows no significant enhancement, but some DNTs exhibit a narrow enhancing rim that can mimic high-grade glioma or an abscess. PET, SPECT, and spectroscopy suggest a benign lesion, but the findings are not specific for DNT. The choline/creatine and N-acetyl-aspartate/creatine ratios in DNTs are often lower than those of malignant gliomas.

Pathological Characteristics

Typically, DNTs form blister-like nodules with a mucoid texture on the surface of the cerebral cortex. Perpendicular sections of the surgical specimen reveal a blurred gray–white matter junction. Thinning of the overlying skull is commonly noticed intraoperatively.

Microscopically, DNTs are multinodular and multicystic with both glial (oligodendrocyte-like) and neuronal (ganglion-like) components. There is minimal cytologic atypia, and the adjacent cortex shows dysplastic elements. The initial description of DNT included three architectural elements: (i) the nodular element, (ii) the glioneuronal element, and (iii) a region of cortex with dysplastic elements (17). The nodular element is composed of oligodendroglia-like cells. The nodules are patternless, but may have a steaming or circumferential pattern, and invariably contain isolated "floating" ganglion cells within their myxoid matrix (Fig. 2D). The glioneuronal element is composed of small cells similar to oligodendrogliomas with a more infiltrative architecture than the nodular element. The vertical columns of small mature cells forming files and chains arrange themselves along delicate vascular structures. The floating neurons without obvious cytological abnormality are also observed in the glioneuronal element. Cytologically abnormal neurons are commonly identified on the fringes of the glioneuronal element or in the adjacent cortex. This region represents the cortical dysplasia or the third element. DNT can harbor more complex patterns, including compact elongated cells with microcysts, Rosenthal fibers, and EGBs, simulating a pilocytic astrocytoma. Some DNTs exhibit a linear pattern of glomeruloid vascular proliferation that can be attributed to cystic change, degeneration, and rarely infarction. This linear pattern of proliferating vessels corresponds to the contrast-enhancing rim on MRI. Calcifications in the cortical tissue adjacent to the lesion as well as within the lesion are common, and confirm the radiological impression. DNTs typically have no mitoses, but some tumors may have scattered mitotic figures.

Other patterns have been described as nonspecific forms of DNT (18). These observations have led to the concepts of "simple" and "complex" forms of DNT. It remains to be seen whether all nonspecific or complex forms can be considered within the DNT category. Rare cases of coexisting DNT and ganglioglioma further expand the complex form.

Immunohistochemically, the oligodendroglia-like cells of DNT are positive for antibodies against S-100 protein and NSE. A variable percentage of cells are positive for Olig-2, Neu-N, class III ß-tubulin, and neurofilament. Synaptophysin staining is largely negative but highlights a granular background and scattered floating neurons. A small number of cells stain positively with antibodies against GFAP, but this staining is variable. The generally slow growth and relatively benign nature of DNT is reflected by their low Ki-67 index, but rare tumors can exhibit higher percentages.

Ultrastructurally, while neurosecretory granules and clear vesicles can be found in some cases, synapses are rarely encountered, and the cells often show no specific differentiation. A morphologically obvious distinction between DNT and oligodendrogliomas involves absence of LOH in chromosomes 1p, 17p, and 19q in the former. Currently no specific genetic alteration has been associated with DNT.

Treatment and Prognosis

The primary treatment of DNT is gross total resection, without adjuvant therapy. Among the 39 cases originally reported by Daumas-Duport et al., there was no clinical or radiological evidence of progression, even in subtotally resected tumors (17). However, recurrence of seizures can be seen in subtotally resected tumors after a long stable period. It has been suggested that resection of the epileptic focus in addition to the complete removal of DNT is necessary to control seizures. Exceptionally rare is a "malignant transformation" of DNT with or without prior history of radiation therapy. We have yet to observe a typical DNT progress into a malignant glioma in the absence of history of radiation treatment.

DESMOPLASTIC INFANTILE ASTROCYTOMA AND GANGLIOGLIOMA

The original descriptions of desmoplastic infantile astrocytoma (DIA) as "superficial cerebral astrocytoma" by Taratuto et al. (19) and the desmoplastic infantile ganglioglioma (DIG) by VandenBerg et al. (20) define a unique group of large supratentorial tumors in infants that exhibit extensive desmoplasia and a relatively good outcome. These two groups of tumors are essentially identical except for the absence of evidence for neuronal differentiation in the DIA. Due to their striking resemblance for all clinical and radiological aspects, these two entities are considered within the same category. Furthermore, it has been suggested that tumors previously reported as gliofibroma should be considered within this category.

Clinical/Radiological Characteristics

DAI/DIG are rare, exclusively supratentorial, voluminous, and cystic tumors that present primary within the first 18 months of life, and have very favorable prognosis. They comprise less than 1% of all brain tumors, and reportedly occur more commonly in males. Tumors with identical clinical, radiological, and pathological features have been reported in older children.

DIA/DIG occupy multiple lobes, and most commonly the frontal and parietal regions. Patients commonly present with a rapid enlargement of the head with bulging fontanels, seizures, and hemiparesis with a history of symptoms ranging from a few weeks to six months.

Radiological Characteristics

The salient imaging features of DIA/DIG are large size, involvement of two or more lobes, contrast enhancement along the meninges, and a large cystic component. On CT, the tumors are heterogeneous with cystic hypodense portion and a solid-enhancing component. Calcifications and the thinning of the skull overlying the tumor may be seen. On MRI, the tumors are as hypointense cystic masses with an isointense peripheral solid component on T1-weighted images. The peripheral solid component enhances after gadolinium administration (Fig. 1E). On T2-weighted MRI, the cystic component is hyperintense and the solid portion is either isointense or heterogeneous.

Pathological Characteristics

The tumors often contain large cysts with small amounts of clear or xanthochromic fluid. The solid component is gray–white with a rubbery consistency sharply demarcated from the surrounding tissues, but may be partly, attached to the adjacent parenchyma. The main histological feature is the striking degree of "desmoplasia" that gives the tumor a fibroblastic rather than a neuroepithelial character (Fig. 2E). The tumor is highly cellular, wavy, or whirly on low-power magnification, and may display a storiform pattern. The rigid streaming pattern is typically highlighted by a reticulin stain that demonstrates the extent of desmoplasia. Typically, the tumor exhibits a compact pattern of growth, and occasionally infiltrates into neuropil or the Virchow–Robin spaces. Local leptomeningeal dissemination is common, and the tumor cells attain a more spindled appearance once within the leptomeningeal space. The principal cell type observed in DIA/DIG is a spindle cell with elongated and pleomorphic nuclei and eosinophilic cytoplasm. In addition, particularly for DIG, there are numerous ganglion-like cells, representing the neuronal component. Typically, mitoses are rare, and glomeruloid vascular proliferation or necrosis is absent. However, there are rare examples with increased mitoses, vascular proliferation, or necrosis. In some tumors, there is a small undifferentiated cell component with numerous mitoses and hypervascularity. The prognostic significance of these "anaplastic" features is still not clear, but such tumors do not necessarily have an aggressive clinical course. The glial cells of DIA/DIG are strongly positive with antibodies against GFAP, vimentin, and S-100 protein. Some cells also show positive staining with β-tubulin and NSE. Synaptophysin and neurofilament as well as anti-Hu protein highlight the pleomorphic cells and occasionally smaller cells with neuronal qualities. Collagen type IV antibodies highlight the extensive basement membrane material. The Ki-67 labeling index is low, and is often less than 2%.

Ultrastructurally, the spindle tumor cells with lobulated nuclei and highly condensed chromatin constitute the glial component. The cytoplasm of these cells contains numerous intermediate filaments, mitochondria, ribosomes, and granular endoplasmic reticulum (20). The glial cells are also partly covered by a basal lamina, and some exhibit small stacks of rough endoplasmic reticulum and neuroendocrine granules.

Existing studies of DIA/DIG demonstrate absence of genetic aberrations typically seen in common infiltrating astrocytomas. Studies found no evidence of p53 gene mutations or chromosome 10 or 17 alterations. Comparative genomic hybridization analysis of two DIGs revealed a loss on 8p22-pter in one tumor and a gain on 13q21 in another (21).

Treatment and Prognosis

Despite their often-worrisome histological and radiological appearance, DIA/DIG have an excellent prognosis, but can present formidable surgical challenges. Surgery can provide cure without adjuvant therapy even after incomplete resection. In the case of recurrence or subtotal resection, a second surgery should be considered instead of adjuvant therapy. Postoperative regression of subtotally removed DIGs has been recognized.

RECENTLY DESCRIBED GLIONEURONAL TUMORS

In addition to the currently recognized entities, recent studies describe neoplasms that are only partially similar to the entities described above, yet may be distinctly unique tumors. Currently, data on these tumors are limited, and there is uncertainty about their exact designations. Nevertheless, some of these reports describe tumors that are worthy of recognition and are described below.

Extraventricular Neurocytoma

Extraventricular neurocytoma (EVN) is defined as a pure neuronal tumor that is outside the ventricular system. These rare neoplasms containing neuronal as well as ganglion-like cells arise within the parenchyma, but some may abut the ventricles (22). Previously reported tumors such as cystic ganglioneurocytoma or pseudopapillary neurocytoma are most likely in this category (23,24). EVN is not in the current WHO classification scheme. EVNs have been reported at all ages, but the lesions generally favor young adults with a median of 34 years (22). EVN can present with symptoms such as diplopia, headaches, weakness, nausea, and vomiting, while some patients present with seizures. MRI characteristics reportedly show a solid component that is hyperintense on both T1- and T2-weighted images, without appreciable contrast enhancement. Like the typical CN, EVNs contain oligodendrocyte-like cells that are arranged in sheets, clusters, ribbons, or rosettes, in association with a neuropil-like background (22). The tumors resemble oligodendrogliomas with their fried-egg appearing cells. The neoplasm is infiltrative in certain regions, and is architecturally and cytologically more complex than CN, with ganglion-like cells more common than in CNs. The tumors often contain psammomatous calcifications. Only rarely do neurocytic neoplasms exhibit malignant cytologic features or contain neuroblastic cells. In a recent study, EVNs with geographic necrosis, vascular proliferation, or mitoses greater than 3 per 10 high-power fields constituted an "atypical" group (22). The tumor typically shows granular synaptophysin positivity and focal staining with Neu-N and anti-Hu antibodies. Chromogranin may be negative. Astrocytes, either reactive or neoplastic, are GFAP positive. The principal goal for treatment of EVN is gross total resection. In one of the larger series published, none of the gross totally resected tumors recurred (22). EVN may have a long recurrence-free survival even after subtotal resection.

Papillary Glioneuronal Tumor

Komori et al. described the clinicopathologic features of a unique papillary glioneuronal tumor within the cerebrum exhibiting astrocytic and extensive neuronal differentiation (25). This neoplasm may represent either a variant of ganglioglioma or a complex variant of EVN with divergent differentiation. The tumor can occur at any age, and presents with mild neurologic symptoms such as headache or visual symptoms. MRI shows a well-demarcated solid/cystic mass that is hyperintense on T2-weighted images. Most tumors do not show enhancement with gadolinium, but rare cases with focal enhancement were reported. Overall, cellularity is moderate with minimal atypia. No mitotic activity, vascular proliferation, or necrosis was recorded in any of the reported examples. Microscopically, tumors have a compact pseudopapillary component with hyalinized vessels covered by a single layer of GFAP-positive astrocytes, and a synaptophysin-positive neuronal component. Immunostains for Olig-2 stained a small population of tumor cells, while chromogranin was negative (26). The Ki-67 labeling is low, and p53 staining is often negative. Ultrastructurally, neuronal cells show microtubule-containing processes, aberrant synaptic terminals, and rare dense-core granules. Most tumors were totally resected, which resulted in a favorable outcome. All patients reported to date showed no evidence of tumor recurrence, confirming the indolent behavior of this tumor (27).

Rosetted Glioneuronal Tumor of the Fourth Ventricle

In 2002, Komori et al. described a distinctive tumor of the posterior fossa as a novel glioneuronal CNS neoplasm (28). The patients presented with headache and/or ataxia, and were found to have relatively discrete, focally enhancing tumors primarily involving the fourth ventricle. Rare cases were incidental. All patients were adults, and a wide age range was recorded. Due to the tumor location, most patients presented with hydrocephalus, but occasionally headaches and cervical pain were noted. MRI demonstrated ventriculomegaly and a solid tumor that was hyperintense on T2- and hypointense on T1-weighted images with occasional contrast enhancement (Fig. 1F). Microscopically, the tumors exhibited two components: neurocytes forming rosettes or perivascular pseudorosettes and an astrocytic component with EGBs resembling pilocytic astrocytoma. The tumors were partly invested in a rich neuropil-like matrix, with small neuronal cells forming rosettes, hyalinized vessels, and microcalcifications (Fig. 2F). Rare ganglion cells were also present. Immunohistochemically, the tumors demonstrated a divergent differentiation with GFAP- and synaptophysin-positive cells. The rosettes were primarily synaptophysin and MAP-2 positive, while the spindle cells were S-100 protein and GFAP positive. None of the tumors had mitoses, and Ki-67 labeling was low. Ultrastructurally, the neurocytic cells featured processes containing microtubules, occasional dense-core granules, and rare mature synapses. The natural history of rosette-forming glioneuronal tumors of the fourth ventricle is not yet fully understood, and the prognosis is uncertain.

Glioneuronal Tumor of the Adult Cerebrum with Neuropil-Like (Including "Rosetted") Islands

Glioneuronal tumors with neuropil-like islands (rosetted glioneuronal tumors) have been reported as a unique entity with characteristic clinico-pathological features (29). These tumors affect adults and are located within the cerebral hemisphere, and rarely in the spinal cord. Symptoms include seizures, weakness, as well as manifestations of raised intracranial pressure. CT scans reveal a hypodense mass without calcification. MRI shows a solid T1-hypointense and T2-hyperintense tumor with moderate mass effect, and without contrast enhancement. Tumors are infiltrative microscopically, with a prominent glial component similar to infiltrating astrocytomas, but also contain sharply delimited, neuropil-like islands with intense synaptophysin staining. The nuclei of the neuronal cells are Neu-N and anti-Hu positive. Mitoses and increased proliferation rate can be seen in the glial component, with occasional tumors exhibiting Ki-67 (MIB-1) indices as high as 8%. The outcome of patients is highly variable with rare cases proving fatal in a relative short time. In one case, there was gain of chromosome 7q and a loss on chromosome 9p suggestive of an aggressive neoplasm (30). Recurrence and poor outcome of some these tumors distinguish this group from most other glioneuronal tumors (31).

Cerebellar Liponeurocytoma

Ellison et al. described a posterior fossa tumor characterized histologically by bland, oval cells with fibrillary cytoplasm and by small groups of lipo-cytes (32). The tumor demonstrated expression of synaptophysin and NSE, and a few cells also expressed GFAP. Subsequent studies confirmed the presence of a well-differentiated lesion with clear adipose differentiation and a small cell component with neuronal differentiation. On CT scans, the tumor is hypointense with foci exhibiting the attenuation values of adipose tissue. On MRI, the tumor is hypointense on T1-weighted images with scattered foci of hyperintense signal and moderate contrast enhancement.

A recent study revealed missense p53 gene mutations in cerebellar liponeurocytomas at a frequency higher than in medulloblastomas, but found no mutations in PTCH, APC, or beta-catenin, or evidence of isochromosome 17q (33). A cDNA array analysis suggested that the tumors were closer to CNs rather than medulloblastomas. Typically, cerebellar liponeurocytomas are associated with a favorable outcome, but exceptions to this clinical course have reported. Current recommended treatment is total resection, and the benefit of adjuvant therapy is unclear.

REFERENCES

1. Blumcke I, et al. Evidence for developmental precursor lesions in epilepsy-associated glioneuronal tumors. Microsc Res Tech 1999; 46(1):53–58.
2. Kleihues P, Cavenee WK. Pathology and Genetics of Tumours of the Nervous System. In: World Health Organization Classification of Tumours. Lyon: IARC Press, 2000.
3. Rickert CH, Paulus W. Epidemiology of central nervous system tumors in childhood and adolescence based on the new WHO classification. Childs Nerv Syst 2001; 17(9):503–511.
4. Tampieri D, et al. Intracerebral gangliogliomas in patients with partial complex seizures: CT and MR imaging findings. AJNR Am J Neuroradiol 1991; 12(4): 749–755.
5. Aronica E, et al. Glioneuronal tumors and medically intractable epilepsy: a clinical study with long-term follow-up of seizure outcome after surgery. Epilepsy Res 2001; 43(3):179–191.
6. Jallo GI, Freed D, Epstein FJ. Spinal cord gangliogliomas: a review of 56 patients. J Neurooncol 2004; 68(1):71–77.
7. Ventureyra E, et al. Temporal lobe gangliogliomas in children. Child Nerv Syst 1986; 2(2):63–66.
8. Liu GT, et al. Gangliogliomas involving the optic chiasm. Neurology 1996; 46(6):1669–1673.
9. Otsubo H, et al. Evaluation, surgical approach and outcome of seizure patients with gangliogliomas. Pediatr Neurosurg 1990; 16(4–5):208–212.
10. Tihan T, et al. Glioneuronal tumors with malignant histological features. J Neuropathol Exp Neurol 1999; 58:509.
11. Hassoun J, et al. Central neurocytoma. An electron-microscopic study of two cases. Acta Neuropathol 1982; 56(2):151–156.
12. Schild SE, et al. Central neurocytomas. Cancer 1997; 79(4):790–795.
13. Soylemezoglu F, et al. Atypical central neurocytoma. J Neuropathol Exp Neurol 1997; 56(5):551–556.
14. Sharma MC, et al. Intraventricular neurocytoma: a clinicopathological study of 20 cases with review of the literature. J Clin Neurosci 1999; 6(4):319–323.
15. Abel TW, et al. Lhermitte-Duclos disease: a report of 31 cases with immunohistochemical analysis of the PTEN/AKT/mTOR pathway. J Neuropathol Exp Neurol 2005; 64(4):341–349.

16. Nelen MR, et al. Novel PTEN mutations in patients with Cowden disease: absence of clear genotype-phenotype correlations. Eur J Hum Genet 1999; 7(3): 267–273.
17. Daumas-Duport C, et al. Dysembryoplastic neuroepithelial tumor: a surgically curable tumor of young patients with intractable partial seizures. Report of thirty-nine cases. Neurosurgery 1988; 23(5):545–556.
18. Daumas-Duport C, et al. Dysembryoplastic neuroepithelial tumors: nonspecific histological forms—a study of 40 cases. J Neurooncol 1999; 41(3):267–280.
19. Taratuto AL, et al. Superficial cerebral astrocytoma attached to dura: report of six cases in infants. Cancer 1984; 54:2505–2512.
20. VandenBerg SR, et al. Desmoplastic supratentorial neuroepithelial tumors of infancy with divergent differentiation potential ("desmoplastic infantile gangliogliomas"). Report on 11 cases of a distinctive embryonal tumor with favorable prognosis. J Neurosurg 1987; 66(1):58–71.
21. Kros JM, et al. Desmoplastic infantile astrocytoma and ganglioglioma: a search for genomic characteristics. Acta Neuropathol (Berl) 2002; 104(2):144–148.
22. Brat DJ, et al. Extraventricular neurocytomas: pathologic features and clinical outcome. Am J Surg Pathol 2001; 25(10):1252–1260.
23. Giangaspero F, et al. Extraventricular neoplasms with neurocytoma features. A clinicopathological study of 11 cases. Am J Surg Pathol 1997; 21(2):206–212.
24. Kim DH, Suh Y-L. Pseudopapillary neurocytoma of temporal lobe with glial differentiation. Acta Neuropathol 1997; 94:187–191.
25. Komori T, et al. Papillary glioneuronal tumor: a new variant of mixed neuronal-glial neoplasm. Am J Surg Pathol 1998; 22(10):1171–1183.
26. Tanaka Y, et al. A distinct pattern of Olig2-positive cellular distribution in papillary glioneuronal tumors: a manifestation of the oligodendroglial phenotype? Acta Neuropathol (Berl) 2005.
27. Borges G, et al. Long term follow-up in a patient with papillary glioneuronal tumor. Arq Neuropsiquiatr 2004; 62(3B):869–872.
28. Komori T, Scheithauer BW, Hirose T. A rosette-forming glioneuronal tumor of the fourth ventricle: infratentorial form of dysembryoplastic neuroepithelial tumor? Am J Surg Pathol 2002; 26(5):582–591.
29. Teo JG, et al. A distinctive glioneuronal tumor of the adult cerebrum with neuropil-like (including "rosette") islands: report of 4 cases. Am J Surg Pathol 1999; 23(5):502–510.
30. Keyvani K, et al. Rosetted glioneuronal tumor: a case with proliferating neuronal nodules. Acta Neuropathol (Berl) 2001; 101(5):525–528.
31. Prayson RA, Abramovich CM. Glioneuronal tumor with neuropil-like islands. Hum Pathol 2000; 31(11):1435–1438.
32. Ellison DW, Zygmunt SC, Weller RO. Neurocytoma/lipoma (neurolipocytoma) of the cerebellum. Neuropathol Appl Neurobiol 1993; 19(1):95–98.
33. Horstmann S, et al. Genetic and expression profiles of cerebellar liponeurocytomas. Brain Pathol 2004; 14(3):281–289.

14

Pineal Parenchymal Tumors

Daizo Yoshida and Akira Teramoto

Department of Neurosurgery, Nippon Medical School, Tokyo, Japan

INTRODUCTION

Pineal region tumors are derived from cells located in and around the pineal gland. The principal cell of the pineal gland is the pineal parenchymal cell or pinocyte. This cell is a specialized neuron related to retinal rods and cones. The pinocyte is surrounded by a stroma of fibrillary astrocytes, which interact with adjoining blood vessels to form part of the blood–pial barrier. The pineal gland is a neuroendocrine transducer that synchronizes hormonal release with phases of the light–dark cycle by means of its sympathetic input. However, the exact relationship between the pineal gland and human circadian rhythm remains unclear and is an active area of investigation (1).

In the early part of the 20th century, pineal region surgery had poor outcomes, with operative mortality rates approaching 90%. If a pineal tumor did not respond to radiation, a surgical procedure was performed. The algorithm of cerebrospinal fluid (CSF) diversion, radiation, and observation was sometimes successful, but patients with benign lesions were exposed to unnecessary and ineffective radiation. The advent of microsurgical techniques and stereotactic procedures in the later part of the 20th century obviated the need for empiric radiotherapy without tissue diagnosis. Therapeutic decision-making is now based on tumor histology rather than on response to radiation. The current standard of care for patients with pineal parenchymal tumors (PPT) consists of initial surgical management, both for diagnosis and for possible resection (2).

EPIDEMIOLOGY

Tumors of the pineal cell origin are much less common than those of germ cell origin and usually occur in the first and early in the second decade of life. PPT account for less than 1% of primitive central nervous system (CNS) tumors. The revised World Health Organization (WHO) Classification of CNS tumors divides PPT into well-differentiated pineocytoma (PC), poorly differentiated pineoblastoma (PB), and mixed pineocytoma and pineoblastoma (PC–PB) or PPT with intermediate differentiation. PCs (WHO grade II) are slow-growing pineal parenchymal neoplasms, comprising approximately 45% of all PPT, which occur primarily in young adults, aged 25 to 35 years. There are no specific cytogenetic abnormalities or molecular genetics for this tumor. The five-year survival rate has been reported to be as high as 86%. PBs (WHO grade IV) are highly malignant primitive embryonal tumors of the pineal gland, comprising approximately 45% of all PPT, which manifest primarily in children. There are no specific cytogenetic abnormalities or molecular genetics. Tumors similar in appearance to PBs have been observed in patients with familial (bilateral) retinoblastoma (3). PPT of intermediate differentiation are monomorphous tumors exhibiting moderately high cellularity, mild nuclear atypia, occasional mitosis, and absence of large pineocytomatous rosettes. They comprise approximately 10% of all PPT and occur in all age groups. Clinically, PPT have unpredictable growth and clinical behavior. Briefly, PCs are generally benign lesions of the pineal parenchyma occurring predominantly in adults, whereas PBs are quite rare in adults, usually occurring before the age of 20, and are slightly more common in males (4).

Due to the rarity of PPT, there are a limited number of case series reporting the histological features of these neoplasms. In addition, most of the large retrospective series have focused on the clinical and therapeutic aspects of these tumors. The incidence of mixed/intermediate PPT varies, which may reflect the difficulty in classifying intermediate-type tumors. However, accurate histological diagnosis is critical for appropriate management of this disease. The spectrum of pineal region tumors includes two possible groups of lesions: tumors arising from the pineal gland and tumors extending to the pineal region from adjacent regions. The first group can be subdivided into neoplastic derivatives of multipotential embryonic germ cells such as PBs and PCs. The second group, tumors extending to the pineal region from adjacent regions, includes various types of lesions, in particular astrocytomas and meningiomas. Magnetic resonance imaging (MRI) has markedly improved the preoperative delineation of benign and malignant pineal masses and has distinguished true pineal masses from parapineal masses impinging into the region of the gland. While pineal tumors are uncommon overall, accounting for 12% of all intracranial masses, they are relatively more frequent in children (38%). Germinomas are the most common type of pineal tumor, accounting for more than two-thirds of pineal region masses, followed by teratomas and pineal gland tumors (15%), and PCs/PBs (15%) (5).

SPECIFIC CLINICAL FEATURES

The clinical syndromes associated with pineal region tumors are related directly to normal pineal anatomical structures, as well as to tumor histology. Mass lesions in the pineal region that compress adjacent structures induce typical clinical syndromes. One of the most common clinical manifestations is headache, nausea, and vomiting caused by aqueductal compression and resultant obstructive hydrocephalus. Untreated, hydrocephalus may lead progressively to lethargy, obtundation, and death. Compromise of the superior colliculus, either through direct compression or through tumor invasion, results in a syndrome of vertical gaze palsy that can be associated with pupillary or oculomotor nerve paresis. This eponymic syndrome was first described by the French ophthalmologist Henri Parinaud in the late 1800s and has become virtually pathognomonic for lesions involving the quadrigeminal plate. Further compression of the periaqueductal gray region may cause mydriasis, convergence spasm, pupillary inequality, and convergence or retractory nystagmus. Impairment of downgaze becomes more pronounced with tumors involving the ventral midbrain. Patients also can present with motor impairment, such as ataxia and dysmetria, resulting from compromise of cerebellar efferent fibers within the superior cerebellar peduncle. Indications for neurosurgical intervention relate to the severity and chronicity of clinical presentation. The symptoms of pineal region tumors can be as varied as their diverse histology. Prodromal periods can last from weeks to years. Therefore, a rigorous and uniform preoperative workup is a requisite for all patients thought to harbor pineal region tumors (6).

DIAGNOSIS IN MRI

MRI can distinguish true pineal masses from parapineal masses impinging into the region of the gland. The surgical approach depends upon the size of the pineal mass and its precise localization relative to the tentorium, because the infratentorial approach is considered preferable unless there is a large component extending supratentorially. Common pineal region tumors include pineal cell tumors (PCs and PBs), germ cell tumors (germinomas, choriocarcinomas, and teratomas), gliomas, and meningiomas, as well as pineal cysts. MRI signal characteristics are usually unable to differentiate among these tumors. However, large size (> 4 cm) and irregular shape are highly indicative of PB or malignant teratoma. Pineal cysts are common as incidental necropsy findings, and have been reported in up to

40% of routine autopsies. These incidental lesions went virtually undetected prior to routine MRI employing direct sagittal imaging to evaluate plausible brain pathology. Even large pineal cysts with apparent compression of the dorsal midbrain are usually asymptomatic, but occasionally pineal cysts can bleed internally or be so large that they may be a cause of aqueductal compression with secondary hydrocephalus and gaze disorders. The role of the radiologist in this entity is to distinguish pineal cysts from pineal neoplasms and to recognize the former as a benign and probably noncontributory factor to a patient's clinical symptoms (7).

The specific diagnosis of the histopathologic type of pineal cell tumors is often not achievable with MRI alone. MRI, however, can differentiate between pineal neoplasms and pineal cysts. On MRI, pineal neoplasms appear as lobulated, solid tumors, which are densely enhanced with contrast. In most cases, cystic lesions should be regarded as pineal cysts. PCs, with a higher degree of cytoplasm, should have relatively higher signal intensities on T2-weighted images (Fig. 1A). Signal intensities vary, but generally PBs essentially appear as iso- or higher-intense to gray matter on T1-weighted images (Fig. 2B), a typical pattern shared by other primitive neuroectodermal tumors (PNET) and perhaps related to the known scarcity of cytoplasm and overall dense cellularity (i.e., low water content) seen in these lesions. Pineal germinomas can appear identical to PBs on MRI. Although both PBs and PCs can calcify, intratumoral calcifications have been noted more commonly in PCs. The MR diagnosis of a pineal cyst is usually based on both shape and signal intensity. It is advisable, therefore, to routinely include a gradient-echo sequence for the detection of calcification as well as postcontrast imaging, when evaluating pineal region masses with MRI. Of course, the clinical history and serum β-human chorionic gonadotropin (HCG), placental alkaline phosphate (PLAP), or α-Fetoprotein (AFP) level are also extremely helpful in the differential diagnosis of germinal tumors, because the latter are usually absent in PCs and PBs. MRI with intravenous contrast is a very sensitive and perhaps more specific imaging tool and should be very useful in the preoperative evaluation and treatment planning of masses in this region (2).

PATHOLOGY

PCs can be differentiated from PBs based on the presence in the former of small cells with a moderate amount of cytoplasm, rare to very few mitoses, strong staining for synaptophysin (Fig. 1B), and obvious synapses on electron microscopy. Glial neoplasms tend to stain strongly with glial fibrillary acidic protein (GFAP), while PBs demonstrate inconsistent positivity. PBs are highly cellular tumors composed of poorly differentiated, immature cells with very scant cytoplasm (Fig. 2B). These tumors often show focal hemorrhage and microscopic necrosis. PBs can be classified as a type of PNET, because they appear histopathologically identical to other primitive, undifferentiated neoplasms, including retinoblastomas and cerebellar medulloblastomas, and

(A)

(B)

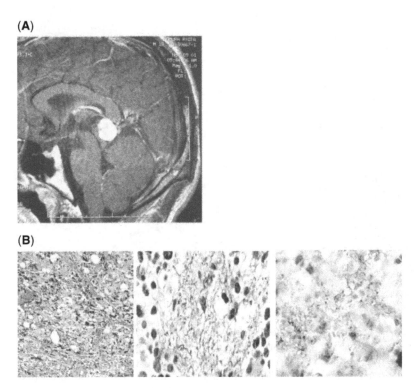

Figure 1 (A) A 39-year-old female suffered from ataxia of gait and dizziness as well as intermittent headache for five years. These impairments were slowly progressive. In the pineocytomas, T1-weighted images reveal rounded, sometimes or slightly lobulated low-signal masses with strong, homogeneous contrast enhancement. Their margin is usually clear, without invasion of adjacent structures. (B) In this case, the pineocytoma consists of small round cells set in a fibrillary background. The cells may form Homer Wright (neuroblastoma) rosettes, but the nuclear/cytoplasmic ratio is much lower in this tumor, and the mitoses are not evident. Histological hallmarks of neuronal differentiation in pineocytomas are large atypical ganglion cells and a regular pattern of large mature rosettes. These are composed of cells with small round nuclei and scanty cytoplasm surrounding delicate fibrillary processes revealed by silver impregnation techniques specific for axons. Occasionally, the cytoplasm was vacuolated. There were small amounts of an eosinophilic matrix between the tumor cells in a central location. resembling neuropil (*left*). Immunohistochemical studies revealed few mitoses and there was no necrosis. The tumor showed few microcalcifications and was bounded by a fibrous capsule, in which a network of neurites could be visualized here and along vessels and septae by Bodian silver impregnation (*center*), synaptophysin was positive in the neuropil islands in a fine granular distribution (*right*).

exhibit similar biological behavior. Differential diagnosis includes PCs, mixed PBs/PCs, glial neoplasms such as glioblastoma multiforme, and primary CNS germ cell tumors. Some features of each of these malignancies may be useful in distinguishing among them. Primary germ cell neoplasms can usually be

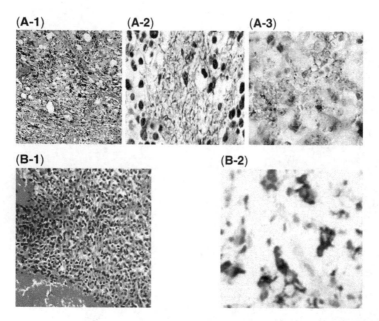

Figure 2 (**A**) Case: Seven-year-old boy who presented with a short history of upward gaze palsy with rapid progression. In the pineoblastomas, T1-weighted images disclose multilobulated tumors with heterogeneous contrast enhancement. They have poorly defined margins with adjacent structures such as the posterior thalamus or corpus callosum, suggesting a more invasive nature. (**B**) In the current case, hematoxylin and eosin staining revealed the presence of clusters of highly atypical cells, some large with pleomorphic large hyperchromatic nuclei, moderate amounts of eosinophilic cytoplasm and inconspicuous nucleoli. Scattered small cells with dense small nuclei and little cytoplasm were also seen neighboring intratumoral bleeding (*left*). Immunostaining for glial fibrillary acidic protein (data not shown) and synaptophysin (*right*) showed inconsistent but sometimes numerously positive in large cells, but pineocytic rosettes are much fewer.

differentiated from PBs histologically, but special stains for β-HCG, PLAP, or AFP, which react positively with various types of germ cell neoplasms but negatively with PBs, may be used to rule out the presence of PB (8).

PROGNOSIS AND MANAGEMENT

PBs tend to disseminate early to the subarachnoid space, with leptomeningeal and subependymal seeding often found at the time of initial diagnosis. The prognosis in children with this tumor is generally still poor. Stereotactic biopsy has the benefit of relative ease and minimal morbidity, but it may be associated with greater likelihood of diagnostic inaccuracy compared with open surgery, where more extensive tissue sampling is possible. Meanwhile, there is no agreement on whether PCs have a potential for seeding into the

CSF space. Some investigators believe that PCs cannot spread metastases and that, if they do so, they are not PCs. Other investigators, however, have reported that PCs can spread metastases throughout the CSF, but this occurs less frequently than with PBs. Seeding of PCs has been observed mostly in infantile cases. Therefore, it should be carefully considered if radiation therapy of the entire neuroaxis is necessary for all patients with PCs. High-risk children with PCs should be considered for postoperative radiation of the entire neuroaxis. It is essential, however, that these patients be followed up extensively by neuroimaging evaluation. The role of surgical debulking is clearly defined for some pineal tumors but is less evident for others. The one-third of pineal tumors that are benign or of low-grade malignancy can be managed by complete surgical resection, which is optimal in these tumors and associated with excellent long-term recurrence-free survival. In other, more malignant tumor types, however, the benefits of aggressive surgical resection are less clear, but several studies have shown that surgery improves overall outcome, which is correlated to the extent of tumor removal. Although developments in surgical technique, intraoperative monitoring, and postoperative care have minimized surgical complications, all surgical procedures in the pineal region, including both stereotactic biopsy and open surgery, are potentially hazardous. Advanced judgment, experience, and expertise are necessary to achieve rates of success sufficient to justify aggressive management. Treatment tactics employing stereotactic biopsy, endoscopy, and radiosurgery can also provide favorable outcomes in selected cases. Selective incorporation of these innovations may improve the already highly favorable outcomes for all patients with pineal region tumors (9).

In 2005, data from the Brain Tumor Registry of Japan (BTRJ) were analyzed to determine patient, tumor, and treatment characteristics associated with increased survival in adults with PBs. The BTRJ contained 34 adults with PBs diagnosed from 1969 to 1998. These patients had a median age of 35 years (range, 16–66 years), and 22 were males. Median survival from diagnosis was 25.7 months, with a median follow-up of 20.5 months. Median surgical resection was 75% to 94%, and 5 of the 34 patients (15%) had gross total resection. Twenty-nine of the 34 patients (85%) received cranial irradiation therapy with a median dose of 50 Gy (range 30–70 Gy). In the final multivariate model, cranial irradiation > 40 Gy and gross total resection were associated with significantly improved survival. There was a trend toward improved survival for women (10).

In another report, 16 patients who had undergone radiosurgery as the primary or adjuvant treatment for PPT were retrospectively evaluated. Ten patients (62.5%) had PCs, two (12.5%) had mixed PC and PB, and four (25%) had PBs. The mean marginal dose was 15 Gy, and the mean tumor volume was 5.0 cm. The mean follow-up periods from the time of diagnosis and the time of radiosurgery were 61 and 52 months, respectively. The overall actuarial two- and five-year survival rates after diagnosis were 75.0% and

66.7%, respectively. In 14 patients who were evaluated with imaging, 4 (29%) demonstrated complete remission, 8 (57%) had partial remission, 2 (14%) had no change, and no patient had local progression. The local tumor control rate (complete remission, partial remission, or no change) was 100%. Five patients died during follow-up, including one patient with a PC and three patients with PBs, all of whom died secondary to leptomeningeal or extracranial spread tumor. No cause of death was established for one patient. Two patients showed adverse effects to radiosurgery. The authors concluded that stereotactic radiosurgery is a valuable primary management modality for patients with PCs. As adjuvant therapy, radiosurgery may be used to boost local tumor dose during multimodal management of malignant PPT (7).

REFERENCES

1. Bruce JN, Ogden AT. Surgical strategies for treating patients with pineal region tumors. J Neurooncol 2004; 69:221–236.
2. Deshmukh VR, Smith KA, Rekate HL, et al. Diagnosis and management of pineocytomas. Neurosurgery 2004; 55:349–355.
3. Jan JE, Tai J, Hahn G, et al. Melatonin replacement therapy in a child with a pineal tumor. J Child Neurol 2001; 16:139–140.
4. Fauchon F, Jouvet A, Paquis P, et al. Parenchymal pineal tumors: a clinicopathological study of 76 cases. Int J Radiat Oncol Biol Phys 2000; 46:959–968.
5. Konovalov AN, Pitskhekauri DI. Principles of treatment of the pineal region tumors. Surg Neurol 2003; 59:250–268.
6. Amendola BE, Wolf A, Coy SR, et al. Pineal tumors: analysis of treatment results in 20 patients. J Neurosurg 2005; 102(Suppl):175–179.
7. Hasegawa T, Kondziolka D, Hadjipanayis CG, et al. The role of radiosurgery for the treatment of pineal parenchymal tumors. Neurosurgery 2002; 51:880–889.
8. Parwani AV, Baisden BL, Erozan YS, et al. Pineal gland lesions: a cytopathologic study of 20 specimens. Cancer 2005; 105:80–86.
9. Yamini B, Refai D, Rubin CM, et al. Initial endoscopic management of pineal region tumors and associated hydrocephalus: clinical series and literature review. J Neurosurg 2004; 100:437–441.
10. Lee JY, Wakabayashi T, Yoshida J. Management and survival of pineoblastoma: an analysis of 34 adults from the brain tumor registry of Japan. Neurol Med Chir (Tokyo) 2005; 45:132–141.

15

Embryonal Tumors

Roger J. Packer

*Departments of Neurology and Pediatrics, Children's National Medical Center,
The George Washington University, Washington, D.C.; Department of
Neurosurgery, University of Virginia, Charlottesville, Virginia; and Department of
Neurology, Georgetown University, Washington, D.C., U.S.A.*

Tobey MacDonald

*Department of Oncology, Children's National Medical Center,
and Department of Pediatrics, The George Washington University,
Washington, D.C., U.S.A.*

Gilbert Vezina

*Department of Neuroradiology and Radiology, Children's National Medical Center,
The George Washington University, Washington, D.C., U.S.A.*

INTRODUCTION

Embryonal tumors, predominantly arising in pediatric patients, are categorized in the most recent World Health Organization (WHO) classification as lesions that demonstrate an undifferentiated round cell tumor background and divergent patterns of differentiation (1) Tumor types within this classification include medulloblastoma—the most common form of embryonal tumor, supratentorial primitive neuroectodermal tumor (sPNET), medulloepithelioma, ependymoblastoma, medullomyoblastoma, and melanotic medulloblastoma (Table 1) (1). The atypical teratoid/rhabdoid tumor (ATRT), a newly categorized lesion occurring primarily in very young children, is also classified as an embryonal tumor. The pineoblastoma, histologically similar to the medulloblastoma and sPNET, has been categorized by the WHO as a

Table 1 Embryonal Tumors

Medulloblastoma
  Classical
  Desmoplastic
  Medullomyoblastoma
  Melanocytic medulloblastoma
Supratentorial primitive neuroectodermal tumors
  Cerebral neuroblastoma
  Ganglioneuroblastoma
  Pineoblastoma
Atypical teratoid/rhabdoid tumors
Ependymoblastoma
Medulloepithelioma

pineal parenchymal tumor. Although embryonal tumors share common light microscopy features, they seem to evolve by different genetic pathways (2). Principles of management for embryonal tumors are relatively similar as all are aggressive and have a proclivity to disseminate the central nervous system early in the course of illness. However, the intensity of therapy required for disease control and prognosis is variable within and among tumor subtypes, and is dependent not only upon the histology of the embryonal tumor, but also its molecular genetic make up, the age of the patient, and possibly the location of the tumor within the nervous system.

MEDULLOBLASTOMA

Medulloblastoma is the most common malignant childhood brain tumor, comprising approximately 20% of all primary central nervous system tumors occurring in patients less than 18 years of age (3). They have a somewhat bimodal distribution, peaking at three to four years and then again between eight and nine years. By present definition, medulloblastomas must arise in the posterior fossa and are predominantly composed of densely packed cells with round-to-oval, hyperchromatic nuclei (1). Melanocytic medulloblastoma and medullomyoblastoma are rare and are usually considered variants of medulloblastoma. Medulloblastomas can arise in adults and, if so, tend to occur more frequently in young adults, constituting 1% to 2% of all adult primary nervous system tumors (3).

The etiologies of medulloblastoma are unknown for most patients. There have not been conclusive links between parental occupations or exposures in the development of medulloblastoma, although in some studies parental pesticide use and occupational contact with hydrocarbons and metals, as well as exposure to *N*-nitroso compounds, have been linked with a higher likelihood of development of medulloblastoma (4,5). Several familial cancer syndromes predispose to an increase in risk of developing medulloblastoma in childhood, including TP53 germline mutation syndromes, the nevoid basal cell carcinoma syndrome (NBCCS), Gorlin's syndrome, and Turcot's syndrome (6).

In the current WHO classification of medulloblastoma, the tumor has been broadly histologically divided into two subsets, classical and desmoplastic (1). Nondesmoplastic medulloblastomas are more frequent, and within that grouping, an anaplastic phenotype, that seems to overlap with a large cell variant, has received increasing attention (7). Retrospective studies have suggested that the large cell/anaplastic variant may carry a poorer prognosis (8). Desmoplastic medulloblastomas, probably arising more commonly in older patients, including adults, may carry a somewhat better prognosis and within that subtype there is an extensive nodular variant that is associated both with younger age and possibly a more favorable prognosis (9).

Molecular Biology

Over the past decade, the molecular profile of medulloblastoma and possibly its cell of origin, or cells of origin, have been increasingly identified. Medulloblastomas may be comprised of multiple biologically distinct tumor types with individual subtypes arising from different progenitors Desmoplastic medulloblastomas express markers of granule cell lineage (of the cerebellum), while classical tumors are more likely to express markers associated with non-granule cell lineage neurons and may originate from the cerebellar ventricular zone (10). Expression of the neurotrophin-3 receptor (TRKC), which regulates proliferation, differentiation, and cell death of GCPs, was the first molecular alteration shown to have clinical significance in embryonal tumors (11). Its expression level in medulloblastoma directly correlates with favorable outcome (12).

The NBCCS, which is caused by inherited germline mutations of the PTCH gene on chromosome 9q22, accounts for 2% of medulloblastomas. PTCH encodes the sonic-hedgehog (Shh) receptor Patched1 (Ptc1), which normally represses Shh signaling (13). Studies have shown that somatic mutations of Ptc1 and other members of the Shh pathway that similarly result in constitutive activation of Shh signaling are associated with 10% of sporadic medulloblastomas (14–17). Medulloblastomas arising from either NBCCS or sporadic Shh pathway mutations are predominantly the desmoplastic variant; however, there is overlap, with 9q22 loss also being seen in some nondesmoplastic tumors (18). These molecular alterations have potential clinical relevance, because Ptc1 $(+/-)$ heterozygous mice spontaneously develop medulloblastomas, which can be induced to regress with Shh pathway antagonists (19,20). Furthermore, inactivation of the Shh target gene Gli1 has also been shown to significantly reduce medulloblastoma formation in this tumor model (21).

Approximately 10% of medulloblastomas harbor amplification of the MYCC oncogene, which has been associated with the large cell anaplastic (LCA) variant and poor prognosis (9) MYCC expression is more common, observed in 30% to 50% of tumors, including other histological subtypes of medulloblastoma (22). Similarly, expression of the tyrosine kinase receptor ERBB2 has been demonstrated in 40% of medulloblastomas, most frequently LCA type, and is also an independent poor prognostic indicator (23). Most recently, amplification of the OTX2 homeobox gene, whose product can be targeted by retinoids, was identified in LCA medulloblastoma, suggesting that OTX2 is another potential therapeutically susceptible oncogene in medulloblastoma (24,25).

Gene expression profiling has also provided some important insight into the biology of embryonal tumors. For example, microarray analysis of metastatic (M+) and nonmetastatic (M0) medulloblastomas at the time of diagnosis found the platelet-derived growth factor receptor beta (PDGFR-β) and members of the Ras/MAP kinase pathways to be significantly upregulated in the M+ tumors (26). These results suggest that this growth factor–mediated signal pathway may be critical in the control of metastasis of these tumors. Similarly, ERBB2 was found to upregulate S100A4 and other prometastatic genes, including several targets of the PDGFR pathway, in medulloblastoma (27). Microarray profiling also revealed that morphologically identical tumors such as medulloblastoma and sPNET could be separated based solely on their specific patterns of gene expression and that the desmoplastic type of medulloblastoma was molecularly distinct from classic appearing medulloblastoma, predominantly due to the differential expression of the Shh pathway (28).

Loss of genetic material from the short arm of chromosome 17p is the most common cytogenetic abnormality in medulloblastoma, occurring in 35% to 50% of tumors, most commonly as an isochrome 17q. The remainder of 17p deletions is confined to distal markers near 17p13.3. Among the genes localized to the common breakpoint at 17p13.3, HIC-1 is the leading candidate to be the tumor suppressor gene inactivated by 17p deletion. HIC-1 encodes for a zinc finger transcriptional repressor, whose expression is upregulated by p53 and is silenced by hypermethylation (28).

Diagnosis

The diagnosis of medulloblastoma is usually not difficult (29). Children classically present with the signs and symptoms of obstruction of cerebrospinal fluid flow and cerebellar dysfunction. Morning headaches, often associated with vomiting and lethargy, are present in the majority of patients at the time of diagnosis, usually with associated midline cerebellar defects and some degree of unsteadiness. Symptoms are usually present for less than three months before diagnosis. Cranial nerve deficits, except for abducens palsies due to increased intracranial pressure, usually are not present. The development of a stiff neck or head tilt suggests tonsillar involvement and possible impending herniation. Infants with medulloblastoma may present less characteristically and have intermittent vomiting, macrocephaly, and nonspecific signs of ventricular dilatation, including the "sun-setting" sign, where there is an inability to elevate the eyes. Older children and adults tend to have more cerebellar pontine angle symptomatology, including sixth, seventh, and eighth nerve involvement early in the course of illness. Although a significant number of children, and to a lesser extent adults, have disseminated disease at the time of diagnosis, few will have symptoms or signs associated with such dissemination.

Neuroimaging characteristically discloses a relatively well-defined mass lesion that arises in the inferior medullary velum/roof of the fourth ventricle, and grows anteriorly into the fourth ventricle; it can invade the middle cerebellar peduncle or the dorsal brain stem. In older children and adolescents, medulloblastomas have a tendency to present either in the lateral cerebellar hemisphere or near the cerebellopontine angle cistern (29–33). The tumor is iso to hyperdense compared to cortex on computed tomography (CT); calcifications are present in 10% to 20% of cases.

On magnetic resonance imaging (MRI), medulloblastomas are usually homogeneous with low T1 signal and intermediate (between gray matter and white matter) T2 signal; signal is often isointense to gray matter on fluid-attenssated inversion recovery (FLAIR) images and hyperintense on diffusion-weighted images (Fig. 1) (29,30,33). In about 75% of cases, the solid portions of the tumors enhance completely and intensely (31,33). Approximately 5% to 10% of patients will have nonenhancing tumors;

(A)   **(B)**

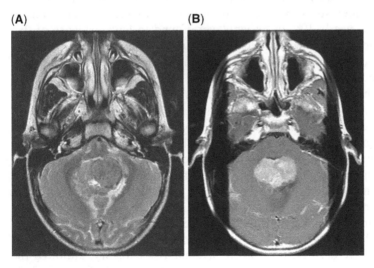

Figure 1 Axial T2 (**A**) and contrast-enhanced T1 (**B**) images of a three-year-old child with a medulloblastoma. The tumor arises from the anterior midline cerebellum and fills the fourth ventricle. It displays low T2 signal and near-complete enhancement. Surrounding edema is evident.

nonenhancing tumors are notoriously difficult to evaluate for extent of tumor dissemination.

Magnetic resonance spectroscopy findings are similar for all the embryonal tumors. In general, these tumors have very high levels of choline and very low or absent NAA peak (decreased NAA to creatine ratio). High choline levels indicate a high degree of membrane metabolism, which usually takes place in rapidly proliferating malignant tumors. Lactate and lipid peaks can also be identified as a result of metabolic acidosis and tissue breakdown.

Staging

Staging studies are critical in the evaluation of most embryonal tumors, including medulloblastoma (29). Neuroimaging of the entire neuroaxis coupled with sampling of the cerebrospinal fluid for evidence of tumor dissemination is complimentary and is a standard component of medulloblastoma management, because as high as 30% of younger patients and 10% of older patients and adults will have disseminated disease at the time of diagnosis (29,34,35). Subarachnoid dissemination along the spinal cord is most common, although intracranial spread may be present. Although evidence for tumor spread is a component of basic management of medulloblastoma, interpretation can be difficult and be complicated by postoperative changes. If possible, to avoid such artifacts, patients with presumed medulloblastoma undergo neuroaxis neuroimaging prior to surgery. In a recent multicenter study of over 400 children with medulloblastoma, in central review, nearly 10% of patients were found to have evidence of dissemination not appreciated by their referring institution and in another 10%, images were considered inadequate to determine the extent of disease (36).

The management of medulloblastoma is dependent on the result of staging studies and age of the patient. Increasingly, molecular genetic results are being used to supplement the results of staging studies, and based on all these parameters, children are usually separated into high- and average-risk disease groupings (Table 2) (23,29). Children with average-risk disease include those with totally or near-totally resected tumors and no evidence of dissemination on staging studies (29). Brain stem involvement at the time of diagnosis was found to be a factor predictive or poorer outcome in older series of patients treated with radiation therapy alone, but has not been found to be of significance in more recent series that utilize both radiation and chemotherapy (34,36). Children with less than 1.5 cm^2 of residual disease have been included in the average-risk category, although the 1.5-cm^2 parameter is arbitrary (36). Patients with high-risk disease include those with disseminated tumor at the time of diagnosis and subtotally resected lesions. Molecular genetic parameters found to be associated with poorer prognosis include increased ERBB2, high MYCC expression, and

Table 2 Risk Stratification for Medulloblastoma

	Average risk	? Intermediate risk[a]	Poor risk[b]
Extent of disease	Localized	? Positive cytology only	Disseminated
Extent of resection	Total/ near-total	Brainstem involvement; ? partial resection (if no adjuvant radiotherapy plus chemotherapy)	Subtotal (? $>1.5\,cm$ at residual)
Pathology	? Desmoplastic/ nodular variant	? Large cell/ anaplastic (despite total resection)	? Large cell/ anaplastic
Biologic parameter	Elevated neurotrophin-3 receptor (even in child less than 3 yr)	? Amplified MYCC ? Upregulated ERBB2 ↑ p53 accumulation	? Upregulated ERBB2 ? ↑ p53 accumulation
Age at diagnosis (years)	Greater than 3		3 or less

[a]? Does one factor put patient at increased risk?
[b]One positive factor necessary.

possibly p53 accumulation (22,23,37–39). Recent work has questioned the utility of any single marker and has suggested that gene profile expression classification based on a multigene model may be more useful (2,23). Anaplastic/large cell variants have been predominantly linked with more extensive and/or disseminated tumors and associated in retrospective series with poorer outcome (8,9). Thus, although the stratification of medulloblastoma has in the past been relatively straightforward, the identification of molecular markers that predict outcome has blurred such separations and raises the possibility that an intermediate risk group may exist (Table 2) (23,29,38).

The impact of treatment on the validity of separation of patients into risk groups is an important issue. Some parameters such as brain stem involvement and extent of surgical resection may be less predictive of outcome as therapy is intensified. Infants and young children are also a difficult subgroup of patients to assign risk, as for such patients radiotherapy may be altered or omitted, due to the concerns of the long-term risk of such therapy. The staging system utilized for children with medulloblastoma is usually applied to adults, although its validity has been demonstrated only in relatively small patient populations (29). However, in every study to date, the single, most-predictive clinical factor is extent of disease at the time of diagnosis, because independent of age, patients with disseminated disease fare less well.

Surgery

Surgery remains a critical component of the treatment of medulloblastoma (40). The extent of surgical resection has been associated with outcome in most series, and patients with subtotal resections, especially biopsies, fare less well than those who have undergone a total or near-total resection (40). Factors that may preclude a complete surgical resection include brain stem invasion, leptomeningeal spread at diagnosis, and proximity of the tumor to the cranial nerves. Hydrocephalus is seen in approximately 75% to 80% of patients with medulloblastoma at the time of diagnosis, and most patients are treated with an external ventriculostomy followed by surgery to the primary site. The drainage catheter is usually placed at the time of resection. Third ventriculostomy is increasingly being employed to avoid permanent ventriculoperitoneal shunts. Approximately 30% of patients will ultimately require a permanent external ventricular drainage.

A major concern after surgery has been the increasing diagnosis of the posterior fossa mutism syndrome. This is a constellation of findings in which a patient seems to be recovering postoperatively and then 6 to 24 hours following surgery becomes mute and is found to have marked irritability, supranuclear cranial nerve palsies, usually with associated hypotonia and cerebellar deficits (41). Initially considered a rarity, the posterior fossa mutism syndrome has been identified in nearly one-quarter of all patients undergoing surgery for medulloblastoma (42).

Radiotherapy

Following surgery, radiotherapy remains the single most effective means of treatment for medulloblastoma (34,43). Even in patients without frank evidence of dissemination, medulloblastoma is considered, similar to childhood leukemia, to have some degree of neuroaxis dissemination, and craniospinal radiation therapy supplemented with local boost radiotherapy to the primary tumor site is a component of conventional treatment. The dose of craniospinal radiation therapy required for disease control has not been demonstrated by randomized studies and for decades, the "standard" dose of craniospinal radiation therapy has been 3600 cGy delivered on a daily basis in 180 cGy dose fractions (34,43). In a study comparing 3600 to 2400 cGy of craniospinal radiation without chemotherapy in patients with nondisseminated disease, the lower dose of radiotherapy was found to be associated with a higher incidence of disease relapse within three years of diagnosis, although the difference in survival at five to six years was of borderline significance (44). Five-year survival in children with average-risk disease after 3600 cGy of craniospinal radiotherapy, without chemotherapy, is 50% to 60% (45). In a recently completed study of over 400 children with nondisseminated medulloblastoma, between the ages of 3 and 21 years of age, treated with 2400 cGy of radiation and chemotherapy, survival was greater than 80% at three years, and seemed comparable to that historically obtained with higher doses of craniospinal radiation plus adjuvant chemotherapy (36). The 2340 cGy dose of craniospinal radiation therapy has been demonstrated to result in inferior (40%) five-year survival, if given after chemotherapy (46). Prospective randomized studies are presently underway in children between three and seven years of age, attempting to determine if a further reduction of the craniospinal radiotherapy dose to 1800 cGy will result in similar disease control as the 2340-cGy dose, as long as chemotherapy is given during and after radiation therapy.

For patients with disseminated disease at the time of diagnosis, the conventional dose of craniospinal radiation therapy remains at 3600 cGy, with local boosts of radiotherapy to sites of disseminated disease. After such therapy, even if given with chemotherapy, there is a significant incidence of leptomeningeal disease relapse.

The volume of local radiotherapy required for disease control is also under evaluation. In the past, local radiotherapy consisted of whole posterior fossa radiotherapy. With conformal radiotherapy techniques, more precise tumor delivery is possible and studies are underway to determine if radiotherapy delivered to the primary tumor site with a 1- to 2-cm margin will be adequate for disease control. Limiting the volume of local radiotherapy will often spare the cochlea and possibly result in less long-term hearing sequelae.

The primary rationale for decreasing the dose of craniospinal radiotherapy, and for that matter the volume of local radiotherapy, is to decrease long-term radiotherapy-related sequelae. After craniospinal radiotherapy, children, especially those less than seven years of age, will have significant intellectual compromise, related predominantly, but not completely, to whole brain radiotherapy (47,48). Full-scale intelligence quotients have been demonstrated to drop by 20 to 30 points two to three years after radiotherapy (49). Reducing the dose of radiotherapy seems to result in a somewhat lesser degree of cognitive sequelae. Also, doses less than 2400 to 2900 cGy of radiotherapy to the hypothalamic and pituitary region may result in less endocrine sequelae (50,51). However, reductions in dose and volume are being done cautiously, because of the concern over increased disease relapse. There is no specific age when radiotherapy is contraindicated or, alternatively, when radiotherapy is entirely safe, including adulthood. However, there is significant reluctance to irradiate very young children, especially those less than three years of age, with craniospinal treatment. In children as young as six months of age, however, there are studies underway evaluating both the efficacy and the toxicity of utilizing radiotherapy to the primary tumor site alone for those with nondisseminated disease.

Chemotherapy

Since the mid-1980s, chemotherapy has taken on a prominent role in the treatment of children with medulloblastoma. Initially, randomized studies demonstrated that chemotherapy, when added to radiotherapy, resulted in improved survival for children with "poor-risk disease," as compared to treatment with radiotherapy alone (34,43). It then became evident that the survival rates for children with poor-risk disease treated with radiotherapy and chemotherapy matched, or exceeded, those obtained after the use of radiotherapy alone for children with nondisseminated or average-risk disease (52). In addition, as these studies and studies in patients with recurrent disease documented the relative chemosensitivity of medulloblastoma, it became evident that many long-term survivors treated with craniospinal radiation therapy had severe sequelae. Chemotherapy was evaluated as a means to allow a reduction in the dose of craniospinal radiation therapy required for disease control (53). Chemotherapy, at least for children, is now considered a standard component of management for all patients with medulloblastoma (29).

A variety of different chemotherapeutic agents have been shown to be effective in children with medulloblastoma, either at the time of diagnosis or at the time of recurrence. Such agents include cisplatin, cyclophosphamide, carboplatin, and oral etoposide. In addition, drug combinations such as the three-drug regimen of CCNU, cisplatinum, and vincristine and the two-drug regimen of higher dose carboplatin and etoposide have been shown to be active regimens (29). One of the most widely tested regimens for children with newly diagnosed disease has been vincristine during radiotherapy followed by eight cycles of cisplatin, CCNU, and vincristine. When coupled with 3600 cGy of craniospinal radiation therapy and 5480 cGy of local radiotherapy, such combination treatment resulted in a nearly 90%, five-year disease-free survival in children with nondisseminated disease, who were considered to be of poor risk because of brain stem involvement or subtotal resection, and a 60% five-year, progression-free survival rate in patients with disseminated disease (53). The same drug regimen, coupled with 2400 cGy of craniospinal radiation, resulted in a greater than 80% three-year disease control rate in children with nondisseminated disease in a multicentered prospective trial (52). An alternative regimen of cyclophosphamide, vincristine, and cisplatin was found to be equally efficacious in a subsequent trial (36).

Preradiation chemotherapy is of more questionable utility in children with medulloblastoma. In one of the earliest trials, the use of an eight-drug-in-one-day regimen prior to radiotherapy was found to be inferior to radiotherapy and postradiotherapy adjuvant chemotherapy (54). In an international trial, preradiotherapy chemotherapy was not found to be of benefit for any subgroup of patients with medulloblastoma, and for those children treated with reduced dose of 2500 cGy of craniospinal radiation therapy, the use of preradiation chemotherapy with procarbazine, vincristine, and methotrexate resulted in only 40% three- to five-year progression-free survival (46). An international study using a more aggressive approach also could not demonstrate benefit for preradiation chemotherapy and inferior results as compared to radiation plus vincristine during radiation therapy and CCNU and vincristine and cisplatinum after radiotherapy in children with nondisseminated disease (54). Preradiation chemotherapy with the combination of vincristine, etoposide, carboplatin, and cyclophosphamide prior to full-dose craniospinal radiation therapy of 3600 cGy was found to be more effective (three-year, event-free survival 78.5% vs. 68.4%) compared to treatment with similar doses of radiotherapy alone (45). However, preirradiation chemotherapy did not result in better overall survival. Thus, to date, although preradiation chemotherapy plus radiotherapy may be superior to radiotherapy alone, the majority of studies have resulted in inferior outcome as compared to treatment with radiotherapy supplemented with chemotherapy during and after radiotherapy.

The excellent survival rates demonstrated with craniospinal radiation therapy and adjuvant chemotherapy during and after radiation open promising avenues for future therapy. Multiple studies are presently underway attempting to improve survival by either increasing the intensification of postradiation chemotherapy, such as the use of higher doses of chemotherapy supported by peripheral stem cell rescue, or attempting to take advantage of the potential radiosensitization properties of some chemotherapeutic agents, such as carboplatin, by delivering more aggressive chemotherapy during radiation (55,56).

The utility of chemotherapy for adults with medulloblastoma has never been clearly proven. Studies in adults, usually involving only a small number of patients with medulloblastoma who are treated with radiotherapy alone, have demonstrated a survival rate of 60% to 65% at five years (39, 57,58) This is inferior to that now being reported in most radiotherapy plus chemotherapy pediatric trials (58). However, the chemotherapeutic approaches utilized for children with medulloblastoma, namely the protracted use of vincristine and cisplatin, have not been well tolerated in adults (59).

Because of the reluctance to use radiotherapy, especially craniospinal radiation therapy in young children, chemotherapy has been extensively explored in children less than three years, and in some studies in children less than six years, with medulloblastoma (60–62). A variety of different chemotherapeutic regimens have been employed and most have utilized an alkylator (cyclophosphamide or ifosfamide), cisplatin and/or carboplatin, oral or intravenous VP-16, and vincristine. Outcome with such treatment has been relatively disappointing, and resulting in disease control in only 20% to 30% of patients. In some of the earlier studies, craniospinal and local boost radiotherapy were utilized after completion of chemotherapy or when the child reached three years of age (60). Despite this, overall disease control still remained only in the 30% to 35% range. The majority of children who had long-term benefit were those who had nondisseminated, totally resected disease.

In attempts to make chemotherapy even more effective, other drugs have been added to these multiagent approaches, including intravenous and intraventricular methotrexate and intraventricular and intralumbar mafosfamide, an activated cyclophosphamide derivative (63). In patients who had nondisseminated tumors that were completely resected, five-year progression-free survival after the addition of methotrexate was approximately 60%. Similarly, improved survival rates have been recently demonstrated for the same subset of children with the use of higher dose chemotherapy without the use of methotrexate, supported by peripheral stem cell rescue. Methotrexate remains a problematic drug to incorporate in treatment of children with medulloblastoma given its potential neurotoxicity, and in the recent study, which utilized high-dose methotrexate and intraventricular methotrexate; a high incidence of leukoencephalopathy was found, although the significance of such leukoencephalopathy as regards long-term neurocognitive outcome was unclear (63). There does seem to be a subset of patients who can be treated with chemotherapy alone, and it is likely that the wider availability and application of molecular genetic markers will, in time, better identify this subset.

Outcome

With present means of surgery, radiotherapy, and chemotherapy, between 75% and 90% of children greater than three years of age with nondisseminated medulloblastoma are likely to be alive five years after treatment, the majority of whom are cured of their disease (29,36). Even for those children with high-risk disease, survival rates of 60% to 70%, at five years, are now being reported. For infants, overall survival remains poor, although some subsets of infants, primarily those with nondisseminated localized disease and favorable molecular genetic markers have a relatively good prognosis, with survival ranging between 50% and 60% five years following diagnosis (63). A major concern is the quality of life of long-term survivors.

It has been repeatedly shown that children surviving medulloblastoma are at high-risk for neurologic, neurocognitive, endocrinologic, and psychological sequelae (29,48). Although radiotherapy has been incriminated as the primary cause of neurocognitive sequelae, it is now becoming clear that other factors including preoperative neurologic damage, hydrocephalus, postoperative complications such as the posterior fossa mutism syndrome, possibly the use of neurotoxic chemotherapy, and poorly understood host factors significantly impact outcome. Progressive intellectual deterioration has been noted in both younger and older children. Even if there are no demonstrable decreases in overall intelligence, more subtle deficits in memory and executive function abilities are evident. It is likely that adults also have sequelae, although this has not been formally assessed in a large cohort of survivors. Endocrinological dysfunction is common after 3600 cGy of radiation therapy, with the majority of prepubertal patients having demonstrable growth hormone insufficiency and other endocrinopathies such as hypothyroidism, hypogonadism, and hypoadrenal function may occur, but somewhat less commonly (51). The combination of detrimental direct effects of radiation on vertebral growth and hypothalamic dysfunction put prepubertal children at high risk for moderate-to-severe growth retardation. Growth hormone use, although demonstrated to be safe in this patient population, is often delayed or not used at all due to concerns that it may cause disease relapse (50).

SUPRATENTORIAL PRIMITIVE NEUROECTODERMAL TUMORS

sPNETs, by definition occurring in the cerebrum or suprasellar region, are composed of undifferentiated or poorly differentiated neuroepithelial cells which may show differentiation along various cell lines (1) Cerebral neuroblastoma is considered a subtype of sPNET with marked neuronal differentiation; if ganglion cells are present, the term ganglioneuroblastoma is utilized. sPNETs are infrequent, accounting for approximately 2.5% of childhood brain tumors and less than 1% of adult primary central nervous system tumors. These tumors seem to peak in the first three years of life. Some have contended that such tumors should be considered to be medulloblastomas; however, cytogenetic and molecular genetic studies have now demonstrated that sPNETs are distinct (2,64). For example, the most common molecular alteration in medulloblastoma, 17p deletion, has not been commonly found in sPNET (64). Further evidence that these tumors are molecularly distinct has been provided by microarray gene expression profiling studies and the finding that the loss of the tumor suppressor gene, PTEN, observed in about 30% medulloblastomas, has not been detected in sPNET (2,65).

Presentation and Diagnosis

sPNETs commonly present as focal cortical lesions with associated mass effect. Symptoms prior to diagnosis are usually present for less than six months (66). Seizures may occur, but not as frequently as focal neurologic deficits and symptoms and signs of increased intracranial pressure (66). Very young children may present with macrocephaly. Neuroimaging studies usually disclose large, well-defined masses most often located in the frontoparietal region; sPNETs can arise either cortically or in the deep periventricular white matter (30,67). Hemorrhage, necrosis, calcifications, and cyst formation are common; the tumors may be associated with large cystic areas (Fig. 2). Calcification occurs in up to 70% of patients. Thus, MRI and CT features are heterogeneous. On MRI, solid tumor tissue is often isointense to gray matter on fluid-attenuated inversion recovery (FLAIR) images and hyperintense on diffusion-weighted images and characteristically enhances intensely. Peritumoral edema is common, though often mild or minimal given the large size of the tumor and often minimal as compared to glial tumors of similar size.

Management

As is the case for medulloblastomas, sPNETs require staging for identification of subarachnoid dissemination at the time of diagnosis. In most series, 20% or less of patients are disseminated at time of diagnosis. Obtainment of cerebrospinal fluid for analysis may not be possible due to intracranial mass effect.

The degree of surgical resection in series of patients with sPNETs has varied, and in most series, the majority of patients, whether infants or young children, have had subtotal resections (66,68,69). The extent of surgical resection has not been shown to correlate with outcome in children treated with radiotherapy, with or without chemotherapy. The presence of leptomeningeal dissemination at the time of diagnosis does portend a poorer rate of survival.

Postsurgical therapy has been similar to that for children with poor-risk medulloblastomas (66,68,69). The volume of radiation therapy required for disease control has not been clearly delineated, although in most series patients have been treated with craniospinal and local boost radiation therapy at doses similar to those given for children with medulloblastoma. There may be a subgroup of cortical PNETs, especially cystic lesions, which can be successfully treated with postsurgical local radiotherapy alone.

Preradiation chemotherapy has not been demonstrated to improve survival (69). Treatment with chemotherapy alone, predominantly evaluated in children less than five years of age at the time of diagnosis, has resulted in a poor rate of survival. Outcome may be somewhat better after the use of higher dose chemotherapy supported by autologous bone marrow transplantation or peripheral stem cell rescue (70). In studies using chemotherapy alone, patients who had total or near-total resections fared better than those whose tumors were subtotally resected or biopsied.

Outcome

The overall outcome for children with sPNETs is relatively poor. In series of older patients, who have received craniospinal radiation therapy plus local

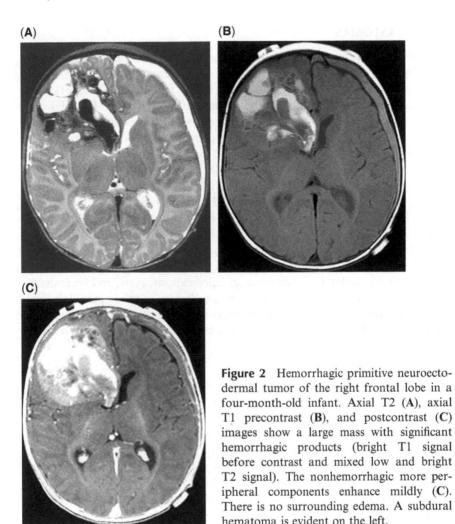

Figure 2 Hemorrhagic primitive neuroecto-dermal tumor of the right frontal lobe in a four-month-old infant. Axial T2 (**A**), axial T1 precontrast (**B**), and postcontrast (**C**) images show a large mass with significant hemorrhagic products (bright T1 signal before contrast and mixed low and bright T2 signal). The nonhemorrhagic more per-ipheral components enhance mildly (**C**). There is no surrounding edema. A subdural hematoma is evident on the left.

boost radiotherapy and adjuvant chemotherapy, survival at five years is approximately 50% (66,68). After treatment with chemotherapy alone, children less than five years of age have a 30% or less chance of five-year survival. As is the case for children with medulloblastoma, children with sPNETs are at high risk for long-term neurocognitive sequelae. This is not only due to the whole brain radiation therapy these children are often treated with, but also due to the local effects of the tumor and the need for higher dose boost radiotherapy to the primary tumor site, which results in the sur-rounding brain receiving doses of radiotherapy ranging between 4500 and 5500 cGy.

PINEOBLASTOMAS

Dependent on series, 1% to 4% of all pediatric brain tumors occur in the pineal region, and approximately 25% of such tumors are pineoblastomas. Although classified with the pineal parenchymal tumors, these tumors share histological features with medulloblastomas and other forms of sPNETs (1). In most series, the ratio of sPNETs to pineoblastomas is approximately 4–5:1 (68,71). These tumors present as other pineal region masses and are characterized by a relatively short period between onset of symptoms and diagnosis. Presenting symptoms include those secondary to increased intracranial pressure and associated hydrocephalus, such as impaired upgaze, nystagmus, ataxia, and tremor. Parinaud's syndrome may be present. Although these tumors may occur all through childhood and rarely in adulthood, they tend to be more frequent in younger patients.

On MRI, pineoblastoma are large, lobulated, heterogeneous tumors (30,67). They are often isointense on T1. On T2-weighted images, the lesions are heterogeneous due to the presence of calcifications, cysts, and necrosis; the solid components tend to be hypointense, a reflection of the hypercellular nature of the tumors. Malignant pineal tumors are occasionally encountered in patients with bilateral retinoblastoma; the condition is designated a trilateral retinoblastoma.

Management

Staging is a component of management of pineoblastomas, and dissemination at the time of diagnosis occurs in 20% to 30% of patients (68–71). Due to tumor location, total resections are uncommon with many patients having only a biopsy prior to the initiation of postsurgical therapy. Therapy is usually similar to that given for patients with poor-risk medulloblastoma. Although numbers are small, the reported progression-free survival rate for patients treated with craniospinal plus local boost radiotherapy and chemotherapy (60% at five years) has been equal to, or somewhat superior to, survival rates for children with sPNETs. Outcome for patients treated with conventional chemotherapy alone has been quite poor. The use of radiotherapy and higher dose chemotherapy supported by autologous bone marrow rescue or peripheral stem cell support has shown somewhat better survival rates, albeit in quite small series (55,56).

ATYPICAL TERATOID/RHABDOID TUMORS

The ATRT is an increasingly diagnosed lesion that was first fully characterized in the 1980s (72). These lesions are composed of rhabdoid cells usually intermixed with variable components of primitive neuroectodermal, mesenchymal, and epithelial cells. The rhabdoid cell is a medium-sized, round-to-oval cell, with distinct borders, an eccentric nucleus, and a prominent nucleolus. The primitive neuroectodermal component of the atypical teratoid tumors is indistinguishable from cells found in sPNETs. Unlike medulloblastomas or sPNETs, ATRTs display a wide range of immuno-reactivity on immunohistochemical staining, with clusters of cells usually positive for epithelial membrane antigen and vimentin. There is also frequent reactivity for glial fibrillary acidic protein, cytokeratin and, to a lesser extent, for smooth muscle actin and neurofilament protein. The rhabdoid cells are negative for germ cell markers. Molecular genetic investigations have demonstrated that ATRTs are distinct from other embryonal tumors, in that the vast majority demonstrates monosomy 22 or deletions of chromosome band 22q11. Inactivating deletions or mutations of the tumor suppressor gene hSNF5/INI-1, located in the chromosomal region 22q11.2, are now regarded as a crucial step in the molecular pathogenesis of most ATRTs. However, at least 20% of cases do not have genomic alterations of INI-1, despite showing loss of immunostaining for the INI-1 protein (73,74). INI-1 encodes a subu-nit of the SWI/SNF family of chromatin-remodeling complexes, although its direct tumor suppressor function remains unknown.

Presentation and Diagnosis

ATRTs usually present early in life where they may constitute as many as 20% of all embryonal tumors. However, the ATRTs have been reported all throughout childhood and into early adulthood.

The clinical presentation of ATRTs is indistinguishable from that of medulloblastomas or sPNETs. About 50% of ATRTs arise in the posterior fossa, 40% are supratentorial, and the rest are pineal, spinal, or multifocal (72). Their location can be intra-axial, extra-axial, or both, as they often invade through the meningeal and ependymal boundaries. Leptomeningeal spread occurs in one-third of cases at presentation.

Radiological features are heterogeneous due to the frequent presence of cystic and necrotic areas, calcifications, and hemorrhage. The CT findings of ATRTs are relatively characteristic but not diagnostic. They are usually hyperdense and enhance intensely. Calcifications may occur but are not as common as in sPNETs. With MRI, T1-weighted images often feature hyper-intense foci within the lesion, due to the hemorrhagic components (Fig. 3). On T2-weighted images, the lesions are often heterogeneous; the solid com-ponents are iso- to hypointense on T2-weighted images, hemorrhagic and necrotic foci are usually hyperintense. Most ATRTs enhance intensely with gadolinium. Distinction between sPNET and ATRT is not possible due to their shared propensity to display necrotic and hemorrhagic foci.

Management

The management of ATRTs, as is the case with other embryonal tumors, begins with staging. Approximately one-third of patients will have disseminated

(A)   (B)

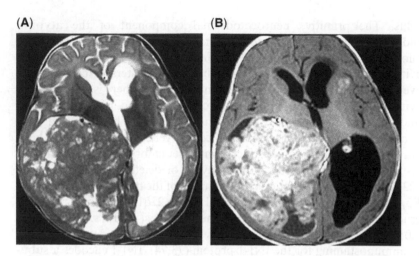

Figure 3 Axial T2 (A) and contrast-enhanced T1 (B) images of an eight-month-old with a large rhabdoid tumor arising in the posterior right lateral ventricle. The mass shows intense enhancement, and has low T2 signal with small islands of high T2 signal that do not enhance (small cysts or necrotic foci). A metastatic lesion is evident deep to the left anterior insula. Hydrocephalus results from posterior third ventricular compression by the tumor.

disease at the time of diagnosis. The utility of surgery, radiotherapy, and chemotherapy for children, especially infants with ATRT, is under active study (72). Overall survival rates for children less than three years of age treated with surgery and chemotherapy, independent of the type of chemotherapy utilized, have been poor, with survival occurring in less than 20% of patients at 12 months from diagnosis. Children have been primarily treated with chemotherapy regimens utilized for children with medulloblastoma or sPNETs. The use of other types of regimens, including those utilized for patients with sarcomas and regimens including high-dose and intrathecal methotrexate, have demonstrated questionable increased efficacy. In general, the results of chemotherapeutic studies have shown that a variety of chemotherapeutic regimens may result in tumor stabilization, and in some cases objective tumor shrinkages, but have not resulted in long-term disease control, especially in patients with disseminated disease at the time of diagnosis or in those with subtotal resections. Older patients who have survived have been treated with extensive resections, radiotherapy (craniospinal and local boost), and chemotherapy (75). It is unclear whether the better survival in older patients is due to the more aggressive treatment they received or age-related biologic differences. Because of the poorer survival rates in infants, approaches are now focusing on treatment combining aggressive resection with high-dose chemotherapy utilizing both methotrexate and, if possible, peripheral stem cell support. In patients with localized disease at the time of diagnosis, chemotherapy is usually given for a relatively short period of time (two to four months) and followed by focal radiotherapy.

OTHER EMBRYONAL TUMORS

The presentation and optimal management for other forms of embryonal tumors are poorly characterized. Medullomyoblastoma and melanocytic medulloblastomas are extremely rare tumors, which predominantly arise in children but rarely may arise in adults. Interestingly, in both subtypes, a male predominance has been noted (1). The majority of these variants of medulloblastoma tend to occur in the posterior fossa and reported survival has been quite poor.

Ependymoblastoma is now also characterized as an embryonal tumor occurring predominantly in the first and second year of life (1). Ependymoblastomas, although more common supratentorially, may occur throughout the brain. Therapy is usually similar to that for children with poor-risk medulloblastomas or sPNETs, and overall survival is usually quite poor (76).

Medulloepitheliomas, also occurring both infrantentorially and supratentorially, are histologically fascinating tumors that seem to mimic the embryonic neural tube (1). They are characterized by papillary, tubular, or trabecular arrangement of neoplastic neuroepithelial cells with an external limiting membrane. As is the case with other embryonal tumors, medulloepitheliomas may also display cellular differentiation. The tumor is rare and tends to occur predominantly in very young children. It has been diagnosed not only in the cerebral cortex, but also in the cauda equina, presacral area, and outside the central nervous system along nerve trunks. They are often quite large at the time of diagnosis, but interestingly are usually relatively well circumscribed. Outcome for children with medulloepitheliomas is quite poor, although information is predominantly based on case reports or small retrospective series (77). Management, for lack of a better understanding of the tumor, is similar to that for children with poor-risk medulloblastomas or sPNETs.

REFERENCES

1. Kleihues P et al. Tumours of the Nervous System. World Health Organization IARC Press, Classification of Tumors, Pathology and Genetics. Lyon, France: 2000.
2. Pomeroy SL et al. Nature 2002; 415:436–442.
3. Primary Brain Tumours in the United States CBTRUS 2002:1995–1999 Statistical Report.
4. Bunin GR et al. N Engl J Med 1993; 329:536–541.
5. Colt JS et al. Environ Health Perspect 1996; 106:909–925.
6. Stavrou T et al. J Pediatr Hematol/Oncol 2001; 23(7):431–436.

7. Brown HG et al. J Neuropathol Exp Neurol 2000; 59:857–865.
8. Eberhart C et al. Cancer 2002; 94(2):552–560.
9. Eberhart CG et al. J Neuropathol Exp Neurol 2004; 63:441–449.
10. Read T-A, Hegedus B, Wechsler-Reya R, and Gutmann DH, The Neurobiology Ann Neurol 2006; 60:3–11.
11. Segal RA et al. Proc Natl Acad Sci USA 1994; 91:12867–12871.
12. Grotzer MA et al. J Clin Oncol 2000; 18:1027–1035.
13. Rubin JB et al. Cancer Cell 2002; 2:7–8.
14. Zurawel RH et al. Genes Chromosomes Cancer 2000; 27:44–51.
15. Hallahan AR et al. Cancer Res 2004; 64:7794–7800.
16. Taylor MD et al. Nat Genet 2002;31:306–310.
17. Raffel C et al. Cancer Res 1997; 57:842–845.
18. Dong J et al. Hum Mutat 2000; 16:89–90.
19. Berman DM et al. Science 2002; 297:1559–1561.
20. Romer JT et al. Cancer Cell 2004; 6:229–240.
21. Kimura H et al. Oncogene 2005; 24:4026–4036.
22. Herms J et al. 2000; 89:395–402.
23. Gajjar A et al. J Clin Oncol 2004; 22:984–993.
24. Boon K et al. Cancer Res 2005; 65:703–707.
25. Di C et al. Cancer Res 2005; 65:919–924.
26. MacDonald TJ et al. Nat Genet 2001; 29:143–152.
27. Hernan R et al. Cancer Res 2003; 63:140–148.
28. Rood BR et al. Cancer Res 2002; 62:3794–3797.
29. Packer RJ et al. Neurooncology 1999; 1:232–250.
30. Zimmerman RA et al. Neuroradiology 2001; 43:927–933.
31. Vezina LG et al. Neuroimaging Clin N Am 1994; 4:423–426.
32. Zimmerman RA et al. Radiology 1978; 126:137–141.
33. Zimmerman RA et al. Pediatr Neurosurg 1992; 18:58–64.
34. Evans AE et al. J Neurosurg 1990; 72:572–582.
35. Gajjar A et al. J Clin Oncol 1999; 17:1825–1828.
36. Packer RJ et al. Ann Neurol 2004; 56(S8):89–90.
37. Gilbertson RJ, Pearson Ad, Perry RH, et al. Br J Cancer 1995; 71:473–477.
38. Lamont JM et al. Clin Cancer Res 2004; 10:5482–5493.
39. Ray A et al. Clin Cancer Res 2004; 10:7613–7620.
40. Albright AL et al. Neurosurgery 1996; 38:265–271.
41. Pollack IF et al. Neurosurgery 1995; 37:885–893.
42. Robertson PL et al. Ann Neurol 2002; 52(S1):S115.
43. Tait DM et al. Eur J Cancer 1990; l26:464–469.
44. Thomas PR et al. J Clin Oncol 2000; 18:3004–3011.
45. Taylor RE et al. J Clin Oncol 2003; 21:1581–1591.
46. Bailey CC et al. Med Pediatr Oncol 1995; 25:166–178.
47. Walter AW et al. J Clin Oncol 2003; 21:1581–1591.
48. Ris MD et al. J Clin Oncol 2001; 19:3470–3476.
49. Radcliffe J et al. Ann Neurol 1992; 32:551–554.
50. Packer RJ et al. J Clin Oncol 2001; 19:480–487.
51. Shalet SM et al. J Pediatr 1977; 90:920–923.
52. Packer RJ et al. J Clin Oncol 1999; 17(7):2127–2136.

53. Packer RJ et al. J Neurosurg 1994; 81:690–698.
54. Kuhl J et al. Klin Padiatr 1998; 210:227–233.
55. Strother D et al. J Clin Oncol 2001; 19:2696–2704.
56. Mason WP et al. J Clin Oncol 1998; 16:210–221.
57. Carrie C et al. Cancer 1994; 74:2352–2360.
58. Prados MD et al. Int J Radiat Oncol Biol Phys 1994; 32:1145–1152.
59. Greenberg HS et al. Neurooncology 2001; 3:29–34.
60. Duffner PK et al. N Engl J Med 1993; 328:1725–1731.
61. Geyer JR et al. J Clin Oncol 1994; 12:1607–1615.
62. Dupuis-Girod S et al. J Neurooncol 1996; 27:87–98.
63. Rutkowski S et al. N Engl J Med 2005; 352: 978–986.
64. Fruhwald MC et al. Genes Chromosomes Cancer 2001; 30:38–47.
65. Inda MM et al. Oncol Rep 2004; 12:1341–1347.
66. Reddy AT et al. Cancer 2000; 88:2189–2193.
67. MacDonald TJ et al. Oncologist 2003; 8:174–186.
68. Cohen BH et al. J Clin Oncol 1995; 13(7):1687–1696.
69. Marec-Berard P et al. Med Pediatr Oncol 2002; 38(2):83–90.
70. Gururangan S et al. J Clin Oncol 2003; 21(11):2187–2191.
71. Jakacki RI et al. J Clin Oncol 1995; 13(6):1377–1383.
72. Packer RJ et al. J Ped Hem/Onc 2002; 24:337–342.
73. Zhang F et al. Cancer 2002; 34:398–405.
74. Judkina AR et al. J Neuropathol Exp Neurol 2005; 64:391–397.
75. Tekautz TM et al. J Clin Oncol 2005; 23:1491–1499.
76. Robertson PL et al. J Neurosurg 1995; 88:695–703.
77. Malloy PT et al. J Neurosurg 1996; 84:430–436.

16

Peripheral Neuroblastic Tumors

Sajeel Chowdhary and Marc Chamberlain
*Department of Interdisciplinary Oncology, H. Lee Moffitt Cancer Center,
University of South Florida, Tampa, Florida, U.S.A.*

Amyn M. Rojiani
*Departments of Interdisciplinary Oncology and Pathology, H. Lee Moffitt
Cancer Center, University of South Florida,
Tampa, Florida, U.S.A.*

INTRODUCTION

The term "neuroblastoma" is commonly used to refer to a spectrum of neuroblastic tumors (including neuroblastomas, ganglioneuroblastomas, and
ganglioneuromas) that arise from primitive sympathetic ganglion cells.
Olfactory neuroblastoma (ONB), a malignancy of the olfactory epithelium,
has a different cell of origin, presentation, and treatment than neuroblastoma. ONB is often known to represent a well-differentiated primitive
peripheral neuroectodermal tumor (PNET).

Ewing's sarcoma (ES) and primitive PNET were originally described
as distinct clinicopathologic entities. In 1918, Stout described a tumor of
the ulnar nerve with the gross features of a sarcoma, but composed of small
round cells, focally arranged as rosettes; this entity was subsequently designated neuroepithelioma, and then PNET. ES was described by James Ewing
in 1921 as an undifferentiated tumor involving the diaphysis of long bones
that, in contrast to osteosarcoma, was radiation sensitive. Although most
often a primary bone tumor, ES was also reported to arise in soft tissue
[extraosseous ES (EES)]. However, over the last several decades, it has

become clear that these entities are actually part of a spectrum of neoplastic diseases known as the ES family of tumors (EFT), which also includes adult neuroblastoma, malignant small-cell tumor of the thoracopulmonary region (Askin's tumor), paravertebral small-cell tumor, and atypical ES (1). Because of their similar histologic and immunohistochemical characteristics and shared nonrandom chromosomal translocations, these tumors are considered to be derived from a common cell of origin (2). Although the histogenetic origin has been debated over the years, evidence from immunohistochemical, cytogenetic, and molecular genetic studies supports a neuroectodermal origin for all EFTs.

OLFACTORY NEUROBLASTOMA

ONB and esthesioneuroblastoma arise from the olfactory epithelium that lines the superior one-third of the nasal septum, cribriform plate, and superior turbinates (3). ONB occurs over a broad age range (three to 88 years) with a mean age of 45 years. About 20% of these tumors occur in children and adolescents. There is no gender predilection.

Clinical Presentation

The most common symptom is unilateral nasal congestion or obstruction. In one series of 22 patients, the most common symptoms were nasal congestion (64%), anosmia (55%), and recurrent epistaxis and pain (36% each) (4). Other symptoms included frontal headache and diplopia. The symptoms are related both to the site and to the local extent of the tumor. Anosmia is caused by penetration into the cribriform plate, while epistaxis reflects the marked vascularity of the tumor. Pain, proptosis, and excessive lacrimation are induced by orbital extension. Ear pain and otitis media result from obstruction of the eustachian tube. Frontal headache accompanies involvement of the frontal sinus. Physical examination usually reveals a red-brown, polypoid mass located high in the nasal cavity (5). At initial diagnosis, tumors tend to be quite large as early symptoms are nonspecific.

Diagnosis

Plain radiographs may reveal an intranasal soft tissue mass, giving rise to bone destruction and opacification of paranasal sinuses. Computed tomography (CT) and magnetic resonance imaging (MRI) can help to differentiate tumor from other causes of nasal obstruction and are useful for tumor staging (5). CT allows for detailed assessment of bony erosion or destruction, particularly of the cribriform plate. MRI defines the extent of intracranial tumor growth and invasion into adjacent soft tissue areas such as the retromaxillary space (Fig. 1). Radiographic findings are nonspecific and distinction from other tumors such as squamous cell carcinoma,

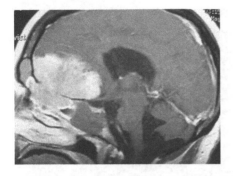

Figure 1 An olfactory neuroblastoma is demonstrated arising from the superior nasal meatus and extending intracranially through the cribriform plate (T1-weighted magnetic resonance imaging with gadolinium).

undifferentiated lymphoma, amelanotic melanoma, or embryonal rhabdomyosarcoma requires histopathological examination.

On macroscopic examination, the tumor is polypoid, soft, and hemorrhagic. Microscopically, it is composed of sheets, discrete nests, or lobules of small round cells, often compartmentalized into nodules by thin fibrous septa (Fig. 2A) (6). The tumor cells have hyperchromatic nuclei with uniform chromatin distribution, small inconspicuous nucleoli, and sparse cytoplasm. The stroma is typically pink, neurofibrillary or edematous, and well vascularized. Mitotic activity is variable (Fig. 2B). Homer-Wright pseudorosettes composed of tumor cells surrounding a central pink fibrillary material are seen in one-half of ONBs (Fig. 2C); true rosettes (Flexner type) composed of tumor cells surrounding a central lumen are infrequent. The tumors invade bone. Necrosis, dystrophic calcification, and vascular or lymphatic invasion are not uncommon (Fig. 2D). In rare instances, a few admixed ganglion cells may be seen. Cytoplasmic glycogen is absent and reticulin fibers surround the tumor lobules, rather than individual tumor cells. Electron microscopy of ONBs demonstrates cytoplasmic neurofilaments, neurotubules, mitochondria, and dense-core neurosecretory granules (100–200 nm in diameter) (3,7). A variety of other small cell tumors can present in the sinonasal region. Many can be distinguished from ONB on light microscopic features alone, but in some instances, additional techniques such as immunohistochemistry may be of value. Immunohistochemically, ONBs typically exhibit positive staining for neuron-specific enolase; approximately 65% of tumors stain for synaptophysin, and a lesser proportion for chromogranin. In some cases, tumor cells may be positive for neurofilament or cytokeratin (7,8). The supporting or sustentacular cells may be positive for S-100 protein or glial fibrillary acidic protein. Tumor cells are negative for a variety of other markers such as epithelial membrane antigen, leukocyte common antigen, kappa and lambda light chains, HMB45, desmin, myoglobin, vimentin, and MIC2 (CD99), the ES marker.

The Hyams histologic grading system distinguishes four tumor grades based upon pathologic features such as mitotic activity and necrosis (3).

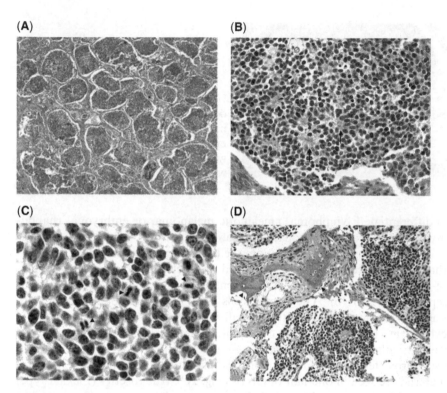

Figure 2 (**A**) Although olfactory neuroblastomas may display a range of architectural arrangements, from sheets to lobules, most tumors will have at least some areas of well-circumscribed, round lobules. This lobular pattern is reminescent of the "Zellballen" pattern seen in paragangliomas. The lobules are formed by a monolayer of cells, often S-100 immunoreactive, that surrounds groups of cells. Hematoxylin- and eosin-stained section. Original magnification 40x. (**B**) At high magnification, tumor nuclei are round to ovoid and present with a stippled nuclear chromatin. Mitotic activity is not infrequent, as seen in this example (*arrows*). Hematoxylin- and eosin-stained section. Original magnification 400x. (**C**) In tune with their "neural" origin, well-differentiated tumors will often form rosettes, typically Homer-Wright rosettes, where tumor cells are arranged in a circle with fibrillary processes pointing towards the center (*arrows*). Other areas of the tumor consist of ill-defined clusters or sheets of cells. Hematoxylin- and eosin-stained section. Original magnification 200x. (**D**) The tumor typically enlarges within the nasal cavity and frequently encroaches upon and destroys the cribriform plate. In this example, the tumor can be seen surrounding irregular fragments of displaced bone (*arrows*). (H&E ×100).

Grade I tumors are characterized by a prominent fibrillary matrix, tumor cells with uniform nuclei and absence of nuclear pleomorphism, mitotic activity, or necrosis. Grade II tumors have some fibrillary matrix and exhibit moderate nuclear polymorphism with some mitotic activity. There is no necrosis. Grade III tumors have minimal fibrillary matrix and Flexner type rosettes are present. There is prominent mitotic activity and nuclear pleomorphism, and some necrosis may be seen. Grade IV tumors have no fibrillary matrix or rosettes, and show marked nuclear pleomorphism and increased mitotic activity with frequent necrosis.

Most studies report a good correlation of Hyams grade with prognosis (6,7,9,10). As an example, in one series of 49 patients, the only significant predictor for overall survival, disease-free survival, and local control was the Hyams grade. Low-grade lesions were associated with a significantly better five-year survival than high-grade tumors (73% vs. 38%).

There is no uniformly accepted staging system for ONB. The Kadish clinical staging system, a three-tier classification based upon disease extent, has traditionally been used and correlated with survival (4,5). Stage A tumors are confined to the nasal cavity (five-year survival rate 90%). When one or more paranasal sinuses are involved, five-year survival rate is reduced to 71%. Stage C tumors extend beyond the nasal cavity and paranasal sinuses (five-year survival 47%). Another staging system in use, the Dulguerov system, is based upon a TNM type of classification and uses CT scanning and MRI to ascertain the local disease extent. Cerebrospinal fluid analysis may be required to rule out leptomeningeal spread.

Treatment

The rarity of this tumor and its often prolonged natural history complicate the assessment of therapeutic efficacy, particularly for those with advanced disease (11). Management has evolved over the years, and there is no consensus as to the best treatment approach, neither for localized nor for advanced disease.

A combined otolaryngologic and neurosurgical craniofacial approach followed by postoperative radiotherapy to tumor bed and cervical lymph nodes is the treatment of choice at many centers for patients with ONB (10,12,13). However, the rate of local failure is high, and late recurrences (which developed beyond two years in four of 11 patients with recurrent disease in one report) are not uncommon (14). Many series report higher local recurrence rates with craniofacial resection alone, although several have found no difference in survival between surgical resection with negative margins, and surgical resection with adjuvant radiation (10,12,15). In one series, combined surgery and radiation resulted in recurrence-free status in 92% of patients, compared to 14% and 40% for those treated with surgery or radiation alone, respectively. Additional support for the combined modality approach is derived from a review of the published literature, in which 68% of 898 reported cases were treated with combined surgery and radiotherapy; at five-year follow-up of 234 cases, 68% were alive and recurrence-free (12). The contribution of treatment modality to outcome was also evaluated in a more contemporary review of 390 cases of ONB that were published between 1990 and 2000 (11). The following five-year survivals were reported, stratified according to modality of treatment: surgery alone ($n = 87$) 48%, surgery plus radiation ($n = 169$) 65%, surgery plus radiotherapy and chemotherapy ($n = 48$) 47%, radiation alone ($n = 49$) 37%, and radiation plus chemotherapy ($n = 26$) 51%. Although none of these reports represent randomized trials, and are thus subject to selection and publication bias, they support the benefit of combined surgery and radiation compared to single modality therapy. Other series suggest further benefit from the addition of chemotherapy to radiation therapy following craniofacial resection (16,17). However, the contribution of chemotherapy in this setting is difficult to assess, and its role remains unclear (10,14).

The value of induction or neoadjuvant therapy (i.e., chemotherapy plus radiation) prior to craniofacial resection remains a matter of debate. A retrospective review of 34 patients treated at a single institution found that two-thirds had a significant reduction in tumor burden with neoadjuvant therapy (18). The five- and 10-year disease-free survival rates were 81% and 55%, and the average time to recurrent disease was more than six years. Six percent of patients presented with cervical metastatic disease and ultimately 26% developed at least one episode of metastatic disease. In an attempt to avoid craniofacial resection, treatment protocols combining chemotherapy and irradiation have been developed with encouraging results. One regimen combines two cycles of cisplatin and etoposide (E) before and after combined photon and stereotactic fractionated proton beam radiation therapy, with radical surgery reserved for nonresponders. In a series of 19 patients with ONB or neuroendocrine carcinoma involving the sinonasal tract, 13 patients had a response to induction chemotherapy, which was complete in three. One patient failed to respond, and received surgery followed by postoperative radiation. At a mean follow-up of 45 months, 15 patients were free of recurrence, four of whom had radiation damage to the frontal or temporal lobe, and all of whom had preservation of vision (19). A minimally invasive approach, combining endoscopic sinus surgery with stereotactic radiosurgery, appears promising (20). The average time interval before recurrent disease developed was more than six years in one series, far greater than expected for other sinonasal malignancies.

The benefit of systemic chemotherapy for advanced ONB is difficult to ascertain because chemotherapy is rarely used as a single treatment modality. Cisplatin-based combination regimens (particularly cisplatin and E) have often been chosen but experience is limited to small case series (21–24). Benefit is usually of short duration (one to nine months). In at least one of these reports, chemotherapy was only efficacious in patients with high-grade tumors (23).

Leptomeningeal spread is a serious complication of ONB. Patients may benefit from radiotherapy to symptomatic sites or intrathecal chemotherapy.

Prognosis

Histologic grade, clinical stage, and DNA ploidy may be important prognostic indicators in ONB (9,10). Patients with low histologic grade appear to have a better survival than those with higher-grade tumors (9). In one review of 26 published studies involving 390 patients with ONB, the five-year survival rates for patients with and without cervical nodal metastases were 29% versus 64%, respectively (10). DNA ploidy as determined by flow cytometry has been a useful prognostic indicator in some but not all studies (7). DNA ploidy may simply represent a surrogate for histologic grade. Mutations of the p53 tumor suppressor gene do not appear to play a role in the early development of ONB. However, overexpression of wild-type p53 appears to correlate with local aggressive behavior and a tendency to recurrence (25).

PERIPHERAL PRIMITIVE NEUROECTODERMAL TUMOR

ES and primitive PNET (pPNET) are now considered part of a spectrum of neoplastic diseases known as the EFT derived from a common cell of origin. Although their histogenesis has been debated over the years, evidence from immunohistochemical, cytogenetic, and molecular genetic studies supports a neuroectodermal origin for all EFTs. These neoplasms can develop in almost any bone or soft tissue, but are most common in flat and long bones where they give rise to localized pain and swelling. Although overt metastatic disease is found in fewer than 25% at the time of diagnosis, subclinical metastatic disease is assumed to be present in nearly all patients because 80% to 90% relapse if local therapy alone is provided. As a result, systemic chemotherapy has evolved as an essential component of treatment.

Clinical Presentation

ES most often arises in the long bones of the extremities (predominantly the femur, but also the tibia, fibula, and humerus), and the bones of the pelvis. The spine, hands, and feet are affected less frequently (26,27). On the other side, pPNET and EES arise within the axial skeleton (26,28). In approximately 25%, the primary tumor is located in the soft tissue.

Patients with EFT present with localized pain or swelling of a few weeks or months duration (29,30). A minor trauma may be the initiating event that calls attention to the lesion. The pain is mild at first, but intensifies rapidly and is aggravated by exercise and the supine position. A distinct soft tissue mass is sometimes appreciated in a swollen and erythematous limb. When present, it is firmly attached to the bone and tender to palpation. Patients with juxta-articular lesions present with loss of joint motion, while lesions involving the ribs are associated with direct pleural extension and large extraosseous masses. Tumors involving the axial skeleton result in localized back pain or radicular symptoms. Spinal cord compression is heralded by loss of bowel or bladder control. Constitutional symptoms or signs, such as fever, fatigue, weight loss, or anemia, are present in 10% to 20% of patients at presentation (29). Fever arises from cytokine production by tumor cells and, along with other systemic symptoms, is associated with advanced disease.

Approximately 80% of patients present with seemingly localized disease. Overt metastases may become evident within weeks to months, if the diagnosis is delayed and effective therapy is not provided. Patients with primary pelvic tumors are more likely to present with metastatic disease compared to other sites (25% vs. 16%) (27). Metastases are found in lung and bone, especially the vertebral column (31). Lung metastases represent the first site of distant spread in 70% to 80% of cases, and are the leading cause of death for patients with EFT. Lymph node, liver, and brain involvement are distinctly uncommon (30,32).

Differential diagnosis of EFT presenting as primary bone tumor includes both benign and malignant conditions. Subacute osteomyelitis may have given rise to a similar clinical syndrome (fever, elevated sedimentation rate, and localized pain), and is associated with intense radiotracer uptake on bone scan, and a soft tissue mass on other imaging studies. EES and soft tissue pPNETs must be distinguished from a variety of benign and malignant soft tissue tumors.

Staging evaluation includes a CT scan of chest, abdomen and pelvis, and a radionuclide bone scan. PET is less sensitive than bone scan in the detection of osseous metastases from bone sarcomas but is used to assess the response to neoadjuvant chemotherapy (33–35). A commonly used staging system has not been established for EFT. Initial laboratory studies should include a complete blood count, serum chemistries, and lactate dehydrogenase (LDH), which is a known prognostic factor in patients with EFT (27). When neuroblastoma is considered in the differential diagnosis, urine catecholamine levels may be useful, because they are elevated in neuroblastoma but normal in EFT.

Adequate amounts of tissue are necessary in order to provide sufficient diagnostic material. A detailed pathologic evaluation is often required to establish the correct diagnosis within the group of "small round blue cell tumors"; these samples may require special handling. The microscopic appearance of EFTs is devoid of any typical architectural feature. The tumors cells are arranged in patternless sheets of cells. Individual cell borders are poorly defined, hence the tumor takes on a syncytial appearance. Nuclei are round, with small nucleoli (Fig. 3A). Mitoses are not infrequent. Unlike ONB, the tumor is usually not divided into lobules and rosettes are uncommon. Tumor cells are rich in glycogen, best demonstrated by a Periodic-Acid Schiff stain with diastase digestion. Immunohistochemistry

(A)

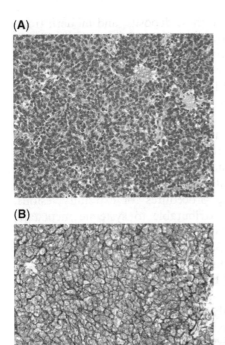

(B)

Figure 3 (**A**) Ewing's sarcoma presents with sheet-like arrangement of tumor cells, with ill-defined cell borders, resulting in a syncytial pattern. Rosettes are rarely seen and the tumor may also have variable areas of necrosis. Hematoxylin- and eosin-stained section. Original magnification 100x. (**B**) CD99 immunoreactivity, while not exclusive to EFT, is nonetheless seen in over 95% of tumors. Staining is widespread throughout the tumor and is readily evident as cytoplasmic membrane positivity. (CD99 immunohistochemistry×200)

provides further evidence of neuroepithelial differentiation with markers such as neuron specific enolase, Leu7, protein-gene-product 9.5 and neurofilaments. EFT frequently expresses CD99 (O13, MIC2) and while this feature is not restricted exclusively to this family of tumors, it remains perhaps the most widely used and specific marker (Fig. 3B). Molecular genetic changes are seen in the vast majority of cases (>95%) and typically consist of the reciprocal translocation 11;22 (q24;q12), with resultant fusion of either FL1 or ERG genes with the ES gene (36,37). In most but not all studies, neither the presence of neural differentiation (as in PNETs) nor extraosseous origin has a significant adverse influence on outcome (28,38,39). In fact, EFTs that arise in skin or subcutaneous sites have a generally favorable prognosis (40).

Treatment

General Treatment Principles

The treatment of peripheral PNET is similar to that of other tumors within the EFT family. EFT has to be considered a systemic disease due to the high incidence of subclinical metastatic disease at the time of diagnosis.

Chemotherapy can successfully eradicate these deposits, and modern treatment schedules all include chemotherapy, usually administered prior to and following local therapy. For patients with localized disease, the addition of several months of intensive polychemotherapy to local therapy has had a dramatic impact on survival. Five- and 10-year survival rates now approach 70% and 50%, respectively (41,42).

Chemotherapy: Most modern treatment plans utilize initial (induction or neoadjuvant) chemotherapy followed by local treatment and additional chemotherapy. Reduction of local tumor volume is accomplished in the majority of patients, and this can facilitate resection. This is particularly important with regard to limb-sparing procedures for extremity lesions. Because most treatment failures are attributable to systemic metastatic disease, local therapy considerations should never compromise the administration of effective systemic therapy. Both EES and PNET respond to the same chemotherapy regimens as osseous ES, and there is no evidence to suggest that these EFT variants should be treated differently (38). Adjuvant treatment has evolved, largely due to the efforts of several cooperative groups. In the first Intergroup ES Study (IESS-I), the combination of vincristine, doxorubicin, cyclophosphamide, and actinomycin D was associated with a better five-year relapse-free survival than vincristine, actinomycin D, and cyclophosphamide (VAC) alone or VAC plus adjuvant bilateral pulmonary irradiation (60% vs. 24% vs. 44%, respectively) (42). Increasing the doxorubicin dose intensity during the early months of therapy further improved response, and in the second intergroup ES study (IESS-II), the five-year relapse-free survival rates using intermittent high-dose four-drug therapy improved to 73% for nonpelvic lesions (43). Because of concerns about limiting the dose intensity of doxorubicin in regimens containing actinomycin D, this drug was omitted from most trials thereafter, with no adverse impact on long-term outcome. Adding alternating cycles of ifosfamide (I) and E to a vincristine, doxorubicin, cyclophosphamide (VDC) backbone provided further benefit. As a result of these data, current standard chemotherapy for EFT in the United States includes vincristine, doxorubicin, and cyclophosphamide alternating with I and E. Typically, four to six cycles of chemotherapy are given before local therapy. As long as there is a response to preoperative chemotherapy, additional cycles of the same treatments are given postoperatively, and the total duration of therapy is approximately 48 weeks. Relief of pain, decrease in tumor size, fall in LDH level, radiologic improvement, or evidence of necrosis in the resected specimen all argue for continued chemotherapy for those who can tolerate its sometimes considerable side effects.

The sensitivity of EFT to alkylating agents, which have a steep dose–response curve, has prompted the evaluation of dose intense regimens in patients with poor-risk disease. The majority of patients in these studies have relapsed or metastatic disease. The benefit of dose-intensive therapy for patients with poor-risk localized disease is unclear. Concerns for an increased risk of secondary malignancies in patients receiving dose-intense therapy have tempered enthusiasm for this approach.

Local Treatment: Local control for EFT can be achieved by surgery, radiation, or both. The choice of radiation or surgery usually represents a trade-off between functional result and the risk of secondary radiation-induced malignancy. Patients who lack a function-preserving surgical option because of tumor location or extent may be recommended radiation therapy. However, surgery is preferred for potentially resectable lesions, and for those arising in dispensable bones (e.g., fibula, rib, small lesions of the hands, or feet). Such an approach avoids the risk of secondary radiation-induced sarcomas, for which the estimated risk is between 10% and 30% at 20 years. An analysis of the degree of necrosis in the excised tumor can permit refinements in the estimate of prognosis. Furthermore, in the skeletally immature child, resection may be associated with less morbidity than radiation, which can retard bone growth and cause deformity. Although there are no randomized trials comparing surgery with radiation therapy for local control, multiple retrospective series suggest superior local control and survival for surgery compared to radiation alone. Selection bias may account for at least some of these results (i.e., smaller, more favorably situated peripheral tumors are more likely to be resected while larger, axial lesions are radiated). Radiation dose and proper field planning are important factors in local control. There were no local failures among tumors less than 8 cm in size treated with at least 40 Gy in one report. Radiation is an essential component of therapy for patients undergoing resection if the surgical margins are inadequate, although effective chemotherapy can also reduce the risk of local failure in such patients.

Treatment for Advanced Disease: Patients with overt metastatic disease at presentation have a less favorable outcome than those with localized disease. However, aggressive multimodality therapy can relieve pain, prolong the progression-free interval, and cure some patients of their disease. In a review of 12 different series in which patients with metastatic EFT were predominantly treated with chemotherapy, five-year event-free and overall survival rates averaged 25 (range 9 to 55), and 33 (range 14–61%, respectively). The small numbers of patients in each series, and the heterogeneity in location and extent of metastatic disease probably account for these wide variations in outcome.

Recurrent Disease: The majority of relapses occur within five years. In general, survival after the first relapse is poor, with few survivors among those who relapse within two years of therapy. In contrast, up to 15% to 20% of those who relapse later may survive for long term.

Patients with ES family tumors require referral to centers that have multidisciplinary teams of sarcoma specialists. With rare exception, systemic combination chemotherapy and definitive local therapy is required in all patients, and care should be coordinated among the medical oncologist, surgeon, and radiation therapist. In most cases, treatment will begin with chemotherapy. The primary tumor can then be treated with surgery, radiation, or a combination, with the choice being dictated by the age of the patient, the location and size of the primary tumor, and functional as well as long-term consequences of therapy (i.e., radiation-induced growth inhibition or secondary malignancy). Postoperatively, chemotherapy is usually continued, typically for several months. Thus, the total duration of therapy ranges from 10 to 12 months. Treatment of patients with clinically detectable metastatic disease, and those who relapse after initial therapy also requires multimodality therapy. All patients with advanced disease should be approached with potentially curative treatment. Up to 40% of patients with limited pulmonary metastatic disease who undergo intensive chemotherapy and pulmonary resection may be long-term survivors. The prognosis for other subsets of patients with advanced disease is less favorable. There is no conclusive evidence that high-dose therapy with or without hematopoietic stem cell infusion at any point during treatment is beneficial for patients with poor-risk localized and metastatic EFT. Most patients with advanced or recurrent disease need new approaches to improve outcomes, and participation in clinical trials should be encouraged. Long-term follow-up is needed following therapy because disease relapse, treatment-related complications, and second malignancies are all common beyond five years after treatment is initiated.

REFERENCES

1. Askin FB, Rosai J, Sibley RK, et al. Malignant small cell tumor of the thoracopulmonary region in childhood: A distinctive clinicopathologic entity of uncertain histogenesis. Cancer 1979; 43(6):2438–2451.
2. Ambros IM, Ambros PF, Strehl S, et al. MIC2 is a specific marker for Ewing's sarcoma and peripheral primitive neuroectodermal tumors. Evidence for a common histogenesis of Ewing's sarcoma and peripheral primitive neuroectodermal tumors from MIC2 expression and specific chromosome aberration. Cancer 1991; 67(7):1886–1893.
3. Hyams VJ, Batsakis JG, Michaels L. Tumors of the upper respiratory tract and ear. Atlas of Tumor Pathology, Armed Forces Institute of Pathology, 1988.
4. Kadish S, Goodman M, Wang CC. Olfactory neuroblastoma. A clinical analysis of 17 cases. Cancer 1976; 37(3):1571–1576.
5. Pickuth D, Heywang-Kobrunner SH, Spielmann RP. Computed tomography and magnetic resonance imaging features of olfactory neuroblastoma: an analysis of 22 cases. Clin Otolaryngol Allied Sci 1999; 24(5):457–461.
6. Dias FL, Sa GM, Lima RA, et al. Pattterns of failure and outcome in esthesioneuroblastoma. Arch Otolaryngol Head Neck Surg 2003; 129(11):1186–1192.

7. Hirose T, Scheithauer BW, Lopes MB, et al. Olfactory neuroblastoma. An immunohistochemical, ultrastructural, and flow cytometric study. Cancer 1995; 76(1):4–19.
8. Frierson HF Jr., Ross GW, Mills SE, Frankfurter, A. Olfactory neuroblastoma. Additional immunohistochemical characterization. Am J Clin Pathol 1990; 94(5):547–553.
9. Morita A, Ebersold MJ, Olsen KD, et al. Esthesioneuroblastoma: prognosis and management. Neurosurgery 1993; 32(5):706–714.
10. Dulguerov P, Allal AS, Calcaterra TC. Esthesioneuroblastoma: a meta-analysis and review. Lancet Oncol 2001; 2(11):683–690.
11. Simon JH, Zhen W, McCulloch TM, et al. Esthesioneuroblastoma: the University of Iowa experience 1978-1998. Laryngoscope 2001; 111(3):488–493.
12. Broich G, Pagliari A, Ottaviani F. Esthesioneuroblastoma: a general review of the cases published since the discovery of the tumour in 1924. Anticancer Res 1997; 17(4A):2683–2706.
13. Lund VJ, Howard DJ, Wei WI, Cheesmna, AD. Craniofacial resection for tumors of the nasal cavity and paranasal sinuses a 19-year experience. Head Neck 1998; 20(2):97–105.
14. Argiris A, Dutra J, Tseke P, Haines, K. Esthesioneuroblastoma: The Northwestern University experience. Laryngoscope 2003; 113(1):155–160.
15. Gruber G, Laedrach K, Baumert B, et al. Esthesioneuroblastoma: irradiation alone and surgery alone are not enough. Int J Radiat Oncol Biol Phys 2002; 54(2):486–491.
16. Eich HT, Hero B, Staar S, et al. Multimodality therapy including radiotherapy and chemotherapy improves event-free survival in stage C esthesioneuroblastoma. Strahlenther Onkol 2003; 179(4):233–240.
17. Zappia JJ, Carroll WR, Wolf GT, et al. Olfactory neuroblastoma: the results of modern treatment approaches at the University of Michigan. Head Neck 1993; 15(3):190–196.
18. Polin RS, Sheehan JP, Chenelle AG, et al. The role of preoperative adjuvant treatment in the management of esthesioneuroblastoma: the University of Virginia experience. Neurosurgery 1998; 42(5):1029–1037.
19. Fitzek MM, Thornton AF, Varvares M, et al. Neuroendocrine tumors of the sinonasal tract. Results of a prospective study incorporating chemotherapy, surgery, and combined proton-photon radiotherapy. Cancer 2002; 94(10):2623–2634.
20. Walch C, Stammberger H, Anderhuber W, et al. The minimally invasive approach to olfactory neuroblastoma: combined endoscopic and stereotactic treatment. Laryngoscope 2000; 110(4):635–640.
21. Sheehan JM, Sheehan JP, Jane JA Sr., Polin, RS. Chemotherapy for esthesioneuroblastomas. Neurosurg Clin N Am 2000; 11(4):693–701.
22. Mishima Y, Nagasaki E, Terui Y, et al. Combination chemotherapy (cyclophosphamide, doxorubicin, and vincristine with continuous-infusion cisplatin and etoposide) and radiotherapy with stem cell support can be beneficial for adolescents and adults with estheisoneuroblastoma. Cancer 2004; 101(6):1437–1444.
23. McElroy EA Jr., Buckner JC, Lewis JE. Chemotherapy for advanced esthesioneuroblastoma: the Mayo Clinic experience. Neurosurgery 1998; 42(5):1023–1027.
24. Chamberlain MC. Treatment of intracranial metastatic esthesioneuroblastoma. Cancer 2002; 95(2):243–248.

25. Papadaki H, Kounelis S, Kapadia SB, et al. Relationship of p53 gene alterations with tumor progression and recurrence in olfactory neuroblastoma. Am J Surg Pathol 1996; 20(6):715–721.
26. Ginsberg JP, Woo SY, Hicks MJ, Horowitz ME. Ewing's sarcoma family of tumors: Ewing's sarcoma of bone and soft tissue and the peripheral primitive neuroectodermal tumors. In: Pizz PA, Poplack DG, eds. Principles and Practice of Pediatric Oncology. Philadelphia: Lippincott, Williams & Wilkins, 2002.
27. Cotterill SJ, Ahrens S, Paulussen M, et al. Prognostic factors in Ewing's tumor of bone: Analysis of 975 patients from the European Intergroup Cooperative Ewing's Sarcoma Study Group. J Clin Oncol 2000; 18(17):3108–3114.
28. Raney RB, Asmar L, Newton WA Jr., et al. Ewing's sarcoma of sort tissues in childhood: A report from the Intergroup Rhabdomyosarcoma Study, 1972 to 1991. J Clin Oncol 1997; 15(2):574–582.
29. Rud NP, Reiman HM, Pritchard DJ, et al. Extraosseous Ewing's sarcoma. A study of 42 cases. Cancer 1989; 64(7):1548–1553.
30. Parasuraman S, Langston J, Rao BN, et al. Brain metastases in pediatric Ewing sarcoma and rhabdomyosarcoma: The St. Jude Children's Research Hospital experience. J Pediatr Hematol Oncol 1999; 21(5):370–377.
31. Wilkins RM, Pritchard DJ, Burgert EO Jr., Unni, KK. Ewing's sarcoma of bone. Experience with 140 patients. Cancer 1986; 58(11):2551–2555.
32. Cangir A, Vietti TJ, Gehan EA, et al. Ewing's sarcoma metastatic at diagnosis. Results and comparisons of two intergroup Ewing's sarcoma studies. Cancer 1990; 66(5):887–893.
33. Hawkins DS, Rajendran JG, Conrad EU III, et al. Evaluation of chemotherapy response in pediatric bone sarcomas by [F-18]-fluorodeoxy-D-glucose positron emission tomography. Cancer 2002; 94(12):3277–3284.
34. Franzius C, Sciuk J, Brinkschmidt C, et al. Evaluation of chemotherapy response in primary bone tumors with F-18 FDG positron emission tomography compared with histologically assessed tumor necrosis. Clin Nucl Med 2000; 25(11):874–881.
35. Franzius C, Sciuk J, Daldrup-Link HE, et al. FDG-PET for detection of osseous metastases from malignant primary bone tumours: Comparison with bone scintigraphy. Eur J Nucl Med 2000; 27(9):1305–1311.
36. Delattre O, Zucman J, Plougastel B, et al. The Ewing family of tumors–a subgroup of small-round-cell tumors defined by specific chimeric transcripts. N Engl J Med 1994; 331:294.
37. May WA, Gishizky ML, Lessnick SL, et al. Ewing sarcoma 11; 22 translocation produced a chimeric transcription factor that requires the DNA-binding domain encoded by FLI1 for transformation. Proc Natl Acad Sci USA 1993; 90(12):5752–5756.
38. Jurgens H, Bier V, Harms D, et al. Malignant peripheral neuroectodermal tumors. A retrospective analysis of 42 patients. Cancer 1988; 61(2):349–357.
39. Bacci G, Ferrari S, Bertoni F, et al. Neoadjuvant chemotherapy for peripheral malignant neuroectodermal tumor of bone: Recent experience at the istituto rizzoli. J Clin Oncol 2000; 18(4):885–892.
40. Chow E, Merchant TE, Pappo A, et al. Cutaneous and subcutaneous Ewing's sarcoma: An indolert disease. Int J Radiat Oncol Biol Phys 2000; 46(2):433–438.

41. Craft A, Cotterill S, Malcolm A, et al. Ifostamide-containing chemotherapy in Ewing's sarcoma: The Second United Kingdom Children's Cancer Study Group and the Medical Research Council Ewing's Tumor Study. J Clin Oncol 1998; 16(11):3628–3633.
42. Nesbit ME Jr., Gehan EA, Burgert EO Jr., et al. Multimodal therapy for the management of primary, nonmetastatic Ewing's sarcoma of bone: A long-term follow-up of the First Intergroup study. J Clin Oncol 1990; 8(10):1664–1674.
43. Burgert EO Jr., Nesbit ME, Garnsey LA, et al. Multimodal therapy for the management of nonpelvic, localized Ewing's sarcoma of bone: Intergroup study IESS-II. J Clin Oncol 1990; 8(9):1514–1524.

17

Meningiomas

Marcus L. Ware, Anita Lal, and Michael W. McDermott

*Departments of Neurological Surgery, Radiation Oncology,
and The Brain Tumor Research Center, University of California,
San Francisco, California, U.S.A.*

INTRODUCTION

Meningiomas are common tumors seen in neurosurgical practice. We review the common literature regarding the epidemiology, histopathology, molecular mechanisms of tumorigenesis, diagnosis, and treatment of benign, atypical, and malignant meningiomas. Moreover, we discuss the current literature supporting the current pathological classification of these tumors and propose a rational scheme for tumor treatment.

EPIDEMIOLOGY

Meningiomas arise from arachnoid cells or arachnoid cap cells, and account for 20% to 26% of all primary intracranial neoplasms and 25% of all intraspinal tumors (1). They account for 20% of all intracranial tumors in males and 38% in females (2). The incidence of meningiomas in the general population varies between 2 and 15 per 100,000 people, and increases with age (1); the prevalence of meningioma is estimated to be approximately 97.5 in 100,000 in the United States (3). The age-adjusted incidence rates are similar for Caucasians, African Americans, and Hispanics (3.78, 3.77, and 3.45, respectively) (2). Thus, meningiomas are the most common primary tumors of the central nervous system. Approximately 94% of meningiomas are considered benign, 4% are atypical, and 1% is malignant. Benign meningiomas are more prevalent in women, but atypical and anaplastic forms appear to be more common in men (4,5). Up to 2% of all benign meningiomas will transform into malignant forms (6) and up to 28.5% of all recurrent benign meningiomas will be found to be atypical or anaplastic (6–8). In several large series, the 10-year survival rate after complete resection of benign meningiomas has been estimated between 43% and 77% (9,10). In contrast, atypical and malignant meningiomas are much more aggressive with shorter median survival times (8,11). The five-year mortality rate is 21% for atypical meningiomas (12); median survival for anaplastic meningiomas is 1.5 years (12).

MENINGIOMA CLASSIFICATION

In 1938, Cushing and Eisenhardt (13) described a variant of meningioma in patients with a mean survival time of 2.5 years. These authors noted other variants that were not as aggressive and introduced a classification scheme that divided meningiomas into mesenchymatous, angioblasic, meningotheliomatous, psammomatous, osteoblastic, chondroblastic, fibroblastic, melanoblastic, and lipomatous types (13). Based on the criteria of Jaaskelainen et al. (8), six parameters were used to grade tumors according to the degree of anaplasia: benign (I), atypical (II), anaplastic (III), and sarcomatous (IV). Based on these tumor grades, five-year recurrence rates of 3% for benign meningiomas, 38% for atypical meningiomas, and 78% for malignant meningiomas have been reported (8).

The World Health Organization (WHO, 1993) classified meningiomas into four types: (i) classic (meningotheliomatous, fibroblastic, and transitional subtypes); (ii) angioblastic (hemangiopericytoma); (iii) aggressive (papillary subtype); and (iv) malignant (14). According to this classification system, malignant meningiomas were defined as tumors demonstrating histological anaplasia, invasion of brain parenchyma, or metastasis. The second WHO classification provided a more objective system of classification in which proliferation indices, such as MIB-1 labeling, and brain invasion are not criteria for the diagnosis of atypical and malignant meningiomas (15). This change was based largely on the experience at the Mayo Clinic (5,12), which correlated six histological parameters with recurrence. These studies found that histological anaplasia, subtotal resection, 20 mitoses per 10 high-power fields (HPF), and nuclear atypia were associated with poor survival (12). Taken together, these are presently the best data for features of meningiomas associated with recurrence and are thus the basis for the WHO II classification system, which is used to classify meningiomas (Table 1).

Molecular Mechanisms of Meningioma Tumorigenesis

All tumors are thought to develop from the clonal expansion of a single cell with mutations that provide a growth or survival advantage. Cells formed

Table 1 World Health Organization II Classification (2000) of Meningiomas

WHO Grade 1	WHO Grade 2	WHO Grade 3
Meningothelial	Atypical	Anaplastic
Fibrous (fibroblastic)	Chordoid	Papillary
Transitional (mixed)	Clear cell	Rhabdoid
Psammomatous		
Angiomatous		
Microcystic		
Secretory		
Lymphoplasmacyte-rich		
Metaplastic		

Abbreviation: WHO, World Health Organization.

from this expansion may then gain further growth advantages through the accumulation of additional mutations. Models of this process have been described for a number of different tumor types. Meningiomas have increasing grades that correspond to more aggressive tumors with larger numbers of mutations. Loss of neurofibromatosis 2 gene (*NF2*) is associated with benign meningiomas and is therefore an early event in meningioma tumorigenesis. Progression from benign to atypical meningioma is associated with losses on chromosomes 1p, 6q, 10, 14q, and 18q, and gain on 1q, 9q, 12q, 15q, 17q, and 20 (16); progression from atypical to malignant meningioma with losses on 9p and 17q.

Many cytogenetic and molecular genetic studies have shown loss of chromosome 22 in 40% to 70% of all meningiomas (17–19). The loss of the NF2 on 22q12 is thought to be critical for meningioma tumorigenesis in virtually all NF2 syndrome related and 20% to 30% of sporadic meningiomas (Table 3) (20). The frequency of this mutation varies among meningioma subtypes with 10% to 20% in meningothelial types and 60% to 80% in fibroblastic and transitional types (21). These mutations are accompanied by loss of the wild-type allele suggesting that the complete loss of merlin is the major mechanism leading to meningioma tumorigenesis (19,22,23).

The NF2 tumor suppressor gene product, merlin or schwanomin, belongs to the protein 4.1 family of structural proteins that link the cytoskeleton to several proteins of the cytoplasmic membrane (24). Wild-type merlin overexpression has been shown to reverse the Ras-induced malignant phenotype of transformed NIH3T3 cells. Merlin restores the contact inhibition of cell growth by suppressing the SRE-dependent transcription by inhibiting the activation of the Ras–ERK pathway (25). Thus, merlin may act by providing proliferative arrest in response to cell–cell interactions.

Monosomy 1p is the most frequent chromosomal aberration associated with meningioma progression (26). Fluorescent in situ hybridization

Table 2 World Health Organization II Criteria for Meningioma Grading

Meningioma grade	Criteria
Atypical meningiomas	≥ 4 mitosis/10 HPF ($\geq 2.5/\text{mm}^2$)
	Or at least three of the following features:
	Sheeting
	Macronuclei
	Small cell formation
	Hypercellularity (≥ 53 nuclei/HPF; $>118/\text{mm}^2$)
	Brain invasion
Anaplastic meningiomas	≥ 20 mitotic figures/10 HPF ($>12.5/\text{mm}^2$)
	Odds ratio
	Focal or diffuse loss of meningothelial differentiation resulting in carcinoma-, sarcoma-, or melanoma-like appearance

Abbreviation: HPF, high power field.

(FISH) studies on meningioma show monosomy 1p in 70% of atypical meningiomas and nearly all anaplastic meningiomas (27). The alkaline phosphatase gene, *ALPL*, is a candidate tumor suppressor gene located on chromosome 1p. However, the mechanism of this gene in tumor progression and the mechanism of inactivation of the second allele have not been explained. Deletions on chromosome 14q are frequently seen in more aggressive meningiomas.

Table 3 Genes Involved in Meningioma Progression

Chromosome	Gene	Association
22q	*NF2*	Merlin, the NF2 gene product, is a tumor suppressor that interacts with the cytoskeleton.
1p	*ALPL*	*ALPL* is a possible tumor suppressor gene. 1p mutations are most frequently seen in atypical and malignant meningioma.
14q	Unknown	14q deletions are seen in malignant tumors and are associated with poor outcome.
18q	Unknown	18q is also associated with more malignant tumors.
18p	DAL-1	DAL-1 is in the same protein family as merlin and has been found to be deficient in 60–70% of meningiomas

Abbreviations: NF2, neurofibromatosis 2; ALPL, alkaline phosphatase; DAL-1, differentially expressed in adenocarcinoma of the lung.

Mutations on 18q have been associated with atypical and malignant meningiomas in a number of studies (16,28,29). Although previous cytogenetic investigations rarely found mutations in 18q in meningiomas, a more recent study shows partial or complete loss of chromosome 18 in 43% of atypical meningiomas (16). Three tumor suppressor genes, *DCC*, *DPC4*, and *JV18-1*, were identified on 18q and found to be deleted in other types of tumors. However, a number of candidate genes from this region have been shown not to be involved in meningioma tumor progression (30).

Although most genes identified on 18q have not shown to be of pathogenetic relevance, differentially expressed in adenocarcinoma of the lung (*DAL-1*), located on 18p11.3, has been implicated in meningioma progression. *DAL-1*, a gene in the same family as merlin, encodes a membrane-associated protein with a potential ATP/GTP binding motif (31). The protein product of this gene suppresses lung and breast cancer cell line growth when introduced into cell lines deficient in this protein. DAL-1 expression is lost in 60% to 70% of meningiomas (32). A more recent study showed that loss of merlin or DAL-1 was present in 92% of tumors with 58% of tumors having combined losses (33). These findings suggest that members of this tumor suppressor family are likely important early events in meningioma pathogenesis.

A number of other chromosomal changes and candidate genes have been associated with atypical meningiomas. Atypical meningiomas have frequent losses on chromosome 6. Cytogenetic studies have shown structural abnormalities or monosomy of chromosome 6 in a number of patients (34,35). In addition, there is loss of heterozygosity on 10q in 27% to 50% of atypical meningiomas (36,37). However, no specific genes have been directly implicated on 10q. There are at least two genomic alterations associated with anaplastic meningiomas, which do not appear in lower grade tumors: losses on 9p and amplification of 17q. The most important candidate for the gene on 9q is CDKN2A, a tumor suppressor gene that encodes the G1 progression regulator p16 (38). However, there is evidence that there is an additional tumor suppressor gene on 9p (16). Comparative genomic hybridization analysis showed high-level amplification of chromosome 17 in 48% of anaplastic meningiomas (16). In contrast, this amplification is rarely seen in benign or atypical meningiomas, suggesting that mutation may be important in malignant progression.

p53

p53 has been shown in a number of studies to play an important role in the control of cellular proliferation, differentiation, and apoptosis. Mutations and loss of *p53* are the most common molecular findings in a variety of human tumors. Surprisingly, mutations in *p53* in meningiomas are rare. Loss of *p53* has not been implicated in meningioma progression. However, there is an association between higher *p53* immunoreactivity and tumor recurrence in both benign and malignant meningiomas (39).

Role of Hormones in Meningioma Progression

The role of steroid hormones in meningioma tumorigenesis has been subject to numerous studies (40). The most-promising hormone in these studies is progesterone, whose receptor is absent in normal meninges, but strongly expressed in benign meningiomas. The progesterone receptor is reduced or absent in higher-grade tumors. However, progesterone receptor immuno-reactivity, although associated with lower-grade tumors, has not been definitively found to be a favorable prognostic factor (33).

Imaging and Diagnosis of Meningiomas

The imaging modalities used to characterize meningiomas include plain roentgenograms, computed tomography (CT), magnetic resonance imaging (MRI), and cerebral angiography. Although plain roentgenograms are rarely used to diagnose meningiomas in the modern era, there are character-istic findings that may be observed secondary to changes in bony architec-ture caused by meningiomas. Osteoblastic changes, such as hyperostosis or sclerosis, are common manifestations of meningioma involvement in the cranial vault. Hyperostosis denotes increase in bone density and thick-ness of the inner table of the skull, while sclerosis refers to the increase in bone density without an increase in bone thickness. Sclerosis of the outer table and lytic bone lesions may indicate greater bone involvement.

CT scans are useful in the diagnosis of meningiomas in that they can provide information regarding the size, consistency, bone involvement, and the presence of mass effect on the adjacent brain. On nonenhanced scans, meningiomas are almost always hyperdense or isodense to the surrounding brain. Upon administration of iodinated dye, these tumors often display intense enhancement. Meningiomas appear well encapsulated with distinct borders between tumor and brain. A recent study found that meningiomas without calcification on CT scan are likely to grow exponentially, whereas those with calcification have linear or no growth (41). Thus, findings on CT scans may be predictive of tumor behavior. In addition, hyperostosis, bone invasion, and bone erosion are best seen on CT scans and may be critical in planning surgery at the skull base.

MRI is the most sensitive modality in the detection of meningiomas and the most important for determining the size and location of these tumors. In addition, MRI provides information about the anatomy of the surrounding brain, cranial nerves, and vascular structures. Meningiomas are isointense on T1-weighted images. On T2-weighted images, 50% are iso-intense, 40% are hyperintense, and 10% are hypointense to brain (42). Most meningiomas strongly enhance with the administration of gadolinium on T1-weighted images. One of the characteristic findings seen on MRI with contrast in 50% to 60% of meningiomas is hyperintensity of the dura adja-cent to a meningioma (43), termed the "dural tail," a nonspecific finding seen in other forms of dural pathology. Malignant degeneration of meningiomas cannot be determined with any certainty by characteristics seen on CT or MRI (44,45). However, a few studies suggest that more aggressive meningeal tumors have heterogeneous enhancement, irregular margins, and increased edema (46–48).

Prior to the development of CT and MRI technology, cerebral angiography was helpful in establishing the diagnosis of meningiomas. Meningiomas are characterized by a dual blood supply: there is always a meningeal-based blood supply and a pial blood supply. Thus, angiographic evidence of tumor with a meningeal blood supply and a delayed blush was highly suggestive of meningiomas. In the modern era, cerebral angiography may be helpful in defining fine vascular detail of structures near the tumor and to assess for vessels supplying the tumor that may be embolized. Interruption of the meningeal-based blood supply prior to resection of the tumor by embolization has been shown to decrease surgical blood loss and operative times (49,50).

Treatment of Meningiomas

Observation

Because the vast majority of meningiomas are benign and slow growing, observation should always be considered an option in the treatment of meningiomas. Many tumors are discovered incidentally, and clinical and radiographic follow-up of patients with meningiomas reveal that some of these tumors are very slow growing or do not grow at all (51–53). It is reasonable to follow asymptomatic patients with serial imaging and clinical evaluation. However, special attention should be paid to younger patients because in those, tumors are more likely to grow and become symptomatic (51). Early intervention is often required in patients with petroclival meningiomas, because even minimal progression may cause disability (54). Elderly patients with meningiomas also comprise a special group in that meningiomas in these patients often do not grow rapidly (53). Importantly, elderly patients often do not tolerate surgical treatment (55) or radiation therapy as well as younger individuals, thus care should be taken when deciding to treat the patients in this population. Cases in whom observation is considered, we recommend an interval follow-up MRI be obtained three months after the diagnostic scan to exclude other more-aggressive dural-based tumors and then at six months to assess the growth rate of the tumor.

Surgical Resection

In patients with larger symptomatic meningiomas, we recommend surgical resection. The extent of surgical resection is the most important factor in meningioma tumor recurrence (9) and is best described by the Simpson grading system [Table 4, (9)]. Although surgery is the mainstay of treatment, the goals of surgery may differ depending on tumor location and the patient's

Table 4 Simpson Grade of Meningioma Resection

Simpson grade	Extent of resection
I	Macroscopic complete removal of tumor with excision of its dural attachment or any abnormal bone.
II	Macroscopic complete removal of tumor and its visible extensions with coagulation of its dural attachments.
III	Macroscopic complete removal of intradural tumor without resection or coagulation of its dural attachment or extradural extensions.
IV	Partial removal leaving intradural tumor in situ.
V	Simple decompression.

condition. When complete resection is feasible without harm to vital structures, gross total resection should be attempted. Choosing the approach, performing a careful dissection around vital structures, and deciding when and when not to leave tumor behind are the keys in the art of meningioma surgery. Thus, gross total removal of tumors of the convexity, olfactory groove, and meningiomas involving the anterior third of the sagittal sinus would appear to be possible and beneficial to the patient, while for tumors of the medial sphenoid wing, clivus and cavernous sinus, subtotal removal may be appropriate. Adjuvant therapy should be considered for atypical or malignant meningiomas or for cases in whom gross total removal of tumor is not achieved and progressive disease would likely result in disability.

The choice of surgeon and surgical institution should also weigh into the treatment of meningiomas. Large-volume centers have lower mortality rates for patients who underwent craniotomy for meningioma (odds ratio 0.74, 95% confidence interval 0.59–0.93, $p = 0.01$) (56). In addition, high-volume hospitals have fewer patients with adverse discharge disposition suggesting a decreased morbidity associated with patient care in this population. This study also showed lower rate of mortality after surgery when higher-caseload providers were involved. Although this study was not definitive, it suggests that neurosurgeons with more experience with patients with meningiomas are better care providers to patients with meningiomas.

Radiation Therapy

Complete surgical resection is the standard therapy for meningiomas and results in excellent control rates at 5 years and 10 years (9). Subtotal resection results in much lower rates of local tumor control, although patients may remain asymptomatic from tumor for a prolonged period of time (9). Conventional radiation therapy for benign meningioma with subtotal resection increases local control to levels of control similar to gross total resection (57–61).

However, because of the indolent behavior of benign meningiomas and the side effects of radiation therapy, many authors argue that radiation therapy should be reserved for tumor progression (62–66).

The role of radiation therapy remains controversial in patients whose atypical tumors are completely resected (67,68). There is little data to support the use of radiation therapy immediately after a Simpson Grade I resection of an atypical meningioma. The relatively small number of cases, difficulty in determining the extent of surgical resection, and the lack of prospective studies render the definition of a standard of care problematic. Patients with atypical convexity meningiomas do well after Simpson Grade I resections, suggesting that a true total resection of tumor may be curative for atypical meningioma (69). In cases of subtotal resection of atypical meningioma, postoperative radiation therapy improves local tumor control rates (61). Maximum resection and postoperative adjuvant radiotherapy are independent predictors of patient and disease-free survival in the treatment of malignant meningioma (70). However, because of the high rate of local recurrence, a number of authors have advocated radiation therapy after resection of malignant meningiomas regardless of extent of resection (63,64,70).

Stereotactic Radiosurgery

More recent studies have supported the use of stereotactic radiosurgery (SRS) in the treatment of meningiomas. A number of studies have shown excellent local tumor control after treatment of benign meningiomas with SRS (Table 5). Tumor control rate at five years was reported as 89.3% in a series of 127 patients with all grades of meningioma (72). In a series of patients treated for benign meningiomas at the University of Pittsburgh, a tumor reduction of 88% eight to ten years after treatment was achieved. Another study showed three- and seven-year actuarial progression-free survival of 100% and 95%, respectively (83). There were no statistically significant differences between tumor control between SRS and Simpson Grade I resection at that institution. Taken together, these studies suggest that for small benign meningiomas, radiosurgery is a viable option for treatment of residual tumor after surgical resection.

The data for treatment of atypical and anaplastic meningioma are not as definitive as that for treatment of benign meningiomas (Table 5). In a cohort of 22 patients with atypical and anaplastic meningioma who underwent gamma knife radiosurgery, 37 lesions were treated with two- and five-year progression-free survival rates of 48% and 34%, respectively (82). Age and tumor volume were predictors of time to progression and survival. Five patients (23%) developed radiation necrosis in this series. In another study including 13 patients with atypical and nine patients with anaplastic meningiomas, a five-year control rate of 68% and a five-year survival rate of 76% was achieved for atypical tumors whereas all patients with malignant

Table 5 Summary of Stereotactic Radiosurgery for Benign, Atypical, and Malignant Meningiomas

Author (year)	Pathology	No. of patients	Follow-up in months	Marginal dose (Gy)	Control rate
Kondziolka et al. (2003) (71)	Benign	85	31 (median)	15 (median)	85% at 5 yr
Hakim et al. (1998) (72)	Benign	106	37 (median)	15 (median)	89% at 5 yr
Subach et al. (1998) (73)	Benign	62	37 (median)	15 (mean)	87% at 8 yr
Morita and Kelly (1999) (74)	Benign	88	35 (median)	16 (median)	95% at 5 yr
Roche et al. (2000) (75)	Benign	92	30.5 (median)	15 (median)	93% at 5 yr
Kobayashi et al. (2001) (76)	Benign	87	30 (mean)	14.5 (median)	90% at 7 yr
Stafford et al. (2001) (77)	Benign	168	40 (median)	16 (median)	93% at 5 yr
Shin et al. (2001) (78)	Benign	40	42 (median)	18 (median)	86% at 3 yr
Lee et al. (2002) (79)	Benign	159	35 (median)	13 (median)	93% at 5 yr
Nicolato et al. (2002) (80)	Benign	122	48.9 (median)	14.6 (mean)	97% at 4 yr
Eustacchio et al. (2002) (81)	Benign	121		13 (median)	98.3% at 5–9.8 yr
Hakim et al. (1998) (72)	Atypical	26	22.9 (median)	15 (median)	22.9 mo FFP
Hakim et al. (1998) (72)	Malignant	18	22.9 (median)	15 (median)	22.9 mo FFP
Ojemann et al. (2000) (82)	Malignant	22	22.6 (median)	15.5 (median)	26% at 5 yr
Kobayashi et al. (2001) (76)	Malignant	12	30 (mean)		
Stafford et al. (2001) (77)	Atypical	13	40 (median)	16 (median)	68% at 5 yr
Stafford et al. (2001) (77)	Malignant	9	40 (median)	16 (median)	0% at 5 yr

neoplasms died within the same period of time (77). These studies suggest that there may be some benefit of SRS in patients with more aggressive meningiomas. However, these patients are still at high risk for recurrence and should be observed closely after treatment.

Brachytherapy

After atypical and malignant tumor resection and treatment with radiation therapy, there are few options available for larger tumor recurrences. In 2004, we reviewed our series of patients with recurrent atypical and malignant meningiomas treated with repeat surgical resection and brachytherapy (84). In a series of 22 patients, the median time to progression after brachytherapy was 11.6 months for patients with malignant meningioma and 10.4 months for the combined group. Survival from the time of resection and brachytherapy was 2.4 years for the combined group. Radiation necrosis occurred in 27% of patients in this series. These results suggest that brachytherapy may be useful as a salvage treatment after the recurrence of atypical and malignant meningiomas.

Chemotherapy

Adjuvant chemotherapy has been explored in a limited number of series with mixed results. In patients with unresectable meningiomas, hydroxyurea showed a 15% to 74% reduction in the size of meningiomas on serial imaging (85). However this series was very small and included only one patient with malignant meningioma. Data from another small series in which patients with malignant meningiomas were given cyclophosphamide, Adriamycin, and vincristine after tumor resection, indicated that 3 of 14 patients had a partial response with reduction of tumor size; 8 of 14 patients had stable disease with a median time to tumor progression of 4.8 years (86). Furthermore, in a small series of patients with recurrent unresectable and malignant meningiomas, interferon alpha-2B was shown to be of limited efficacy with five of the six tumors treated in this study showing a positive response that lasted from 6 to 14 months (87).

Proposed Treatment Algorithm of Meningiomas

At our institution, all lesions suspected of being meningiomas are evaluated by MRI sequences. Prior to any other treatment, patients undergo surgical resection of their tumors (Fig. 1). All efforts are made to safely achieve gross total resection at the time of surgery. Samples are sent for pathological evaluation. In cases of patients with benign meningiomas, Simpson Grade 1 and Grade 2 resections are considered curative; thus, these patients receive a postoperative MRI to verify complete resection and then receive yearly follow-up. In cases of patients with benign meningiomas after Grade 3

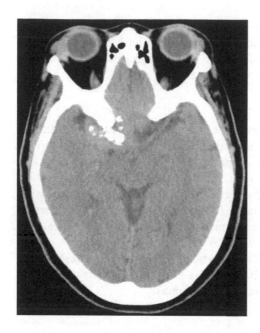

Figure 1 Axial computed tomography scan without contrast of clinoid meningioma showing speckled calcification in the periphery of the clinoid process. At surgery, the tumor had a gritty, sandy consistency. Pathological evaluation revealed a meningioma with numerous psammoma bodies.

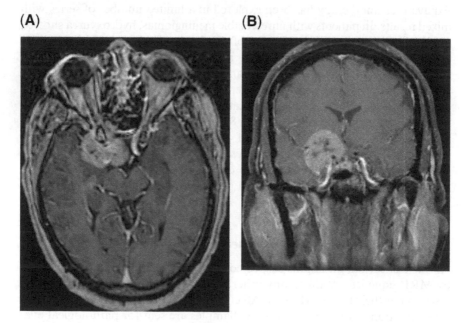

Figure 2 Axial (**A**) and coronal (**B**) T-1 weighted phase contrast magnetic resonance images with intravenous contrast of same tumor as in Fig. 1. Note areas of low signal within tumor bulk, which correspond to areas of calcification seen on computed tomography. The carotid arteries are best seen on coronal images. Cerebral angiography confirmed displacement rather than invasion of carotid by tumor.

(A) (B)

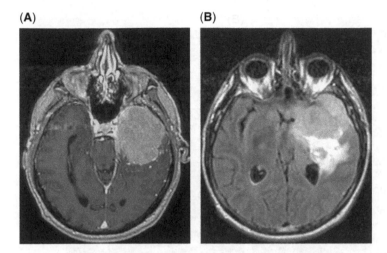

Figure 3 Axial T-1 postcontrast (**A**) and FLAIR sequences (**B**) of an atypical sphenoid wing meningioma.

to 5 resections, recurrence is more likely, but often takes years to occur. We follow these patients with MRIs at 6 and 12 months after resection and then yearly. In cases of tumor progression, patients are treated with repeat resection in cases of large recurrences (when surgical resection is practical, given

(A) (B)

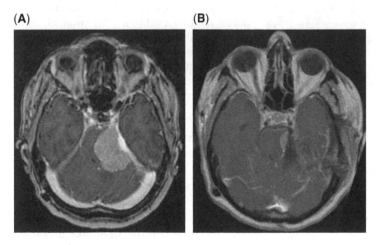

Figure 4 Preoperative magnetic resonance imaging of petroclival meningioma (**A**). Residual tumor attached to the pial surface (**B**) could not be removed without sacrificing perforating arteries on the cerebral peduncle. The residual tumor was treated with fractionated stereotactic radiotherapy.

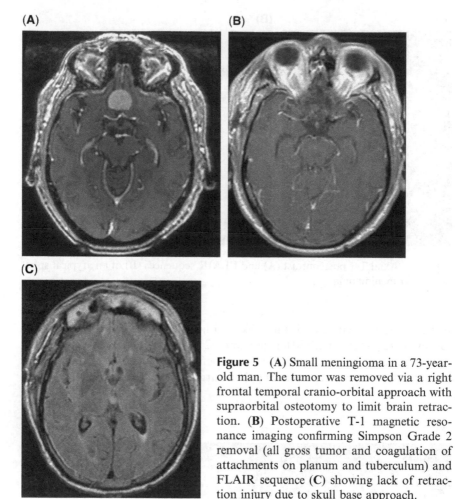

Figure 5 (**A**) Small meningioma in a 73-year-old man. The tumor was removed via a right frontal temporal cranio-orbital approach with supraorbital osteotomy to limit brain retraction. (**B**) Postoperative T-1 magnetic resonance imaging confirming Simpson Grade 2 removal (all gross tumor and coagulation of attachments on planum and tuberculum) and FLAIR sequence (**C**) showing lack of retraction injury due to skull base approach.

patient age and general condition). In cases of small recurrences (<8 cc) patients may be treated with GKS. In cases of larger recurrences of tumor (>8 cc), patients may be treated effectively with conformal radiation and then followed with serial MRIs every six months.

In patients with atypical or anaplastic meningiomas, we recommend maximum resection of tumor possible followed by conformal fractionated radiation. We follow these patients closely given the high likelihood of recurrence, with MRIs at one month, three months, and every six months thereafter. At recurrence, we treat these patients with radiosurgery for small tumors (<8 cc) and resection followed by brachytherapy for larger ones (>8 cc).

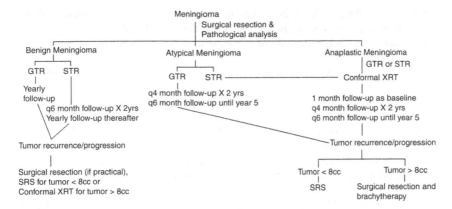

Figure 6 Algorithm for meningioma treatment.

CONCLUSION

Meningiomas are the most common primary tumors of the central nervous system. Although the vast majority of meningiomas are considered benign, more malignant variants exist containing chromosomal and molecular aberrations associated with this aggressive behavior. MRI and CT scans are critical in the diagnosis of meningiomas, and surgical resection remains the mainstay of treatment for meningiomas. When complete surgical resection cannot be achieved or in cases of atypical or anaplastic meningiomas, adjuvant radiotherapy is warranted.

REFERENCES

1. Rachlin J, Rosenblum M. Etiology and biology of meningiomas. In: Al-Mefty O, ed. New York: Raven, 1991:22–37.
2. Claus EB, Bondy ML, Schildkraut JM, et al. Neurosurgery 2005; 57:1088–1095.
3. Davis FG, Kupelian V, Freels S, et al. Neurooncol 2001; 3:152–158.
4. Loven D, Hardoff R, Sever ZB, et al. J Neurooncol 2004; 67:221–226.
5. Perry A, Stafford SL, Scheithaucr BW, et al. Am J Surg Pathol 1997; 21: 1455–1465.
6. Al-Mefty O, Kadri PA, Pravdenkova S, et al. J Neurosurg 2004; 101:210–218.
7. Jaaskelainen J, Haltia M, Laasonen E, et al. Surg Neurol 1985; 24:165–172.
8. Jaaskelainen J, Haltia M, Servo A. Surg Neurol 1986; 25:233–242.
9. Simpson D. J Neurol Neurosurg Psychiatry 1957; 20:22–39.
10. Mirimanoff RO, Dosoretz DE, Linggood RM, et al. J Neurosurg 1985; 62: 18–24.
11. Palma L, Celli P, Franco C, et al. J Neurosurg 1997; 86:793–800.
12. Perry A, Scheithauer BW, Stafford SL, et al. Cancer 1999; 85:2046–2056.
13. Cushing HW, Eisenhardt L. Meningiomas: their classification, regional behavior, life history, and surgical end results. ILL: Springfield, 1938.

14. Kleihues P, Burger PC, Scheithauer B. Histological typing of tumours of the central nervous system, in. Berlin: Springer-Verlag, 1993:28–31.
15. Kleihues P, Louis DN, Scheithauer BW, et al. J Neuropathol Exp Neurol 2002; 61:215–225.
16. Weber RG, Bostrom J, Wolter M, et al. Proc Natl Acad Sci USA 1997; 94: 14719–14724.
17. Dumanski JP, Carlbom E, Collins VP, et al. Proc Natl Acad Sci USA 1987; 84: 9275–9279.
18. Doco-Fenzy M, Cornillet P, Scherpereel B, et al. Anticancer Res 1993; 13:845–850.
19. Ruttledge MH, Sarrazin J, Rangaratnam S, et al. Nat Genet 1994; 6:180–184.
20. Dumanski JP, Kraus JA, Lenartz D, et al. Cancer Res 1995; 50:827–832.
21. Hitotsumatsu T, Iwaki T, Kitamoto T, et al. Acta Neuropathol (Berl) 1997; 93: 225–232.
22. Lekanne Deprez RH, Bianchi AB, Groen NA, et al. Am J Hum Genet 1994; 54: 1022–1029.
23. De Vitis LR, Tedde A, Vitelli F, et al. Hum Genet 1996; 97:632–637.
24. Rouleau GA, Merel P, Lutchman M, et al. Nature 1993; 363:515–521.
25. Lim JY, Kim H, Kim YH, et al. Biochem Biophys Res Commun 2003; 302: 238–245.
26. Bello MJ, de Campos JM, Kusak ME, et al. Genes Chromosomes Cancer 1994; 9:296–298.
27. Muller P, Henn W, Niedermayer I, et al. Clin Cancer Res 1999; 5:3569–3577.
28. Shoshan Y, Chernova O, Juen SS, et al. J Neuropathol Exp Neurol 2000; 59: 614–620.
29. Arslantas A, Artan S, Oner U, et al. Acta Neurol Belg 2002; 102:53–62.
30. Buschges R, Bostrom J, Wolter M, et al. Int J Cancer 2001; 92:551–554.
31. Tran YK, Bogler O, Gorse KM, et al. Cancer Res 1999; 59:35–43.
32. Gutmann DH, Donahoe J, Perry A, et al. Hum Mol Genet 2000; 9:1495–1500.
33. Perry A, Cai DX, Scheithauer BW, et al. J Neuropathol Exp Neurol 2000; 59: 872–879.
34. Lekanne Deprez RH, Riegman PH, van Drunen E, et al. J Neuropathol Exp Neurol 1995; 54:224–235.
35. Biegel JA, Parmiter AH, Sutton LN, et al. Genes Chromosomes Cancer 1994; 9:81–87.
36. Rempel SA, Schwechheimer K, Davis RL, et al. Cancer Res 1993; 53:2386–2392.
37. Simon M, von Deimling A, Larson JJ, et al. Cancer Res 1995; 55:4696–4701.
38. Liggett WH Jr., Sidransky D. J Clin Oncol 1998; 16:1197–1206.
39. Kamei Y, Watanabe M, Nakayama T, et al. J Neurooncol 2000; 46:205–213.
40. Sanson M, Cornu P. Acta Neurochir (Wien) 2000; 142:493–505.
41. Nakasu S, Fukami T, Nakajima M, et al. Neurosurgery 2005; 56:946–955.
42. Zimmerman RD, Fleming CA, Saint-Louis LA, et al. Am J Neuroradiol 1985; 6:149–157.
43. Goldsher D, Litt AW, Pinto RS, et al. Radiology 1990; 176:447–450.
44. Verheggen R, Finkenstaedt M, Bockermann V, et al. Acta Neurochir Suppl (Wien) 1996; 65:66–69.
45. Shapir J, Coblentz C, Malanson D, et al. AJNR Am J Neuroradiol 1985; 6:101–102.
46. Younis GA, Sawaya R, DeMonte F, et al. J Neurosurg 1995; 82:17–27.

47. Drape JL, Krause D, Tongio J. J Neuroradiol 1992; 19:49–62.
48. Mahmood A, Caccamo DV, Tomecek FJ, et al. Neurosurgery 1993; 33:955–963.
49. Chun JY, McDermott MW, Lamborn KR, et al. Neurosurgery 2002; 50: 1231–1235.
50. Hekster RE, Matricali B, Luyendijk W. J Neurosurg 1974; 41:396–398.
51. Nakamura M, Roser F, Michel J, et al. Neurosurgery 2003; 53:62–70.
52. Bindal R, Goodman JM, Kawasaki A, et al. Surg Neurol 2003; 59:87–92.
53. Niiro M, Yatsushiro K, Nakamura K, et al. J Neurol Neurosurg Psychiatry 2000; 68:25–28.
54. Van Havenbergh T, Carvalho G, Tatagiba M, et al. Neurosurgery 2003; 52:55–62.
55. Bateman BT, Pile-Spellman J, Gutin PH, et al. Neurosurgery 2005; 57:866–872.
56. Curry WT, McDermott MW, Carter BS, et al. J Neurosurg 2005; 102:977–986.
57. Barbaro NM, Gutin PH, Wilson CB, et al. Neurosurgery 1987; 20:525–528.
58. Condra KS, Buatti JM, Mendenhall WM, et al. Int J Radiat Oncol Biol Phys 1997; 39:427–436.
59. Jaaskelainen J. Surg Neurol 1986; 26:461–469.
60. Taylor BW Jr., Marcus RB Jr., Friedman WA, et al. Int J Radiat Oncol Biol Phys 1988; 15:299–304.
61. Pourel N, Auque J, Bracard S, et al. Radiother Oncol 2001; 61:65–70.
62. al-Mefty O, Kersh JE, Routh A, et al. J Neurosurg 1990; 73:502–512.
63. Chan RC, Thompson GB. J Neurosurg 1984; 60:52–60.
64. Mesic JB, Hanks GE, Doggett RL. Am J Clin Oncol 1986; 9:337–340.
65. Miralbell R, Linggood RM, de la Monte S, et al. J Neurooncol 1992; 13:157–164.
66. Newman SA: Meningiomas. J Neurosurg 1994; 80:191–194.
67. Modha A, Gutin PH. Neurosurgery 2005; 57:538–550.
68. Goyal LK, Suh JH, Mohan DS, et al. Int J Radiat Oncol Biol Phys 2000; 46:57–61.
69. Palma L, Celli P, Franco C, et al. Neurosurg Focus 1997; 2:e3.
70. Dziuk TW, Woo S, Butler EB, et al. J Neurooncol 1998; 37:177–188.
71. Hakim R, Alexander E III, Loeffler JS, et al. Neurosurgery 1998; 42:446–453.
72. Pollock BE, Stafford SL, Utter A, et al. Int J Radiat Oncol Biol Phys 2003; 55:1000–1005.
73. Ojemann SG, Sneed PK, Larson DA, et al. J Neurosurg 2000; 93(suppl 3):62–67.
74. Stafford SL, Pollock BE, Foote RL, et al. Neurosurgery 2001; 49:1029–1037.
75. Ware ML, Larson DA, Sneed PK, et al. Neurosurgery 2004; 54:55–63.
76. Schrell UM, Rittig MG, Anders M, et al. J Neurosurg 1997; 86:840–844.
77. Chamberlain MC. J Neurosurg 1996; 84:733–736.
78. Kaba SE, DeMonte F, Bruner JM, et al. Neurosurgery 1997; 40:271–275.
79. Kondziolka D, Nathoo N, Flickinger JC, et al. Neurosurgery 2003; 53:815–821.
80. Subach BR, Lunsford LD, Kondziolka D, et al. Neurosurgery 1998; 42:437–443.
81. Morita A, Kelly PJ. Neurosurgery 1993; 32:920–926.
82. Roche PH, Regis J, Dufour H, et al. J Neurosurg 2000; 93(suppl 3):68–73.
83. Kobayashi T, Kida Y, Mori Y. Surg Neurol 2001; 55:325–331.
84. Shin M, Kurita H, Sasaki T, et al. J Neurosurg 2001; 95:435–439.
85. Lee JY, Niranjan A, McInerney J, et al. J Neurosurg 2002; 97:65–72.
86. Nicolato A, Foroni R, Alessandrini F, et al. Int J Radiat Oncol Biol Phys 2002; 53:992–1000.
87. Eustacchio S, Trummer M, Fuchs I, et al. Acta Neurochir 2002; 84(suppl):71–76.

18

Malignant Central Nervous System Neoplasms of Mesenchymal Origin

Evanthia Galanis

Mayo Clinic College of Medicine, Rochester, Minnesota, U.S.A.

INTRODUCTION

Mesenchymal neoplasms of the central nervous system (CNS), included as mesenchymal nonmeningothelial tumors in the current World Health Organization (WHO) classification of CNS tumors (1), usually arise from the meninges, or from mesenchymal elements of the CNS parenchyma. Their histologic features are those of corresponding extracranial soft-tissue tumors. The most frequent malignant mesenchymal tumors of the CNS are hemangiopericytomas (HPCs) and CNS sarcomas. Benign tumors include chondromas, osteochondromas, osteomas, leiomyomas, rhabdomyomas, and lipomas.

MENINGEAL HEMANGIOPERICYTOMA

HPC is a highly vascular meningeal malignancy (2). It is a rare tumor, with an incidence of less than 1% of all CNS tumors (3). Meningeal HPC was first described in 1928 by Bailey et al. who considered the tumor as an angioblastic variant of meningioma (4). Its soft-tissue counterpart described in 1942 by Stout and Murray was termed HPC (5). Finally, in 1954, Begg and Garret recognized the similarities between these two entities and suggested that the angioblastic meningioma was in fact a HPC arising within the meninges (6). Since then, numerous clinicopathologic, immunohistochemical, ultrastructural, and genetic studies have confirmed the similarities between meningeal HPC and its soft-tissue counterpart, as well as the distinction of HPC from the various forms of meningioma (3,7–13). The current WHO classification of CNS tumors distinguishes HPCs as a separate entity in the group of mesenchymal nonmeningothelial tumors (14). HPCs are thought to arise from pericytes, which are leiomyoblastic cells spiraling around capillaries and postcapillary venules (15–17).

Epidemiology

HPCs, unlike meningiomas, are more common in males, with a male to female ratio ranging from 1.1:1 to 1.5:1 (3,8,15,18–21). Average age in diagnosis ranges from 38 to 51 years (3,18,22,23). Less than 10% of HPC tumors occur in children and infants (15,24–27); the infantile form appears to have a better prognosis (25,26) however. The most common location of HPCs is supratentorial, usually in the parasagittal plane (15,19). In some series, up to 15% of the HPCs are located in the posterior fossa or in the spine (3,23,28,29). Unusual locations such as orbit (30), lateral ventricles (31), cellular/supracellular areas (32), pineal body (33), and the brain parenchyma have also been described. Multicentricity is very unusual and has been attributed to cerebrospinal fluid (CSF) seeding (15).

Presentation

Presenting symptoms depend on tumor location with a mean duration of symptoms prior to diagnosis ranging from 3.1 to 7.5 months (3,21,34–36). Focal neurologic deficits are more common than seizures (20,35), the latter being present in 15% or less of the patients. Other less common presentations include intratumoral or intracerebral hemorrhage (15), cranial nerve deficit (37), hyperprolactinemia, and bitemporal hemianopsia (18).

Imaging

Meningeal HPCs resemble hemangiomas on imaging studies. In plain films, there is absence of hyperostosis. Bone changes are rare and if present, they consist of bone erosion (3,21). On computed tomography (CT) imaging, HPCs are dense, dural-based lesions, with heterogeneous enhancement (3,21,34,38–40). Unlike meningiomas, calcification is extremely rare (39,40). They usually have a broad dural attachment and tend to show features such as irregular or lobulated borders, "mushrooming," indicating parenchymal invasion, and a more heterogeneous contrast enhancement compared to meningiomas. HPCs show strong contrast enhancement on magnetic resonance imaging (MRI) imaging (Fig. 1). Occasionally, prominent internal serpentine signal voids are also observed (39–41), suggesting presence of large vessels, which can be associated with substantial intraoperative

(A)   (B)

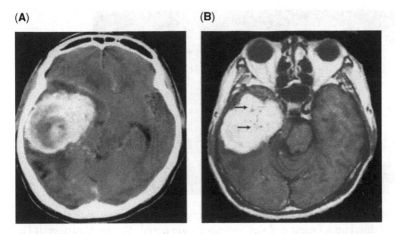

Figure 1 Hemangiopericytoma. **(A)** Axial contrast-enhanced CT shows a large, irregular, middle cranial fossa mass with heterogeneous enhancement. **(B)** Axial contrast-enhanced T1-weighted image demonstrates prominent signal voids suggesting the presence of large vessels (*arrows*). *Source*: From Ref. 40.

bleeding. In angiography, a characteristic finding is the presence of small corkscrew vessels arising within the tumor mass (42), although this typical appearance is observed only in a minority of cases (3,38,40).

Pathology

At resection, meningeal HPCs are usually well demarcated from adjacent brain tissue. Cut surfaces are fleshy and grayish to red-brown, often with a number of visible vascular spaces (Fig. 2). HPCs are usually cellular tumors composed of small, although slightly spindled cells. Their turbulent architecture is occasionally associated with vague whirling or with collagen deposition. They are characterized by numerous branching thin wall vessels of varying caliber, which is the basis of the characteristic staghorn vascular pattern (Fig. 3). A commonly used grading scheme is the one described by Mena et al. (32); in this scheme, high-grade or anaplastic HPCs are defined as tumors having either at least 5 mitoses per 10 high-powered fields or necrosis in addition to at least two of the following features: hemorrhage, nuclear atypia, and hypercellularity. The differential diagnosis includes benign tumors such as meningioma, solitary fibrous tumor, paraganglioma, as well as malignant tumors such as anaplastic meningioma, malignant solitary fibrous tumor, and primary CNS sarcomas such as fibrosarcoma, leiomyosarcoma, malignant fibrous histiocytoma, and neurofibrosarcoma (43). HPCs stain positive for vimentin, but they are negative for epithelial membrane antigen, cytokeratins, glial fibrillary acidic protein, and S-100 protein (32). Lack of staining for the epithelial membrane antigen and S-100

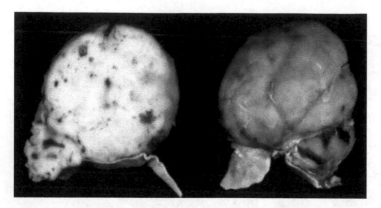

Figure 2 Macroscopic appearance of resected hemangiopericytoma, with the characteristic broad dural attachment and rich vascularity are noted. *Source*: Courtesy of Dr. B. Scheithauer, Mayo Clinic.

protein can be helpful in differentiating HPCs from fibrous meningiomas, while the CD34 stain can assist in the distinction between HPC and solitary fibrous tumor. Solitary fibrous tumors usually exhibit a strong diffuse CD34 positivity in contrast to both HPCs and meningiomas showing either no or only weak patchy CD34 reactivity in approximately 33% of the cases (43).

Treatment

Surgery

Surgical management represents the mainstay of treatment of meningeal HPCs. Although older surgical series have reported significant perioperative mortality ranging between 9% and 27% (3,21,23), the use of microsurgery techniques and preoperative embolization has significantly decreased operative morbidity and mortality (18,34). Preoperative embolization decreases operative blood loss as compared to nonembolized patients (18). Nevertheless,

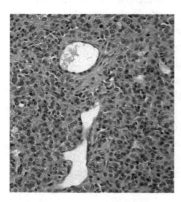

Figure 3 Microscopic appearance of anaplastic hemangiopericytoma with characteristic "staghorn" shaped vasculature. *Source*: From Ref. 49.

because meningeal HPCs also receive blood supply from cerebral vasculature, embolization of meningeal feeders may not be as effective in preventing hemorrhage as it is for ordinary meningiomas (20). The ability to perform a complete tumor resection rate also differs among different surgical series, ranging between 50% and 83% (18,34).

Adjuvant Radiation Therapy

Several retrospective patient series have supported the role of postoperative adjuvant radiation therapy in decreasing the risk of local recurrence (32,44). Doses in the range of 5000 to 5500 cGy are usually employed (3). In a large retrospective series, patients receiving adjuvant radiation therapy developed recurrent disease at a median time of 75 months with a 5-year and 10-year recurrence rate of 38 and 64%. In contrast, those treated with surgery alone suffer recurrence at a median time of 29 months with a five-year recurrence rate of 90% (3). Although preoperative radiation therapy has also been advocated by some investigators (45,46), the role of this approach in the management of HPC remains unproven.

Management of Recurrent Disease

HPCs tend to recur both locally (19,20,47,48) and systemically (20). Surgical resection of recurrent CNS lesions or isolated extraneural metastasis is appropriate if the lesions are amenable to surgery and the extent of the patient's disease justifies surgical management. HPC patients frequently require multiple resections in the long-term management of their disease. Palliative external beam radiation therapy can also be employed if the threshold dose for normal tissue has not been exceeded or if the recurrence occurred outside the prior radiation field. Stereotactic radiosurgery has been successfully employed to treat recurrent HPCs after failure of external beam radiation therapy (49–52). Its use can result in tumor regression (partial or complete response) in more than 80% of appropriate candidates (49,51,52). The usual margin dose in these series varied from 15 Gy to 20 Gy. Rate of tumor regression is slow, and maximum tumor response is rarely seen before 6 to 10 months after treatment. The majority of patients, however, eventually progress in median time intervals ranging from less than 12 to 21 months. Patients with smaller tumors (<3 cm) appear to have longer lasting tumor control in response to stereotactic radiosurgery and represent ideal candidates for this treatment modality (49,52). The chemotherapy experience in the management of recurrent meningeal HPC is limited and indicates low efficacy. In a small series of seven patients, who received doxorubicin-containing regimens, only one patient receiving a doxorubicin/dacarbazine combination accomplished a partial response lasting for eight months, while three patients had stable disease with a median duration of six months. This is in contrast to the higher response rate of soft-tissue HPCs in response to chemotherapy (53,54) and may in part represent a reflection of the location of metastatic disease in CNS HPC patients, since a significant percentage of these patients have bone metastases. Novel therapeutic approaches including small molecule inhibitors and monoclonal antibodies with antiangiogenic properties represent research directions with potential promise in the management of this disease.

Prognosis

Prognosis of HPC patients is affected by tumor grade; patients with anaplastic HPCs have a worse prognosis as compared to patients with well-differentiated tumors (32). In addition, extraneural recurrences confer an adverse prognosis (49) (Fig. 4). Five-year recurrence rate ranges from 36.4% to 65% (3,18), with calculated 10- and 15-year recurrence rates of 76% and 87%, respectively (3). In a comprehensive literature review, a median recurrence-free interval of 50 months (range 1 to 26 years) was reported (23). After the first recurrence, HPCs tend to recur at shorter intervals (3). In one series, the average time to second, third, and fourth operation for recurrence was 38, 35, and 17 months, respectively.

A significant percent of HPC patients develop extracranial metastases. The incidence of systemic metastases at 5, 10 and 15 years from diagnosis has been reported to be 13%, 33%, and 64%, respectively (3) with the mean time interval ranging from 4.5 to 8 years (3,18,34). Therefore, and in contrast to other malignancies, a five-year disease-free interval is not equivalent to cure, and continuous surveillance is recommended. Location of extracranial metastases can include bone, liver, lungs, abdominal cavity, lymph nodes,

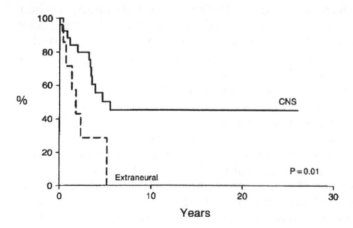

Figure 4 Kaplan-Meier survival curves for patients with meningeal hemangiopericytoma. Those who suffered their first relapse within the central nervous system survived longer than those with extracranial recurrence ($p = 0.01$). *Abbreviation*: CNS, central nervous system. *Source*: Galanis et al., 1998 (ref. 49), with permission.

skeletal muscles, kidney, pancreas, skin and subcutaneous tissue, breast, adrenal glands, gallbladder, diaphragm, retroperitoneum, and heart (18,49).

Five-year survival ranges from 65% to 81% in different series (3,18,23) with reported 10- and 15-year survival rates of 40% to 45% and 15% to 23%, respectively (3,23). The significant variability in reported outcomes reflects the relative rarity of intracranial HPCs along with the lack of standardized treatment protocols. Furthermore, improvement in the reported outcomes in more recent series likely reflects development of better neurosurgical techniques and the advent of newer treatment modalities such as stereotactic radiosurgery.

PRIMARY CENTRAL NERVOUS SYSTEM SARCOMAS

Primary CNS sarcomas are rare, representing less than 0.1% of intracranial tumors (14,55–58). The higher incidence of CNS sarcomas reported in the past likely resulted from overdiagnosis based upon older histologic classification schemes. The cell of origin of these tumors represents a matter of controversy. The most widely accepted theory advocates their origin from pluripotent primitive mesenchymal cells located in the dura, leptomeninges, or the pial extension into the brain and the spinal cord, or along the periadventitial spaces, the tela choroidea, and the stroma of the choroid plexus (55,59–66). The etiology of primary CNS sarcomas is also poorly understood. A known causative factor is prior CNS radiation therapy; while inversely correlated with age, risk is a direct function of dose (67). Latent periods between radiation and development of secondary sarcoma can range from years to decades (68). Increased risk of postirradiation CNS tumors, including sarcomas, is observed in children with neurofibromatosis or neuroblastoma (69), suggesting that genetic factors may also play a role. The Epstein–Barr virus is considered an etiologic factor in the development of intracranial leiomyosarcomas in HIV patients (70).

EPIDEMIOLOGY

Primary CNS sarcomas can occur at any age, but are more common in children (61,64). Malignant fibrous histiocytomas and fibrosarcomas are more frequent in adults (58,71), while sarcomas showing muscle differentiation are more prevalent in children (56). Congenital primary CNS sarcomas have also been described (72). No difference in incidence based on gender has been reported (56–58). Primary CNS sarcomas are commonly located in the parietal and temporal lobe (32,55,58,73,74). Posterior fossa sarcomas, spinal sarcomas, and intraventricular sarcomas have also been reported (55,75). There is high incidence of leptomeningeal dissemination (up to 40% of cases in some series) (55,56,61,73,76); systemic spread occurs to lungs, bone, and liver.

PRESENTATION

Clinical presentation depends on tumor location. Not uncommonly, they present as vascular masses with intracranial hemorrhage (61,77,78). A careful clinical exam and staging studies should be performed at presentation to exclude the possibility of an extracranial sarcoma, presenting with a cerebral metastasis.

IMAGING

The appearance of primary brain sarcomas on CT or MRI is nonspecific. They usually enhance after contrast administration, both on CT and on MRI imaging (Fig. 5). Occasionally they have cystic appearance (Fig. 6), or show signs of intratumoral hemorrhage (76,79–81). The high incidence of leptomeningeal spread mandates imaging of the entire neuraxis at the time of diagnosis.

PATHOLOGY

The differentiation of CNS sarcomas is variable resembling fibrous tissue (fibrosarcoma, malignant fibrous histiocytoma) (Fig. 7), cartilage (chondromas, chondrosarcomas, and mesenchymal sarcomas), striated muscles (rhabdomyosarcoma), bone (osteosarcoma) (Fig. 8), smooth muscles (leiomyosarcoma) (Fig. 9), or blood vessels (angiosarcoma). Malignant fibrous histiocytoma is the most common subtype. In addition to tumor morphology, immunohistochemistry can be helpful in establishing the diagnosis. For example, myoglobin staining can be positive in 50% to 89% of rhabdomyosarcomas (82), while factor XIIIa staining is common in angiosarcomas. Electron microscopy can also assist in establishing the diagnosis of rhabdomyosarcoma by

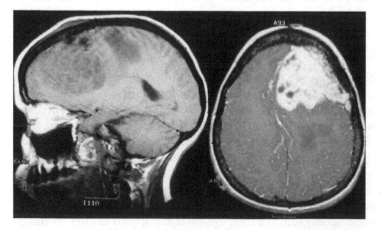

Figure 5   Chondroblastic osteosarcoma, Grade 4 [T1-weighted MRI, sagittal (*left*) and axial view]. There is significant enhancement after gadolinium administration (*right*).

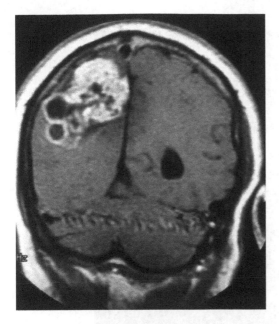

Figure 6 T1-weighted, gadolinium-enhanced MRI of a patient with an intracranial Grade 1 chondrosarcoma demonstrates a characteristic cystic appearance.

demonstrating thick and thin band filaments or Z-bands (83), while cytogenetic abnormalities with the presence of the (11,22) (q24; q12) translocation is pathognomonic for the Ewing's sarcoma family of tumors.

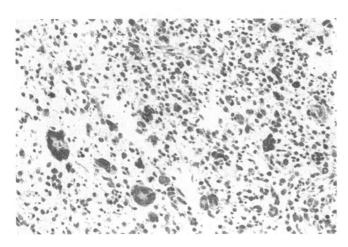

Figure 7 High-grade malignant fibrous histiocytoma of the CNS showing high degree of pleomorphism. The tumor was positive for vimentin and negative for glial fibrillary acid protein, S-100, cytokeratin CAM 5.2, and desmin. *Source*: Reprinted with permission from Oliveira et al., 2002.

(A)

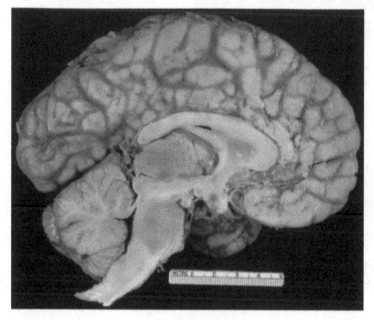

(B)

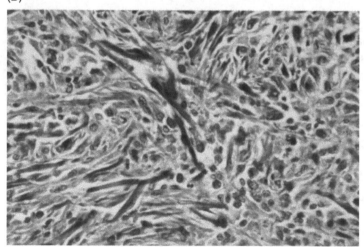

Figure 8 Macroscopic (**A**) and microscopic (**B**) appearance of a rhabdomyosarcoma of the pineal region. Histopathologically, the tumor is characterized by small, undifferentiated cells, intermingled with rhabdomyoblastoma and strap-like cells. *Source*: Courtesy of Dr. B. Scheithauer, Mayo Clinic.

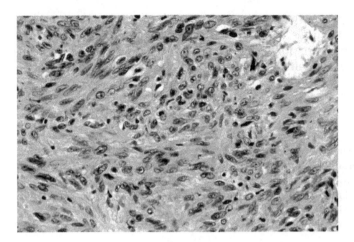

Figure 9   Leiomyosarcoma of the dura in a patient with the AIDS showing fascicles of spindle cells with characteristic cigar-shaped nuclei. *Source*: Courtesy of Dr. B. Scheithauer, Mayo Clinic.

Primary meningeal sarcomatosis refers to diffuse involvement of the leptomeninges by a sarcomatous process in the absence of a localized tumor. Primary meningeal sarcomatosis is most frequent in infants and children; cellular features are frequently those of polymorphic cell sarcoma, although features of fibrosarcoma may occasionally predominate (56). Cerebrospinal fluid cytology is usually positive for malignant cells.

TREATMENT

Given the rarity of primary intracranial sarcomas, a standard of care approach based on prospective studies cannot be established. Treatment recommendations are based on experience with similar sarcoma histologies outside the central nervous system. Management depends on the extent of disease, location of the primary tumor, neuraxis involvement, and presence of systemic metastases. Surgery, if feasible, represents the mainstay of treatment, usually followed by involved field radiation therapy (76). If the neuraxis is involved at presentation, craniospinal radiation should be administered. Systemic chemotherapy is frequently added, employing agents and treatment protocols appropriate for the specific sarcoma histology although the impact of this practice on patients' outcome and survival is uncertain (61,76).

PROGNOSIS

Data on prognosis of primary CNS sarcomas are mostly derived from small retrospective series. Reported survival ranges from 1 month to 16 years

(61,76). Adverse prognostic factors include CSF dissemination, age less than one year at diagnosis, and subtotal tumor resection (76). Long-term sequelae of treatment in long-term survivors including neurobehavioral problems, learning difficulties, and endocrine abnormalities are similar to other childhood brain tumors.

REFERENCES

1. Kleihues P, Burger PC, Scheithauer BW. (1991) World Health Organization International Histological Classification of Tumours: Histological Typing of Tumours of the Central Nervous System. Springer, Berlin, Heidelberg, New York, Tokyo, pp. 38.
2. Enzinger FM, Smith BH. Hemangiopericytoma. An analysis of 106 cases. Hum Pathol 1991; 7:61–82.
3. Guthrie BL, Ebersold MJ, Scheithauer BW, Shaw EG. Neurosurgery 1989; 25:514–522.
4. Bailey P, Cushing H, Eisenhardt LA. Angioblastic meningiomas. Arch Pathol 1928; 6:953–990.
5. Stout AP, Murray MR. Hemangiopericytoma: a vascular tumor featuring Zimmermann's pericyte. Ann Surg 1942; 116:26–33.
6. Begg CF, Garret R. Hemangiopericytoma occuring in the mengines. Cancer 1954; 7:602–606.
7. D'Amore ES, Manivel JC, Sung JH. Soft-tissue and meningeal hemangiopericytomas: an immunohistochemical and ultrastructural study. Hum Pathol 1990; 21:414–423.
8. Goellner JR, Laws ER Jr., Soule EH, Okazaki H. Hemangiopericytoma of the meninges. Mayo Clinic experience. Am J Clin Pathol 1978; 70:375–380.
9. Henn W, Wullich B, Thonnes M, Steudel WI, Feiden W, Zang KD. Recurrent t(12;19)(ql3;ql3.3) in intracranial and extracranial hemangiopericytoma. Cancer Genet Cytogenet 1993; 71:151–154.
10. Iwaki T, Fukui M, Takeshita I, Tsuneyoshi M, Tateishi J. Hemangiopericytoma of the meninges; a clinicopathologic and immunohistochemical study. Clin Neuropathol 1988; 7:93–99.
11. Moss TH. Immunohistochemical characteristics of haemangiopericytic meningiomas: comparison with typical meningiomas, haemangioblastomas and haemangiopericytomas from extracranial sites. Neuropathol Appl Neurobiol 1987; 13:467–480.
12. Pena CE. Meningioma and intracranial hemangiopericytoma. A comparative electron microscopic study. Acta Neuropathol (Berl) 1977; 39:69–74.
13. Winek RR, Scheithauer BW, Wick MR. Meningioma, meningeal hemangiopericytoma (angioblastic meningioma), peripheral hemangiopericytoma, and acoustic schwannoma. A comparative immunohistochemical study. Am J Surg Pathol 1989; 13:251–261.
14. Kleihues P, Cavenee WK. The World Health Organization Classification of Tumours. Lyon: IARC Press, 2000.
15. Brunori A, Delitala A, Oddi G, Chiappetta F. Recent experience in the management of meningeal hemangiopericytomas. Tumori 1997; 83:856–861.

16. Muller J, Mealey J Jr. The use of tissue culture in differentiation between angioblastic meningioma and hemangiopericytoma. J Neurosurg 1971; 34: 341–348.
17. Pena CE. Intracranial hemangiopericytoma: ultrastructural evidence of its leiomyoblastic differentiation. Acta Neuropathol (Berl) 1975; 33:279–284.
18. Fountas KN, Kapsalaki E, Kassam M, et al. Management of intracranial meningeal hemangiopericytomas: outcome and experience. Neurosurg Rev 2006; EPub (Jan) 4:1–9.
19. Berger MS, Kros JM. Sarcomas and neoplasms of blood vessels: hemangiopericytomas (angioblastic meningioma). In: Youmans JR, ed. Neurological Surgery. Philadelphia: Saunders, 1996:2700–2703.
20. Kaye AH, Laws ER. Brain Tumors. Tokyo: Livingstone, 1995:705–711.
21. Jaaskelainen J, Servo A, HaltiaM, WahlstromT, Valtonen S. Intracranial hemangiopericytoma: radiology, surgery, radiotherapy, and outcome in 21 patients. Surg Neurol 1985; 23:227–236.
22. Kochanek S, Schroder R, Firsching R. Hemangiopericytoma of meninges I. Histopathological variability and differential diagnosis. Zentralbl Neurochir 1986; 47:183–190.
23. Schroder R, Firsching R, Kochanek S. Hemangiopericytoma of meninges. II. General and clinical data. Zentralbl Neurochir 1986; 47:191–199.
24. Aouad N, Vital C, Rivel J, Ramsoubramanian K, Santosh S, Chowdry O. Giant supratentorial meningeal haemangiopericytoma in a newborn. Acta Neurochir (Wien) 1991; 112:154–156.
25. Cole JC, Naul LG. Intracranial infantile hemangiopericytoma. Pediatr Radiol 2000; 30:271–273.
26. Herzog CE, Leeds NE, Bruner JM, Baumgartner JE. Intracranial hemangiopericytomas in children. Pediatr Neurosurg 1995; 22:274–279.
27. Huisman TA, Brandner S, Niggli F, Kael G, Willi UV, Martin E. Meningeal hemangiopericytoma in childhood. Eur Radiol 2000; 10:1073–1075.
28. Younis GA, Sawaya R, DeMonte F, Hess KR, Albrecht S, Bruner JM. Aggressive meningeal tumors: review of a series. J Neurosurg 1995; 82:17–27.
29. Cappabianca P, Maiuri F, Pettinato G, Di Prisco B. Hemangiopericytoma of the spinal canal. Surg Neurol 1981; 15:298–302.
30. Fu ER, Goh SH, Fong CM. Case report of primary orbital hemangiopericytoma. Ann Acad Med Singapore 1993; 22:966–968.
31. Hattingen E, Pilatus U, Good C, Franz K, Lanfermann H, Zanella FE. An unusual intraventricular haemangiopericytoma: MRI and spectroscopy. Neuroradiology 2003; 45:386–389. Epub 2003 Apr 2018.
32. Mena H, Ribas JL, Pezeshkpour GH, Cowan DN, Parisi IE. Hemangiopericytoma of the central nervous system: a review of 94 cases. Hum Pathol 1991; 22:84–91.
33. Olson JR, Abell MR. Haemangiopericytoma of the pineal body. J Neurol Neurosurg Psychiatry 1969; 32:445–449.
34. Alen JF, Lobato RD, Gomez PA, et al. Intracranial hemangiopericytoma: study of 12 cases. Acta Neurochir (Wien) 2001; 143:575–586.
35. Borg MF, Benjamin CS. Haemangiopericytoma of the central nervous system. Australas Radiol 1995; 39:36–41.

36. Tsou H, Wang Y, Yang D, Wei S. Intra-extracranial hemangiopericytoma: clinical manifestations, histopathological feature, diagnosis, treatment, and outcomes. Chin Med J (Taipei) 2002; 65:314–319.
37. Tan I, Soo MY, Ng T. Haemangiopericytoma of the trigeminal nerve. Australas Radiol 2001; 45:350–353.
38. Guthrie BL. Meningeal hemangiopericytomas. In: AH K, ed. Brain Tumours. Edinburgh: Churchill Livingstone, 1995:705–711.
39. Chiechi MV, Smirniotopoulos JG, Mena H. Intracranial hemangiopericytomas: MR and CT features. AJNR Am J Neuroradiol 1996; 17:1365–1371.
40. Akiyama M, Sakai H, Onoue H, Miyazaki Y, Abe T. Imaging intracranial haemangiopericytomas: study of seven cases. Neuroradiology 2004; 46:194–197. Epub 2004 Feb 2027.
41. Barba I, Moreno A, Martinez-Perez I, et al. Magnetic resonance spectroscopy of brain hemangiopericytomas: high myoinositol concentrations and discrimination from meningiomas. J Neurosurg 2001; 94:55–60.
42. Marc JA, Takei Y, Schechter MM, Hoffman JC. Intracranial hemangiopericytomas. Angiography, pathology and differential diagnosis. Am J Roentgenol Radium Ther Nucl Med 1975; 125:823–832.
43. Perry A, Scheithauer BW, Nascimento AG. The immunophenotypic spectrum of meningeal hemangiopericytoma: a comparison with fibrous meningioma and solitary fibrous tumor of meninges. Am J Surg Pathol 1997; 21:1354–1360.
44. Uemura S, Kuratsu J, Hamada J, et al. Effect of radiation therapy against intracranial hemangiopericytoma. Neurol Med Chir (Tokyo) 1992; 32:328–332.
45. Wara WM, Sheline GE, Newman H, Townsend JJ, Boldrey EB. Radiation therapy of meningiomas. Am J Roentgenol Radium Ther Nucl Med 1975; 123: 453–458.
46. Fuki M, Kitamura K, Nakagaki H. Irradiated meningiomas: a clinical evaluation. Acta Neurochir 1980; 54:33–43.
47. Bruner JM, Tien RD, Enterline DS. Tumors of the meninges and related tissues: hemangiopericytomas of the meninges. In: Bigner DD, Mclendon RE, Bruner JM, eds. Russell and Rubinstein's pathology of tumors of the nervous system. Arnold: London, 1998:112–117.
48. Palkovic S. Multiple recurrence of an intracranial hemangiopericytoma. Neurosurg Rev 1987; 10:233–236.
49. Galanis E, Buckner JC, Scheithauer BW, Kimmel DW, Schomberg PJ, Piepgras DG. Management of recurrent meningeal hemangiopericytoma. Cancer 1998; 82:1915–1920.
50. Coffey RJ, Cascino TL, Shaw EG. Radiosurgical treatment of recurrent hemangiopericytomas of the meninges: preliminary results. J Neurosurg 1993; 78:903–908.
51. Payne BR, Prasad D, Steiner M, Steiner L. Gamma surgery for hemangiopericytomas. Acta Neurochir (Wien) 2000; 142:527–536; discussion 536–527.
52. Sheehan J, Kondziolka D, Flickinger J, Lunsford LD. Radiosurgery for treatment of recurrent intracranial hemangiopericytomas. Neurosurgery 2002; 51:905–910; discussion 910–901.
53. Beadle GF, Hillcoat BL. Treatment of advanced malignant hemangiopericytoma with combination adriamycin and DTIC: a report of four cases. J Surg Oncol 1983; 22:167–170.

54. Wong PP, Yagoda A. Chemotherapy of malignant hemangiopericytoma. Cancer 1978; 41:1256–1260.
55. Tomita T, Gonzalez-Crussi F. Intracranial primary nonlymphomatous sarcomas in children: experience with eight cases and review of the literature. Neurosurgery 1984; 14:529–540.
56. Russell DS, Rubinstrein LJ. Pathology of Tumours of the Central Nervous System. Baltimore, MD: Williams & Wilkins, 1989.
57. Zulch KJ. Histologic Typing of Tumours of the Central Nervous System. WHO: Geneva, 1979, 53–58.
58. Paulus WF, Slowik L, Jellinger K. Primary intracranial sarcomas: histopathological features of 19 cases. Histopathology 1991; 18:395–402.
59. Arumugasamy N. Some neuropathologic aspects of intracranial sarcomas. Med J Malaya 1969; 23:169–173.
60. Bahr AL, Gayler BW. Cranial chondrosarcomas. Report of four cases and review of the literature. Radiology 1977; 124:151–156.
61. Dropcho EJ, Allen JC. Primary intracranial rhabdomyosarcoma: case report and review of the literature. J Neurooncol 1987; 5:139–150.
62. Lam RM, Malik GM, Chason JL. Osteosarcoma of meninges: clinical, light, and ultrastructural observations of a case. Am J Surg Pathol 1981; 5:203–208.
63. Legier JF, Wells HA Jr. Primary cerebellar rhabdomyosarcoma, Case report. J Neurosurg 1967; 26:436–438.
64. Mena H, Ribas J, Enzinger FM, Parisi JE. Primary brain sarcomas: light and electron miniscopic features. Cancer 1978; 42:1289–1307.
65. Min KW, Gyorkey F, Halpert B. Primary rhabdomyosarcoma of the cerebrum. Cancer 1975; 35:1405–1411.
66. Onofrio BM, Kernohan JW, Uihlein A. Primary meningeal sarcomatosis. A review of the literature and report of 12 cases. Cancer 1962; 15:1197–1208.
67. Moppett J, Oakhill A, Duncan AW. Second malignancies in children: the usual suspects? Eur J Radiol 2001; 38:235–248.
68. Amirjamshidi A, Abbassioun K. Radiation-induced tumors of the central nervous system occurring in childhood and adolescence. Four unusual lesions in three patients and a review of the literature. Childs Nerv Syst 2000; 16:390–397.
69. Wong FL, Boice JD, Jr., Abramson DH, et al. Cancer incidence after retinoblastoma. Radiation dose and sarcoma risk. JAMA 1997; 278:1262–1267.
70. Brown HG, Burger PC, Olivi A, Sills AK, Barditch-Crovo PA, Lee RR. Intracranial leiomyosarcoma in a patient with AIDS. Neuroradiology 1999; 41:35–39.
71. Malat J, Virapongse C, Palestro CJ, Richman AH. Primary intraspinal fibrosarcoma. Neurosurgery 1986; 19:434–436.
72. Zwartverwer FL, Kaplan AM, Hart MC, Hertel GA, Spataro J. Meningeal sarcoma of the spinal cord in a newborn. Arch Neurol 1978; 35:844–846.
73. Gaspar LE, Mackenzie IR, Gilbert JJ, et al. Primary cerebral fibrosarcomas. Clinicopathologic study and review of the literature. Cancer 1993; 72:3277–3281.
74. Kubota T, Hayashi M, Yamamoto S. Primary intracranial mesenchymal chondrosarcoma: case report with review of the literature. Neurosurgery 1982; 10:105–110.
75. Rueda-Franco F, Lopez-Corella E. Sarcomas in the central nervous system of children. 1982 [classical article]. Pediatr Neurosurg 1995; 22:49–55.

76. Al-Gahtany M, Shroff M, Bouffet E, et al. Primary central nervous system sarcomas in children: clinical, radiological, and pathological features. Childs Nerv Syst 2003; 19:808–817.
77. Heros RC, Martinez AJ, Ahn HS. Intracranial mesenchymal chondrosarcoma. Surg Neurol 1980; 14:311–317.
78. McDonald P, Guha A, Provias J. Primary intracranial fibrosarcoma with intratumoral hemorrhage: neuropathological diagnosis with review of the literature. J Neurooncol 1997; 35:133–139.
79. Cybulski GR, Russell EJ, D'Angelo CM, Bailey OT. Falcine chondrosarcoma: case report and literature review. Neurosurgery 1985; 16:412–415.
80. Lee YY, Van Tassel P, Raymond AK. Intracranial dural chondrosarcoma. AJNR Am J Neuroradiol 1988; 9:1189–1193.
81. Reusche E, Rickels E, Reale E, Stolke D. Primary intracerebral sarcoma in childhood: case report with electron-microscope study. J Neurol 1990; 237:382–384.
82. Brooks JJ. Immunohistochemistry of soft tissue tumors. Myoglobin as a tumor marker for rhabdomyosarcoma. Cancer 1982; 50:1757–1763.
83. Enzinger FM, Weiss SW. Soft Tissue Tumors. MV Mosby: St. Louis, 1988.

19

Primary Lymphoma of the Central Nervous System

Joachim M. Baehring

Yale University School of Medicine, New Haven, Connecticut, U.S.A.

Fred H. Hochberg

Pappas Center for Neuro-Oncology, Massachusetts General Hospital, Boston, Massachusetts, U.S.A.

EPIDEMIOLOGY

The brain, eye, cerebrospinal fluid (CSF), and nerves are prone to invasion by primary extranodal Non-Hodgkin lymphoma (NHL). Primary central nervous system lymphoma (PCNSL) represents 2% to 3% of all primary brain tumors and a like number of extranodal NHL. The neurologic tumor, after increasing three-fold two decades ago, has remained stable in frequency in the last 10 years (1). Based upon data from the Central Brain Tumor Registry of the United States of America, up to 1200 new cases were expected during the year 2004 (2). In general, immunosuppression- or acquired immunodeficiency syndrome (AIDS)-related PCNSL afflicts younger patients (38 years) than immunocompetent patients (59 years); but many patients with PCNSL have experienced subtle forms of immunosuppression from cancer or connective tissue diseases, or have had prior therapy with corticosteroids or immunosuppressive agents. Although acquired and congenital immunodeficiencies precede PCNSL, the introduction of highly active antiretroviral therapy (HAART) has resulted in a declining incidence of disease (3,4).

Primary brain lymphoma, as a post-transplant lymphoproliferation (PTLD), arises in up to 7% of organ transplant recipients. The extent of immunosuppression is the major risk factor. Risk is lowest in recipients of renal allografts. As for systemic PTLD, the majority of cases is associated with infection by the Ebstein–Barr virus (EBV) and occurs within 6 to 10 months after transplantation. In 20% of patients, EBV infection is absent. EBV-negative PTLD tends to occur later (four to five years after transplantation) (5).

PATHOGENESIS

Ninety-eight percent of primary nervous system lymphomas are diffuse large B-cell lymphomas (DLBCL) (World Health Organization classification). However there also exist examples of polyclonal B-cell neoplasms of the brain as well as rarer intermediate or lower grade lymphomas. These tumors must be separated from the neurologic involvement in up to 17% of patients with systemic NHL in the setting of age more than 60, elevated plasma concentrations of lactate dehydrogenase, and significant lymph node burden. It remains uncertain whether there is an in situ transformation of reactive B-cells drawn to the nervous system by an antigenic stimulus or extraneural evolution of the malignant lymphocyte clone, which then homes to the central nervous system (CNS), based on its display of certain surface "addressins" (6). As with many diffuse large B-cell lymphomas, PCNSL likely originates from cells that have undergone maturation in lymph nodes. These cells exhibit findings characteristic of germinal centers: clonal rearrangement and somatic hypermutation of immunoglobulin genes (6,7). BCL6 rearrangements—frequently detected in systemic DLBCL—are rarely found in PCNSL. Aberrant somatic hypermutation in proto-oncogenes such as c-MYC, PIM1, RhoH/TTF, and PAX5 can be detected (8,9), but it remains unknown if this finding is of pathogenetic relevance. CDKN2A is inactivated either by gene deletion or by promotor methylation (10). Loss of human leukocyte antigen expression may help tumor cells to evade elimination by the immune system (11). Infectious agents have long been suspected of playing a role in the pathogenesis of PCNSL through either direct transforming capabilities or chronic stimulation of the immune system. EBV is commonly detected in PCNSL arising in immunocompromised patients but rarely in immunocompetent individuals (12). A temporal evolution from a polyclonal to an oligoclonal and ultimately a clonal process has been described outside the nervous system in the setting of PTLD but likely also occurs in the CNS and the immunocompetent host (13). For example, we have seen polyclonal masses within brain in at least seven patients and others whose benign dural-based "follicular" lymphoma extended as more aggressive histologies into the subarachnoid space.

CLINICAL PRESENTATION

Sixty percent of afflicted individuals present with parenchymal brain lesions, while invasion of eye (10%) and leptomeninges (<5%) is less common (14,15). Reportable are examples of primary lymphomatous infiltration of cranial or spinal nerves (16). Spread to extraneural systemic sites is a feature of advanced disease. The infiltrative nature of the tumor cells likely accounts for premonitory nonspecific symptoms such as personality change and cognitive decline. Mass effect from the tumor(s) produces focal neurological deficits, headache, hiccoughs, emesis, and imbalance not distinguishable from symptoms associated with other primary or secondary brain tumors. Seizures are uncommon. Diencephalic infiltrates surrounding the third ventricle give rise to diabetes insipidus or syndrome of inappropriate antidiuretic hormone secretion (SIADH), sexual dysfunction, hyperphagia, and psychiatric symptoms. Less common are infratentorial manifestations with alteration of conjugate gaze, vertigo, ataxia, and intractable vomiting, but cranial nerve deposits may appear without obvious parenchymal brainstem or meningeal involvement. A predisposing systemic disease or viral infection should be suspected in PCNSL patients with "B symptoms" (weight loss, fever, and anorexia). Rarer still is spinal cord lymphoma, indistinguishable from other causes of transverse myelopathy with leg weakness and hyperactivity of reflexes. Often the clinician elicits a prodrome of months to years, which antedates PCNSL. Presumably, during this time cells evolve clonally. In leptomeningeal lymphomatosis, signs of meningeal irritation including headache and sequential asymmetric cranial neuropathies may be absent and subacute dementia coexists with SIADH. Dural lymphoma should be suspected in the setting of a rapidly evolving headache or focal neurological signs in a patient with radiographic findings resembling meningioma or with bone destruction in continuity with dural infiltration. Intravascular lymphoma, a systemic lymphoma with frequent nervous system involvement, produces acute, small vessel strokes (17). The subacute clinical syndrome includes blunting of personality and memory, myelopathy, or peripheral neuropathic presentations. Lymphomatous infiltration of cranial or spinal nerve roots (neurolymphomatosis) is usually painful and characterized by isolated then widespread neuropathies. Rare is the absence of pain or affliction of a single peripheral nerve (16). Ocular lymphoma must be considered in the setting of steroid and cyclosporine-resistant vitritis or retinal infiltration accompanied by ocular "floaters" and blurred vision. Although these patients present to ophthalmologists, neurologic care is soon mandated as a result of the rapid progression of involvement of both eyes and then brain (18). Indeed little separates the survival of patients with this disorder and those with PCNSL. Although eye lymphoma is often diagnosed of inflammatory or infectious origin (sarcoid, rheumatoid, viral origin, or Behcet's disease), these disorders are excluded by drug resistance and demonstration of malignant cells or molecular markers of clonality.

DIAGNOSIS

The lesions of PCNSL are solitary and supratentorial masses within the hemispheric white matter and the basal ganglia. Spread occurs along intra-hemispheric white matter tracts, projection, or commissural fibers. At initial presentation, 20% to 40% of patients have multifocal lesions that become the majority as the disease progresses. In immunocompetent patients, the masses enhance homogeneously whereas central necrosis is observed in the setting of immunosuppression or after corticosteroid use (Figs. 1 and 2). The tumor infiltrates are well represented on T2-weighted or fluid attenuation inversion recovery (FLAIR) sequences. Rare examples of none-nhancing PCNSL, assumed to be demyelinating disease or gliomatosis, account for fewer than 2% of lesions in our experience; but lack of enhancement is encountered in up to one-third of immunocompromised patients. The cellular tumors are hyperdense on computed tomography (CT) and iso- to hyperintense on T1- and diffusion-weighted magnetic resonance (MR) images (Fig. 3). Diffusion abnormalities reflecting small vessel

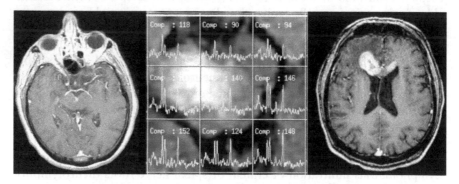

Figure 1 A 63-year-old man complained of fatigue, "dizziness" and intermittent horizontal diplopia. *Left*: Magnetic resonance imaging (MRI) revealed enhancement overlying the ventral surface of the midbrain and surrounding vasogenic edema extending rostrally into the diencephalon. *Middle*: Multivoxel magnetic resonance spectroscopy showed an increased choline to creatine ratio and a decreased N-acetyl-aspartate peak consistent with a neoplasm. Cerebrospinal fluid analysis showed only a mildly increased protein level, and cytopathology was normal. His symptoms resolved on corticosteroid treatment. One month later, he returned with recurrence of symptoms and imbalance. *Right*: MRI demonstrated a large mass lesion within the white matter of the right frontal lobe extending through the genu of the corpus callosum to the other hemisphere. Stereotactic biopsy revealed diffuse large B-cell lymphoma.

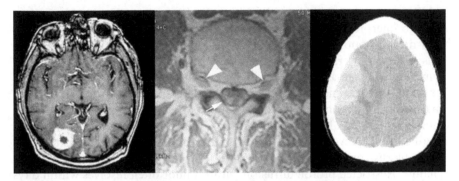

Figure 2 Unusual presentations of primary nervous system lymphoma. *Left*: A heterogeneously enhancing mass lesion is seen within the right occipital lobe. This appearance is typical in patients with acquired or congenital immunodeficiency (here: status post–kidney transplantation; T1-weighted MRI with gadolinium). *Middle*: Axial cut through the L2 nerve roots. There is enhancement of both L2 nerve roots and the cauda equina (T1-weighted MRI with gadolinium). *Right*: A dural-based mass lesion displays homogeneous contrast enhancement (contrast-enhanced computed tomography). Histopathology revealed marginal zone lymphoma.

ischemia accompany intravascular and leptomeningeal lymphoma (Fig. 3) (19). MR spectroscopy may reveal the typical "fingerprint" of a malignant brain neoplasm: decreased *N*-acetyl-aspartate peak and accentuated ratios (>3:1) of choline to creatine (Fig. 1). MR perfusion studies are useful

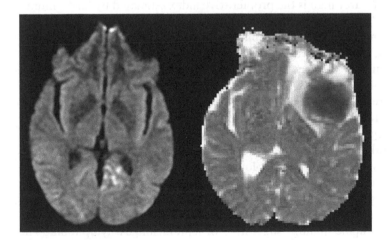

Figure 3 Diffusion-weighted magnetic resonance imaging in nervous system lymphoma. The left image shows small areas of restricted proton diffusion within the left occipital lobe consistent with acute small vessel ischemia. Biopsy revealed intravascular lymphoma. The apparent diffusion coefficient map on the right side demonstrates a hypointense mass within the left frontal lobe. Histopathological evaluation reveale diffuse large B-cell lymphoma.

additions to anatomic images. Lacking experience, physicians find it challenging to interpret these radiographic features of the early poorly enhancing and diffuse tumor infiltrates (Fig. 1). Evading histopathological diagnosis, this disease pattern is underrepresented in the literature. Leptomeningeal lymphoma is seen as linear or nodular enhancement within the intracranial or spinal subarachnoid space, Virchow-Robin spaces, and the subependymal layer. Lymphoma of the dura mater is indistinguishable from meningioma (Fig. 2). Neurolymphomatosis diagnosis rests upon imaging studies, which reveal diffuse enlargement and enhancement of extradural root, plexus, or nerve (Fig. 2) (16). Following therapy, the MRI lesions change. Restricted proton diffusion within tumor often resolves within days of treatment, and contrast-enhanced lesions diminish in both density and size and then disappear (20). Resolution of contrast-enhancing foci is accompanied by reduction, but not resolution of T2 or FLAIR changes. Diagnosis rests upon histopathologic confirmation after brain or eye biopsy using CT- or MRI-guided stereotactic approaches. Lack of confirmation in up to 10% of cases reflects the preoperative use of corticosteroids or the selection of biopsy targets containing few infiltrating tumor cells. Tumors are often viewed as mixtures of neoplastic cells and histologically "reactive" lymphocytes surrounding vessels or diffusely infiltrating white matter. The B-cell origin of tumor cells is disclosed by immunohistochemical studies using monoclonal antibodies targeting CD19-, CD20, or CD79a. The clonality of these B-cells can be confirmed with antibodies to light chains (κ- and λ) or with analysis of immunoglobulin heavy chain gene rearrangement (IGHR). Invariably high is the proliferative index estimated by Ki-67 immunostaining. Cytomorphologic examination of fluid is the basis for diagnosis of leptomeningeal and ocular lymphoma. These studies are thwarted by low cell numbers, poor preservation of cells after storage for several hours, morphologic similarity to "reactive lymphoproliferation," and the commixture of reactive T-lymphocytes. Automated fluorescent cell sorting is more specific but requires at least 40,000 cells. IGHR analysis is useful in paucicellular specimens but has not been widely adapted to evaluation of CSF. Spinal fluid analysis using polymerase chain reaction primers to identify EBV genes has proven useful in the diagnosis of PCNSL in patients with AIDS or PTLD, but its positive predictive value is low (21).

The patient with newly diagnosed PCNSL should receive a formal ophthalmologic evaluation including a slit lamp examination of the eye. CSF cytopathological evaluations are seldom of value in the absence of clinical or radiographic findings suggestive of leptomeningeal lymphoma. The cells identified may be termed "reactive" or may represent responding T-lymphocytes. Of limited value are "screening" studies for systemic lymphoma including body CT or bone marrow biopsy. An examination of the testes is warranted as testicular dissemination is reported. Testing for human immunodeficiency virus infection is always performed.

MANAGEMENT

Surgical therapy of patients with PCNSL is limited to diagnostic stereotactic or open biopsy. The role of resection is limited to reduction of mass causing herniation or brainstem compression. At the present time external beam radiation therapy to the whole brain is no longer the standard of care for PCNSL. The short duration of response and the devastating neurocognitive sequelae of whole brain radiation have supported the deferral of radiotherapy in favor of chemotherapy (22). In clinical practice, whole brain radiation is provided upon failure of systemic chemotherapy and focal radiosurgery to small symptomatic recurrences in the setting of otherwise stable disease. The introduction of methotrexate (MTX) at doses exceeding $3 \, g/m^2$ in treatment regimens for PCNSL led to a profound increase in relapse-free and overall survival. As a result, most protocols now include MTX in addition to agents drawn from the treatment of systemic lymphoma. Current trials investigate the use of new agents (rituximab) in combination with MTX, thio-TEPA, and temozolomide.

The early positive benefits of preirradiation MTX at doses of $3.5 \, g/m^2$ gave rise to current provision of the drug at $8 \, g/m^2$ (23–28). The drug, provided by vein at 10 to 14 day intervals, produces a complete response in over 50% of patients within two months. Thereafter monthly consolidation treatments continue for one year (29). High-dose MTX is well tolerated even by elderly patients and often by the immunosuppressed. As of this date, combination therapies are united in similarities of response rates and median duration of survival. Fully two-thirds of patients will likely respond to chemotherapy with survival durations approaching six years for MTX and multidrug recipients. These therapies include high-dose MTX, procarbazine, vincristine, cytarabine (30,31), M-BACOD (32), high-dose MTX, lomustine, procarbazine, and methylprednisolone, and intrathecal chemotherapy with MTX and cytarabine (33), or MTX with cyclophosphamide, ifosfamide, vincristine/vindesine, dexamethasone, cytarabine and intrathecal chemotherapy (34) as well as MTX mono- or combination chemotherapy in combination with external beam irradiation (35–37). Virtually all reports underscore the neurocognitive sequelae of concomitant irradiation. A variant of MTX administration has been the use of intra-arterial application of chemotherapy preceded by mannitol-induced blood–brain barrier disruption (BBBD) to facilitate drug delivery to the brain tumor. Although provision of BBBD MTX with intravenous cyclophosphamide and etoposide produced high rates of response (38), the benefits of this approach may be no better than those from MTX by vein. The BBBD regimen requires monthly triple vessel angiography and is associated with procedure-related complications.

The incidence of spinal fluid spread of PCNSL likely is no higher than 15% but varies by institutional biases in morphological analysis and interobserver variability. As a general rule, high-dose intravenous MTX provides higher and more sustained levels of drug in the CSF than does intrathecal administration. Thus sustained remission of disease has been associated with provision or omission of intrathecal chemotherapy. Our approach has been to treat meningeal disease with parenteral MTX before providing intrathecal chemotherapy. In this way, the clinician may avoid placement of an Ommaya reservoir or repeated lumbar puncture access to the CSF.

Approximately 50% of patients will recur after having achieved a complete disappearance of tumor and having ceased chemotherapy. At relapse, PCNSL remains chemosensitive, and remission can again be achieved with MTX or MTX-based regimens (39). The use of topotecan for relapsed PCNSL provides responses in 20% of patients with notable hematologic toxicities; temozolomide is better tolerated and one-quarter of patients experience responses, while case series demonstrate the efficacy of procarbazine, lomustine, vincristine (PCV) and VIA (etoposide, ifosfamide, and cytarabine). As optimistic experience has followed rituximab by systemic or intrathecal routes, this drug is increasingly used off-label in combination with temozolomide to treat recurrent disease. The role of whole brain radiation therapy for chemoresistant disease is undisputed, and we have provided focal therapy of unresponsive nodules using radiosurgical approaches.

High-dose chemotherapy with autologous stem cell transplantation has been used in single institutions in the United States and France. Promising results achieved in the setting of relapsing and refractory disease (40) were not supported in a formal clinical trial including patients with newly diagnosed PCNSL (41).

Most forms of chemotherapy, provided in advance of irradiation, include patients whose survival exceeds five years. This success has been associated with MTX-based therapies inclusive of alkylating agents with radiation therapy. As a general rule, protocols, which include whole brain irradiation in excess of 36 Gy in standard fractions, report neurocognitive complications in survivors over two years. Similar cognitive changes, progressive over time, are associated with whole brain radiation therapy followed by intrathecal MTX therapy (42). As few studies are available that prospectively assess the effects of chemotherapy and radiation (43), there is consensus that future trials should incorporate serial neurocognitive testing such as the functional assessment of cancer therapy-brain (FACT-BR) or 36-item short-form health survey (SF-36) batteries. Leukoencephalopathy has been seen in a minority of recipients of solely high-dose MTX (44). With rare exceptions, the neurocognitive effects are not significant.

Patients with the AIDS syndrome develop PCNSL in the advanced stage of their disease. Whole brain radiation therapy provided to severely immunocompromised patients has been associated with responses lasting less than six months. The few patients eligible for systemic chemotherapy or combined modality treatment can receive MTX or PCV therapy (45). The introduction of HAART has led to a marked reduction in the incidence of PCNSL, an increase in the number of patients eligible for chemotherapy, and a dramatic increase in survival of chemotherapy recipients (4,46). Of the data available regarding treatment of PCNSL in PTLD, chemo- and radiation therapy is associated with a poor prognosis (47). As a general rule, physicians pursue reduction or discontinuation of immunosuppression at the risk of rejection of the donor organ. Rituximab has been successfully used in systemic post-transplant lymphoproliferative disorder but its efficacy in central nervous system lymphoma is unknown and many tumors do not express CD20 epitopes. The efficacy of antiviral agents in this almost invariably EBV-mediated disorder remains unclear because in the majority of patients treated with these drugs immunosuppression was simultaneously reduced or discontinued (48). Rarely suitable is chemotherapy with MTX or combination chemotherapy.

Patients with eye and eye/brain involvement are often provided systemic chemotherapy to achieve control of microscopic widespread deposits before launching into local therapy of the eye. Therapeutic concentrations of MTX are reached within the vitreous fluid using systemic chemotherapy (49). Local treatment consists of either direct injection of chemotherapy into the vitreous or irradiation of the orbit.

Long-term survival and, in selected cases, even a cure is possible in PCNSL. However late relapses are common. Treatment should be provided in specialized multidisciplinary centers. Our most robust experience is with monotherapy MTX ($8 \, g/m^2$), but regimens combining MTX and alkylating agents with or without radiation have been used by others. Obscure is the future therapy of this unusual neoplasm because the disease is seldom truly curable and often misdiagnosed. Molecular markers such as IGHR may prove to be more sensitive and specific than morphological or flow-cytometric analysis. The validation of this technology is underway for paucicellular specimens. Novel diagnostic tools should provide a means of identifying early stages or minimal residual disease in brain, eye, or blood pools. This knowledge will influence treatment because smaller tumor burdens carry improved therapeutic response and prognosis. Additional studies should provide insights into the proclivity of specific B-cell subtypes to enter the eye, nerve, and brain vessels as well. These approaches will expand the role for new cytotoxic chemotherapeutic agents and targeted tumor therapy including radioactively labeled antibodies binding to B-lymphocyte epitopes or anti-idiotype cytotoxic T-lymphocytes. New strategies will have to take into account peculiar aspects applicable to the mostly elderly patient population. With increasing life expectancy of PCNSL patients, long-term treatment-related toxicity will be an important outcome variable.

REFERENCES

1. Olson JE, Janney CA, Rao RD, et al. The continuing increase in the incidence of primary central nervous system non-Hodgkin lymphoma: a surveillance, epidemiology, and end results analysis. Cancer 2002; 95(7):1504–1510.

2. Statistical Report. Primary Brain Tumors in the United States, 1997–2001. CBTRUS, Central Brain Tumor Registry of the United States, 2004.
3. Chow KU, Mitrou PS, Geduldig K, Helm EB, Hoelzer D, Brodt HR. Changing incidence and survival in patients with aids-related non-Hodgkin's lymphomas in the era of highly active antiretroviral therapy (HAART). Leuk Lymphoma 2001; 41(1–2):105–116.
4. Newell ME, Hoy JF, Cooper SG, et al. Human immunodeficiency virus-related primary central nervous system lymphoma: factors influencing survival in 111 patients. Cancer 2004; 100(12):2627–2636.
5. Leblond V, Dhedin N, Mamzer Bruneel MF, et al. Identification of prognostic factors in 61 patients with posttransplantation lymphoproliferative disorders. J Clin Oncol 2001; 19(3):772–778.
6. Larocca LM, Capello D, Rinelli A, et al. The molecular and phenotypic profile of primary central nervous system lymphoma identifies distinct categories of the disease and is consistent with histogenetic derivation from germinal center-related B cells. Blood 1998; 92(3):1011–1019.
7. Thompsett AR, Ellison DW, Stevenson FK, Zhu D. V(H) gene sequences from primary central nervous system lymphomas indicate derivation from highly mutated germinal center B cells with ongoing mutational activity. Blood 1999; 94(5):1738–1746.
8. Pasqualucci L, Neumeister P, Goossens T, et al. Hypermutation of multiple proto-oncogenes in B-cell diffuse large-cell lymphomas. Nature 2001; 412(6844): 341–346.
9. Montesinos-Rongen M, Van Roost D, Schaller C, Wiestler OD, Deckert M. Primary diffuse large B-cell lymphomas of the central nervous system are targeted by aberrant somatic hypermutation. Blood 2004; 103(5):1869–1875.
10. Zhang SJ, Endo S, Ichikawa T, Washiyama K, Kumanishi T. Frequent deletion and 5' CpG island methylation of the p16 gene in primary malignant lymphoma of the brain. Cancer Res 1998; 58(6):1231–1237.
11. Jordanova ES, Riemersma SA, Philippo K, Giphart-Gassler M, Schuuring E, Kluin PM. Hemizygous deletions in the HLA region account for loss of heterozygosity in the majority of diffuse large B-cell lymphomas of the testis and the central nervous system. Genes Chromosomes Cancer 2002; 35(1):38–48.
12. Hochberg FH, Miller G, Schooley RT, Hirsch MS, Feorino P, Henle W. Central-nervous-system lymphoma related to Epstein-Barr virus. N Engl J Med 1983; 309(13):745–748.
13. Seiden MV, Sklar J. Molecular genetic analysis of post-transplant lymphoproliferative disorders. Hematol Oncol Clin North Am 1993; 7(2):447–465.
14. Akpek EK, Ahmed I, Hochberg FH, et al. Intraocular-central nervous system lymphoma: clinical features, diagnosis, and outcomes. Ophthalmology 1999; 106(9):1805–1810.
15. Freilich RJ, DeAngelis LM. Primary central nervous system lymphoma. Neurol Clin 1995; 13(4):901–914.
16. Baehring JM, Damek D, Martin EC, Betensky RA, Hochberg FH. Neurolymphomatosis. Neuro-oncol 2003; 5(2):104–115.
17. Glass J, Hochberg FH, Miller DC. Intravascular lymphomatosis. A systemic disease with neurologic manifestations. Cancer 1993; 71(10):3156–3164.
18. Buggage RR, Chan CC, Nussenblatt RB. Ocular manifestations of central nervous system lymphoma. Curr Opin Oncol 2001; 13(3):137–142.

19. Baehring JM, Henchcliffe C, Ledezma CJ, Fulbright R, Hochberg FH. Intravascular lymphoma: magnetic resonance imaging correlates of disease dynamics within the central nervous system. J Neurol Neurosurg Psychiatry 2005; 76(4):540–544.
20. Moffat BA, Chenevert TL, Lawrence TS, et al. Functional diffusion map: a noninvasive MRI biomarker for early stratification of clinical brain tumor response. Proc Natl Acad Sci USA 2005; 102(15):5524–5529.
21. Cingolani A, De Luca A, Larocca LM, et al. Minimally invasive diagnosis of acquired immunodeficiency syndrome-related primary central nervous system lymphoma. J Natl Cancer Inst 1998; 90(5):364–369.
22. Nelson DF, Martz KL, Bonner H, et al. Non-Hodgkin's lymphoma of the brain: can high dose, large volume radiation therapy improve survival? Report on a prospective trial by the Radiation Therapy Oncology Group (RTOG): RTOG 8315. Int J Radiat Oncol Biol Phys 1992; 23(1):9–17.
23. Gabbai AA, Hochberg FH, Linggood RM, Bashir R, Hotleman K. High-dose methotrexate for non-AIDS primary central nervous system lymphoma. Report of 13 cases. J Neurosurg 1989; 70(2):190–194.
24. Hochberg FH, Loeffler JS, Prados M. The therapy of primary brain lymphoma. J Neurooncol 1991; 10(3):191–201.
25. Glass J, Gruber ML, Cher L, Hochberg FH. Pre-irradiation methotrexate chemotherapy of primary central nervous system lymphoma: long-term outcome. J Neurosurg 1994; 81(2):188–195.
26. Glass J, Shustik C, Hochberg FH, Cher L, Gruber ML. Therapy of primary central nervous system lymphoma with pre-irradiation methotrexate, cyclophosphamide, doxorubicin, vincristine, and dexamethasone (MCHOD). J Neurooncol 1996; 30(3): 257–265.
27. Cher L, Glass J, Harsh GR, Hochberg FH. Therapy of primary CNS lymphoma with methotrexate-based chemotherapy and deferred radiotherapy: preliminary results. Neurology 1996; 46(6):1757–1759.
28. Guha-Thakurta N, Damek D, Pollack C, Hochberg FH. Intravenous methotrexate as initial treatment for primary central nervous system lymphoma: response to therapy and quality of life of patients. J Neurooncol 1999; 43(3):259–268.
29. Batchelor T, Carson K, O'Neill A, et al. Treatment of primary CNS lymphoma with methotrexate and deferred radiotherapy: a report of NABTT 96–07. J Clin Oncol 2003; 21(6):1044–1049.
30. Abrey LE, Yahalom J, DeAngelis LM. Treatment for primary CNS lymphoma: the next step. J Clin Oncol 2000; 18(17):3144–3150.
31. Freilich RJ, Delattre JY, Monjour A, DeAngelis LM. Chemotherapy without radiation therapy as initial treatment for primary CNS lymphoma in older patients. Neurology 1996; 46(2):435–439.
32. Boiardi A, Silvani A, Pozzi A, Fariselli L, Broggi G, Salmaggi A. Chemotherapy is effective as early treatment for primary central nervous system lymphoma. J Neurol 1999; 246(1):31–37.
33. Hoang-Xuan K, Taillandier L, Chinot O, et al. Chemotherapy alone as initial treatment for primary CNS lymphoma in patients older than 60 years: a multicenter phase II study (26952) of the European Organization for Research and Treatment of Cancer Brain Tumor Group. J Clin Oncol 2003; 21(14):2726–2731.
34. Pels H, Schmidt-Wolf IG, Glasmacher A, et al. Primary central nervous system lymphoma: results of a pilot and phase II study of systemic and intraventricular chemotherapy with deferred radiotherapy. J Clin Oncol 2003; 21(24):4489–4495.

35. DeAngelis LM, Seiferheld W, Schold SC, Fisher B, Schultz CJ. Combination chemotherapy and radiotherapy for primary central nervous system lymphoma: Radiation Therapy Oncology Group Study 93–10. J Clin Oncol 2002; 20(24): 4643–4648.
36. O'Brien P, Roos D, Pratt G, et al. Phase II multicenter study of brief single-agent methotrexate followed by irradiation in primary CNS lymphoma. J Clin Oncol 2000; 18(3):519–526.
37. Poortmans PM, Kluin-Nelemans HC, Haaxma-Reiche H, et al. High-dose methotrexate-based chemotherapy followed by consolidating radiotherapy in non-AIDS-related primary central nervous system lymphoma: European Organization for Research and Treatment of Cancer Lymphoma Group Phase II Trial 20962. J Clin Oncol 2003; 21(24):4483–4488.
38. Doolittle ND, Miner ME, Hall WA, et al. Safety and efficacy of a multicenter study using intraarterial chemotherapy in conjunction with osmotic opening of the blood-brain barrier for the treatment of patients with malignant brain tumors. Cancer 2000; 88(3):637–647.
39. Plotkin SR, Betensky RA, Hochberg FH, et al. Treatment of relapsed central nervous system lymphoma with high-dose methotrexate. Clin Cancer Res 2004; 10(17):5643–5646.
40. Soussain C, Suzan F, Hoang-Xuan K, et al. Results of intensive chemotherapy followed by hematopoietic stem-cell rescue in 22 patients with refractory or recurrent primary CNS lymphoma or intraocular lymphoma. J Clin Oncol 2001; 19(3):742–749.
41. Abrey LE, Moskowitz CH, Mason WP, et al. Intensive methotrexate and cytarabine followed by high-dose chemotherapy with autologous stem-cell rescue in patients with newly diagnosed primary CNS lymphoma: an intent-to-treat analysis. J Clin Oncol 2003; 21(22):4151–4156.
42. Lai R, Abrey LE, Rosenblum MK, De Angelis LM. Treatment-induced leukoencephalopathy in primary CNS lymphoma: a clinical and autopsy study. Neurology 2004; 62(3):451–456.
43. Harder H, Holtel H, Bromberg JE, et al. Cognitive status and quality of life after treatment for primary CNS lymphoma. Neurology 2004; 62(4):544–547.
44. Fliessbach K, Urbach H, Helmstaedter C, et al. Cognitive performance and magnetic resonance imaging findings after high-dose systemic and intraventricular chemotherapy for primary central nervous system lymphoma. Arch Neurol 2003; 60(4):563–568.
45. Forsyth PA, Yahalom J, DeAngelis LM. Combined-modality therapy in the treatment of primary central nervous system lymphoma in AIDS. Neurology 1994; 44(8):1473–1479.
46. Skiest DJ, Crosby C. Survival is prolonged by highly active antiretroviral therapy in AIDS patients with primary central nervous system lymphoma. AIDS 2003; 17(12):1787–1793.
47. Penn I, Porat G. Central nervous system lymphomas in organ allograft recipients. Transplantation 1995; 59(2):240–244.
48. Roychowdhury S, Peng R, Baiocchi RA, et al. Experimental treatment of Epstein-Barr virus-associated primary central nervous system lymphoma. Cancer Res 2003; 63(5):965–971.
49. Batchelor TT, Kolak G, Ciordia R, Foster CS, Henson JW. High-dose methotrexate for intraocular lymphoma. Clin Cancer Res 2003; 9(2):711–715.

20

Tumors of the Sellar Region: Craniopharyngioma and Pituitary Adenoma

Oren N. Gottfried and William T. Couldwell
Department of Neurosurgery, University of Utah School of Medicine, Salt Lake City, Utah, U.S.A.

Martin H. Weiss
Department of Neurological Surgery, University of Southern California, Los Angeles, California, U.S.A.

CRANIOPHARYNGIOMA

Craniopharyngiomas are slow-growing, benign epithelial neoplasms of the sellar region that arise from embryonic squamous cells of the hypophysio-pharyngeal duct (Rathke's pouch). Although Erdheim originally described this lesion in 1904, in 1932, Cushing introduced the term "craniopharyngioma" to denote its origin from the embryological remnant. Histologically benign, these tumors nonetheless display insidious growth to involve important neurovascular structures. Endocrine, visual, and mental disturbances are frequently seen at presentation and are secondary to involvement of the hypothalamus–pituitary axis, optic pathways, thalamus, and frontal lobes. Early attempts at surgical resection were associated with a high risk of damage to the local neuroanatomy. Although advances in microsurgical and skull base techniques, radiation therapy, chemotherapy, and hormonal replacement have provided better long-term survival and longer recurrence-free intervals, controversies remain as to the optimal treatment of this tumor.

Craniopharyngiomas have an annual incidence of 0.5 to 2 cases per million population per year (1). They exhibit a bimodal age distribution, with the first peak at age 5 to 10, and a second peak between ages 50 and 60. Two subtypes, *adamantinomatous* and *papillary*, have been defined, with the classic type, the adamantinomatous variety, occurring 10 times as often and mainly in children (2). In contrast, the papillary subtype affects mainly adults (2). Typically, craniopharyngiomas occur sporadically and do not follow a direct pattern of familial inheritance, although rare cases have demonstrated inheritance.

Craniopharyngiomas of both subtypes are thought to derive from Rathke's cleft/pouch because of the occasional ability of some tumor cells to express one or more pituitary hormones (2). It has also been suggested that the adamantinomatous craniopharyngioma may arise from embryonic rests with enamel organ potential (2). Interestingly, papillary craniopharyngiomas may share a similar origin or represent a spectrum of a similar disease process with Rathke's cleft cysts as evidenced by the fact that these two disease entities are occasionally very similar on pathology (2,3). Papillary craniopharyngiomas may have focal ciliation of epithelium or goblet cells, whereas some Rathke's cleft cysts have extensive squamous metaplasia of their cyst wall resulting in a solid component, and these cysts may have an associated higher rate of recurrence more similar to papillary craniopharyngiomas (2,3).

Molecular Markers

A subset of craniopharyngiomas has been shown to have increased insulin-like growth factor (IGF)-1 receptor expression, and these tumors display growth arrest with IGF-1R inhibitors (4). Select craniopharyngiomas express estrogen and progesterone receptors (~30%), and it has been found that the incidence of regrowth after surgery is higher in patients negative for these receptors because of loss of differentiation (5). Also, a high Ki-67 index suggests a high possibility of tumor regrowth and was significantly higher in patients who progressed to have a recurrence than in patients without regrowth (5). An elevated beta human chorionic gonadotrophin level has been reported in the cerebrospinal fluid (CSF) of patients with craniopharyngioma, and the tumor has been found to stain positive for this hormone.

Clinical Features

Presentation

In craniopharyngioma, the usual interval between symptom onset and presentation is one to two years (6). Clinical manifestations depend on origin, direction of growth, degree of tumor extension, and involvement of surrounding neural structures. Patients may present with symptoms related to increased intracranial pressure from mass effect, hydrocephalus, or compression of the optic apparatus, pituitary/hypothalamus axis, or cerebrum. Headache is one of the most common complaints prompting medical attention in all age groups; however, children are more apt to present with headache and vomiting and complain less of visual difficulties than adults (6,7).

Visual Symptoms: Although approximately 20% of children have papilledema at presentation (6), adults appear to be more sensitive to visual deficits than children. Eighty percent of adults demonstrate visual disturbance as a presenting symptom as compared with 20% to 30% of children (6). Visual disturbance may manifest as a decrease in visual acuity (1), diplopia, blurred vision, bitemporal hemianopia, homonymous hemianopia, various quadrantanopsias, or seesaw nystagmus, which is present in only 5% to 10% of cases (8). Rare cases of unilateral or even bilateral blindness have been reported.

Endocrine Abnormalities: Although endocrine dysfunction is not a frequent cause of medical consultation, 80% to 90% of individuals harbor abnormalities at presentation (6,7,9). Children commonly present with short stature and delayed linear growth, whereas adolescents may complain of delayed or arrested puberty. Men may observe a loss of libido; women may present with secondary amenorrhea. The most common hormonal deficiencies include growth hormone (GH) (75%), followed by luteinizing hormone (LH) or follicle-stimulating hormone (FSH) (40%), adrenocorticotropic hormone (ACTH) (25%), and thyroid-stimulating hormone (TSH) (25%). Hyperprolactinemia (20%) in some patients indicates impingement of areas within the hypothalamus or pituitary stalk that normally exert an inhibitory influence on prolactin release ("stalk section" effect). Diabetes insipidus (DI) is less frequent at presentation but is present in 9% to 17% of patients before surgery (9).

Behavioral Changes: Some patients come to medical attention as a result of changes in mental status or behavior. Although unusual in children, mental disturbance is present in approximately 25% of adults (8). Psychological or intellectual manifestations are to a large extent due to the direction of tumor expansion. Tumor growth involving the frontal lobes may cause dementia, apathy, abulia, or psychomotor slowing (6). Complex psychomotor seizures and amnesia have been documented with tumor extension into the temporal lobe and hippocampus (6).

Imaging

Plain radiographs of the skull have largely been replaced by computed tomography (CT) or magnetic resonance imaging (MRI) as the initial imaging studies for diagnosis of craniopharyngioma, although calcification is apparent on plain skull radiographs in many patients (6). CT demonstrates calcification and the degree of secondary skull base bone changes. Calcifications are seen in most childhood craniopharyngiomas. Similarly, while cystic components are identified in more than half of all craniopharyngiomas, they are found in almost all pediatric craniopharyngiomas. The cyst fluid is iso- or hypodense on CT but may appear hyperdense if sufficient calcification is present. Intravenous contrast on CT enhances the solid portion of the tumor as well as the cyst capsule. MRI is the neuroimaging modality of choice, precisely demonstrating the extent and location of the tumor as well as the tumor's relationship to important surrounding neurovascular structures. On MRI, the cyst exhibits a hyperintense signal on T1-weighted images. The solid component is isointense but enhances on administration of intravenous gadolinium. MRI or CT angiography provides anatomic detail of the cerebral vasculature in relation to the tumor, which is important in surgical planning.

Typically, craniopharyngiomas are located in the parasellar region. Approximately 5% to 15% manifest within the confines of the sella; another 20% present as a suprasellar mass (6,10). They may arise from within the third ventricle. Craniopharyngiomas may extend anteriorly to involve the frontal lobes (30%), laterally to involve the temporal lobe and structures of the middle cranial fossa (25%), or posteriorly and inferiorly, encroaching on the brain stem and extending into the cerebellopontine angle or foramen magnum (20%) (10).

Radiographically, craniopharyngiomas may be described in relation to the optic chiasm; craniopharyngiomas are characterized as prechiasmatic, retrochiasmatic, or subchiasmatic. Prechiasmatic tumors grow forward between the optic nerves, displacing the optic chiasm upward and backward as well as displacing the A-1 segment of the anterior cerebral artery (10). In contrast, retrochiasmatic craniopharyngiomas displace the chiasm forward and have a propensity to fill the third ventricle, resulting in obstructive hydrocephalus. With posterior and inferior extension, retrochiasmatic tumors may displace the basilar artery (10).

Management

Surgical Treatment

Cushing referred to craniopharyngiomas as "the most baffling problem which confronts the neurosurgeon." The role of aggressive surgical removal of these tumors is still somewhat controversial. Some authors contend that total resection offers the best chance for tumor-free survival (11,12). With advances in microsurgical and skull base techniques, safe gross total or near-total excision of these tumors has become possible in most cases with low rates of morbidity and mortality. In more recent series, the percentage of patients with complete resections has increased from 69% to 90%, but it is well established that tumors can still return even after a radical resection (11). We agree that complete microsurgical removal, when safe, is the treatment of choice to offer the best chance of long-term control. Other authors support a more conservative approach consisting of subtotal resection combined with postoperative radiation, because of an increased risk of hypothalamic, pituitary, and visual complications with radical resection in some cases. For primarily cystic tumors, drainage and injection of radioactive isotopes or a chemotherapeutic agent may be an alternative to surgical resection (13). The goal of surgery is decompression of the optic and ventricular pathways regardless of whether a total or subtotal resection is undertaken.

Surgical Approaches

Subfrontal Approach: The subfrontal approach is a versatile approach for removing craniopharyngiomas that are midline with extension along the anterior skull base and suprasellar cistern, because it offers a straight frontal trajectory with good visualization of both optic nerves and internal carotid arteries. It also has the advantage of accessing the anterior third ventricle via the lamina terminalis if the tumor extends intraventricularly. This approach is commonly used for resection of pre-chiasmatic craniopharyngiomas and for some retrochiasmatic tumors that extend anteriorly and fill the third ventricle. This approach may not be suitable for patients with a prefixed chiasm.

Frontotemporal Approach: The pterional (frontotemporal) approach may be used for large retrochiasmatic craniopharyngiomas with significant anterior and posterior extension. It is the workhorse for approaching cranio-pharyngiomas involving primarily the suprasellar cistern because it provides the shortest distance to the suprasellar region via a transcranial approach. This is the preferred method in patients with a prefixed chiasm, because the tumor can be resected beneath the chiasm. A combined pterional and subfrontal approach allows access to both anterior and posterior portions of the tumor.

For craniopharyngiomas with significant suprasellar extension or superior extension into the third ventricle, the orbitozygomatic variation offers an improved inferior-to-superior ("looking-up") view to the hypothalamic and suprasellar regions. By removing the orbital rim and lateral sphenoid region, the bony obstruction that typically limits adequate superior exposure is circumvented. The angle of exposure, based on the fulcrum of the inferior frontal lobe, is significantly improved. Removal of the zygomatic arch allows more inferior mobilization of the temporalis muscle and reduces the muscle bulk that may otherwise obstruct visualization.

Trans-Sphenoidal Approach: Craniopharyngiomas that occupy both sellar and suprasellar regions are favorable for trans-sphenoidal resection if the sella is enlarged. This approach is associated with a lower surgical morbidity and a lower incidence of postoperative DI than conventional craniotomy. In a series of 68 tumors, 90% were totally resected via a trans-sphenoidal approach (14). Intrasellar craniopharyngiomas frequently lack the intimate adherence to vital neurovascular structures such as the hypothalamus, thus facilitating surgical removal (6). However, the surgeon must be aware of the nearby cavernous sinus. Although rare, intraoperative hemorrhage has been reported. The trans-sphenoidal approach also has a potential for CSF leak. This approach is contraindicated for large calcified craniopharyngiomas with significant suprasellar or lateral extension as well as tumors demonstrating adherence to the optic nerves or hypothalamus (6). The trans-sphenoidal approach may be more difficult in young children who do not have a pneumatized sphenoid sinus. In these cases, access to the sella requires additional drilling of the sphenoid bone with the aid of stereotactic CT guidance.

Transcallosal Approach: The transcallosal approach is advocated primarily for craniopharyngiomas arising from within the third ventricle or those with marked superior extension within the third ventricle. The transcallosal route may also be applied for the planned staged resection of the superior component of a large tumor extending superiorly into the third or lateral ventricles in conjunction with a pterional or subfrontal approach.

Surgical Complications

Since the advent of hormone replacement therapy, the surgical mortality rate has dropped to less than 2% in recent series (11,12,15). Surgical complications may involve visual, hormonal, behavioral, or vascular sequelae. DI is the most frequently encountered complication, with postoperative incidence ranging from 76% to 94%. In almost 75% of patients, the DI is transient (16). Other complications include panhypopituitarism, memory deficits, and psychological abnormalities. These complications can be attributed to manipulation of the pituitary stalk and hypothalamus at surgery. Vascular complications resulting from attempts at radical resection have also been reported. Although rare, intraoperative laceration or delayed formation of a fusiform dilation of the internal carotid artery may occur from dissection of the tumor.

Radiation Therapy: Radiation was first used in the treatment of craniopharyngioma in 1937 (8). Radiation following subtotal resection is associated with a better long-term, recurrence-free survival than is subtotal resection alone. Regine et al. documented a 20-year survival rate of 60% in patients treated with adjuvant radiotherapy following subtotal removal (17).

Radiation therapy in children may negatively impact neurocognitive development, and the rate of IQ decline is typically associated with several risk factors, including younger age at treatment, higher radiotherapy dose, and greater volume of brain receiving treatment. Technical advances in radiotherapy hold promise for lowering the frequency of neurocognitive sequelae.

A fractionated approach with conventional external beam treatment or with radiosurgery will result in fewer and less severe radiation-related sequelae, and a higher total radiation dose can be more safely delivered. Optimum response occurs with radiation doses ranging from 50 Gy to 65 Gy in fractionated doses of 180 to 200 cGy/d (17). Although notable long-term survival rates exist, complications include radiation necrosis, optic neuritis, dementia, calcification of the basal ganglia, radiation-induced vasculopathy, hypothalamic–pituitary dysfunction, and a decrease in intellectual performance in the very young. This latter complication has led to the avoidance of fractionated field radiation therapy by most authors for tumors in early childhood. Additionally, neoplasms, including meningiomas, sarcomas, and gliomas, have all been reported at varying latencies following radiation therapy. In one study with a median follow-up of 17 years after treatment, radiation-related complications occurred in 58% of children and 46% of adults (18).

Stereotactic radiosurgery (SRS) allows accurate and precise application of multiple convergent beams of ionizing radiation to a focally distinct volume of tissue with a single dose. The use of multiple beams of ionizing radiation results in a sharp dose falloff beyond the target area, which spares normal adjacent tissue (19). Typically, SRS has been used as a treatment for recurrent disease. In one study of 10 patients who underwent stereotactic gamma-knife radiosurgery (GKRS), seven patients had considerable shrinkage of the tumor and the remaining three patients had no overall change in tumor size after median 14-month follow-up; however, follow-up MRI showed central low-intensity signal changes consistent with central necrosis (19). In another series of 10 patients treated with GKRS, four patients had complete regression and another four had tumor shrinkage at last follow-up at a median of 63 months (20). Although the mean marginal tumor dose was 16.4 Gy and 14.3 Gy in these series, in one series in which 13 patients were treated with 6 Gy, 11 patients suffered tumor progression at a mean of 17 years follow-up (21). In another study, 23 patients with recurrent craniopharyngioma were treated with GKRS with a mean of 10.8 Gy and 61% of patients had tumor reduction (at a mean of 22.6 months), but interestingly, local control was achieved in another 13% after a second radiosurgical intervention (22). SRS is generally contraindicated in craniopharyngiomas with solid components of larger than 2.5 to 3 cm, primarily cystic tumors, tumors involving the hypothalamus and brain stem, as well as tumors less than 3 to 5 mm in distance from the optic apparatus, although a single fractionated dose less than 8 to 10 Gy to the optic apparatus is considered to be safe (19).

Fractionated stereotactic radiotherapy (SRT) is a technique that uses fractionated irradiation under stereotactic guidance. SRT allows multiple doses of fractionated radiation to focal areas and offers the advantage of treating tumors greater than 3 cm in size and those adjacent to critical neural structures, in which the application of SRS is normally limited (23). One group noted excellent relapse-free survival without any evidence of radiation-induced optic neuropathy (23).

Intracavitary irradiation was first introduced by Leksell in 1951 and has been primarily recommended for solitary cystic craniopharyngioma or cystic components of a mixed tumor. Intracavitary irradiation employs placement of beta-emitting isotopes (^{32}P or ^{90}Y) into the cyst cavity following stereotactic aspiration of the cyst contents. Results have demonstrated stabilization or a decrease in the size of the cyst in more than 75% of patients treated with primary cystic craniopharyngiomas (24). Side effects include decreased visual acuity or decrease in visual fields, which typically occurs in one third of patients (24). Of note, unlike these beta-emitting isotopes, interstitial irradiation with 125-Iodine may be useful in patients with solid tumors.

Chemotherapy: The role of chemotherapy in the treatment of craniopharyngioma has yet to be clearly defined, and most articles are limited to case reports. The use of intracavitary bleomycin injection into cystic craniopharyngiomas has aroused some interest. In a small series, 11 patients with cystic craniopharyngiomas were treated and followed up for 3 to 16 years; in three patients, the cyst resolved completely; in four patients, the size of the cyst decreased by 80% to 90% and the patients were observed with serial imaging; in three patients, the size decreased 60% to 70% and the patients were also treated with radiosurgery; and one patient died of hormone insufficiency (25). In another study, 24 craniopharyngiomas were treated with only bleomycin; nine tumors completely resolved whereas 15 cysts decreased in size by 50% to 70%, and at a median of five years, no recurrences were reported (26). The most serious problem associated with intralesional injection of bleomycin relates to the neurotoxic effects of drug leakage on normal neural tissue, in particular the hypothalamus.

In contrast to predominantly cystic tumors, intralesional injection of bleomycin into solid or mixed craniopharyngiomas has demonstrated minimal or no effect (13). A substitute for bleomycin might be interferon (IFN)-α, which has low neurotoxicity. Its intralesional use was described in nine patients with cystic craniopharyngiomas and resulted in disappearance of the tumor in seven and partial tumor reduction in the other two at a mean of 20 months of follow-up (27).

Recurrence

Although craniopharyngiomas are histologically benign, they are characterized by a high incidence of tumor recurrence. The pathogenesis of recurrence is unclear. One hypothesis contends that "brain invasion" is the most likely nidus for tumor regrowth. This invasion, seen in some specimens of craniopharyngioma, represents in fact islets of tumor cells surrounded by neural tissue and does not represent true invasion (6).

Recurrence rates approach 28%, with the average interval to recurrence of two to five years (1,6). The extent of surgical resection is the most significant factor associated with recurrence. Recurrence rates of 7% to 34% have been reported following gross total resection (6,12,15). In contrast, 63% to 90% of the tumors subtotally removed increased in size (7). This rate was reduced to 30% when subtotal removal was combined with adjuvant radiation (6). Most authors agree that an attempt at gross total resection offers the best long-term outcome. However, radical surgery is not without risk, especially in those patients with tumor adherent to vital visual pathway structures and the hypothalamus, damage to which may have disastrous consequences. On the other hand, radiation therapy has its own inherent risks that are compounded in the developing nervous system.

Various modalities exist for the treatment of recurrent tumor. Most authors still advocate surgery for recurrent disease, if accessible, with radiation reserved for those tumors deemed not amenable to surgery (6). Reoperation for tumor regrowth carries a higher morbidity and the possibility of total removal is decreased (6,11). Age and location of tumor are important factors for consideration in the surgical treatment for recurrent disease. The deleterious effects of irradiation on the developing nervous system warrant an attempt at radical resection in children. Similarly, patients harboring residual tumor in accessible areas are good candidates for reoperation.

Outcome

In a literature review, the 5- and 10-year survival rates were found to be 58% to 100% and 24% to 100% for total resection, 37% to 71% and 31% to 52% for subtotal excision, and 69% to 95% and 62% to 84% for subtotal resection and postoperative radiotherapy (28). In a study of 75 patients treated with surgery alone or with subtotal resection plus radiotherapy, no significant difference was observed in overall survival (29).

Craniopharyngioma is one of the main causes of hypothalamic–pituitary dysfunction in childhood and may arise from the tumor itself or as a result of the treatment (30). Some authors have argued that the incidence of endocrine dysfunction is greater after total resection than after subtotal resection (7,9). Radiotherapy after partial resection may result in less endocrine dysfunction than a total resection does and may not be as harmful on the pituitary–hypothalamic axis (7,30). Others have noted no difference between the extent of resection and endocrine dysfunction with the exception of an increased incidence of DI after a radical dissection (11).

Multiple endocrinopathies occur in 84% to 97% of patients after treatment (29). In one series of 66 children with craniopharyngiomas, the most frequent hypothalamic dysfunctions after treatment were GH deficiency (100%), gonadotropin deficiency (80%), and thyroid deficiency (74%) (30). Adrenal insufficiency increased from 18% at diagnosis to 57% after treatment, DI from 17% to 52%, hypothyroidism from 15% to 74%, and hyperprolactinemia from 8% to 21% (30). The need for long-term hormone replacement occurred in 60% to 100% of patients (11,12,16).

Morbidity can be considerable even when the tumor can be resected completely. Patients with a childhood craniopharyngioma often suffer from severe obesity, which significantly affects the quality of life (31). Hypothalamic damage can also result in defective short-term memory, limited concentration span, defective thirst sensation, and sleep disturbance.

Poor functional outcomes were associated with large tumors infiltrating or displacing the hypothalamus, the occurrence of hydrocephalus, young age at diagnosis, and multiple surgeries because of tumor recurrence. Patients with craniopharyngiomas rated their health-related quality of life considerably lower than healthy controls, and their social and emotional functioning were particularly affected. Cognitive dysfunction and disability occurred frequently in patients with craniopharyngiomas. Neurocognitive dysfunction, including difficulties with concentration, learning, and memory, were well-known complications of radical craniopharyngioma surgery. The incidence of epilepsy ranged from 7% to 17%. Visual complications, including decreased visual acuity or constriction of the visual field, occurred in approximately 30% to 50% (11).

Conclusions

Advances in neurosurgical technique, radiation therapy, and adjuvant endocrine treatment have provided a better prognosis, but craniopharyngiomas still present a difficult management problem. The surgeon must consider the goals of therapy and the possible sequelae of treatment. Therapy should be individualized for each patient to achieve the best overall management retaining quality of life, with a solid understanding of limitations and risks of treatment.

PITUITARY ADENOMA

Benign adenomas of the anterior pituitary gland are common, accounting for almost 10% of surgically removed intracranial neoplasms and approximately 20% of all surgeries performed for primary brain tumors (32). Endocrinologically active tumors may secrete any of the hormones usually produced by the anterior pituitary gland, although 25% of pituitary adenomas are not associated with clinical evidence of endocrine hyperfunction (32). Pituitary adenomas are classified on the basis of size and endocrinologic function. Microadenomas are those tumors less than 10 mm in diameter; larger tumors are identified as macroadenomas.

Clinical Features

Presentation

Visual Abnormalities: Pituitary tumors cause neuro-ophthalmologic or visual changes more often than do other tumor types because the proximity of the pituitary gland to the optic chiasm allows compression of the optic nerves via mass effect, resulting in temporary or permanent visual deficit. Loss of peripheral vision (bitemporal hemianopsia) is noted most often. Superior quadrantanopsia is the most common presentation, whereas patients with craniopharyngiomas most commonly present with inferior quadrantanopsia.

A comprehensive visual field examination is highly recommended for all pituitary tumor patients, especially those with macroadenomas. Visual fields often improve after resection of the tumor but improvement may be minimal in cases with extensive periods of visual loss before surgical or medical treatment.

Endocrine Abnormalities: Any patient with a presumptive pituitary tumor should have a comprehensive endocrine evaluation of all major pituitary hormones to establish the secretory status of the tumor, provide an evaluation of baseline pituitary function, and identify those patients in whom efficacious medical therapy should be initiated (e.g., prolactinoma). Preoperative endocrine evaluation should include measurement of serum GH and IGF-1, prolactin, cortisol, ACTH, thyroxine, triiodothyronine and TSH, FSH, LH, and serum testosterone in men. In larger tumors, mild hyperprolactinemia ($<200\,\text{ng/mL}$) may be a result of hypothalamo-hypophysial disconnection, or the "stalk effect."

Pituitary tumors can manifest various endocrinopathies depending on their respective cell type. The most common subtypes of adenomas include prolactinomas and nonfunctional tumors, which present with no apparent hypersecretory syndrome. Prolactinomas, the most common functional adenomas, may present with symptoms of hypogonadism and galactorrhea and can be diagnosed by measuring morning prolactin levels. Other tumors require different techniques for identifying their subtype. For example, acromegaly may be identified by a lack of plasma GH suppression during the oral glucose tolerance test and elevation of IGF-1 levels. Signs and symptoms of hypercortisolism may suggest ACTH-secreting adenomas.

Imaging

T1-weighted MRI, with and without gadolinium enhancement, is the best method of delineating sellar pathology. MRI is superior to CT because of its inherently greater soft-tissue contrast, which allows clear visualization of the optic chiasm, optic nerves, carotid arteries, and cavernous sinuses (33). MRI is also valuable for planning the surgical approach. For smaller tumors, dynamic MRI imaging with intravenous gadolinium contrast may offer better resolution.

Management

Pituitary tumors typically produce symptoms by way of mass effect (including "stalk-section" effect or direct compression of visual apparatus) or hypersecretion of hormone. The objectives of treatment are primarily to eliminate mass effect and its symptoms or normalize hormone secretion, to address effects on pituitary function, and to prevent tumor recurrence.

Incidental nonfunctional microadenomas should be managed conservatively, as they follow a benign course in most cases. In elderly patients, nonfunctional tumors may also be followed if they cause no clinically relevant symptoms. The age of the patient and associated comorbidities, which would determine the surgical risk, should have the primary effect on the decision to treat the tumor more aggressively.

Surgical Treatment

Surgery for pituitary tumors aims to (i) eliminate tumor mass; (ii) normalize hormonal hypersecretion; (iii) preserve normal pituitary function; and (iv) eliminate potential for recurrence (34). A common indication for surgery of pituitary adenomas is a macroadenoma that produces progressive visual loss from mass effect (35).

Trans-sphenoidal removal of GH-secreting adenomas remains the primary treatment of choice in acromegaly (36,37). Successful removal results in a prompt decrease in GH levels. Large tumors in which a "chemical cure" may not be achieved may require additional medical or radiation therapy. Trans-sphenoidal extirpation of a microadenoma in Cushing's disease is also superior to medical management in obtaining prompt and long-term remission (38). Failure of prior medical or radiation therapy may warrant surgical intervention to treat recurrences. Prolactinomas shrink dramatically with medical management (dopamine agonist therapy, usually bromocriptine or cabergoline), although some may be refractory to medical treatment and maintain persistently high levels of prolactin. Additionally, some patients may not tolerate the medical therapy.

Surgery is most often performed via the transnasal trans-sphenoidal route and is very safe in experienced hands, with mortality approaching zero and morbidity related mostly to the risk of CSF leak and postoperative endocrine dysfunction, most commonly transient DI.

Surgical Approaches

The Endonasal Trans-sphenoidal Approach: The trans-sphenoidal approach to the sella, based on the foundations of Hirsch and Cushing, continues to be the preferred method in treating most sellar lesions. We usually employ the endonasal approach. In comparison with the sublabial approach, the endonasal approach produces less patient discomfort and avoids postoperative numbness of the anterior teeth. Although the surgeon gives up some superior trajectory and viewing angle, which slightly limits the visualization of the suprasellar cistern (39), this is more than offset by the ease of performing the endonasal approach and the decreased patient discomfort. The endoscope may be used to facilitate suprasellar exposure from any approach used (40). The details of the surgical approach used by the authors have recently been described in detail (41).

Modifications of the Trans-sphenoidal Approach: The standard trans-sphenoidal approach is used in most cases of pituitary tumors with sellar and suprasellar extension. Occasionally, tumor will be located wholly suprasellar or have significant lateral extension to the parasellar cavernous sinus region. In the last two decades, the classical trans-sphenoidal approach has undergone further transformation. Regions of the skull base that were once thought only accessible "from above" are now being approached transfacially. With better knowledge of microsurgical anatomy and modern microinstrumentation, neurosurgeons have modified the trans-sphenoidal approach to gain better access to regions such as the cavernous sinus and the suprasellar cisterns.

The senior authors have recently described extended trans-sphenoidal approaches to gain additional exposure of the skull base for lesions of the parasellar and clival region (42). By manipulating the patient's head and repositioning the self-retaining speculum, various portions of the skull base may be exposed and bone resection can be extended. The surgeon may successfully extend the standard trans-sphenoidal approach anteriorly to resect suprasellar lesions, inferiorly to expose clival lesions, and inferolaterally to access cavernous sinus lesions (Figs. 1–3) (42). These variations on the trans-sphenoidal approach provide a minimally invasive technique that avoids prolonged surgery and brain retraction.

Endoscope-Assisted Trans-sphenoidal Approach: Technological advances in endoscope-assisted microneurosurgery have been applied to the classical trans-sphenoidal operation to decrease morbidity and mortality risks further. Jho et al. (43) have reported a series of 50 patients who underwent endoscopic endonasal trans-sphenoidal surgery with encouraging results. This approach involves only one nostril (Fig. 4). The endoscope is held in the surgeon's nondominant hand and surgical instruments in the dominant hand. Once the anterior sphenoidotomy is made, the endoscope is mounted, freeing both hands to maneuver instruments. Some surgeons use the endoscope for the initial sphenoidotomy, which is then converted to a microsurgical approach for the tumor resection (45). Others use the endoscope to inspect for residual tumor that may be out of view (46). One of the main advantages of this approach is excellent panoramic visualization of the sellar and suprasellar anatomy with increased illumination and magnification.

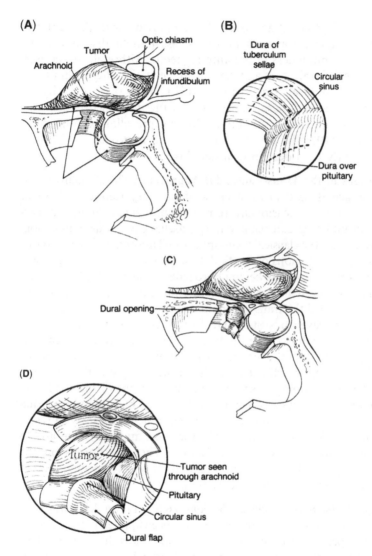

Figure 1 (**A–D**) Modification of the trans-sphenoidal approach: exposure of the anterior skull base (extended trans-sphenoidal). A pure suprasellar tumor may be approached by extending the bony resection anteriorly over the tuberculum sellae, thus exposing the dura mater lying anterior to the circular sinus. An incision is made in the dura anteriorly and inferiorly to the circular sinus. The sinus is then coagulated and transected to gain a direct view of the suprasellar cistern without disturbing the pituitary gland. *Source*: From Ref. 42.

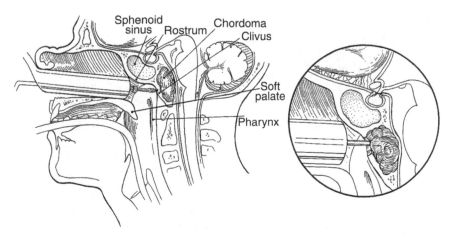

Figure 2 Modifications of the trans-sphenoidal approach: inferior exposure of the clivus. Exposure of the clivus is facilitated by slight flexion of the patient's head and repositioning of the nasal self-retaining retractor to point inferiorly. The upper clivus lies directly posterior to the sphenoid sinus, but additional exposure to the mid- and lower clivus requires more inferior exposure. *Source*: From Ref. 42.

Anatomic studies have demonstrated that the endoscope provides a volume of exposure superior to that of the operating microscope (40). Major drawbacks include the lack of stereoscopic vision and the lack of adequate instrumentation. Working through the limited space of one nostril can also pose potential conflicts, especially between the surgeon's hands and the endoscope (47). Moreover, this technique has a learning curve. Nevertheless, the endoscopic technique offers many advantages of a minimally invasive procedure with satisfying preliminary results. Whether these techniques will lead to more effective management of sellar lesions awaits longer follow-up studies and additional experience.

Pterional Approach: The pterional approach described by Yasargil (48) has become the most widely used approach to access the circle of Willis for treating anterior circulation aneurysms. With removal of the sphenoid wing, a straight trajectory to the parasellar structures provides excellent visualization for removing pituitary tumors with minimized brain retraction. It represents the shortest transcranial trajectory to the suprasellar cistern. This should be the method of choice when a transcranial approach is used in a patient with a prefixed chiasm because the tumor can be resected beneath the chiasm.

Anterior Subfrontal Approach: The anterior subfrontal approach, although used less than the pterional approach, has the advantage of a

(A) **(B)**

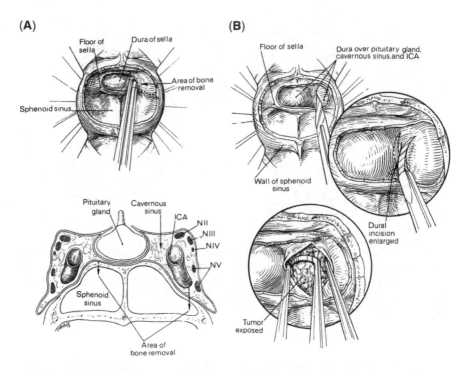

Figure 3 Modification of the trans-sphenoidal approach: inferolateral exposure of the cavernous sinus. (**A**) After exposure of the dura overlying the sella, the bone overlying the cavernous sinus, including that overlying the carotid grooves, is carefully removed. This removal defines the lateral extent of the exposure limited by the cavernous cranial nerves. (**B**) The dura medial to the internal carotid artery is first incised with a size 11 blade and opened with curved alligator microscissors. Removal of the intracavernous portion of the tumor is carried out with a microcurette. *Source:* From Ref. 42.

(A) **(B)**

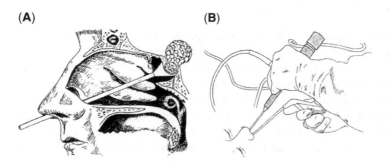

Figure 4 (**A**) Drawing illustrating an endonasal endoscopic approach to the sella. The absence of septal or alar incisions is noted. No speculum or retractor is used. (**B**) Endoscope is held in surgeon's nondominant hand and instruments are held in the dominant hand until anterior sphenoidotomy is made. *Source:* From Ref. 44 with permission from Elsevier.

straight frontal trajectory with direct visualization to the tumor as it is being removed between the optic nerves. The disadvantages include the potential violation of the frontal sinus and damage to olfactory nerves. This procedure is usually not performed in patients with a prefixed chiasm.

Radiation Therapy

Local invasion of the cavernous sinus presents an impediment to successful surgery for many pituitary tumors, which subsequently recur. Persistently elevated pituitary hormones may also be noted after complete resection has apparently been achieved. In these cases, postoperative radiation therapy may offer a resolution. It can be administered postoperatively to prevent regrowth or given after recurrence. Radiation therapy is usually employed as an adjuvant treatment with subtotal resection or in instances of tumor recurrence. It has been proven effective and radiosurgery is being used more frequently. Conventional fractionated radiation therapy successfully controls more than 90% of nonfunctioning adenomas followed up for at least five years; hormone-secreting tumors demonstrate a slightly less favorable response, taking several years to normalize hormone levels. Poor results for GH- and ACTH-producing tumors may suggest that higher radiation doses using newer techniques are needed for effective clinical tumor (and hormonal) control. Many authors have recommended a total dose of 45 Gy, which remains the lowest dose with proven efficacy.

Current high-energy photon techniques have few associated negative symptoms, but administration of ionizing radiation therapy carries the risk of damage to surrounding structures. The most common late complication is hypopituitarism, but other late sequelae can be minimized if the total and daily doses are kept below 50 Gy and 2 Gy, respectively. Radiation may also injure the optic chiasm and nerve, usually producing delayed visual difficulty 9 to 24 months following completion of treatment. Some reports have also suggested radiation-induced arterial occlusion in patients with pituitary adenomas treated with doses over 50 Gy.

Stereotactic radiation techniques can minimize the dose to the adjacent normal tissue by sharply focusing on the dose distribution. Pituitary tumors are particularly well suited to stereotactically focused treatment because of their localized nature and their proximity to radiosensitive structures (hypothalamus and optic chiasm). Because of this benefit, the use of stereotactic radiation will likely supersede field radiation therapy techniques for most small residual or recurrent pituitary tumors. The control rate for tumor growth after linear accelerator (LINAC) or GKRS is comparable with that of published traditional radiation techniques.

In cases where the cavernous sinus has been invaded and residual tumor is expected, pituitary transposition (hypophysopexy) away from the tumor in the cavernous sinus and interposition of a fat graft between the normal gland and the tumor in the cavernous sinus can be performed in anticipation of

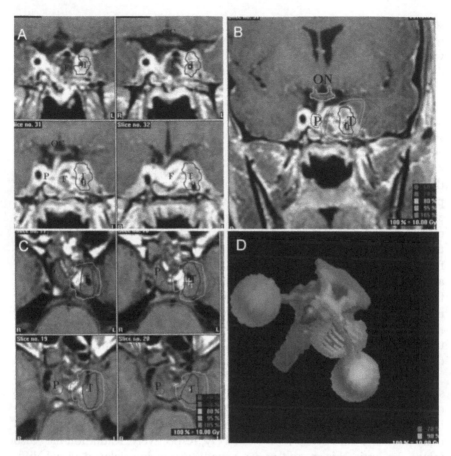

Figure 5 Pituitary transposition (hypophysopexy) with planned radiosurgical treatment of residual cavernous sinus tumor. Acromegalic young woman with residual
tumor within the cavernous sinus following hypophysopexy. Coronal (**A**) T1-weighted
gadolinium-enhanced magnetic resonance images demonstrating the relationship of the
cavernous sinus tumor (*T*), fat graft (*F*), optic chiasm (*OC*), and transposed pituitary
gland (*P*). Isodose curves on coronal image demonstrating doses delivered to surrounding tissues on coronal (**B**) and axial (**C**) images. Lateral displacement of the gland by the
interposed fat graft is noted on coronal image. Diagram representing dosimetry target
in relationship to brainstem and optic apparatus with transposed pituitary in green (**D**).
Source: From Ref. 49 with kind permission of Springer Science and Business Media.

postoperative radiosurgical treatment. This increases the distance between
the pituitary gland and the residual tumor to reduce the effective biological
dose to the normal pituitary gland (Fig. 5). The reduction of radiation exposure to the gland decreases the likelihood of developing hypopituitarism.

Medical Therapy

Prolactin-secreting adenomas comprise 30% to 50% of endocrinologically active neoplasms of the pituitary. Dopamine agonist therapy (bromocriptine and more recently cabergoline) offers the preferred treatment of prolactinomas and it is highly effective. In those rare patients who cannot tolerate side effects of medication or in those in whom the tumor has demonstrated resistance to medical therapy, surgery remains an option.

Medical therapy is also often a component of treatment of GH-secreting adenomas and some ACTH-secreting adenomas. The description of the medical therapy for each of the hypersecretion syndromes is beyond the scope of this chapter, but the reader is referred to an excellent recent review of the topic (50).

Conclusions

Pituitary tumors are common in the general population; prevalence rates approach 20%. Indications for treatment include endocrinopathy and visual disturbances. The majority of symptomatic pituitary tumors are managed with surgical resection, or in cases of prolactin-secreting tumors, very effective medical therapy. Medical therapy for GH- or ACTH-secreting adenomas is less effective, and surgery is indicated in most cases as a component of multimodal therapy. Newer radiotherapy modalities, including shaped-beam LINAC or gamma-knife treatment, are increasingly used in the management of residual or recurrent tumors.

ACKNOWLEDGMENTS

The authors would like to thank Kristin Kraus for her superb editorial assistance.

REFERENCES

1. Adamson TE, Wiestler OD, Kleihues P, et al. Correlation of clinical and pathological features in surgically treated craniopharyngiomas. J Neurosurg 1990; 73(1):12–17.
2. Burger PC, Scheithauer BW, Vogel FS. Surgical Pathology of the Nervous System and its coverings. 4th ed. New York: Churchill Livingstone, 2002.
3. Aho CJ, Liu C, Zelman V, et al. Surgical outcomes in 118 patients with Rathke cleft cysts. J Neurosurg 2005; 102(2):189–193.
4. Ulfarsson E, Karstrom A, Yin S, et al. Expression and growth dependency of the insulin-like growth factor I receptor in craniopharyngioma cells: A novel therapeutic approach. Clin Cancer Res 2005; 11(13):4674–4680.
5. Izumoto S, Suzuki T, Kinoshita M, et al. Immunohistochemical detection of female sex hormone receptors in craniopharyngiomas: Correlation with clinical and histologic features. Surg Neurol 2005; 63(6):520–525; discussion 525.

6. Samii M, Tatagiba M. Craniopharyngioma. In A.H. K, Laws ER Jr., eds. Brain Tumors. New York: Churchill Livingstone, 1995, 873–894.
7. Thomsett M Jr, Conte FA, Kaplan SL, et al. Endocrine and neurologic outcome in childhood craniopharyngioma: Review of effect of treatment in 42 patients. J Pediatr 1980; 97(5):728–735.
8. Cohen ME, Duffner PK. Brain Tumors in Children: Principles of Diagnosis and Treatment. New York: Raven Press, 1994, 285–301.
9. Sklar CA. Craniopharyngioma: Endocrine sequelae of treatment. Pediatr Neurosurg 1994; 21(Suppl 1):120–123.
10. Harwood-Nash DC. Neuroimaging of childhood craniopharyngioma. Pediatr Neurosurg 1994; 21(Suppl 1):2–10.
11. Yasargil MG, Curcic M, Kis M, et al. Total removal of craniopharyngiomas. Approaches and long-term results in 144 patients. J Neurosurg 1990; 73(1):3–11.
12. Fahlbusch R, Honegger J, Paulus W, et al. Surgical treatment of craniopharyngiomas: Experience with 168 patients. J Neurosurg 1999; 90(2):237–250.
13. Takahashi H, Nakazawa S, Shimura T. Evaluation of postoperative intratumoral injection of bleomycin for craniopharyngioma in children. J Neurosurg 1985; 62(1):120–127.
14. Chakrabarti I, Amar AP, Couldwell W, et al. Long-term neurological, visual, and endocrine outcomes following transnasal resection of craniopharyngioma. J Neurosurg 2005; 102(4):650–657.
15. Van Effenterre R, Boch AL. Craniopharyngioma in adults and children: A study of 122 surgical cases. J Neurosurg 2002; 97(1):3–11.
16. Caldarelli M, Massimi L, Tamburrini G, et al. Long-term results of the surgical treatment of craniopharyngioma: The experience at the Policlinico Gemelli, Catholic University, Rome. Childs Nerv Syst 2005; 21(8–9):747–757.
17. Regine WF, Kramer S. Pediatric craniopharyngiomas: Long term results of combined treatment with surgery and radiation. Int J Radiat Oncol Biol Phys 1992; 24(4):611–617.
18. Regine WF, Mohiuddin M, Kramer S. Long-term results of pediatric and adult craniopharyngiomas treated with combined surgery and radiation. Radiother Oncol 1993; 27(1):13–21.
19. Kobayashi T, Tanaka T, Kida Y. Stereotactic gamma radiosurgery of craniopharyngiomas. Pediatr Neurosurg 1994; 21(Suppl 1):69–74.
20. Chiou SM, Lunsford LD, Niranjan A, et al. Stereotactic radiosurgery of residual or recurrent craniopharyngioma, after surgery, with or without radiation therapy. Neuro-oncol 2001; 3(3):159–166.
21. Ulfarsson E, Lindquist C, Roberts M, et al. Gamma knife radiosurgery for craniopharyngiomas: Long-term results in the first Swedish patients. J Neurosurg 2002; 97(5 Suppl):613–622.
22. Mokry M. Craniopharyngiomas: A six year expericence with gamma knife radiosurgery. Stereotact Funct Neurosurg 1999; 72(Suppl 1):140–149.
23. Kalapurakal JA, Goldman S, Hsieh YC, et al. Clinical outcome in children with recurrent craniopharyngioma after primary surgery. Cancer J 2000; 6(6):388–393.
24. Hasegawa T, Kondziolka D, Hadjipanayis CG, et al. Management of cystic craniopharyngioma with phosphorus-32 intracavitary irradiation. Neurosurgery 2004; 54(4):813–820; discussion 820–822.

25. Takahashi H, Yamaguchi F, Teramoto A. Long-term outcome and reconsideration of intracystic chemotherapy with bleomycin for craniopharyngioma in children. Childs Nerv Syst 2005; 21(8–9):701–704.
26. Mottolese C, Stan H, Hermier M, et al. Intracystic chemotherapy with bleomycin in the treatment of craniopharyngiomas. Childs Nerv Syst 2001; 17(12):724–730.
27. Cavalheiro S, Dastoli PA, Silva NS, et al. Use of interferon alpha in intratumoral chemotherapy for cystic craniopharyngioma. Childs Nerv Syst 2005; 21(8–9):719–724.
28. Heideman RL, Packer RJ, Albright LA, et al. Tumors of the central nervous system. In Pizzo PA, Poplak DG, eds. Principles and Practice of Paediatric Oncology. Philadelphia: Lippincott-Raven, 1997, 633–697.
29. Stripp DC, Maity A, Janss AJ, et al. Surgery with or without radiation therapy in the management of craniopharyngiomas in children and young adults. Int J Radiat Oncol Biol Phys 2004; 58(3):714–720.
30. Gonc EN, Yordarn N, Ozon A, et al. Endocrinological outcome of different treatment options in children with craniopharyngioma: A retrospective analysis of 66 cases. Pediatr Neurosurg 2004; 40(3):112–119.
31. Muller HL, Bruhnken G, Emser A, et al. Longitudinal study of quality of life in 102 survivors of childhood craniophryngioma. Childs Nerv Syst 2005; 21(11):975–980.
32. Kovacs K, Horvath E. Tumors of the pituitary gland. Fascicle 21. In: Atlas of Tumor Pathology, Washington, D.C.: Armed Forces Institute of Pathology, 1986.
33. Karnaze MG, Sartor K, Winthrop JD, et al. Suprasellar lesions: Evaluation with MR imaging. Radiology 1986; 161(1):77–82.
34. Laws ER Jr. Pituitary syrgery. Endocrinol Metab Clin North Am 1987; 16(3):647–665.
35. Ebersold ML, Quast LM, Laws ER, Jr., et al. Long-term results in transsphenoidal removal of nonfunctioning pituitary adenomas. J Neurosurg 1986; 64(5):713–719.
36. Davis DH, Laws ER, Jr., Ilstrup DM, et al. Results of surgical treatment for growth hormone-secreting pituitary adenomas. J Neurosurg 1993; 79(1):70–75.
37. Freda PU, Wardlaw SL, Post KD. Long-term endocrinological follow-up evaluation in 115 patients who underwent transsphenoidal surgery for acromegaly. J Neurosurg 1998; 89(3):353–358.
38. Leinung MC, Kane LA, Scheithauer BW, et al. Long term follow-up of transsphenoidal surgery for the treatment of Cushing's disease in childhood. J Clin Endocrinol Metab 1995; 80(8):2475–2479.
39. Das K, Spencer W, Nwagwu CI, et al. Approaches to the sellar and parasellar region: Anatomic comparison of endonasal-transsphenoidal, sublabial-transsphenoidal, and transethmoidal approaches. Neurol Res 2001; 23(1):51–54.
40. Spencer WR, Das K, Nwagu C, et al. Approaches to the sellar and parasellar region: Anatomic comparison of the microscope versus endoscope. Laryngoscope 1999; 109(5):791–794.
41. Couldwell WT. Transsphenodial and transcranial surgery for pituitary adenomas. J Neurooncol 2004; 69(1–3):237–256.

42. Couldwell WT, Weiss MH. The transnasal transsphenoidal approach. In: Apuzzo MLJ, ed. Surgery of the Third Ventricle. 2nd ed. Baltimore: Williams & Wilkins, 1998, 553–574.
43. Jho HD, Carrau RL. Endoscopic endonasal transsphenoidal surgery: Experience with 50 patients. J Neurosurg 1997; 87(1):44–51.
44. Jho HD, Carrau RL, Ko Y. Endoscopic pituitary surgery: an early experience. Surg Neurol 1997; 47:213–223.
45. Yaniv E, Rappaport ZH. Endoscopic transseptal transsphenoidal surgery for pituitary tumors. Neurosurgery 1997; 40(5):944–946.
46. Elias WJ, Laws ER, Jr. Transsphenoidal approaches to lesions of the sella. In Schmidek HH, ed. Operative Neurosurgical Techniques: Indications, Methods, and Results. 4th ed. Philadelphia: W.B. Saunders, 2000, 373–384.
47. Alfieri A. Endoscopic endonasal transsphenoidal approach to the sellar regions: Technical evolution of the methodology and refinement of a dedicated instrumentation. J Neurosurg Sci 1999; 43(2):85–92.
48. Yasargil MG. Microneurosurgery, Vol. 1. Microsurgical Anatomy of the Basal Cisterns and Vessels of the Brain, Diagnostic Studies, General Operative Techniques, and Pathological Considerations of the Intracranial Aneurysms. Stuttgart, Germany: Georg Thieme Verlag, 1984.
49. Couldwell WT, Rosenow JM, Rovit RL, et al. Hypophysopexy technique for a radiosurgical treatment of cavernous sinus pituitary adenoma. Pituitary 2002; 5:169–173.
50. Vance ML. Medical treatment of functional pituitary tumors. Neurosurg Clin N Am 2003; 14(1):81–87.

21

Peripheral Nerve Sheath Tumors

Joachim M. Baehring
*Yale University School of Medicine,
New Haven, Connecticut, U.S.A.*

Serguei Bannykh
*Department of Pathology and Laboratory Medicine, Yale University
School of Medicine, New Haven, Connecticut, U.S.A.*

SCHWANNOMA AND NEUROFIBROMA

Schwannomas and neurofibromas are benign tumors of the peripheral nerve sheath (PNST). Few population-based incidence estimates are available. About 7.9% of primary central nervous system tumors originate from cranial or spinal nerves accounting for 2500 cases per year, but this number does not include tumors arising beyond the intradural nerve root (1). The incidence of schwannomas and neurofibromas is increased in patients with neurofibromatosis type I and II.

Nerve sheath tumors, while commonly found along large nerve trunks, have been described in almost any location in the body. Nearly 40% are located in the brachial plexus (mostly supraclavicular), one-third in the upper extremities (ulnar, median and radial nerves), one quarter in the lower extremities (sciatic nerve and its branches, and femoral nerve), and the remainder in the lumbosacral plexus (2). Schwannomas have a predilection for head, neck, and flexor surfaces of the extremities. Spinal PNSTs are usually extramedullary and either intra- or extradural; they can be located entirely within the spinal canal, paraspinal or extend through the intervertebral foramen. Three quarters of spinal PNST are intradural. The ratio of intradural to extradural tumors increases from the cervical to the lumbosacral level. The vast majority originates from the dorsal rootlets (3). Intracranial schwannomas arise commonly from the sensory branches of cranial nerves such as the acoustic or trigeminal nerves. However, these rarely occur within the cerebral parenchyma.

PNSTs occurring in the neurofibromatoses arise on the background of mutations in two tumor suppressor genes: neurofibromin (NF)1 located on chromosome 17q11.2 (4–6) and NF 2 (Merlin, Schwannomin) on chromosome 22q12.2 (7,8). NF1 contains a domain homologous to the GTPase activating protein family and downregulates activity of the RAS oncogenic pathway. NF2 is structurally related to the ezrin, radixin, and moesin proteins that act as linkers between the plasma membrane and the actin cytoskeleton. NF2 mutations and lack of NF2 expression are also found in sporadic schwannomas (9). The occurrence of melanotic schwannoma in patients with Carney complex, a subset of which carry mutations in PRKAR1A (cAMP-dependent protein kinase regulatory subunit 1α), suggests involvement of this gene in the pathogenesis of this tumor (10).

Patients with PNST complain of pain, paresthesias, numbness, focal weakness, or a slowly expanding, painless mass lesion in the course of a nerve. Transverse myelopathy or cauda equina syndrome from extrinsic compression by an intraspinal PNST occurs late due to the slow growth of these tumors and the compensatory capacity of the affected neural structures. On examination, the masses can be moved laterally, but not longitudinally. Percussion of the tumor elicits paresthesias in the course of the affected nerve. Patients with acoustic schwannomas present with gradual hearing loss and tinnitus, a sensation of fullness in the ear and vertigo. Large tumors give rise to symptoms resulting from compression of brainstem or adjacent cranial nerves. However, the majority is without symptoms and thus undetected.

PNSTs are hypo- to isointense to neural tissue on T1-weighted images. Signal heterogeneity on T2-weighted images reflects myxoid or cystic areas (hyperintense) and fibrous or cellular areas (hypointense). Benign central degenerative changes such as cyst formation, calcification, or hemorrhage give rise to a rim-enhancing appearance of the tumors on gadolinium-enhanced images and should not be mistaken for signs of malignancy (Fig. 1). Paraspinal growth of PNST through the intervertebral foramen into the spinal canal gives rise to a "dumbbell" shape of the tumor. This growth pattern is not unique to PNSTs, but is also seen in paraspinal malignant soft tissue tumors, lymphoma, and lung and renal cell carcinoma. However, only the slow-growing PNSTs result in enlargement of the intervertebral foramen, visible on plain radiographs of the spine (Fig. 2).

Schwannomas are entirely composed of neoplastic Schwann cells. They are encapsulated and grow on the surface of the nerve. Histologic appearance of schwannoma is classically characterized by a biphasic architecture with densely cellular Antoni A and loosely cellular Antoni B areas (Fig. 3).

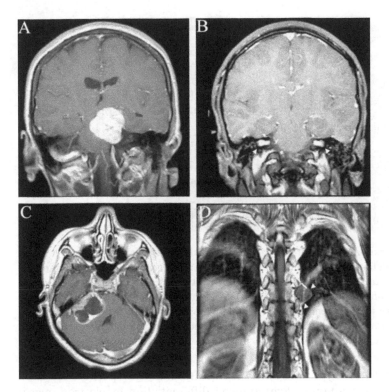

Figure 1 (**A**) Schwannoma of the left trigeminal nerve (coronal T1-weighted magnetic resonance imaging (MRI) of the brain with gadolinium). (**B**) Bilateral acoustic schwannomas in a patient with neurofibromatosis Type II (*arrow heads*; coronal T1-weighted MRI of the brain with gadolinium). (**C**) Cystic acoustic schwannoma. (**D**) Extradural schwannoma of a proximal thoracic spinal nerve (*arrow heads*; coronal T1-weighted MRI of the thoracic spine).

Nuclear palisading (Verocay bodies) are frequent in peripheral but not in central schwannomas. Degenerative changes including cyst formation, characterized by accumulation of lipid-laden macrophages, and "ancient change" nuclear pleomorphism are encountered. The vasculature is typically hyalinized and ectatic. The slightly more aggressive cellular variant of schwannoma lacks Antoni B areas and also Verocay bodies, but retains encapsulation, and often features subcapsular lymphocytic infiltrates. It lacks metastatic potential, but can recur after excision. Attesting to the tumor's origin from the neural crest, a fraction of schwannomas show melanocytic differentiation. Half of melanotic schwannomas contain psammoma bodies, and 50% of those are seen in patients with Carney complex. About 10% of melanotic schwannomas are malignant (11). Another variant of schwannoma growing in a multinodular fashion (plexiform) is frequent in patients with

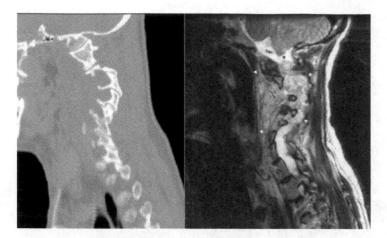

Figure 2 Plexiform neurofibroma in a patient with neurofibromatosis Type I. Sagittal reconstruction of a computed tomography of the cervical and upper thoracic spine demonstrates severe kyphoscoliotic deformity and enlargement of the intervertebral foramina (*left*). Corresponding T2-weighted magnetic resonance imaging (*right*) shows a heterogenous mass lesion (*arrow heads*) extending anteriorly into the retropharyngeal space and posteriorly into the nuchal musculature.

neurofibromatosis Type II. Schwannomas are uniformly positive for S100 and show some features of Schwann cell differentiation by electron microscopy. These include formation of reticulin, collagen IV and laminin-positive basal lamina, and long-spacing collagen (Luse body).

Neurofibromas lack a capsule and are inseparable from the nerve of origin. They are known for their association with von Recklinghausen's disease, although the majority are sporadic. Four variants exist: (i) cutaneous, localized and diffuse type, (ii) intraneural, localized and plexiform, (iii) massive soft tissue type (with its extreme variant elephantiasis neurofibromatosa), and (iv) visceral. All forms of neurofibromas share mixed proliferation of S100-immunoreactive Schwann cells, which are considered to be the only tumor population (12), but also cells of perineurial and fibroblastic differentiation. Mucinous background with "shredded carrots"-type collagen bundles, generally low cellularity, lack of mitotic activity, and occasional "ancient" nuclear atypia characterize typical neurofibroma (Fig. 3). Cellular neurofibromas display increased cellularity with nuclear enlargement, increased mitotic activity, and p53 overexpression; they can be precursor lesions for malignant tumors (MPNST).

Surgical removal is the treatment of choice for PNST and is curative. Schwannomas can be removed with resolution of symptoms and preservation of function in 90% of cases (2,13). Spinal PNSTs can adhere to spinal cord or critical extradural structures such as the vertebral artery rendering complete removal difficult. Transection of the dorsal rootlets rarely results

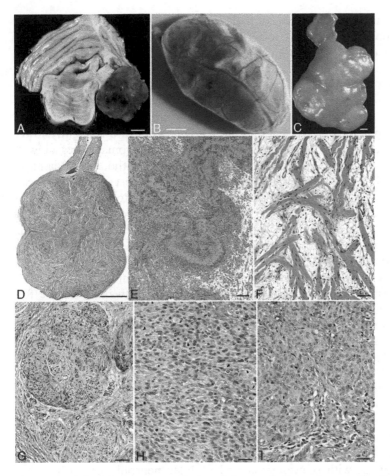

Figure 3 (**A**) Schwannoma of the right cerebellopontine angle. Bar: 0.5 cm.
(**B**) Intradural schwannoma of the thoracic spine. A well-encapsulated bean-shaped
tumor, bulging off the dorsal root, seen at top left. Bar: 0.5 cm. (**C**) This irregularly
shaped, semitranslucent tumor is a neurofibroma. Bar: 0.5 cm. (**D**) Schwannoma of
the lumbar spine appears as a well-encapsulated tumor coming off the dorsal root
(*top*). The tumor is predominantly composed of Antony A areas with prominence
of Verocay bodies. Bar: 0.1 cm. (**E**) Typical morphology of a large schwannoma
showing dense Antony A areas with nuclear palisading (Verocay bodies) and loose
Antony B areas. Bar: 1 mm. (**F**) Histopathologic appearance of neurofibroma.
Paucicellular tumor featuring "shredded carrots"-like collagen bundles composed
of elongated cells sitting in a loose myxoid background. Bar: 0.2 mm. (**G**) Intraneural
perineurioma. A distinct "onion-bulb"-like proliferation of tumor cells involving
several nerve fascicles. Bar: 0.5 mm. (**H, I**) Morphologic appearance of malignant
peripheral nerve sheath tumor (MPNST). (**H**) Inconspicuous but mitotically active
tumors cells form vaguely defined fascicles. Bar: 100 μ. (**I**) Epitheloid areas of
MPNST show lobular arrangements of cells with prominent nucleoli. Bar: 100 μ.

in paresthesias; segmental loss of motor function results from sacrificing the anterior portion of nerve roots at the level of the upper and lower extremities (C5-T1, L3-S1) but is frequently only transient suggesting that nerves afflicted by a nerve sheath tumor are not functional (3,14).

Using an interfascicular approach and neurophysiologic monitoring, gross total removal can also be accomplished in the majority of solitary neurofibromas, although these tumors are not encapsulated and intertwined with their parent and surrounding fascicles. Success rate is slightly lower in NF-related tumors. Treatment of plexiform neurofibromas poses a bigger challenge. Complete resection cannot be accomplished without nerve damage, but subtotal decompressive surgery may relieve pain. Most spinal tumors can be accessed by a posterior or posterolateral approach. More complex approaches including combined anterior–posterior exposure may be required for tumors originating from the anterior rootlets or dumbbell tumors. Thoracoscopy is an alternative for peripherally located tumors (15). An image-guided frameless radiosurgery delivery system is now available, which may have a role in treatment of symptomatic spinal tumors that cannot be resected. Small and stable asymptomatic acoustic schwannomas are followed up with serial magnetic resonance imaging (MRI) scans on an annual basis. Symptomatic tumors are treated with microsurgical resection or stereotactic radiosurgery. Surgical risks include postoperative cerebrospinal fluid leak, facial and trigeminal neuropathy, and deafness. These risks are directly related to tumor size (16). The use of proton radiosurgery or fractionated stereotactic radiation therapy helps achieve tumor "control" without disappearance in over 90% of patients, with hearing complications in approximately 20% (17). The risk of hearing loss has been decreased by limiting the dose to 12 Gy (prescribed to the 50% isodose line).

Complete surgical removal provides long-term local control or cure for the patient with schwannoma and nodular neurofibroma. Malignant degeneration for those tumors is rare. Outcome is less favorable in patients with neurofibromatosis. Transformation into a malignant nerve sheath tumor is more common in plexiform neurofibroma.

PERINEURIOMA

Perineurioma is a rare tumor with distinct perineurial differentiation of the constituent cells. Two forms—intraneural and soft tissue—are distinguished. Intraneural perineurioma affects adolescents and young adults, manifesting as progressive muscle weakness and segmental (2–30 cm) nerve enlargement. Soft-tissue variant predominantly involves the subcutis. Morphology of intraneural perineurioma shows striking "pseudo-onion bulb" proliferations of epithelial membrane antigen (EMA)-positive tumor cells around axons, resembling an appearance of nerve in hypertrophic neuropathies (Fig. 3G). No axons are detected in soft-tissue perineuriomas, and the diagnosis relies on characteristic "bent coin" nuclear morphology, reactivity with EMA, and ultrastructural features. Perineurioma is a benign tumor. Surgical excision of soft tissue variant is curative. Conservative management is advocated for the intraneural perineurioma.

MALIGNANT PERIPHERAL NERVE SHEATH TUMOR

MPNSTs are among the most common malignant mesenchymal tumors of soft tissues, although their overall incidence is low (18,19), largely outnumbered by metastases, benign tumors (neurofibromas and schwannomas), and nontumor lesions.

MPNSTs are derived from Schwann cells, although the diverse phenotype of these tumors suggests derivation from pluripotent cells of the neural crest (20). Most MPNSTs arise from neurofibromas (21–23). Rare occurrences are tumors arising on the background of ganglioneuromas ganglioneuroblastomas, or dermatofibroma protuberans (24–26). There is a genetic predisposition for MPNST in patients with neurofibromatosis type I. About 4% of patients with NF1 develop MPNST compared to an incidence of 0.001% in the general population. About 20% to 60% of MPNSTs are found in the genetic background of NF1 (21–23,27). These tumors can be distinguished from their benign counterparts based on cDNA expression profiling. Plexiform neurofibromas seem to have an intermediate status between dermal neurofibromas and MPNST as they share expression patterns with both. Interestingly, there is no difference in the cDNA expression patterns of sporadic and NF1-related MPNST (28). In contrast to other malignant soft tissue tumors, no pathognomonic chromosomal translocations have been identified in MPNST. Loss of p16^{INK4A} and p53 function seems to play a role in the process of malignant transformation (29). Few patients with Carney complex develop psammomatous melanotic schwannoma, which is malignant in 10% of cases (25). Carney complex is a genetically heterogeneous disorder with linkage to at least two loci.

About 5% to 11% of MPNSTs occur in the brachial or lumbosacral plexus, or the retroperitoneum of patients with Hodgkin's lymphoma, Non-Hodgkin's lymphoma, breast cancer, cancer of the uterine cervix or neuroblastoma between 2 and 41 years after exposure to ionizing radiation (20 Gy and above) (21–23,30,31). Among postradiation sarcomas, MPNST represents a rare histopathological subtype compared to malignant fibrous histiocytoma, osteosarcoma, and fibrosarcoma (0–6%) (32). Tumors arise "de novo" or on the background of benign precursors (neurofibroma and ganglioneuroma).

Brachial plexus, sciatic nerve and spinal nerve roots are the most frequently affected sites (23,26,33). Peripheral nervous system structures with a smaller number of nerve fibers such as spinal nerve roots, and somatic or visceral nerves are less commonly involved. Overall, tumors of the trunk

(46%) are more common than those of extremities (35%) or head and neck (19%) (21). MPNST of the trunk is more common below the diaphragm, and involves one or multiple spinal nerve roots or the lumbosacral plexus. Tumors of the lower extremities arise from the sciatic nerve (52%) followed by the tibial (19%) and femoral (13%) nerve (22). Primary intraspinal location of MPNST is less common than transforaminal extension of a paravertebral tumor. Intracranial MPNST typically involve the trigeminal or the vestibular nerve (34). In half the cases, tumors originate from terminal fibers and thus, a nerve trunk cannot be identified at surgery. Those can be located in almost any location: subcutaneous soft tissue of skin, orbit, esophagus, intestine, liver, prostate, or uterine cervix. Primary intraosseous tumors are located within the mandible or maxilla. Long bones and vertebral bodies are rarely affected. Only a handful cases of primary MPNST of cerebral hemispheres, cerebellum, ventricles, and extradural space have been described (35,36).

MPNSTs most commonly present as a painless, stable or growing mass (36%) (26). Neurological symptoms are encountered at initial manifestation in one-third, most commonly as a painful radiculopathy or plexopathy. Neuropathic pain is almost invariably the defining symptom. Others have strictly localized pain in the area of the mass lesion (21,22,26,37). The rare cases of cerebral MPNST present with seizures. A compressive transverse myelopathy results from transforaminal extension of a brachial plexus tumor. An asymmetric myelopathy or a Brown-Sequard syndrome indicates cord infiltration.

Tumors presenting as bulky masses of the extremities or trunk are easily diagnosed. If not palpable, imaging studies [computed tomography (CT), MRI] reveal large masses with a necrotic center. Imaging characteristics resemble their benign counterparts. T1-weighted MR images depict the tumor as an iso- to hyperintense mass that is markedly enhancing after the application of contrast dye. The margins have an infiltrative appearance. On T2-weighted sequences, MPNST are hyperintense (Fig. 4). CT shows iso- to hypodense (compared to muscle) masses that may contain calcification or cavities (38). MPNSTs involving the most proximal sites of the peripheral nervous system are a diagnostic challenge. Not uncommonly, patients have a longstanding history of neuropathic pain syndromes (radiculopathies and plexopathies), are misdiagnosed with carpal tunnel syndrome or radiculopathies, and even undergo empiric surgical repair for these diagnoses. Early thorough evaluation is crucial in those cases, because centripetal progression with involvement of central neural structures render them unresectable. Workup should include MRI of spine and plexus with coronal sections within the plane of the brachial or lumbosacral plexus. MPNSTs that arise within bony canals can lead to dilatation and ultimately destruction of the bone visible on plain X-ray images. Patients who present with neuropathic pain or a neurological deficit in an area previously irradiated pose another difficult diagnostic problem. MPNST is a rare complication compared to radiation-induced fibrosis or recurrence of

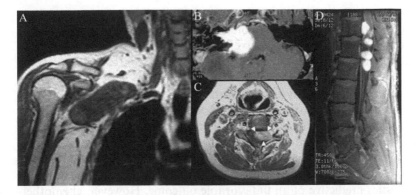

Figure 4 (**A**) Malignant peripheral nerve sheath tumor (MPNST) of the infraclavicular right brachial plexus (coronal T1-weighted MRI). (**B**) Malignant schwannoma of the right vestibulocochlear nerve (axial T1-weighted MRI with gadolinium). (**C**) MPNST of the supraclavicular left brachial plexus. This image demonstrates infiltration (*arrow heads*) and displacement of the cervical spinal cord to the right by the tumor that had grown along the nerve root through the intervertebral foramen (axial T1-weighted MRI with gadolinium). (**D**) Leptomeningeal metastases from MPNST of the eighth cranial nerve (same patient as in **B**). Tumor nodules attached to the cauda equina are shown (sagittal T1-weighted MRI with gadolinium of the lumbosacral spine).

metastatic tumor for which the radiation was given. Pain combined with a Horner's syndrome, tumor location within the lower trunk, and absence of myokymic discharges on electromyography distinguish metastatic brachial plexopathy from brachial neuritis (39). 18-Fluorodeoxyglucose positron emission tomography may be useful, but lacks sensitivity.

MPNSTs are usually large masses at initial resection, ranging in size from 1.5 to 30 cm. Immunohistochemistry demonstrates staining of tumor cells with vimentin, S100, myelin basic protein, and Leu-7. Up to one-third of tumors express glial acidic fibrillary protein. Loss of S100 immunoreactivity may accompany the process of malignant degeneration. A three-tiered grading system based on cellularity, pleomorphism, necrosis, and mitoses is commonly used, but a consensus has not been reached. Up to 20% of MPNSTs contain heterotopic elements such as cartilage, bone, striated muscle (rhabdomyoblastic differentiation, malignant "triton" tumor), gland and other epitheloid tissue, vascular, melanocytic, or perineurial cell differentiation), reflecting the capacity of the neoplastic neuroectoderm for divergent differentiation or metaplasia (Fig. 3) (20).

Wide surgical excision is the mainstay of treatment for MPNST. Gross total resection is a predictor of extended survival (21–23,26,40). Tumor location and involvement of vital structures determine resectability. Gross total removal is accomplished in the vast majority of MPNST of the extremities, but only in one-fifth of paraspinal tumors (23). Adjuvant or neoadjuvant radiation therapy improves outcome. Brachytherapy or intraoperative high-energy electron irradiation have been successfully used in addition to external beam radiation leading to improved local control and increased overall survival. Limb-sparing surgery in combination with external beam radiation therapy or brachytherapy with iridium-192 has been used as an alternative to amputation in MPNST of the extremities (41,42). The role of chemotherapy has not been clearly defined. Commonly used protocols include Mesna, Adriamycin, ifosfamide, dacarbazine, and high-dose methotrexate with leucovorin rescue. A lack of benefit in clinical studies may reflect a selection bias as recipients of chemotherapy generally have tumor characteristics predictive of an unfavorable outcome. However, chemotherapy does not seem to have a role in the initial treatment of localized, resectable MPNST. Whether patients with incompletely resected tumors or metastases benefit from chemotherapy is unclear. New approaches such as the combination of conventional chemotherapy with intratumoral injection of oncolytic viruses have been subject to early clinical studies (43).

Up to two-thirds of patients suffer a local recurrence of their tumor within 6 to 32 months of their initial diagnosis (21,22,26,33,40). Late local recurrences after up to 25 years have been described. Metastases at presentation are exceptional, but occur in at least 20% of patients during the course of their illness. Hematogenous spread to lung and regional lymph nodes predominates over transforaminal extension of paravertebral MPNST. Leptomeningeal seeding is observed in patients with MPNST of cranial nerves (Fig. 4). Patients with NF1 are at risk of developing a second primary MPNST. Median overall survival exceeds four years (26). Gross total resection, provision of adjuvant radiation therapy, and young age at diagnosis are predictors of a favorable outcome.

REFERENCES

1. Statistical Report. Primary Brain Tumors in the United States, 1997–2001. CBTRUS, Central Brain Tumor Registry of the United States, 2004.
2. Kim DH, Murovic JA, Tiel RL, Moes G, Kline DG. A series of 397 peripheral neural sheath tumors: 30-year experience at Louisiana State University Health Sciences Center. J Neurosurg 2005; 102(2):246–255.
3. Jinnai T, Koyama T. Clinical characteristics of spinal nerve sheath tumors: analysis of 149 cases. Neurosurgery 2005; 56(3):510–515.
4. Viskochil D, Buchberg AM, Xu G, et al. Deletions and a translocation interrupt a cloned gene at the neurofibromatosis type 1 locus. Cell 1990; 62(1):187–192.
5. Xu GF, O'Connell P, Viskochil D, et al. The neurofibromatosis type 1 gene encodes a protein related to GAP. Cell 1990; 62(3):599–608.
6. Wallace MR, Marchuk DA, Andersen LB, et al. Type 1 neurofibromatosis gene: identification of a large transcript disrupted in three NF1 patients. Science 1990; 249(4965):181–186.

7. Rouleau GA, Merel P, Lutchman M, et al. Alteration in a new gene encoding a putative membrane-organizing protein causes neuro-fibromatosis type 2. Nature 1993; 363(6429):515–521.
8. Trofatter JA, MacCollin MM, Rutter JL, et al. A novel moesin-, ezrin-, radixin-like gene is a candidate for the neurofibromatosis 2 tumor suppressor. Cell 1993; 72(5):791–800.
9. Twist EC, Ruttledge MH, Rousseau M, et al. The neurofibromatosis type 2 gene is inactivated in schwannomas. Hum Mol Genet 1994; 3(1):147–151.
10. Kirschner LS, Carney JA, Pack SD, et al. Mutations of the gene encoding the protein kinase A type I-alpha regulatory subunit in patients with the Carney complex. Nat Genet 2000; 26(1):89–92.
11. Killeen RM, Davy CL, Bauserman SC. Melanocytic schwannoma. Cancer 1988; 62(1):174–183.
12. Perry A, Roth KA, Banerjee R, Fuller CE, Gutmann DH. NF1 deletions in S-100 protein-positive and negative cells of sporadic and neurofibromatosis 1 (NF1)-associated plexiform neurofibromas and malignant peripheral nerve sheath tumors. Am J Pathol 2001; 159(1):57–61.
13. Tiel R, Kline D. Peripheral nerve tumors: surgical principles, approaches, and techniques. Neurosurg Clin N Am 2004; 15(2):167–75, vi.
14. Kim P, Ebersold MJ, Onofrio BM, Quast LM. Surgery of spinal nerve schwannoma. Risk of neurological deficit after resection of involved root. J Neurosurg 1989; 71(6):810–814.
15. Dorsi MJ, Belzberg AJ. Paraspinal nerve sheath tumors. Neurosurg Clin N Am 2004; 15(2):217–222, vii.
16. Kaylie DM, Gilbert E, Horgan MA, Delashaw JB, McMenomey SO. Acoustic neuroma surgery outcomes. Otol Neurotol 2001; 22(5):686–689.
17. Harsh GR, Thornton AF, Chapman PH, Bussiere MR, Rabinov JD, Loeffler JS. Proton beam stereotactic radiosurgery of vestibular schwannomas. Int J Radiat Oncol Biol Phys 2002; 54(1):35–44.
18. Kransdorf MJ. Malignant soft-tissue tumors in a large referral population: distribution of diagnoses by age, sex, and location. AJR Am J Roentgenol 1995; 164(1):129–134.
19. Enzinger FM, Weiss SW. Soft Tissue Tumors. 3rd St. Louis, Mo: CV Mosby Co, 1995.
20. Woodruff JM. Pathology of tumors of the peripheral nerve sheath in type 1 neurofibromatosis. Am J Med Genet 1999; 89(1):23–30.
21. Ducatman BS, Scheithauer BW, Piepgras DG, Reiman HM, Ilstrup DM. Malignant peripheral nerve sheath tumors. A clinicopathologic study of 120 cases. Cancer 1986; 57(10):2006–2021.
22. Hruban RH, Shiu MH, Senie RT, Woodruff JM. Malignant peripheral nerve sheath tumors of the buttock and lower extremity. A study of 43 cases. Cancer 1990; 66(6):1253–1265.
23. Kourea HP, Bilsky MH, Leung DH, Lewis JJ, Woodruff JM. Subdiaphragmatic and intrathoracic paraspinal malignant peripheral nerve sheath tumors: a clinicopathologic study of 25 patients and 26 tumors. Cancer 1998; 82(11):2191–2203.
24. Drago G, Pasquier B, Pasquier D, et al. Malignant peripheral nerve sheath tumor arising in a "de novo" ganglioneuroma: a case report and review of the literature. Med Pediatr Oncol 1997; 28(3):216–222.

25. Carney JA. The Carney complex (myxomas, spotty pigmentation, endocrine overactivity, and schwannomas). Dermatol Clin 1995; 13(1):19–26.
26. Baehring JM, Betensky RA, Batchelor TT. Malignant peripheral nerve sheath tumor: the clinical spectrum and outcome of treatment. Neurology 2003; 61(5):696–698.
27. Trojanowski JQ, Kleinman GM, Proppe KH. Malignant tumors of nerve sheath origin. Cancer 1980; 46(5):1202–1212.
28. Holtkamp N, Reuss DE, Atallah I, et al. Subclassification of nerve sheath tumors by gene expression profiling. Brain Pathol 2004; 14(3):258–264.
29. Agesen TH, Florenes VA, Molenaar WM, et al. Expression patterns of cell cycle components in sporadic and neurofibromatosis type 1-related malignant peripheral nerve sheath tumors. J Neuropathol Exp Neurol 2005; 64(1):74–81.
30. Foley KM, Woodruff JM, Ellis FT, Posner JB. Radiation-induced malignant and atypical peripheral nerve sheath tumors. Ann Neurol 1980; 7(4):311–318.
31. Newbould MJ, Wilkinson N, Mene A. Post-radiation malignant peripheral nerve sheath tumour: a report of two cases. Histopathology 1990; 17(3):263–265.
32. Hussussian CJ, Mackinnon SE. Postradiation neural sheath sarcoma of the brachial plexus: a case report. Ann Plast Surg 1999; 43(3):313–317.
33. Wong WW, Hirose T, Scheithauer BW, Schild SE, Gunderson LL. Malignant peripheral nerve sheath tumor: analysis of treatment outcome. Int J Radiat Oncol Biol Phys 1998; 42(2):351–360.
34. Akimoto J, Ito H, Kudo M. Primary intracranial malignant schwannoma of trigeminal nerve. A case report with review of the literature. Acta Neurochir (Wien) 2000; 142(5):591–595.
35. Sharma S, Abbott RI, Zagzag D. Malignant intracerebral nerve sheath tumor: a case report and review of the literature. Cancer 1998; 82(3):545–552.
36. Takahashi Y, Sugita Y, Abe T, Yuge T, Tokutomi T, Shigemori M. Intraventricular malignant triton tumour. Acta Neurochir (Wien) 2000; 142(4):473–476.
37. Vege DS, Chinoy RF, Ganesh B, Parikh DM. Malignant peripheral nerve sheath tumors of the head and neck: a clinicopathological study. J Surg Oncol 1994; 55(2):100–103.
38. Beggs I. Pictorial review: imaging of peripheral nerve tumours. Clin Radiol 1997; 52(1):8–17.
39. Kori SH. Diagnosis and management of brachial plexus lesions in cancer patients. Oncology (Williston Park) 1995; 9(8):756–760.
40. Wanebo JE, Malik JM, VandenBerg SR, Wanebo HJ, Driesen N, Persing JA. Malignant peripheral nerve sheath tumors. A clinicopathologic study of 28 cases. Cancer 1993; 71(4):1247–1253.
41. Fein DA, Lee WR, Lanciano RM, et al. Management of extremity soft tissue sarcomas with limb-sparing surgery and postoperative irradiation: do total dose, overall treatment time, and the surgery-radiotherapy interval impact on local control? Int J Radiat Oncol Biol Phys 1995; 32(4):969–976.
42. Mundt AJ, Awan A, Sibley GS, et al. Conservative surgery and adjuvant radiation therapy in the management of adult soft tissue sarcoma of the extremities: clinical and radiobiological results. Int J Radiat Oncol Biol Phys 1995; 32(4):977–985.
43. Galanis E, Okuno SH, Nascimento AG, et al. Phase I-II trial of ONYX-015 in combination with MAP chemotherapy in patients with advanced sarcomas. Gene Ther 2005; 12(5):437–445.

22

Germinoma, Nongerminomatous Germ Cell Tumors

Masao Matsutani

Department of Neurosurgery, School of Medicine, Saitama Medical University, Moroyamamachi, Irumagunn, Saitama, Japan

INTRODUCTION

Their unique growth sites, characteristic subtypes with different histology, and high incidence in Japan render intracranial germ cell tumors fascinating. They grow at various brain sites as solitary masses or multiple foci; mostly occur in the pineal and neurohypophyseal (suprasellar) region; and they are rarely found in the basal ganglia or at other sites in the brain. Characteristically they include subtypes composed of cells that resemble those seen in the embryonic stage of development, i.e., trophoblast (in choriocarcinoma) that appear as early as the stage of blastocyte formation, yolk sac endoderm (in yolk sac- or endodermal sinus tumors), pluripotent stem cells (in embryonal carcinomas), differentiated embryonic cells (in teratomas), and primordial germ cells (in germinomas). Why choriocarcinoma, essentially a female cancer, grows in the brain of boys remains an interesting question. Epidemiologically, there is a difference in the incidence of these germ cell tumors; they represent 3.0% of all primary brain tumors in Japan (1) while the reported incidence in the United States is 0.6% (2). These features, not observed in other neuroectodermal or embryonal tumors of the brain, have attracted the attention of neuropathologists, neurosurgeons, and now tumor biologists.

HISTOLOGICAL CLASSIFICATION

The World Health Organization classifies germ cell tumors as five basic types (i.e., germinoma, teratoma, choriocarcinoma, yolk sac tumor or endodermal sinus tumor, and embryonal carcinoma); tumors consisting of two or more components are classified as mixed germ cell tumors (3).

Germinomas are composed of small lymphocytes that infiltrate along the vascular connective tissue stroma and large polygonal cells with a pale eosinophilic or clear cytoplasm. The polygonal cells stain positive immunohistochemically for placental alkaline phosphatase (PLAP). Antibodies targeting the protein derived from the proto-oncogene c-kit diffusely stain the surface of the polygonal cells, rendering it an important second immunohistochemical marker for germinomas (4). Some germinomas manifest fibrous tissue and a granulomatous reaction.

Germinomas that contain syncytiotrophoblastic giant cells (STGC) staining positive for human chorionic gonadotropin (hCG) are called germinomas with STGC. As the number of germinomas with a high serum titer of hCG or hCG-β but no STGC has been increasing, the term "hCG-β-secreting germinoma" has been proposed to describe these tumors.

Teratomas are divided into three subtypes according to the degree of tumor cell differentiation, i.e., mature- and immature teratomas, and teratomas with malignant transformation. Mature teratomas contain three well-differentiated germ cell layers, the ectoderm, endoderm, and mesoderm. Immature teratomas are composed of incompletely differentiated tissues resembling those of the fetus; some are positive for α-fetoprotein (AFP) or carcinoembryonic antigen. In the past, these tumors were readily diagnosed as mature teratomas without sufficient consideration of the degree of differentiation in the germ cell layers. Because intracranial germ cell tumors have become better understood, fewer of these tumors are diagnosed as mature teratomas and most are now classified as immature teratomas. The rare form of teratoma with malignant transformation is defined as teratoma with carcinomatous or sarcomatous elements. In the Tokyo and Hokkaido University series, 4 of 30 (13.3%) and 4 of 19 (21.1%) teratomas were teratomas with malignant transformation, respectively (5,6). The term "malignant teratoma (MT)" is often used in discussions of the treatment results of immature teratomas and teratomas with malignant transformation.

Choriocarcinomas are composed of two characteristic cell types, syncytiotrophoblast and cytotrophoblast; these are arranged in a bilayered pattern and are strongly immunopositive for hCG or hCG-β.

Yolk sac tumors or endodermal sinus tumors comprise primitive epithelial cells that proliferate in loose-knit reticular networks or compact sheets. Their diagnostic features are Schiller-Duval bodies and placental alkaline phophatase (PAS)-positive, cytoplasmic and extracellular eosinophilic droplets immunopositive for AFP.

Embryonal carcinomas are made of primitive epithelial cells growing in solid sheets or poorly formed glands. Some are positive for AFP, hCG, or hCG-β.

In mixed tumors, the most frequently observed components are germinomatous, followed by teratomatous (mature or immature) components. Among 49 mixed germ cell tumors reported in the Tokyo University series (5), 43% were mixed tumors with germinomatous and teratomatous components, 33% were germinomas, and 24% were teratomas with other components. There were no mixed tumors with other than germinomatous or teratomatous components.

The incidence of these pathological subtypes differs from other reports in which germinomas represented 40% to 60%, teratomas 10% to 20%, pure malignant germ cell tumors (choriocarcinomas, yolk sac tumors, and embryonal carcinomas) approximately 5%, and mixed tumors 15% to 30% (Table 1).

SEX AND AGE DISTRIBUTION

According to a recent statistical analysis of the Committee of Brain Tumor Registry in Japan (1), 1463 patients with intracranial germ cell tumors were registered between 1984 and 1996; of these, 1068 were males (73.0%) and 395 females (27.0%). Only 43 patients (2.9%) were younger than five years and 90 (6.2%) were older than 35 years; 1026 patients (70.1%) were between 10 and 24 years.

Among 252 histologically verified patients assessed by the Japanese Pediatric Brain Tumor Study Group (JPBTSG), 204 were male (81%) and

Table 1 Incidence of Histological Subtypes

	Tokyo University (5) $n=153$	Hokkaido University (6) $n=111$	Japanese Pediatric Brain Tumor Study Group[a] $n=252$
Germinoma	55 (36%)	60 (54%)	142 (56%)
Germinoma with syncytiotrophoblastic giant cells	8 (5%)	14 (13%)	39 (15%)
Teratoma, mature	19 (12%)	6 (5%)	
Malignant[b]	11 (7%)	13 (12%)	10 (4%)
Pure malignant GCT	11 (7%)[c]	4 (4%)[d]	14 (6%)[e]
Mixed tumor	49 (32%)	14 (13%)	47 (19%)

[a]Japanese Pediatric Brain Tumor Study Group (unpublished data).
[b]Including immature teratomas and teratomas with malignant transformation.
[c]Three choriocarcinomas, five embryonal carcinomas and three yolk sac tumors.
[d]Four yolk sac tumors.
[e]Five choriocarcinomas, three embryonal carcinomas and six yolk sac tumors.
Abbreviation: GCT, germ cell tumor.

48 female (19%). Their average age was 16.8 ± 7.0 years (range 2–44); only six patients (2.4%) were younger than five years and seven (2.8%) were older than 35 years; 205 patients (81.3%) were between 8 and 24 years old (unpublished data).

TUMOR LOCATION

Most germ cell tumors arise in the pineal area followed by the suprasellar region (Fig. 1). Some are found in the basal ganglia and thalamus and approximately 10% to 20% occur at multiple sites.

Advances in magnetic resonance imaging (MRI) and ventricular endoscopy have changed conventional notions regarding the location of these tumors. Fujisawa et al. (7) reported germinomas in the suprasellar region, which originated in the neurohypophysis; these tumors exhibited intramedullary growth in a line from the hypothalamus, pituitary stalk, and pituitary posterior lobe (neurohypophysis) (Fig. 2). Their MRI findings were confirmed by autopsy studies. A survey of pituitary function in patients with neurohypophyseal germinomas (8) revealed decreased levels of anterior pituitary hormones [especially growth hormone (GH), follice stimulating hormone (FSH), and luteinizing hormone (LH)] and vasopressin, and elevated prolactin titers; these are features of panhypopituitarism attributable to neurohypophyseal dysfunction. The anatomical and functional characteristics of suprasellar tumors led to the adoption of the term "neurohypophyseal tumors" to describe these neoplasms.

It is now possible to determine more precisely the location of multiple tumors; it is not uncommon to reveal the presence of small tumor nodules in the wall of the third or lateral ventricle in patients with pineal or neurohypophyseal tumors on MRI. In addition, ventricular endoscopy can disclose small tumor nodules or fragments on or beneath the ventricular ependyma that are not detected on MRI scans (Fig. 3) (9).

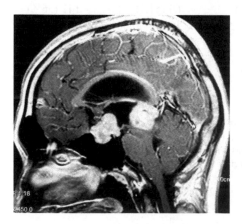

Figure 1 Pineal and neurohypophyseal germinoma is well enhanced by gadolinium (T1-weighted magnetic resonance imaging).

(A)   (B)

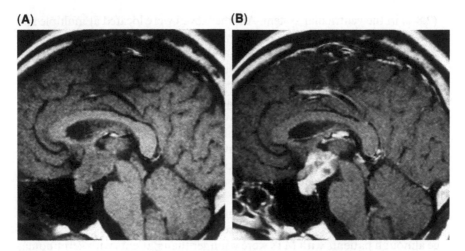

Figure 2 Neurohypophyseal mixed tumor with predominant component of embryonal carcinoma. The tumor occupies hypothalamus, pituitary stalk and pituitary gland suggesting intramedullary growth in the neurohypophysis. It manifests as an irregularly shaped, isointense mass on T1-weighted magnetic resonance imaging (A) with heterogeneous enhancement (B).

Among 252 histologically verified tumors listed in the JPBTSG database, 106 (42.1%) were restricted to the pineal region on MRI and 60 (23.8%) to the neurohypophysis; 43 (17.1%), including multiple tumors, arose in the vicinity of the third or lateral ventricle, 23 (9.1%) in the basal ganglia, and

(A)   (B)

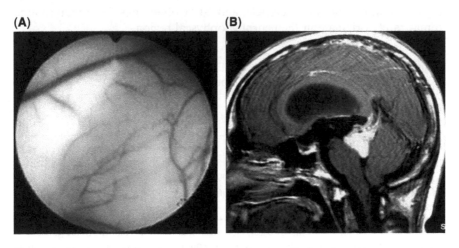

Figure 3 In a case of pineal germinoma, endoscopy disclosed small tumor nodules beneath the ventricular ependyma (A) that was not detected on magnetic resonance imaging scans. (B) Biopsy of the nodule revealed germinoma cells.

7 (2.8%) in the ventricular system. Another seven were located at multiple and six at other sites. None of the tumors were both intracranial and spinal.

With respect to tumor location and sex, only 3 of 106 (2.8%) pineal tumors, 6 of 43 (14.0%) tumors around the third ventricle, and 1 of 23 (4.3%) tumors in the basal ganglia occurred in females. However, slightly more females than males (33 vs. 27) had tumors in the neurohypophysis. It is well known that germ cell tumors develop predominantly in males, and this male predominance is equally found in histological subtypes: the pure germinomas (79.6% of them are in males), hCG or hCG-•- secreting germinomas (84.6%), MTs (70.0%), mixed tumors comprised primarily of germinomatous or teratomatous components (82.4%), and highly malignant tumors including choriocarcinomas, yolk sac tumors, embryonal carcinomas, and mixed tumors mainly consisting or these elements (82.5%). Overall, there was no obvious correlation between the different histological subtypes and patient age although patients with MTs were younger than patients with germinomas or highly malignant germ cell tumors (Table 2).

Before the introduction of diagnostic MRI, it appeared that the incidence of germinomas in the neurohypophyseal region was similar to, or only slightly higher than that of germinomas in the pineal region. The reported distribution of neurohypophyseal and pineal tumors was 58% and 37% (10), 49% and 38% (11), and 45% and 45% (5). However, recent examination of these tumors by MRI and endoscopy led to an increase in the number of cases with multiple tumors along the third ventricle and the designation of these tumors as being of pineal or neurohypophyseal origin became controversial. Among 142 germinomas registered in the JPBTSG database, 51 arose solely from the pineal region, 37 solely in the neurohypophyseal region, 30 along the third ventricle, and 24 at other sites. Pure mature teratomas rarely originate in the neurohypophyseal region.

Table 2 Histological Subtypes and Age Distribution from the Japanese Pediatric Brain Tumor Study Group Database (Unpublished Data)

Histological subtypes	Age mean ± SD	G	hCG-G	MT	MMX	HMT
G ($n = 142$)	17.93 ± 7.10	–	n.s.	0.007	0.006	n.s.
hCG-G ($n = 39$)	15.92 ± 5.97	n.s.	–	0.042	n.s.	n.s.
MT ($n = 10$)	11.00 ± 5.74	0.007	n.s.	–	n.s.	n.s.
MMX ($n = 34$)	14.67 ± 5.74	0.006	n.s.	n.s.	–	n.s.
HMT ($n = 27$)	16.59 ± 8.05	n.s.	n.s.	0.037	n.s.	–

Abbreviations: n.s., not significant by t-test; G, germinoma; hCG, human chorionic gonadotropin; MT, malignant teratoma (immature teratomas and teratomas with malignant transformation); MMX, moderately malignant mixed tumor (mixed tumor with predominant germinoma or teratoma); HMT, highly malignant tumor (pure malignant germ cell tumors and mixed tumors with predominant highly malignant elements); SD, standard deviation.

CLINICAL SYMPTOMS AND SIGNS

Patients with germ cell tumors manifest symptoms and signs attributable to the affected site. Tumors in the pineal region tend to compress and obstruct the cerebral aqueduct, resulting in progressive hydrocephalus with intracranial hypertension. They also compress the tectal plate and produce the characteristic upward- and downward-gaze palsy (Parinaud sign) and Argyll-Robertson pupils. Patients with suprasellar or neurohypophyseal tumors present with bitemporal hemianopsia and decreased visual acuity due to compression of the optic chiasm. Tumor invasion into the neurohypophysis results in panhypopituitarism and diabetes insipidus. A survey of pituitary function revealed decreased levels of anterior pituitary hormones (especially GH, FSH, and LH) and vasopressin and elevated prolactin titers (8). Patients with tumors in both the pineal and the neurohypophyseal region exhibit signs characteristic for tumors at these sites (5). Tumors in the basal ganglia or thalamus invade the pyramidal tract and result in contralateral hemiparesis.

With the exception of hCG-secreting tumors, the clinical signs and symptoms of the different histological subtypes are not tumor specific. Some hCG-secreting tumors manifest with intratumoral hemorrhage that results in acute intracranial hypertension. In sexually immature males, they induce precocious puberty. The induction of precocious puberty by ectopic hCG in only prepubertal males in the absence of elevated LH and FSH levels has been explained as follows: as hCG and LH share structural homology in their β-subunits, hCG, because of its LH-like hormonal action, stimulates Leydig's cells to produce testosterone prematurely. On the other hand, as both LH and FSH are necessary for the production of estradiol, hCG alone does not usually induce precocious puberty in girls. The few instances of precociously pubertal girls (12,13) suggest that hCG has some weak intrinsic FSH-like activity. The rarity of precocious puberty in girls is also explicable by the extremely low incidence of germ cell tumors that secrete a high level of serum hCG or hCG-β in this subpopulation. We counted only three girls younger than eight years among 56 reported patients with histologically verified choriocarcinoma or serum hCG or hCG-β titers exceeding 500 IU/l or 100 IU/l, respectively (14).

RADIOLOGICAL FINDINGS

MRI is useful not only for detecting the tissue components of the tumor but also for revealing its anatomical relationship with adjacent critical structures, and for choosing appropriate surgical strategies. However, because some tumor types manifest few characteristic CT or MRI features, it remains impossible to establish a histological diagnosis based on neuroradiological findings alone (15).

Germinomas are visualized as iso- or slightly low-signal areas on T1-weighted MRI scans; they appear as iso- or high-signal areas on T2-weighted images. They are mostly homogeneously and partly heterogeneously enhanced by gadolinium. They are round, square round, or oval, and their shape is regular in most cases. Some germinomas contain multiple small cysts; large cysts without a solid part are uncommon. In some instances, focal edema is seen. The MRI pattern of hCG- or hCG-β-secreting germinomas is almost identical to that of pure germinomas except for the occasional presence of intratumoral hemorrhage. Although germinomas in the basal ganglia tend to exhibit the same MRI pattern, some present with unusual MRI findings; the T1-weighted images are almost normal, an ill-defined hyperintense area is seen on T2-weighted images, and there is no or very weak gadolinium contrast enhancement. In such cases, high uptake on ^{11}C-methionine positron emission tomographs has been reported (16). An additional common MRI finding in early-stage basal ganglia germinomas is atrophy of the ipsilateral basal ganglia.

Mature teratomas are characterized by their irregular shape with clear margins, mixed signals, and the frequent presence of large cysts and areas of calcification. MRI studies are useful for detecting fatty components. Basically, the images of immature and MTs are identical to those of mature teratomas (Fig. 4). However, their cystic components tend to be smaller and areas of calcification are rarer. The demonstration of perifocal edema, a feature not observed in mature teratomas, is suggestive of immature or malignant components.

Choriocarcinomas appear as isointense masses on T1-weighted and iso- to hyperintense on T2-weighted images; this renders their appearance slightly different from germinomas. Most choriocarcinomas are intensely enhanced by gadolinium. CT scans are useful for detecting intratumoral hemorrhage.

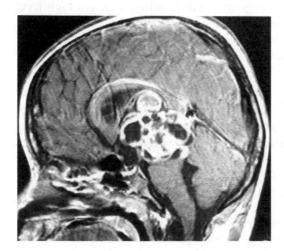

Figure 4 Pineal immature teratoma. An irregularly shaped tumor with multiple cysts extends from the pineal region into the third ventricle. The tumor parenchyma is well enhanced by gadolinium.

The MRI pattern of yolk sac tumors and embryonal carcinomas exhibits identical features. These tumors manifest as an irregularly shaped iso-, hypo-, or hyperintense, homogeneously enhancing mass; cystic components and perifocal edema are also observed.

In mixed tumors, the presence of homogeneous, slightly high- or high-signal areas on MRI suggests a germinomatous component. On the other hand, visualization of multiple calcified areas or multiple medium- to large-sized cysts is strongly suggestive of teratomatous differentiation.

SERUM TITERS OF AFP, HCG (HCG-β), AND PLAP

While a preoperative survey of these tumor markers is essential in patients with germ cell tumors, in most cases, the results are not informative regarding the histological tumor subtype. Some patients with immature teratomas or embryonal carcinomas manifest high hCG (or hCG-β) and AFP serum titers.

In the Tokyo University series (5), among 56 patients with nongerminomatous germ cell tumors, 6 of 11 with MT, 8 of 11 with mixed germinoma and teratoma (MGT), and 6 of 10 with tumors containing embryonal carcinoma had normal AFP or hCG titer. On the other hand, all three choriocarcinomas and one mixed tumor that consisted primarily of choriocarcinoma produced highly elevated serum hCG levels (2120–32,000 and 6000 mIU/ml, respectively). Patients with tumors other than choriocarcinoma manifested serum hCG titers below 770 mIU/ml; they were 40 to 690 mIU/ml in all seven germinomas with STGC, 30 to 590 mIU/ml in four immature teratomas, and 61 to 770 mIU/ml in three mixed tumors. Highly elevated AFP titers were recorded for all three yolk sac tumors (2700–9500 ng/ml) and for three mixed tumors mainly comprising yolk sac tumors (3380–6700 ng/ml); these levels were elevated to a lower degree in three immature teratomas (7.5–500 ng/ml), two embryonal carcinomas (183–700 ng/ml), and 11 mixed tumors consisting of a small part of immature teratoma, embryonal carcinoma, or yolk sac tumor (7.3–1810 ng/ml).

AFP and hCG titers reflect the number of cells secreting these proteins. Thus, when they exceed 2000 ng/ml or 2000 mIU/ml, respectively, they are useful for differentiating between tumors with predominant choriocarcinoma or yolk sac components and other kinds of tumors that secrete these markers such as immature teratomas or germinomas with STGC. Elevated serum and cerebrospinal fluid (CSF) levels of PLAP are characteristic of tumors composed wholly or partly of germinoma; elevated PLAP titers indicate that the tumor contains germinomatous components.

TREATMENT: PAST AND PRESENT

The traditional approach to germinomas consisted of biopsy followed by prophylactic craniospinal irradiation and a boost to the local area because these tumors may disseminate throughout the CSF pathways. According to five reports with more than 30 patients (6,17–20), 87% to 91% of 366 patients with pure germinomas treated primarily with craniospinal radiation therapy alone survived for at least 10 years. Due to advances in imaging technology, the proportion of patients presenting with metastatic disease at the time of germinoma diagnosis is low, and the risk of secondary seeding outside the irradiated volume did not exceed 12% in histologically verified series (5,18,21). In children, irradiation of the neuroaxis resulted in mental retardation, pituitary gland dysfunction, and short stature in later life (22,23). Therefore, the benefits of craniospinal radiotherapy appear questionable, especially in view of the report by the Tokyo University group that the 15-year survival rate of patients with localized germinomas who were treated by extended focal irradiation that included almost the entire ventricular field, i.e., the third and lateral ventricles as well as the sella and pineal region, was 87.9% (5).

After combination chemotherapy with cisplatin was confirmed to be effective in gonadal germ cell tumors, nongerminomatous germ cell tumors in the brain became candidates for chemotherapy. Because platinum-based chemotherapy yielded a complete response rate of 85% to 100% in patients with germinomas (24,25), chemotherapy may eventually replace radiotherapy as the primary treatment modality for central nervous system (CNS) germinomas.

Nongerminomatous tumors proved refractory to conventional treatments with surgery and irradiation. A retrospective survival analysis of 216 patients with intracranial germ cell tumors who had received conventional treatment revealed that most patients with nongerminomatous tumors did not survive beyond three years (10).

According to an analysis of the results obtained in patients with nongerminomatous germ cell tumors treated by radiation therapy with or without chemotherapy (5), the 10-year survival rate of 11 patients with MTs was 70.7%. On the other hand, the three-year survival rate of 11 patients with pure malignant germ cell tumors (PM) choriocarcinoma, yolk sac tumor, and embryonal carcinoma) was 27.3%. In 39 patients with mixed tumors, the three- and five-year survival rates were 94.1% and 84.7%, respectively, for MGT, 70.0% and 52.5% for mixed tumors predominantly comprising germinomatous or teratomatous components and a small portion of pure malignant tumors (MXB), and both 9.3% for mixed tumors mainly consisting of pure malignant elements (MXM). In a retrospective analysis, cisplatin- or carboplatin-based combination chemotherapy delivered before or after radiation therapy was effective in patients with moderate malignancy (MT, MGT, and MXB) but not in those with highly malignant tumors (PM and MXM) (26).

Based on experience gained with radiation therapy and in pilot chemotherapy trials, prospective phase II and phase III studies were designed to assess the effectiveness of combination chemo- and radiation therapy to treat patients with germ cell tumors. Their aim was to reduce the irradiated volume and radiation dose in patients with germinoma, and to prolong the survival of patients with nongerminomatous tumors.

The Japanese Pediatric Brain Tumor Study Group

In 1995, a multi-institutional phase II study was started under the auspices of the JPBTSG (27); it was founded on treatment results obtained in Japanese patients with germ cell tumors. Patients were divided into good prognosis (pure germinoma), intermediate prognosis (moderate malignancy), and poor prognosis (high malignancy) groups (Table 3). Patients with hCG- or hCG-β-secreting germinomas were placed in the intermediate prognosis group because these tumors have a higher recurrence rate than pure germinomas (5).

The treatment strategy included surgical debulking of the tumor and verification of its histological composition, followed by preirradiation chemotherapy and subsequent radiation therapy. Two chemotherapy regimens were studied. The carboplatin–etoposide combination consisted of carboplatin (450 mg/sqm) on day 1 and etoposide (150 mg/sqm) on days 1 to 3. The ifosfamide–cisplatin–etoposide (ICE) combination delivered ifosfamide (900 mg/sqm), cisplatin (20 mg/sqm), and etoposide (60 mg/sqm) on days 1 to 5. Each regimen was repeated every four weeks for three total courses as an induction therapy. Radiation therapy was subsequently delivered to the tumor area, the generous local area, or the whole brain and the whole spine.

Table 3 Therapeutic Classification in the Japanese Pediatric Brain Tumor Study Group

Good prognostic group
Germinoma, pure
Intermediate prognostic group
Germinoma with syncytiotrophoblastic giant cells or, hCG- or hCG-β-secreting germinoma
Immature teratoma
Teratoma with malignant transformation
Mixed tumors composed of predominant germinoma or teratoma
Poor prognostic group
Choriocarcinoma
Yolk sac tumor
Embryonal carcinoma
Mixed tumors composed of predominant choriocarcinoma, yolk sac tumor, or embryonal carcinoma

Abbreviation: hCG, human chorionic gonadotropin.

Patients with pure germinoma received three courses of CARE followed by local irradiation (24 Gy) to the generous local field encompassing the tumor site, the third and lateral ventricles, and the sellar and pineal regions. The choice of a 24 Gy dose was based on data regarding the maximum dose that could be delivered without inducing radiation damage to the anterior pituitary gland in children (28). Patients in the intermediate prognosis group received three courses of CARE followed by 30 Gy irradiation to a generous local field and 20 Gy to the tumor site. They then received additional CARE chemotherapy every three to four months for a total of five cycles. Patients in the poor prognosis group received three courses of ICE followed by whole brain and spinal irradiation with a dose of 30 Gy, and a 30 Gy boost delivered to a generous local field and additional ICE chemotherapy every three to four months for a total of five cycles. However, as four of the initial six patients manifested tumor progression during postoperative chemotherapy, the protocol was modified to start radiation therapy concurrent with chemotherapy.

Entry into the study was closed at the end of 2003. By then, 252 patients had been registered and 228 evaluated (29). The five-year overall survival (OS) rate and event-free survival (EFS) rate in all 123 patients with germinoma were 98.3% and 88.6%, respectively. Of 38 patients with hCG (hCG-β)-secreting germinoma, five suffered recurrence; the five-year OS and EFS rate were 100% and 87.4%, respectively. The five-year OS and EFS rate of 40 patients in the intermediate prognosis group, excluding those with hCG-secreting germinomas, were 94.7% and 81.9%, respectively; the five-year OS rate of 27 patients in the poor prognosis group was 60.2%.

The International CNS Germ Cell Tumor Study Group

This group first conducted a preliminary trial to determine whether irradiation could be avoided by the delivery of four cycles of carboplatin, etoposide, and bleomycin. It encountered a recurrence rate of 49% among 45 patients with germinoma followed for a median of 31 months (30). In the subsequent trial, this group tested the effectiveness and safety of two chemotherapy regimens that consisted of the administration of cisplatin, etoposide, cyclophosphamide, and bleomycin (regimen A) and carboplatin, etoposide, and bleomycin (regimen B). Patients without complete response underwent salvage surgery with or without irradiation. Of 19 germinoma patients, eight remained in complete remission (median follow-up 6.5 years); the five-year EFS rate was 47%. Three patients died of treatment-related toxicity and another died in complete remission from leukoencephalopathy. The study group thus concluded that while the chemotherapeutic strategies used were effective for achieving remission, the long-term outcomes were unsatisfactory due to unacceptably high mortality rates. Of 20 patients with nongerminomatous tumors, eight remained in complete remission and six achieved long lasting second or third complete remission. The five-year EFS- and OS rate were 45% and

75%, respectively. The results obtained in patients with nongerminomatous tumors were considered encouraging (31).

In the third trial, patients were divided into three groups. Group 1 had pure germinomas and was considered low-risk (G-LR group). Group 2 included patients whose germinomas contained hCG-β positive STGC or whose CSF hCG-β titers were less than 50 mIU/ml; these patients were placed in the intermediate-risk group. The third group comprised patients with biopsy-proven nongerminomatous germ cell tumors or elevated serum or CSF AFP levels, elevated serum hCG-β, CSF hCG-β levels greater than 50 mIU/ml, and patients with disseminated disease determined by MRI- or CSF cytology studies; these patients were assigned to the high-risk group (NG-HR group).

Patients in the G-LR group received carboplatin/etoposide in cycles one, three, and five, and cyclophosphamide/etoposide in cycles two, four, and six. Patients in the other two groups were treated with six cycles of car-boplatin/cyclophosphamide/etoposide. Patients with complete response after two or four cycles received two additional cycles after which treatment was considered complete. Patients who did not manifest complete response after four cycles underwent a second-look surgery or were treated with irradiation. Patients in the NG-HR group who failed to respond underwent irradiation or autologous bone marrow transplantation in an effort to obtain a complete radiological response and tumor marker normalization. The two-year OS and EFS rate in all patients in the third trial were 87.7% and 70.1%, respectively; however, the number of patients enrolled in this study was small ($n = 25$) and the follow-up period short (median 28.6 months) (32).

The French Society for Pediatric Oncology

This group conducted a study that combined chemotherapy (alternating courses of etoposide/carboplatin and etoposide/ifosfamide for a recommended total of four courses) with 40 Gy local irradiation to treat 57 patients with localized germinomas. Their three-year EFS rate was 96.4% (33). In their latest report (34), the eight-year OS- and EFS rate in 60 patients were 98% and 83%, respectively. Ventricular dissemination at the margin or outside the field of radiation occurred in 8 of 10 patients.

The Society of International Pediatric Oncology Central Nervous System GCT-96 Trial by the International Society of Pediatric Hematology and Oncology

This group treated 41 patients with germinoma using the French Society for Pediatric Oncology (SFOP) protocol. The five-year EFS rate was 82%, the median follow-up 27 months. In an extended protocol, it used identical chemotherapy regimens; under option A, the patients received craniospinal irradiation with 24 Gy followed by a tumor boost of 16 Gy. Under option B, they received focal irradiation with 40 Gy. The EFS rates were 93% (median follow-up 35 months) and 90% (median follow-up 26 months) in patients treated by option A and B, respectively (35).

A population with nongerminomatous tumors ($n = 122$) comprised patients with localized—including bifocal—disease, received focal radiation therapy (54 Gy) after four courses of cisplatin/etoposide/ifosfamide; patients with dissemination were treated with craniospinal irradiation (54 Gy). The EFS rate was 68% in the absence and 72% in the presence of dissemination, and the median follow-up was 25 months and 33 months, respectively (36).

The Children's Oncology Group

This group performed a phase III study (ACNSO232) of radiation therapy alone (Regimen A) versus chemotherapy followed by response-based reduced radiation therapy (Regimen B) for localized germinomas. Patients subjected to regimen A received 24 Gy to the whole ventricle plus 21 Gy delivered to the involved field. Patients treated by regimen B first underwent chemotherapy with carboplatin/etoposide and cyclophosphamide/cisplatin followed by response-based reduced radiation therapy. In patients in whom a complete response was achieved after two courses of chemotherapy, radiation therapy with 24 Gy to the involved field was followed. Patients with disseminated germinoma either underwent regimen A consisting of craniospinal irradiation (24 Gy) plus 21 Gy delivered to the involved field, or regimen B consisting of 21 Gy craniospinal irradiation plus 9 Gy to the involved field if they manifested a complete response to chemotherapy. The results of this phase III study have not been reported yet (37).

This group also started a phase II study of neoadjuvant chemotherapy with or without second-look surgery to treat nongerminomatous germ cell tumors (ACNSO122). Patients received carboplatin/etoposide/ifosfamide followed by craniospinal irradiation with boost irradiation to the involved field. To date, no Grade 4 toxicity has been encountered in this group of 26 patients (38).

REFERENCES

1. The Committee of Brain Tumor Registry of Japan. Report of Brain Tumor Registry of Japan (1969–1996). 11th ed. Neurol Med Chir (Tokyo) 2003; 43(suppl).
2. Central Brain Tumor Registry of the United States. Primary brain tumors in the United States. Statistical report 1995–1999. CBTRUS, 2002.
3. Kleihues P, Cavenee WK, eds. WHO classificaton of tumours. Pathology & Genetics of Tumours of the Nervous System. Lyon: IARC Press, 2000.
4. Miyanohara O, Takeshima H, Kaji M, et al. Diagnostic significance of soluble c-kit in the cerebrospinal fluid of patients with germ cell tumors. J Neurosurg 2002; 97:177–183.

5. Matsutani M, Sano K, Takakura K, et al. Primary intracranial germ cell tumors: A clinical analysis of 153 histologically verified cases. J Neurosurg 1997; 86: 446–455.

6. Sawamura Y, Ikeda J, Shirato H, et al. Germ cell tumours of the central nervous system: treatment considerations based on 111 cases and their long-term clinical outcomes. Eur J Cancer 1998; 34:104–110.

7. Fujisawa I, Asato R, Okumura R, et al. Magnetic resonance imaging of neuro-hypophyseal germinomas. Cancer 1991; 68:1009–1014.

8. Saeki N, Takami K, Murai H, et al. Long-term outcome of endocrine function in patients with neurohypophyseal germinomas. Endocr J 2000; 47:83–89.

9. Wellons JC, Reddy AT, Tubbs RS, et al. Neuroendoscopic findings in patients with intracranial germinomas correlating with diabetes insipidus. J Neurosurg (Pediatrics) 2004; 100: 430–436.

10. Jennings MT, Gelman R, Hochberg F. Intracranial germ-cell tumors: Natural history and pathogenesis. J Neurosurg 1985; 63:155–167.

11. Bjornsson J, Scheithauer BW, Okazaki H, Leech RW. Intracranial germ cell tumors: Pathological and immunohistochemical aspects of 70 cases. J Neuropath Exp Neurol 1985; 44:32–46.

12. Kitanaka C, Matsutani M, Sora S, et al. Precocious puberty in a girl with an hCG-secreting suprasellar immature teratoma. J Neurosurg 1994; 81:601–604.

13. Starzyk J, Starzyk B, Bartnik-Mikuta A, et al. Gonadotropin releasing hormone-independent precocious puberty in a 5 year-old girl with suprasellar germ cell tumor secreting β-hCG and α-fetoprotein. J Ped Endocrinol Metab 2001; 14:789–796.

14. Shinoda J, Sakai N, Yano H, et al. Prognostic factors and therapeutic problems of primary intracranial choriocarcinoma/germ-cell tumors with high levels of HCG. J Neuro-Oncol 2004; 66:225–240.

15. Fujimaki T, Matsutani M, Funada N, et al. CT and MRI features of intracranial germ cell tumors. J Neuro-Oncol 1994; 19:217–226.

16. Sudo A, Shiga T, Okajima M, et al. High uptake on 11C-methionine positron emission tomographic scan of basal ganglia germinoma with cerebral atrophy. AJNR Am J Neuroradiol 2003; 24:1909–1911.

17. Haddock M, Schild SE, Scheithauer BW, et al. Radiation therapy for histologically confirmed primary central nervous system germinoma. Int J Radiat Oncol Biol Phys 1997; 38:915–923.

18. Aoyama H, Shirato H, Kakuto Y, et al. Pathologically-proven intracranial germinoma treated with radiation therapy. Radiother Oncol 1998; 47:201–205.

19. Shibamoto Y, Sasai K, Oya N, et al. Intracranial germinoma: Radiation therapy with tumor volume-based dose selection. Radiology 2001; 218:452–456.

20. Ogawa K, Shikama N, Toita T, et al. Long-term results of radiotherapy for intracranial germinoma: a multi-institutional retrospective review of 126 patients. Int J Radiat Oncol Biol Phys 2004; 58:705–713.

21. Shirato H, Nishio M, Sawamura Y, et al. Analysis of long-term treatment of intracranial germinoma. Int J Radiat Oncol Biol Phys 1997; 37:511–515.

22. Jenkin D, Berry M, Chan H, et al. Pineal region germinomas in childhood. Treatment considerations. Int J Radiat Oncol Biol Phys 1990; 18:541–545.

23. Matsutani M, Sano K, Takakura K. Long-term follow-up of patients with primary intracranial germinomas. In: Packer R, Bleyer WL, Pochedly C, eds.

Pediatric Oncology. Harwood Academic Publishers: Chur, Paris, Philadelphia, Tokyo; Ped Neuro-Oncol 1992; 254–260.

24. Allen JC, Kim JH, Packer RJ. Neoadjuvant chemotherapy for newly diagnosed germ cell tumors of the central nervous system. J Neurosurg 1987; 67:65–70.

25. Yoshida J, Sugita K, Kobayashi K, et al. Prognosis of intracranial germ cell tumours: effectiveness of chemotherapy with cisplatin and etoposide (CDDP and VP-16). Acta Neurochir (Wien) 1993; 120:111–117.

26. Matsutani M, Sano K, Takakura K, et al. Combined treatment with chemotherapy and radiation therapy for intracranial germ cell tumors. Child's Nerv Syst 1998; 14:59–62.

27. Matsutani M, Ushio Y, Abe H, et al. Combined chemotherapy and radiation therapy for central nervous system germ cell tumors: Preliminary results of a phase II study of the Japanese Pediatric Brain Tumor Study Group. Neurosurg Focus 1998; 7:1–5.

28. Rappaport R, Brauner R. Growth and endocrine disorders secondary to cranial irradiation. Pediat Res 1989; 25:561–567.

29. Matsutani M. Japanese Pediatric Brain Tumor Study Group: Treatment for intracranial germinoma: Final results of Japanese Study Group [abstr]. Neuro-Oncol 2005; 7:519.

30. Balmaceda C, Heller G, Rosenblum M, et al. Chemotherapy without irradiation-a novel approach for newly diagnosed CNS germ cell tumors: results of an international cooperative trial. J Clin Oncol 1996; 14:2908–2915.

31. Kellie SJ, Boyce H, Dunkel IJ, et al. Primary chemotherapy for intracranial nongerminomatous germ cell tumors: results of the second international CNS germ cell study group protocol. J Clin Oncol 2004; 22:846–853.

32. Da Silva N, Finlay J, Cavalheiro S, et al. The third international CNS germ cell tumor study group protocol: Preliminary results [abstr]. Neuro-Oncol 2005; 7:521.

33. Bouffet E, Baranzelli MC, Patte C, et al. Combined treatment modality for intracranial germinomas: results of multicentre SFOP experience. Societe Francaise d'Oncologie Pediatrique. Br J Cancer 1999; 79:1199–1204.

34. Alapetite C, Patte C, Frappaz D, et al. Long-term follow-up of intracranial germinoma treated with primary chemotherapy followed by focal radiation treatment: the SFOP-90 experience [abstr]. Neuro-Oncol 2005; 7: 517.

35. Calaminus G, Alapetite C, Frappaz D, et al. Update of protocol patients with CNS germinoma treated according to slop CNS GCT 96 [abstr]. Neuro-Oncol 2005; 7:518.

36. Calaminus G, Alapetite C, Frappaz D, et al. Update of protocol patients with CNS nongerminoma treated according to slop CNS GCT 96 [abstr]. Neuro-Oncology 2005; 7:526.

37. Allen J, Siffert J, Velasquez L, et al. Review of contemporary North American clinical trials in primary CNS germinoma [abstr]. Neuro-Oncol 2005; 7:517.

38. Goldman S, Bouffet E, Chuba P, et al. A phase II study to assess the ability of neoadjuvant chemotherapy ± second-look surgery to eliminate all measurable disease prior to radiotherapy for NGGCT, Children's Oncology Group Study ACNS0122 [abstr]. Neuro-Oncol 2005; 7:526.

23

Central Nervous System Metastases

Evert C. A. Kaal and Charles J. Vecht

*Department of Neurology, Medical Center Haaglanden,
The Hague, The Netherlands*

INTRODUCTION

The development of brain metastasis greatly influences the outlook for patients with cancer. Brain metastases may be the first sign of metastatic disease or even be the first sign of cancer. Once brain metastases are present, survival is often limited to months. Today, knowledge of prognostic factors—which has been provided by large studies—allows individually tailored treatment. Irradiation of the whole brain is an important therapeutic option for patients with adverse prognostic factors. Others may benefit from surgery or stereotactic radiotherapy (radiosurgery) and survive for up to one year or longer. The increasing availability of therapeutic options such as stereotactic radiotherapy and chemotherapy has offered new opportunities for the treatment of brain metastasis especially in patients with favorable prognostic factors. In this chapter, the current evidence on the proper treatment of brain metastasis is presented while focusing on both survival and quality of life.

The second part of this chapter is dedicated to intramedullary metastasis of the spinal cord. Although relatively rare, intramedullary metastasis is considered a neurological emergency, necessitating instant treatment. Clinical features, differential diagnosis, and the treatment of intramedullary metastasis are discussed.

NATURAL HISTORY OF BRAIN METASTASES

Brain metastases are the most common intracranial tumors and outnumber primary brain tumors at least fourfold. Brain metastases occur in about 25% of all patients with cancer and one estimates that annually over 100.000 patients develop brain metastases in the United States (1).

The majority of brain metastases originate from lung (40–50%), breast (15–25%), melanoma (5–20%) or kidney (5–10%). Tumors that metastasis most frequently to the brain are small cell lung cancer (SCLC), melanoma, germ cell tumors, and choriocarcinoma. Breast cancer, non-SCLC (NSCLC), renal cancer, colorectal, and testicular cancer metastasis less frequently.

Pathophysiology

Brain metastases are located in the cerebral hemispheres in approximately 80%, in the cerebellum in 15%, and in the brainstem in 5% of patients. This distribution depends mainly on tissue volume and blood flow. Terminal arterioles in the gray-white interface ("watershed areas") explain the predominance of brain metastases in this region. Posterior fossa metastasis occurs more frequently with pelvic, renal cell and gastrointestinal tumors, possibly because of dissemination of these tumors via Batson's epidural venous plexus within the vertebral column (2). Molecular characteristics have given new insights into the mechanisms of tumor spread and distribution. Certain metastasis suppressor genes and their level of expression seem to determine the propensity of a primary tumor to metastasis. For example, the metastasis suppressor gene Nm23 is expressed in breast and lung cancer and in melanoma. Patients with cutaneous melanomas expressing low levels of Nm23 have a higher propensity to develop brain metastasis (3). A lower expression of the KISS-1 gene is seen in breast cancer–brain metastasis (4), and experimental studies show that transfecting breast cancer cells with KISS-1 result in suppression of metastasis in vivo (5).

Brain Edema and the Blood–Brain Barrier

Brain metastases are often surrounded by edema, and its presence influences neurological function often substantially. Brain edema in brain metastasis results from leakage of plasma into the parenchyma through dysfunctional cerebral capillaries.

The blood–brain barrier—a highly selective interface separating brain tissue from the blood—is an important intermediate in the formation and prevention of brain edema. Its most important component is the capillary endothelial cell. In contrast to the extracerebral capillaries, cerebral endothelial cells are nonfenestrated, lack intracellular clefts, contain low numbers of pinocytotic vesicles, have high mitochondrial content, and are enclosed by astrocytic foot processes. These capillary cells are connected by tight junctions, which have both high electrical impedance and a low permeability to polar solutes, and in this way contribute to the selective barrier. Vascular endothelial growth factor is an important mediator for the formation of brain edema, probably by reducing expression or function of the tight junction proteins, occludin and claudine, leading to the opening of the tight junction and to the formation of edema (6,7).

CLINICAL FEATURES

The most prominent clinical features of brain metastases are headache, neurological deficit, and seizures. Headache is the presenting symptom in 40% to 50% of patients often secondary to raised intracranial pressure. Papilledema can be seen in 15% to 25% of patients with headache, and seizures are the presenting symptom in 15% to 20%; a similar percentage of patients develop seizures later on. Focal neurological deficits like hemiparesis, aphasia, or hemianopsia occur in 40%, and cognitive dysfunction in 10% or more. Some patients present with a stroke-like onset due to hemorrhage into the tumor, or with symptoms resembling a transient ischemic attack (Table 1).

The frequency of impaired cognitive function is probably underestimated, although its presence can influence the quality of life substantially. Recently, cognitive function in patients with brain metastases has been evaluated together with motor, verbal, executive, and daily functions (9). Despite a good functional status [mean Karnofsky performance score (KPS) of 80 or more], most patients demonstrate impairment in memory and fine motor functions. In one study, the Trailmaking B test, measuring visual-motor and executive mental functions, showed that 36% of patients score below the tenth percentile of normal (9). The investigators advocate the use of a battery of neurocognitive tests, taking no more than 30 minutes of time together with the Barthel index, as indicator of normal daily activities, and question the usefulness of the KPS, as the only measure of daily functioning (9). One study observed impaired function of cognition in 65% of patients before start of treatment (10), and another prospective study showed an approximately 10% decline on mini-mental state examination (MMSE) including 15% of patients having an MMSE of 23 or less,

Table 1 Symptoms in Patients with Brain Metastasis

Headache	40–50%
Seizures	15–40%
Neurological deficits	40%
Stroke-like presentation	5–10%
Cognitive dysfunction	10–65%

Source: From Ref. 8.

indicating dementia (11). Thus, cognitive symptoms are prominent and may critically influence treatment decisions. Its significance as prognostic factor would deserve further study.

DIAGNOSIS AND DIFFERENTIAL DIAGNOSIS

Imaging

In the evaluation of brain tumors, magnetic resonance imaging (MRI) is superior to computed tomography (CT). MRI detects a higher number of brain metastases than CT and better localizes lesions in the posterior fossa. Up to one-third of patients with a single lesion on contrast-enhanced CT have multiple lesions on MRI. In general, metastasis appears hypo- or isointense on T1-weighted MRI with hypointense surrounding edema. On T2-weighted MRI, the tumor and the surrounding edema appear hyperintense. The next step is gadolinium-enhanced MRI (Fig. 1). Although commonly used, a gadolinium dose of 0.1 mMol/kg is probably suboptimal. In a prospective study, 39 patients received both 0.1 and 0.3 mMol/kg gadolinium, identifying 43% more brain metastases with the triple dose (12). Better diagnostic techniques can thus lead to detection of smaller and a higher number of brain metastases. The proportion of multiple brain metastases increases by using triple-dose gadolinium-enhanced MRI and may lead to adaptation of therapy.

(A)   **(B)**   **(C)**

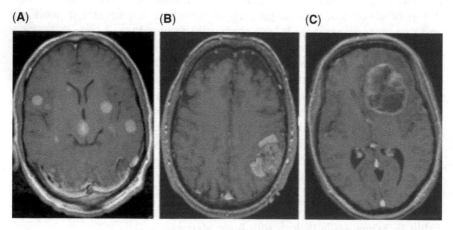

Figure 1 Variety of presentations of brain metastases on gadolinium-enhanced T1 weighted magnetic resonance. (**A**) Typical spherical shape of small brain metastases in a 49-year-old male with cutaneous melanoma. (**B**) Atypical metastasis in 57-year-old male with cutaneous melanoma. Resection revealed metastatic melanoma. (**C**) Large cystic lesion in a 44-year-old female with breast cancer. Differential diagnosis included astrocytoma, abscess, and metastasis. Resection revealed metastatic breast cancer.

Differential Diagnosis of a Single Brain Mass

In patients with a single brain mass, an extensive work-up may reveal its nature and the differential diagnosis includes a primary brain tumor, e.g., glioma or lymphoma, a metastasis, an inflammatory process or necrosis induced by previous radiotherapy. Morphological differences between metastasis and primary brain tumor include that the latter is less spherical in shape and more often showing edema extending into the corpus callosum. A brain abscess usually has a fine and smooth ring of enhancement. In one study, 11% of patients with a suspected single brain metastasis on CT were shown to harbor a glioma, abscess, or inflammation (13). Therefore, as a rule, tissue diagnosis of a single brain mass is indispensable, even if the patient is known to have an extracranial tumor.

When one suspects a brain metastasis in a patient unknown to suffer from cancer, a chest X-ray, a CT of the chest, a CT, or ultrasound of the abdomen, urinary investigation, and in women a mammography is recommended to determine the presence of extracranial disease. Whole-body ^{18}F-fluorodeoxyglucose positron emission tomography (18FDG PET) may greatly facilitate the detection of an unknown primary lesion. In a recent study on 16 patients with histologically confirmed metastatic brain tumor and an unknown primary tumor, whole-body 18FDG PET detected the presence of a lung tumor or lung metastasis in all (14). A diagnostic decision-tree is presented in Figure 2.

The question arises how much effort is mandatory to detect an unknown primary tumor before initiation of the treatment. In other words: Do patients receive suboptimal therapy when a primary neoplasm is not identified? In one study, a primary tumor was found during follow-up in 27 of 33 patients with biopsy-proven brain metastasis, and was located in the lung in 21 (15). Results from a retrospective study did not indicate that an earlier detection of the primary would have resulted in increased survival or an improved quality of life (16). In clinical practice, the search for a potential primary tumor should not unduly delay treatment of single brain metastasis.

Treatment-induced brain changes include postoperative alterations, leukoencephalopathy, or radiation necrosis. These changes, which may occur in areas without prior visible tumor activity, can impair proper evaluation of treatment effects. Particularly, differentiating between radiation necrosis and tumor recurrence on gadolinium-enhanced MR scans can be cumbersome. Single photon emission tomography (SPECT) may help to distinguish radiation necrosis from tumor recurrence following radiotherapy. Increased thallium-201 SPECT uptake was observed in 40 out of 60 patients, in whom tumor recurrence could be confirmed either clinically or by biopsy, and who all had undergone surgery and radiation therapy. In 10 out of 20 cases without increased thallium uptake, patients had small (<1 cm)

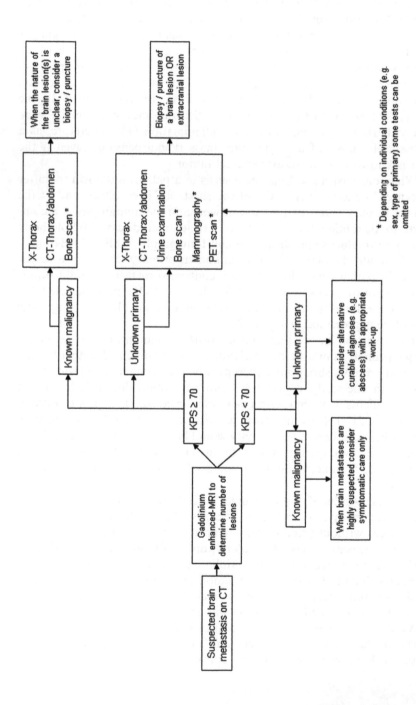

Figure 2 Schedule for diagnostic work-up. *Abbreviations:* CT, computed tomography; KPS, Karnofsky performance score; MRI, magnetic resonance imaging; PET, positron emission tomography.

recurrent lesions, suggesting that SPECT has a high specificity (up to 100%), though a low sensitivity for detecting recurrence of brain metastasis or primary brain tumors of a limited volume (17).

PROGNOSTIC FACTORS

Adequate estimation of independent prognostic factors in the individual patient is essential for deciding on the proper treatment. Studies from the Radiation Therapy Oncology Group (RTOG) constitute the basis for analysis of independent prognostic factors in patients with brain metastases. In 1200 patients from three RTOG trials conducted between 1979 and 1993, recursive partitioning analysis (RPA) identified three groups: Class 1: patients with a KPS ≥ 70, an age < 65 years, a controlled primary tumor and no extracranial disease, with a median survival of 7.1 months. Class 3: patients with a KPS of less than 70 with a median survival of 2.3 months. Class 2: all other patients (median survival: 4.2 months), representing patients with a KPS ≥ 70 and an age ≥ 65 years, or with active extracranial disease. In practice, the majority of patients (65%) belong to Class 2, and approximately 20% of patients to Class 1, and 15% to Class 3 (18). The effects of these prognostic factors are presented in Table 2.

In a retrospective study using uni- and multivariate analysis, concerning 1292 patients who received Whole Brain Radiotherapy (WBRT) and steroids with or without surgery, the strongest independent prognostic factors were performance status and response to steroids, systemic tumor activity, and serum lactate dehydrogenase. Age, number of brain metastases, and primary tumor were—although significant—of lesser importance (21).

Table 2 Prognostic Factors

Recursive partitioning analysis class		Survival (median in months)
	KPS ≥ 70, age < 65 controlled primary tumor, no extracranial disease	7.1
1	Single metastasis	13.5
	Multiple metastases	6.0
	KPS ≥ 70, age ≥ 65 or active extracranial disease	4.2
2	Single metastasis	8.1
	Multiple metastases	4.1
3	KPS < 70	2.3

Abbreviation: KPS, Karnofsky performed score.
Source: From Refs. 19 and 20.

Whether the number of brain metastases is an independent prognostic factor is still unresolved. In a recent study, outcome was better in Class 2 patients with a single metastasis than in Class 1 with multiple metastases. Probably, Class 1 and 2 represent heterogeneous groups (19). In practice, patients with a single brain metastasis receive a different—often more vigorous—treatment than patients with multiple metastases. Thus, the use of the "original" RTOG-RPA classification system, to be combined with subdividing Class 1 and 2 into single and multiple brain metastases, and subdividing Class 2 into patients with or without extracranial tumor control, improves the reliability for predicting the prognosis of the individual patient.

SYMPTOMATIC MANAGEMENT

Corticosteroids

The treatment with the initially strongest effect on neurological symptoms and quality of life is the administration of corticosteroids. In two-thirds of patients, headache and neurological deficit start to improve within one day after start of treatment, and most of the effects can be seen within 48 hours. The main action of corticosteroids is reducing cerebral vasogenic edema. The commonly used agent is dexamethasone. Other corticosteroids such as prednisone have more mineralocorticoid effects band more protein-binding properties than dexamethasone and are therefore considered as second choice (Table 3). Dexamethasone can be given at a starting dose

Table 3 Equivalent Dose of Different Glucocorticoids, Orally or Intravenously

	Glucocorticoid potency	Equivalent glucocorticoid dose (mg)	Plasma half-life (minutes)	Biological half-life (hours)	Physiological replacement dose (mg)
Cortisol (hydro-corti-sone)	1	20	80–115	8–12	30
Cortisone	0.8	25	30	8–12	37.5
Prednisone	4	5	200	12–36	7.5
Predniso-lone	4	5	120–200	12–36	7.5
Methyl-predniso-lone	5	4	80–180	12–36	6
Dexame-thasone	25–30	0.75	110–300	36–54	0.5–0.75

Source: From Ref. 22.

of 4 mg/day orally, divided into two doses. In patients with a metastasis in the brainstem or the cerebellum, or with impaired consciousness or other signs of intracranial pressure, one preferably administers 16 mg/day after a bolus of 10 mg dexamethasone intravenously (23).

Clinically important side effects include proximal myopathy, insomnia, gain of bodyweight, ankle oedema, hyperglycaemia, and psychological changes (hyperactivity and psychosis). Dexamethasone toxicity is dose dependent. In one randomized trial, proximal muscle weakness occurred in 14% receiving 4 mg and in 38% of patients receiving 16 mg/day after four weeks of treatment with dexamethasone. The frequency of Cushingoid facies was reported to be 32% and 65%, respectively. In patients without signs of increased intracranial pressure, lower doses of dexamethasone did not cause inferior therapeutic results as determined by the Karnofsky score (23). Therefore, as a rule, during or after treatment, one tries to prescribe the lowest effective dose of dexamethasone, which is often 4 mg per day and sometimes even lower, resulting in less toxicity.

Seizures

Prophylactic treatment with anticonvulsants does not prevent seizures in patients with brain metastasis. A randomised study (valproic acid vs. placebo) in patients with predominantly brain metastases showed no difference in the occurrence of seizures. Accordingly, the Quality Standards Subcommittee of the American Academy of Neurology recommends that in patients with newly diagnosed brain tumors, prophylactic anticonvulsants should not be used routinely (24,25).

It is clear that patients with symptomatic epilepsy should be treated with anticonvulsants, if possibly starting after the first seizure. The choice of a specific antiepileptic drug, however, is a matter of debate. The use of the "classic" anticonvulsants carbamazepine, phenytoin, and phenobarbital in patients receiving concomitant chemotherapy or dexamethasone may lead to insufficient tumor control. The reason for this is the enzyme-inducing effects of those anticonvulsants on isoenzymes of the hepatic cytochrome P450 system, which also metabolize the majority of chemotherapeutic agents. Alternatively, the enzyme inhibitor valproate may cause enhanced toxicity due to impaired metabolism of concomitantly administered chemotherapeutic drugs, which share 2C metabolic isoenzymes of the hepatic cytochrome P450 system. Novel drugs that do not interact with the P450 system such as levetiracetam, gabapentin, or pregabalin, however, might be preferable. Currently, valproic acid is the preferred anticonvulsant in patients with epilepsy and brain tumors, because of its known effectiveness and relatively good tolerability (26). If insufficient, it is our practice to add levetiracetam, with good results (27).

SURGERY

Surgery has become the standard therapy for patients with a single brain metastasis and good prognostic factors. Data from two randomized studies show that younger patients who are able to care for themselves and with limited extracranial disease benefit from surgery of a single brain metastasis: in these patients survival is extended from approximately three months after WBRT alone, to nine months when WBRT is combined with surgery (13,28). In another study, surgery was not beneficial: inclusion of a higher proportion of patients with active extracranial disease and lower performance score probably explains the failure to demonstrate a positive effect of surgery (Table 4) (29).

Apart from surgery as one means to extend survival, surgery obviously may also be necessary in emergency situations: shunting of obstructive hydrocephalus can restore consciousness, and debulking of a large supratentorial lesion reduces the risk of brain herniation. Surgery of a cerebellar metastasis is often to be preferred over stereotactic radiotherapy or WBRT, because in this location radiation-induced edema may become life threatening (33).

Postoperative Management: WBRT or Observation?

In general, after successful resection of a single brain metastasis, two approaches can be followed: upfront WBRT or observation by MRI follow-up. The latter approach can be followed by salvage WBRT, if necessary. Both approaches were investigated in a prospective study in which 95 patients were randomised between postoperative WBRT or no further treatment. There was no significant difference between the two groups in overall survival or in the length of time that patients remained functionally independent (30). Recurrence of tumor anywhere in the brain was less frequent in the radiotherapy group than in the observation group (18% vs. 70%; $p < 0.001$) and less death rate due to neurological causes was observed in patients treated with postoperative WBRT. Some feel that a neurological cause is the most difficult type of death for patients and their families to deal with, and WBRT reduces the occurrence of neurological death. In cancer patients, especially when providing palliative care, recognition and appropriate application of issues of quality of life are important. The results of an ongoing randomised phase III trial investigating the effects of WBRT versus the omission of WBRT after stereotactic radiotherapy or surgery may hopefully provide the answers (EORTC 22952–26001) (34). We believe that, for now, two approaches can be justified in good prognosis patients: WBRT after surgery, or alternatively, observation with MRI follow-up every three months.

PRIMARY RADIOTHERAPY

Radiotherapy has long been and is still the mainstay of treatment for brain metastases. Radiation of the whole brain in patients displaying multiple

Table 4 Randomized Trials of Whole Brain Radiotherapy With or Without Surgery or Stereotactic Radiotherapy of Brain Metastasis

References	Treatment	Median survival (months)	Comment
Patchell (13)	Biopsy + WBRT	3.4	Surgery improves survival
	Resection + WBRT	9.2	
Vecht, et al. (28)	WBRT	6	Surgery improves
	Resection + WBRT	10	survival
Mintz, et al. (29)	WBRT	6.3	NS; Higher
	Resection + WBRT	5.6	proportion of patients with systemic disease
Patchell, et al. (30)	Resection	11	NS; + WBRT: less
	Resection + WBRT	9.9	death due to neurologic causes
Kondziolka, et al. (31)	WBRT of 2–4 metastases	7.5	NS; Stopped at 60% accrual
	Stereotactic radiotherapy of 2–4 metastases + WBRT	11	
Andrews, et al. (32)	WBRT of 1–3 metastases	6.5	Stereotactic radiotherapy of a
	Stereotactic radiotherapy of 1–3 metastases + WBRT	5.7	single metastasis only improves survival
	WBRT of single metastasis	4.9	
	Stereotactic radiotherapy of single metastasis + WBRT	6.5	

Abbreviations: WBRT, whole brain radiotherapy; NS, not significant.

brain metastases was already in use during the 1950s (35). Today, high-dose radiation of small-specified areas (i.e., stereotactic radiotherapy or radiosurgery) has greatly expanded therapeutic options and has rapidly become one of the most important modalities in treating brain metastasis.

Whole Brain Radiotherapy

WBRT is often considered as the principal treatment for patients with multiple brain metastases in order to reverse neurological deficit and to control tumor progression in the brain. WBRT is more commonly applied in patients with unfavorable prognostic factors. Also, in these patients, WBRT can improve neurological signs and corticoid dependency, and extend survival time from 10 to 14 weeks as compared to steroid treatment only. Several fractionating schemes from 20 Gy in one week to 40 Gy in four weeks have been investigated resulting in median survival times of 3.4 to 4.8 months (36). Today, a standard regimen is a ten-day schedule with daily fractions of 3 Gy (10 × 3 Gy). Shorter radiation schemes with lesser visits to the hospital may be less demanding. In one study, the standard regimen (10 × 3 Gy) was compared in poor prognosis patients with a hypofractionated scheme (2 × 6 Gy), showing no essential differences in survival (37).

Toxicity

Early side effects of WBRT—occurring in almost all patients—include hair loss, fatigue, and scalp erythema or pigmentation. Late toxicity of WBRT, which—if present—would occur after a median latent period of 14 months, exists of progressive dementia, ataxia and urinary incontinence, resembling normal pressure hydrocephalus. Eight of 66 patients treated with surgery and adjuvant WBRT had minor symptoms of late radiation toxicity and three other patients had more severe symptoms, starting approximately nine months after WBRT (38). These data support the notion that WBRT is not associated with significant neurotoxicity in patients with median survival times up to five months. Therefore, in patients with an expectation of longer survival, fraction doses of less than 3 Gy are to be preferred. Prospective studies using cognitive testing would probably better appraise the risk of neurotoxicity after WBRT for patients with good prognostic factors.

Prophylactic Cranial Irradiation

The method of prophylactic cranial irradiation, i.e., irradiation of supposedly subclinical brain metastasis, has been under evaluation for over 30 years. The majority of studies have focused on SCLC. The cumulative risk on intracranial relapse in SCLC treated with systemic chemotherapy approaches 50% to 80% by two years. Data from two meta-analyses show an increased overall survival advantage with relative risk of death of 0.82 to 0.84, and a reduction of the rate of developing brain metastases (relative risk = 0.46–0.48) (39,40).

   In NSCLC, 112 patients with locally advanced disease receiving multimodality treatment, brain metastasis was the first site of failure in 25 patients, especially in the young (41). These observations have led to the suggestion that prophylactic cranial irradiation should also be offered to these patients and some have advocated trials on prophylactic cranial irradiation of highrisk groups with NSCLC (41).

   Prospective studies on SCLC, including two randomized trials on side effects—mainly characterized by cognitive malfunction—have shown that prophylaxis with conventional schedules up to 3 Gy per fraction do not lead to an inferior cognitive outcome (42).

Altogether, present data show a beneficial effect of prophylactic cranial irradiation on the survival and the prevention of brain metastases with SCLC cancer, apparently without a gross negative effect on cognitive function with fraction doses of 3 Gy or lower.

Stereotactic Radiotherapy

Brain metastases with their often-spherical shape make ideal targets for stereotactic radiotherapy or radiosurgery for tumors of small size (4 cm or less). Stereotactic radiotherapy extends survival in patients with a single brain metastasis, as shown in a randomized study in which WBRT was followed by stereotactic radiotherapy or observation. However, this effect was only seen in younger patients with a single brain metastasis without active extracranial disease: median survival increased from 4.9 to 6.5 months after additional stereotactic radiotherapy. In patients with two to four metastases, neurological progression was reduced by applying stereotactic irradiation after WBRT (32), although it is unknown how this affects the quality of life. In selected nonrandomized series, stereotactic radiotherapy results in median survival times of approximately 10 to 15 months.

Apart from enhanced survival in subgroups of patients with brain metastasis, stereotactic radiotherapy has other advantages over WBRT: stereotactic radiotherapy can be repeated in the individual patient with few complications (43). Another advantage is its apparent lack of late toxicity: Unwanted effects as dementia or ataxia as seen following WBRT are less prominent after stereotactic radiotherapy.

Although the radiation can be delivered with surgical precision, stereotactic radiotherapy is not always an alternative for surgery: When immediate mass relief is required, when the diameter of the metastasis exceeds 4 cm or when histological confirmation is needed, surgery is preferred. However, stereotactic radiotherapy would offer new opportunities for lesions in eloquent areas, which are often less suitable for surgery.

The question may thus arise how many metastases can be treated by stereotactic radiotherapy. Often, patients with only a low number of brain metastases (up to three) receive stereotactic radiotherapy. This practice is based on the assumption that the prognosis of patients with multiple brain metastases is too poor to refer them for stereotactic radiotherapy. However, no data from prospective or randomized studies clearly support this approach. In one retrospective study, recursive-partitioning analysis was applied to data from 130 patients treated with stereotactic radiotherapy, in which patients with one to three versus those with four or more metastases were compared. Interestingly, outcome depended on RPA class and not on the number of metastases (44). Thus, there is no evidence justifying a priori exclusion of patients with multiple (four or more) brain metastases from stereotactic radiotherapy. Therefore, patients displaying multiple small brain metastases with no or limited extracranial disease and in a good clinical condition (KPS≥70) may receive stereotactic radiotherapy as an alternative to WBRT.

Stereotactic Radiotherapy Followed by WBRT

The discussion whether or not to apply WBRT after radiosurgery resembles a similar question after surgical removal of a brain metastasis. Several studies have shown that WBRT after stereotactic radiotherapy reduces brain tumor recurrence: local control at one year was 87% after stereotactic radiotherapy only, and 97% after stereotactic radiotherapy and planned WBRT (45). A retrospective study showed that the two-year disease-free survival was 34% after stereotactic radiotherapy alone and 60% after stereotactic radiotherapy if followed by WBRT (46). A prospective study on 36 patients, in which stereotactic radiotherapy followed by planned observation showed a 38% local tumor recurrence anywhere in the brain at a median time of four months (47). In this study, brain tumor recurrence was associated with neurological deficits in 60% of patients. These data indicate that more than half of patients develop recurrent, symptomatic brain metastases after stereotactic radiotherapy alone. The question arises which difference in prognostic factors may help to distinguish between patients, who should or should not receive adjuvant WBRT. Nonrandomized data seem conflicting: In one study, a high recurrence rate was associated with disease limited to the brain (47). However, other prospective data show that a low recurrence rate was associated with the presence of a single brain metastasis (48). From previous studies, we know that metastasis limited to the brain and presence of a single brain metastasis are both favorable prognostic factors. Apparently, both these factors have distinctly different effects on the development of recurrent brain metastasis following treatment. Only randomized studies may clarify this, hopefully to be provided by a presently ongoing EORTC study (surgery or stereotactic radiotherapy either with or without WBRT) (34).

CHEMOTHERAPY

The role of chemotherapy in brain metastases remains largely undefined: In contrast to surgery or WBRT, chemotherapy is not part of the standard treatment and it is unclear whether chemotherapy should be used as primary or adjuvant or rather as salvage therapy. A clinical setting in which chemotherapy can be considered is for patients in good condition presenting with a brain metastasis who display active extracranial disease. In this situation, one can imagine that standard therapy, e.g., WBRT or stereotactic radiotherapy, may be followed by chemotherapy. If chemotherapy for brain metastases is chosen, this should mainly be based on the chemosensitivity of the primary tumor, and preferably drugs with reported cerebral responses should be administered.

The Role of the Blood–Brain Barrier in Chemotherapy

The brain is still often considered a sanctuary for metastases and relatively inaccessible for chemotherapeutic agents. This assumption is largely based on pharmacological considerations that most chemotherapeutics do not cross the blood–brain barrier or only to a minor degree. However, there is ample evidence that in brain metastasis, the blood–brain barrier is dysfunctional, e.g., the presence of contrast-enhanced lesions on CT or MRI indicates that tumor vasculature is at least relatively permeable. Also, objective responses of brain metastasis, following treatment with a variety of chemotherapeutic agents known to be incapable of crossing the blood–brain barrier, have been observed, like response rates up to 60% after cyclophosphamide-based treatment in brain metastases from breast cancer (49). The awareness that the blood–brain barrier may be of lesser importance than previously thought has prompted the suggestion that chemotherapeutic management of brain metastases should therefore mainly be based on the chemosensitivity of the primary tumor (50). Apart from positive results with "non–blood–brain barrier permeable" agents, the development of drugs that easily cross the blood–brain barrier like temozozlomide has contributed to an increased interest to employ chemotherapy for brain metastasis.

Lung Cancer

Treatment of brain metastasis from SCLC is mainly vincristine based, and therapy with this blood–brain barrier impermeable drug results in objective responses of 50% to 60% (51). Treatment with the blood–brain barrier permeable topoisomerase inhibitors, topotecan and teniposide, results in 20% to 30% responses (52,53). The latter two drugs display lesser toxicity but also lesser efficacy. For NSCLC, cisplatin with, e.g., gemcitabine or docetaxel results in 20% to 45% responses (54). Single-agent temozozlomide results in variable results, but temozozlomide combined with WBRT results in objective intracranial responses of 96%, compared to 67% after WBRT alone (55). Therefore, the latter therapy might be worth considering in WBRT-naïve patients.

Breast Cancer

Regarding the large clinical experience and limited side effects, cyclophosphamide-based treatment (e.g., with cyclophosphamide, 5-fluorouracil, and methotrexate) would be the preferential approach in breast cancer–brain metastasis with response rates of 17% to 61% (56). The radiosensitiser RSR13 (efaproxiral) seems promising in WBRT-naïve patients: RSR13 prior to WBRT doubles survival time compared to WBRT alone (9 vs. 4.5 months) (57).

The role of temozozlomide in the treatment of breast cancer–brain metastasis is unclear, and evidence on the efficacy of hormonal therapy for brain metastasis is limited.

Melanoma

Response rates of chemotherapy with DTIC (dacarbazine) or temozozlomide in melanoma brain metastases are low (10–20%) (58,59). An advantage of temozozlomide over other drugs is its low toxicity. Combinations of chemotherapy, e.g., fotemustine or temozozlomide, and WBRT have not resulted in improved response rates. Until now, it is unclear which chemotherapeutic agent should be used—if any—in patients with brain metastasis from melanoma.

THERAPEUTIC STRATEGY FOR BRAIN METASTASIS

A therapeutic strategy for the different categories of brain metastasis is given in a decision-tree in Figure 3. The chart starts at the diagnostic process, dividing patients according to their RPA class (Class 1–3) and subdividing Class 1 and 2 in single or multiple brain metastases, Class 2 is further split into patients with or without active extracranial disease. Class 1 and Class 2 patients without active extracranial disease may be treated with surgery (single metastasis) or radiosurgery (2–4 metastases). This therapy can either be followed by WBRT or, alternatively, by MRI follow-up every three months. Patients with less favorable prognostic factors (e.g., KPS < 70 or active extracranial disease) may benefit from radiosurgery (stereotactic radiotherapy) with one to four brain metastases or from a short course of hypofractionated WBRT, mainly focusing on maintaining or improving quality of life.

INTRAMEDULLARY METASTASIS

Intramedullary metastasis, like epidural and leptomeningeal metastasis, carries a high risk of severe morbidity by causing rapid spinal cord dysfunction with paraparesis or paraplegia as the ultimate consequence. Intramedullary metastasis should be considered a neuro-oncologic emergency, and diagnostic work-up followed by treatment should be started forthwith.

Clinical and Epidemiological Features

Autopsy studies reveal that 1% to 2% of patients with cancer display intramedullary metastatic disease. Intramedullary metastasis usually is seen in the setting of generalized metastatic disease, and 60% to 85% of patients also display concomitant brain metastasis. Nevertheless, in approximately 30% of patients diagnosed with intramedullary metastasis, it has been reported as the first sign of malignancy (60). The most common primary tumors are SCLC, breast cancer, and melanoma.

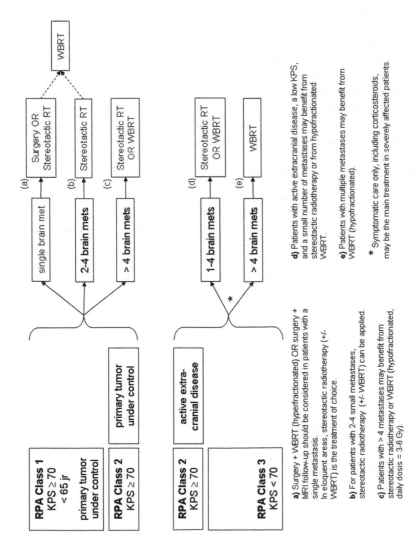

Figure 3 Decision-tree for the treatment of brain metastasis. *Abbreviations:* KPS, Karnofsky performance score; RPA, recursive-partitioning analysis; RT, Radiotherapy; WBRT, whole brain radiotherapy.

The clinical picture consists of a subacute myelopathy with a median duration between start of symptoms and diagnosis of 28 days. This relative long period probably indicates the difficulties in making the diagnosis, although one may expect that nowadays in the era of MR, this time lag has shortened substantially. In contrast to the primary and infiltrating spinal cord tumors like the gliomas, intramedullary metastases are better demarcated on imaging. Over time and at a certain size, the spinal cord blood supply often becomes comprised, resulting in more rapid neurological deterioration (60). Presenting signs are often local back pain, radicular pain with aggravation on coughing. Although these symptoms are also common in extradural spinal cord compression, e.g., by traction on nerve roots, invasion of the dorsal part of the cord may explain sensory symptoms in patients with intramedullary metastasis. In patients with progressive intramedullary disease, three distinct neurological syndromes are characteristic: the most common is a transverse myelopathy with spastic paraparesis. Second, occurring in up to 45% of patients, a Brown-Sequard syndrome with limb paralysis and contralateral spinothalamic sensory loss accompanies unilateral metastasis. Third, an ascending or descending myelopathy may occasionally be the result of necrosis due to vascular compression of the spinal cord becoming clinically manifest (61).

Diagnosis and Differential Diagnosis

The first step in the diagnostic process in patients with a suspected spinal cord compression is contrast-enhanced MRI. An intramedullary metastasis appears hypointense on T1-weighted and iso- or hyperintense on T2-weighted images. After administration of gadolinium, the tumor enhances in a ring-like or regular pattern. However, MRI is not fully sensitive or specific: small metastasis may remain undetected and glioma, infarct, or abscess may resemble a metastasis. In patients known with cancer, mainly cancer of the lung or of the head and neck and previous radiation, a radiation myelopathy may strongly resemble the clinical picture of a growing intramedullary metastasis, although occasionally the course of radiation myelopathy is slower (i.e., over a period of months to years). In 80% radiation myelopathy is associated with tumors of head and neck (62). When differentiating between metastases and spinal cord necrosis or radiation myelopathy, the presence of concomitant brain metastasis favors the presence of metastasis (Fig. 4). PET scanning can be helpful to distinguish necrosis from metastasis, although the small size of the lesion may lead to false negative results; MRI only is often not sufficient in this particular case (63,64).

Treatment of Intramedullary Metastases

Focal radiotherapy is the main mode of treatment for intramedullary metastasis and may result in stabilization or sometimes improvement of spinal cord function. Small retrospective studies indicate that responses depend

(A)　　　　　　　　**(B)**　　　　　**(C)**

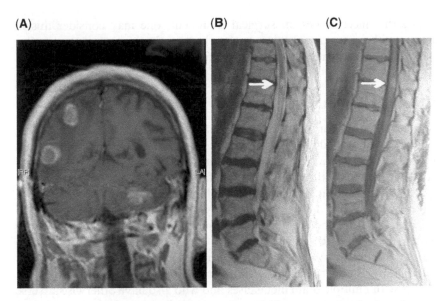

Figure 4　76-year-old man with small-cell urothelial cancer who developed a para-paresis. (**A**) Gadolinium-enhanced magnetic resonance (MR) revealing multiple brain lesions (including a cerebellar lesion) highly suspicious for metastases. (**B**) T2-weighted MR and (**C**) gadolinium-enhanced T1-weighted MR of spinal cord displaying a small metastasis (*arrow*) within the conus of the spinal cord (Th11–Th12).

on neurological function at the time of starting radiation therapy: Patients who are ambulatory often remain so, and patients unable to walk will rarely do so afterwards (60). Untreated, spinal cord metastasis will inexorably lead to paraplegia, and thus radiation therapy should be started as soon as possible. Up to 23% of patients harbor more than one metastasis, and radio-therapy of the complete spinal cord may therefore be considered. Under these circumstances, the risk on bone-marrow suppression should be weighted against the potential benefit of total spinal cord irradiation. Instead, close neurological and MRI follow-up can be recommended to detect new intramedullary metastases outside the radiation field (62).

Reports on surgical treatment of intramedullary metastasis are scarce and its benefit is unclear, also because patients receiving surgery will often receive postoperative radiotherapy as well. Recently, 13 patients receiving surgery for intramedullary metastasis were studied retrospectively. Unex-pectedly, an aggressive surgical approach seemed to be a negative predictive factor for the functional outcome. Tumor histology was identified as a rele-vant predictor for survival with a median survival of 42 weeks in patients with adenocarcinoma in contrast to eight weeks for poorly differentiated carcinoma's (65). Nevertheless, others have advocated a radical resection of intramedullary metastasis (66,67), especially with radioresistant tumors.

Despite the uncertainties on surgical treatment, one may consider this in patients without metastatic disease elsewhere in the nervous system and a well-controlled systemic cancer of a radioresistant nature (68).

CONCLUDING REMARKS

Treatment options for brain metastasis have increased substantially during the last decades. Today, we know from randomized clinical studies that surgery or stereotactic radiotherapy of a single metastasis in addition to WBRT in patients with good prognostic factors results in improved survival (13,28,32). Whether additional WBRT after surgery or stereotactic radiotherapy is beneficial in terms of quality of life or survival is currently unknown. For the time being, two approaches can be justified in good prognostic patients: WBRT after surgery or observation with MRI follow-up every three months. A similar approach may be followed after stereotactic radiotherapy. Patient-friendly, i.e., shorter WBRT schedules prevail in patients with multiple brain metastases and who also have otherwise adverse prognostic factors. Subsets of patients with chemosensitive tumors may benefit from additional chemotherapy.

Finally, small benefits in survival or improved radiological outcome after treatment may not always be the equivalent for better care, especially when side effects of treatment are substantial or when therapy regimens are demanding. Therefore, to achieve optimal standards of care, quality of life including the measurement of cognitive function might be a focus point for future studies. In our opinion, better insight in toxicity issues facilitates decision making on individually tailored treatment, ranging from symptomatic therapy on one side of the spectrum to extensive therapeutic measures on the other.

REFERENCES

1. Landis SH, Murray T, Bolden S, Wingo PA. Cancer statistics, 1998. CA Cancer J Clin 1998; 48:6–29.
2. Delattre JY, Krol G, Thaler HT, Posner JB. Distribution of brain metastases. Arch Neurol 1988; 45:741–744.
3. Sarris M, Scolyer RA, Konopka M, Thompson JF, Harper CG, Lee CS. Cytoplasmic expression of nm23 predicts the potential for cerebral metastasis in patients with primary cutaneous melanoma. Melanoma Res 2004; 14:23–27.
4. Stark AM, Tongers K, Maass N, Mehdorn HM, Held-Feindt J. Reduced metastasis-suppressor gene mRNA-expression in breast cancer brain metastases. J Cancer Res Clin Oncol 2005; 131:191–198.
5. Lee JH, Welch DR. Suppression of metastasis in human breast carcinoma MDA-MB-435 cells after transfection with the metastasis suppressor gene, KiSS-1. Cancer Res 1997; 57:2384–2387.
6. Davies DC. Blood-brain barrier breakdown in septic encephalopathy and brain tumours. J Anat 2002; 200:639–646.

7. Kaal EC, Vecht CJ. The management of brain edema in brain tumors. Curr Opin Oncol 2004; 16:593–600.
8. Kaal EC, Niel CG, Vecht CJ. Therapeutic management of brain metastasis. Lancet Neurol 2005; 4:289–298.
9. Herman MA, Tremont-Lukats I, Meyers CA, et al. Neurocognitive and functional assessment of patients with brain metastases: a pilot study. Am J Clin Oncol 2003; 26:273–279.
10. Mehta MP, Rodrigus P, Terhaard CH, et al. Survival and neurologic outcomes in a randomized trial of motexafin gadolinium and whole-brain radiation therapy in brain metastases. J Clin Oncol 2003; 21:2529–2536.
11. Regine WF, Scott C, Murray K, Curran W. Neurocognitive outcome in brain metastases patients treated with accelerated-fractionation vs. accelerated-hyperfractionated radiotherapy: an analysis from Radiation Therapy Oncology Group Study 91–04. Int J Radiat Oncol Biol Phys 2001; 51:711–717.
12. Van Dijk P, Sijens PE, Schmitz PI, Oudkerk M. Gd-enhanced MR imaging of brain metastases: contrast as a function of dose and lesion size. Magn Reson Imaging 1997; 15:535–541.
13. Patchell RA, Tibbs PA, Walsh JW, et al. A randomized trial of surgery in the treatment of single metastases to the brain. N Engl J Med 1990; 322:494–500.
14. Klee B, Law I, Hojgaard L, Kosteljanetz M. Detection of unknown primary tumours in patients with cerebral metastases using whole-body 18F-fluorodeoxyglucose positron emission tomography. Eur J Neurol 2002; 9:657–662.
15. Ruda R, Borgognone M, Benech F, Vasario E, Soffietti R. Brain metastases from unknown primary tumour: a prospective study. J Neurol 2001; 248:394–398.
16. van de Pol M, van Aalst VC, Wilmink JT, Twijnstra A. Brain metastases from an unknown primary tumour: which diagnostic procedures are indicated? J Neurol Neurosurg Psychiatry 1996; 61:321–323.
17. Lorberboym M, Mandell LR, Mosesson RE, et al. The role of thallium-201 uptake and retention in intracranial tumors after radiotherapy. J Nucl Med 1997; 38:223–226.
18. Gaspar LE, Scott C, Murray K, Curran W. Validation of the RTOG recursive partitioning analysis (RPA) classification for brain metastases. Int J Radiat Oncol Biol Phys 2000; 47:1001–1006.
19. Lutterbach J, Bartelt S, Ostertag C. Long-term survival in patients with brain metastases. J Cancer Res Clin Oncol 2002; 128:417–425.
20. Gaspar L, Scott C, Rotman M, et al. Recursive partitioning analysis (RPA) of prognostic factors in three Radiation Therapy Oncology Group (RTOG) brain metastases trials. Int J Radiat Oncol Biol Phys 1997; 37:745–751.
21. Lagerwaard FJ, Levendag PC, Nowak PJ, Eijkenboom WM, Hanssens PE, Schmitz PI. Identification of prognostic factors in patients with brain metastases: a review of 1292 patients. Int J Radiat Oncol Biol Phys 1999; 43:795–803.
22. Vecht CJ. Clinical management of brain metastasis. J Neurol 1998; 245:127–131.
23. Vecht CJ, Hovestadt A, Verbiest HB, van Vliet JJ, van Putten WL. Dose-effect relationship of dexamethasone on Karnofsky performance in metastatic brain tumors: a randomized study of doses of 4, 8, and 16 mg per day. Neurology 1994; 44:675–680.

24. Glantz MJ, Cole BF, Friedberg MH, et al. A randomized, blinded, placebo-controlled trial of divalproex sodium prophylaxis in adults with newly diagnosed brain tumors. Neurology 1996; 46:985–991.
25. Glantz MJ, Cole BF, Forsyth PA, et al. Practice parameter: anticonvulsant prophylaxis in patients with newly diagnosed brain tumors. Report of the Quality Standards Subcommittee of the American Academy of Neurology. Neurology 2000; 54:1886–1893.
26. Vecht CJ, Wagner GL, Wilms EB. Interactions between antiepileptic and chemotherapeutic drugs. Lancet Neurol 2003; 2:404–409.
27. Wagner GL, Wilms EB, Van Donselaar CA, Vecht CJ. Levetiracetam: preliminary experience in patients with primary brain tumours. Seizure 2003; 12:585–586.
28. Vecht CJ, Haaxma-Reiche H, Noordijk EM, et al. Treatment of single brain metastasis: radiotherapy alone or combined with neurosurgery? Ann Neurol 1993; 33:583–590.
29. Mintz AH, Kestle J, Rathbone MP, et al. A randomized trial to assess the efficacy of surgery in addition to radiotherapy in patients with a single cerebral metastasis. Cancer 1996; 78:1470–1476.
30. Patchell RA, Tibbs PA, Regine WF, et al. Postoperative radiotherapy in the treatment of single metastases to the brain: a randomized trial. JAMA 1998; 280:1485–1489.
31. Kondziolka D, Patel A, Lunsford LD, Kassam A, Flickinger JC. Stereotactic radiosurgery plus whole brain radiotherapy versus radiotherapy alone for patients with multiple brain metastases. Int J Radiat Oncol Biol Phys 1999; 45:427–434.
32. Andrews DW, Scott CB, Sperduto PW, et al. Whole brain radiation therapy with or without stereotactic radiosurgery boost for patients with one to three brain metastases: phase III results of the RTOG 9508 randomised trial. Lancet 2004; 363:1665–1672.
33. Fadul C, Misulis KE, Wiley RG. Cerebellar metastases: diagnostic and management considerations. J Clin Oncol 1987; 5:1107–1115.
34. van den Bent MJ, Stupp R, Brandes AA, Lacombe D. Current and future trials of the EORTC brain tumor group. Onkologie 2004; 27:246–250.
35. Chao JH, Phillips R, Nickson JJ. Roentgen-ray therapy of cerebral metastases. Cancer 1954; 7:682–689.
36. Borgelt B, Gelber R, Kramer S, et al. The palliation of brain metastases: final results of the first two studies by the Radiation Therapy Oncology Group. Int J Radiat Oncol Biol Phys 1980; 6:1–9.
37. Priestman TJ, Dunn J, Brada M, Rampling R, Baker PG. Final results of the Royal College of Radiologists' trial comparing two different radiotherapy schedules in the treatment of cerebral metastases. Clin Oncol (R Coll Radiol) 1996; 8:308–315.
38. Nieder C, Schwerdtfeger K, Steudel WI, Schnabel K. Patterns of relapse and late toxicity after resection and whole-brain radiotherapy for solitary brain metastases. Strahlenther Onkol 1998; 174:275–278.
39. Auperin A, Arriagada R, Pignon JP, et al. Prophylactic cranial irradiation for patients with small-cell lung cancer in complete remission. Prophylactic Cranial Irradiation Overview Collaborative Group. N Engl J Med 1999; 341:476–484.

40. Meert AP, Paesmans M, Berghmans T, et al. Prophylactic cranial irradiation in small cell lung cancer: a systematic review of the literature with meta-analysis. BMC Cancer 2001; 1:5.
41. Ceresoli GL, Reni M, Chiesa G, et al. Brain metastases in locally advanced non-small cell lung carcinoma after multimodality treatment: risk factors analysis. Cancer 2002; 95:605–612.
42. Vines EF, Le Pechoux C, Arriagada R. Prophylactic cranial irradiation in small cell lung cancer. Semin Oncol 2003; 30:38–46.
43. Shuto T, Fujino H, Inomori S, Nagano H. Repeated gamma knife radiosurgery for multiple metastatic brain tumours. Acta Neurochir (Wien) 2004; 146:989–993.
44. Nam TK, Lee JI, Jung YJ, et al. Gamma knife surgery for brain metastases in patients harboring four or more lesions: survival and prognostic factors. J Neurosurg 2005; 102(Suppl):147–150.
45. Hasegawa T, Kondziolka D, Flickinger JC, Germanwala A, Lunsford LD. Brain metastases treated with radiosurgery alone: an alternative to whole brain radiotherapy? Neurosurgery 2003; 52:1318–1326.
46. Chidel MA, Suh JH, Reddy CA, Chao ST, Lundbeck MF, Barnett GH. Application of recursive partitioning analysis and evaluation of the use of whole brain radiation among patients treated with stereotactic radiosurgery for newly diagnosed brain metastases. Int J Radiat Oncol Biol Phys 2000; 47:993–999.
47. Regine WF, Huhn JL, Patchell RA, et al. Risk of symptomatic brain tumor recurrence and neurologic deficit after radiosurgery alone in patients with newly diagnosed brain metastases: results and implications. Int J Radiat Oncol Biol Phys 2002; 52:333–338.
48. Lutterbach J, Cyron D, Henne K, Ostertag CB. Radiosurgery followed by planned observation in patients with one to three brain metastases. Neurosurgery 2003; 52:1066–1073.
49. Boogerd W, Dalesio O, Bais EM, van der Sande JJ. Response of brain metastases from breast cancer to systemic chemotherapy. Cancer 1992; 69:972–980.
50. van den Bent MJ. The role of chemotherapy in brain metastases. Eur J Cancer 2003; 39:2114–2120.
51. Grossi F, Scolaro T, Tixi L, Loprevite M, Ardizzoni A. The role of systemic chemotherapy in the treatment of brain metastases from small-cell lung cancer. Crit Rev Oncol Hematol 2001; 37:61–67.
52. Korfel A, Oehm C, von Pawel J, et al. Response to topotecan of symptomatic brain metastases of small-cell lung cancer also after whole-brain irradiation. A multicentre phase II study. Eur J Cancer 2002; 38:1724–1729.
53. Postmus PE, Haaxma-Reiche H, Smit EF, et al. Treatment of brain metastases of small-cell lung cancer: comparing teniposide and teniposide with whole-brain radiotherapy—a phase III study of the European Organization for the Research and Treatment of Cancer Lung Cancer Cooperative Group. J Clin Oncol 2000; 18:3400–3408.
54. Franciosi V, Cocconi G, Michiara M, et al. Front-line chemotherapy with cisplatin and etoposide for patients with brain metastases from breast carcinoma, nonsmall cell lung carcinoma, or malignant melanoma: a prospective study. Cancer 1999; 85:1599–1605.

55. Antonadou D, Paraskevaidis M, Sarris G, et al. Phase II randomized trial of temozozlomide and concurrent radiotherapy in patients with brain metastases. J Clin Oncol 2002; 20:3644–3650.
56. Fenner MH, Possinger K. Chemotherapy for breast cancer brain metastases. Onkologie 2002; 25:474–479.
57. Stea B, Suh J, Shaw E, et al. Efaproxiral (EFAPROXYN) as an adjunct to whole brain radiation therapy for the treatment of brain metastases originating from breast cancer: updated survival results of the randomized REACH (RT-009) study. 27th Annual San Antonio Breast Cancer Symposium 2004: Poster 4064.
58. Serrone L, Zeuli M, Sega FM, Cognetti F. Dacarbazine-based chemotherapy for metastatic melanoma: thirty-year experience overview. J Exp Clin Cancer Res 2000; 19:21–34.
59. Agarwala SS, Kirkwood JM, Gore M, et al. Temozozlomide for the treatment of brain metastases associated with metastatic melanoma: a phase II study. J Clin Oncol 2004; 22:2101–2107.
60. Schiff D, O'Neill BP. Intramedullary spinal cord metastases: clinical features and treatment outcome. Neurology 1996; 47:906–912.
61. Dunne JW, Harper CG, Pamphlett R. Intramedullary spinal cord metastases: a clinical and pathological study of nine cases. Q J Med 1986; 61:1003–1020.
62. Winkelman MD, Adelstein DJ, Karlins NL. Intramedullary spinal cord metastasis. Diagnostic and therapeutic considerations. Arch Neurol 1987; 44:526–531.
63. Poggi MM, Patronas N, Buttman JA, Hewitt SM, Fuller B. Intramedullary spinal cord metastasis from renal cell carcinoma: detection by positron emission tomography. Clin Nucl Med 2001; 26:837–839.
64. Katz JD, Ropper AH. Progressive necrotic myelopathy: clinical course in 9 patients. Arch Neurol 2000; 57:355–361.
65. Gasser T, Sandalcioglu IE, Hamalawi BE, Nes JA, Stolke D, Wiedemayer H. Surgical treatment of intramedullary spinal cord metastases of systemic cancer: functional outcome and prognosis. J Neurooncol 2005; 73:163–168.
66. Kalayci M, Cagavi F, Gul S, Yenidunya S, Acikgoz B. Intramedullary spinal cord metastases: diagnosis and treatment—an illustrated review. Acta Neurochir (Wien) 2004; 146:1347–1354.
67. Constantini S, Miller DC, Allen JC, Rorke LB, Freed D, Epstein FJ. Radical excision of intramedullary spinal cord tumors: surgical morbidity and long-term follow-up evaluation in 164 children and young adults. J Neurosurg 2000; 93:183–193.
68. Ogino M, Ueda R, Nakatsukasa M, Murase I. Successful removal of solitary intramedullary spinal cord metastasis from colon cancer. Clin Neurol Neurosurg 2002; 104:152–156.

24

Increased Intracranial Pressure and Extradural Compression Syndromes

Scott R. Plotkin and Jeanine T. Grier

Department of Neurology, Massachusetts General Hospital, Boston, Massachusetts, U.S.A.

INCREASED INTRACRANIAL PRESSURE

The most recent classification by the World Health Organization identifies more than 120 types of brain tumors. All central nervous system (CNS) tumors are potential space-occupying lesions. As tumors grow, they can increase intracranial pressure (ICP) or produce extradural compression syndromes (if located outside the CNS). In this chapter, we will review the etiology, presentation, and treatment of increased ICP in patients with CNS tumors as well as extradural compression syndromes. We will begin with a brief discussion of ICP and the Monro–Kellie Doctrine that can be used to understand the effect of mass lesions on ICP.

ICP and the Monro–Kellie Doctrine

The pressure within the cranial cavity at any point in time is termed the ICP. ICP is maintained by the constant secretion of cerebrospinal fluid (CSF) from the choroid plexus. Under normal circumstances, CSF is produced at a rate of 20 mL/h and absorbed at the arachnoid granulations at a similar rate. At any given time, there is approximately 90–150 mL of CSF within the adult ventricular and subarachnoid spaces. At the bedside, ICP can be estimated by inserting a needle into the subarachnoid space and measuring the height of the fluid column within an attached manometer. In normal individuals in the recumbent position, ICP ranges from 5 to 20 cm of water at the level of the lumbar spine (1). Intracranial hypertension, or increased ICP, is generally defined as the situation when ICP exceeds 25 cm of water.

The brain occupies 85% of the cranial volume, with the remainder divided between CSF (10%), and blood (5%) (1). The intracranial contents are held at a constant volume by the rigid structures of the dura mater and skull. The recognition that the total volume (V) of brain, CSF, and blood must remain constant was formulated as the Monro–Kellie doctrine in the 18th century:

$$V_{brain} + V_{CSF} + V_{blood} = constant$$

Thus, any increase in the volume of brain, CSF, or blood must result in a compensatory decrease in the volume of the other compartments. Small increases in intracranial volume are compensated by mobilization of the CSF compartment. Large increases in volume, however, exceed the capacity of the CSF and vascular spaces to compensate and result in increased ICP.

The relationship between ICP and intracranial volume can be represented by the idealized curve in Figure 1. Initially, as intracranial volume rises, ICP rises minimally as the CSF and vascular compartments accommodate the change in volume. As the volume increases, compensatory mechanisms begin to fail and the ICP rises more steeply. For this reason, incremental increases in volume in patients with space-occupying lesions can cause rapid escalation of ICP and lead to brainstem herniation.

Patients with elevated ICP can experience transient increases in ICP caused by changes in position or Valsalva maneuvers. These plateau waves or Lundberg "A-waves" consist of elevations in ICP lasting 5 to 20 minutes, often to levels of 60–130 cm of water. Plateau waves may be accompanied by a wide variety of neurologic symptoms including severe headaches, hiccups, blurred vision, gait difficulty, impaired consciousness, vomiting, or incontinence (2).

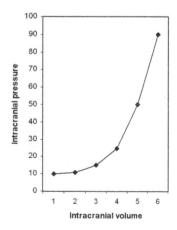

Figure 1 Idealized pressure–volume curve within the cranial vault. A small increase in intracranial volume produces little changes in intracranial pressure (ICP) when intracranial volume is low. When intracranial volume is high, the same increase in volume produces large changes in ICP.

CAUSES OF INCREASED ICP

Any process that expands the brain, CSF, or blood compartments can cause increased ICP. It is important to realize that several causes may exist at the same time. These conditions must be distinguished from pseudotumor cerebri syndromes in which increased ICP exists in the absence of a tumor. The following sections will address the clinical presentation, diagnosis, and management of increased ICP seen in brain tumor patients.

Increased Brain Compartment

Tumor Mass

The most common cause of increased ICP in patients with brain tumors is tumor mass. One of the main goals of surgery is to reduce ICP in symptomatic patients.

Cerebral Edema

The blood–brain barrier (BBB) limits the penetration of blood-borne compounds into the CNS. Anatomic and physiologic specializations of brain endothelial cells subserve this barrier function. Continuous tight junctions between endothelial cells limit the diffusion of large hydrophilic molecules through paracellular pathways. Low rates of pinocytosis in endothelial cells minimize the transport of compounds across capillaries. Efflux proteins actively pump some lipophilic molecules from the abluminal (brain) to luminal (blood) side of cerebral capillaries.

Tumor-related cerebral edema is caused by dysfunction of the BBB, leading to extravasation of plasma into the parenchyma. Ultrastructural studies of microvessels from high-grade astrocytomas reveal loss of tight junctions, increased fenestrations, and increased rates of pinocytosis compared with normal capillaries. For glial tumors, the presence of cerebral edema correlates with histologic grade and, in some studies, with reduced survival (3,4). For meningiomas, the presence of cerebral edema is associated with increasing size, secretory subtype, increased labeling index, and invasion into brain parenchyma (5,6).

The molecular basis of BBB dysfunction is an area of active research. Tumor capillaries have reduced levels and organization of occludin and Claudin, proteins that are required for tight junction function. Furthermore, tumor tissue has increased levels of aquaporin-4, a water channel protein, which correlates with the degree of swelling (7). Increased expression of vascular endothelial growth factor (VEGF), initially known as vascular permeability factor, has been documented in brain tumors (8). VEGF has multiple actions, which serve to increase endothelial cell permeability. These include reduced complexity of tight junctions, increased number in fenestrations and pinocytotic vesicles, and increased functional activity of vesicovacuolar organelles that form channels across endothelial cells (8,9). In addition, the loss of normal astrocytic factors that support the BBB may contribute to BBB dysfunction.

Other factors which can lead to cerebral edema in patients with tumors include radiation and seizures (10,11). Radiation upregulates the expression of VEGF and induces the activity of matrix metalloproteinase-2 and urokinase-type plasminogen activator (12,13). These enzymes act to break down the basement membrane of cerebral microvessels. Ongoing seizure activity can increase blood volume in the brain due to increased metabolic demand. For this reason, attention to seizure control is essential in patients with elevated ICP.

Clinical Presentation: Patients with increased ICP and tumor-related cerebral edema may present with headache, papilledema, nausea, vomiting, abnormal eye movements, or impaired consciousness. Headache is caused by traction or pressure on pain-sensitive structures such as dura mater and blood vessels. Pain is often worse in the morning due to the sustained recumbent position, which reduces vascular drainage. Variables that affect the intensity of pain include the size and location of the tumor (i.e., infratentorial vs. supratentorial), the presence of midline shift, a prior history of headaches, and the amount of edema surrounding the tumor (14). A sudden increase in ICP brought on by change in position or Valsalva maneuver may cause sudden severe headache, visual or gait difficulty, impaired consciousness, or vomiting.

Historically, papilledema was a cardinal sign of long-standing intracranial hypertension. Findings of early papilledema include obscuration or elevation of the optic disc border, blurring of the peripapillary nerve fiber layer, and loss of venous pulsations. However, overreliance on these signs should be avoided. One cannot exclude the presence of intracranial hypertension based on the lack of papilledema because this sign is absent in 75% of patients with tumors (15,16). In addition, patients with preexisting optic atrophy or anomalous optic nerves may not exhibit papilledema despite marked increases in ICP. Congenital abnormalities and optic disc drusen can mimic papilledema caused by increased ICP. The absence of retinal venous pulsations can be suggestive of intracranial hypertension but pulsations are absent in 12% of the normal population under normal circumstances (17).

Vomiting, particularly in the absence of significant nausea, can result from increased ICP. This manifestation is more common in pediatric than in adult patients and is more commonly found with infratentorial rather than with supratentorial tumors. The precise mechanism of ICP-associated vomiting is poorly understood, although involvement of the area postrema in the floor of the fourth ventricle can increase the risk.

Diplopia is reported by some patients with brain tumors and increased ICP. For patients without leptomeningeal metastases, examination typically reveals unilateral or bilateral sixth nerve palsy. In the majority of cases, no direct involvement of the sixth nerve is identified. Thus, the presence of a sixth nerve palsy is often described as a falsely localizing finding.

Impairment of consciousness in patients with brain tumors may result from direct or indirect mechanisms. Direct effects can occur from tumor involvement of structures that subserve memory, intellect, executive function, language, or judgment. Indirect effects occur from pressure on structures that subserve consciousness such as the reticular activating system and its projections through the thalamus to the cortex. In many patients with brain tumors, a progressive decline of consciousness from increased ICP is the ultimate cause of death.

Diagnosis: Cerebral edema is diagnosed by radiological imaging. Cerebral edema presents as regions of low attenuation on computed tomography (CT) and may be confused with other processes such as tumor, infarct, or encephalomalacia. For this reason, CT has low sensitivity for cerebral edema. Magnetic resonance imaging (MRI) has greatly improved the diagnosis of cerebral edema. On T2-weighted images, including fluid attenuation inversion recovery sequences, cerebral edema presents as hyperintense signal predominantly involving white matter (Fig. 2). Diffusion-weighted imaging does not clearly delineate regions of cerebral edema but is helpful in distinguishing cerebral edema from stroke. Postcontrast T1-weighted images can distinguish areas of tumor (which typically enhance) from areas of cerebral edema (which do not enhance).

Treatment: The standard treatment for cerebral edema in brain tumor patients consists of corticosteroids. In 1952, these agents were shown

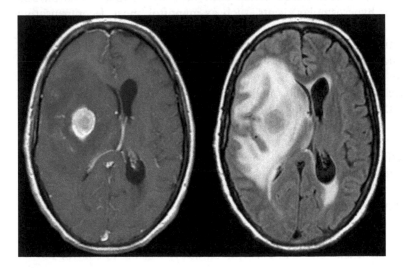

Figure 2 Magnetic resonance imaging scan of a patient with a cerebral metastasis and cerebral edema. The tumor mass (*left*) is visible on T1-weighted sequence after administration of contrast. Cerebral edema is visible on fluid attenuation inversion recovery sequence. Notice how both the tumor volume and the cerebral edema contribute to mass effect with effacement of the lateral ventricle.

to have a remarkable effect on cerebral edema in patients with craniopharyngioma. Gradually, the use of corticosteroids was adopted for treatment of edema caused by primary and metastatic CNS tumors despite their adverse effects and limitation (18). The mechanism of action is still debated but may involve reduced production of VEGF by tumor cells, reduced response of vasculature to VEGF, reduction of CSF production, decrease in free radical production, and cytolytic tumor effect (19).

No randomized trials have compared the efficacy of different corticosteroids for treatment of increased ICP. Traditionally, dexamethasone has been used for tumor-related edema because of its lower mineralocorticoid activity. The typical starting dose for symptomatic lesions is 16 mg/day divided in either three or four daily doses. For patients with metastatic brain tumors and Karnofsky performance status ≤80, 4 mg per day may be as beneficial as 16 mg per day and is associated with less toxicity (20). Clinical response is typically seen within 24 to 48 hours with the maximum response occurring by one week. After a therapeutic response has been achieved, the dose should be slowly tapered with close monitoring of patient's symptoms. Some patients may not tolerate tapered doses, and the clinician may have to weigh quality of life issues versus medication side effects. If no significant response is seen on standard dosing, the amount may be safely doubled every 48 hours up to a dose of 100 mg/day. In patients at risk for cerebral herniation, dexamethasone may be given as a one-time 100-mg bolus followed by 100 mg/day in divided doses. When combined with hyperventilation and intravenous hyperosmolar agents, such as mannitol, most decompensating patients will stabilize and improve.

Corticosteroid-associated toxicity increases with prolonged use. Typical side effects include insomnia, diabetes mellitus, erosive gastritis, myopathy, cushingoid facies, weight gain, and psychiatric disturbances (e.g., psychosis, depression, and mania) (18,20). Corticosteroid levels can be affected by coadministration of other medications commonly prescribed for brain tumor patients (18). For example, phenytoin causes liver enzyme induction, which accelerates metabolism of dexamethasone, thereby reducing its efficacy (21).

Corticosteroids should be avoided when lymphoma is suspected. The oncolytic effects of corticosteroids can cause regression of these tumors and lead to nondiagnostic biopsy specimens. In these patients, corticosteroids should be withheld until adequate tissue has been obtained for diagnosis. For decompensating patients, treatment with mannitol or diuretics should be attempted as long as it is clinically feasible to control ICP.

Other Therapies for Cerebral Edema: Additional therapies for tumor-associated edema include mannitol, hypertonic saline, diuretics, carbonic-anhydrase inhibitors, nonsteroidal anti-inflammatory drugs (NSAIDs), fluid restriction, hyperventilation, and patient positioning.

Mannitol is an inert sugar that increases the osmolality of blood when given intravenously. This leads to a net diffusion of water into the vascular space along an osmolality gradient. A typical loading dose of mannitol is 50–100 g followed by 25–50 g every six hours. A clinical effect usually occurs within 10 to 30 minutes, with maximal ICP reduction occurring within one hour. Serum osmolality should be followed regularly during mannitol treatment. The target for serum osmolality is 300–310 mOsm/L as levels exceeding 320 mOsm/L can increase the risk of renal insufficiency. Long-term treatment with mannitol is generally neither practical nor effective as it is associated with tachyphylaxis with chronic use. Acute discontinuation should be avoided as this can lead to a rapid increase in ICP (rebound effect). Tapering the daily dose by 50% per day is typically safe and well tolerated. Overall, mannitol should not be considered as a first-line agent for tumor-associated brain edema, but may be effective as an adjunctive therapy in certain patients with critically elevated ICP. Side effects include electrolyte disturbances, nonketotic hyperosmolar state, and rebound intracranial hypertension after prolonged use.

Less commonly used antiedema agents include hypertonic saline, loop diuretics, carbonic anhydrase inhibitors, and NSAIDs. However, use of these agents as third-line therapy should be viewed as experimental in most circumstances.

Many clinicians advocate head elevation to reduce ICP. In theory, head elevation reduces ICP by promoting venous drainage. Quantitative studies in patients with occipital or cerebellar tumors suggest that 10° head elevation leads to small decreases in both ICP and mean arterial blood pressure. There is no net change in cerebral perfusion pressure (22). The generally accepted practice is to elevate the head 15° to 30° from horizontal in the immediate postoperative period unless there is risk for tension pneumocephalus (23).

Hyperventilation for increased ICP may be used for short-term management of brain tumor patients. The hypocarbia produced by hyperventilation reduces cerebral blood volume with a rapid effect on ICP. Hypocarbia of 25–35 mmHg is usually effective for a short time period after which ICP returns to baseline despite therapy.

Increased CSF Compartment

Increased CSF Production

Choroid plexus papillomas are rare tumors of the CNS that predominantly affect children. These tumors are derived from the choroid plexus and have been associated with hydrocephalus due to increased production of CSF. Resection is typically curative if total removal is achieved (24).

Decreased CSF Absorption

Hydrocephalus is an enlargement of the CSF spaces of the brain due to an abnormal increase in the proportion of CSF relative to brain tissue. Any

disturbance of normal CSF flow may cause hydrocephalus. When hydrocephalus occurs, a hydrostatic gradient exists between the CSF space and
the brain parenchyma. This pressure gradient leads to flow of CSF into
the extracellular space across the ventricular lining (transependymal flow)
resulting in interstitial edema.

 Obstructive, or noncommunicating, hydrocephalus occurs when there
is blockade along the normal CSF pathways (Fig. 3). The sites of highest
risk for obstruction include the foramen of Monro, which connects the
lateral ventricles to the third ventricle, the cerebral aqueduct, which

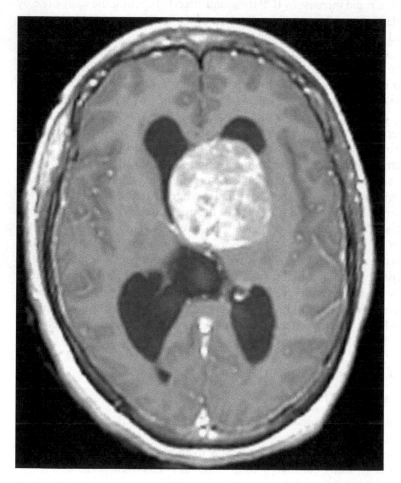

Figure 3 Magnetic resonance imaging scan of a patient with obstructive hydrocephalus due to ependymoma. The tumor mass (*arrow*) is visible on T1-weighted
sequence after administration of contrast. Notice the enlargement of the lateral
ventricles due to obstruction of the foramen of Monroe.

connects the third and fourth ventricles, and the foramina of Luschka and Magendie, which connect the fourth ventricle to the subarachnoid space. For example, preoperative hydrocephalus is reported in approximately 80% of children with posterior fossa tumors, and postoperative treatment may be required for persistent or progressive hydrocephalus (25).

Nonobstructive, or communicating, hydrocephalus occurs when absorption of CSF at the arachnoid granulations is impaired. Communicating hydrocephalus has been reported with malignant gliomas due to leptomeningeal dissemination of tumor cells and subsequent impairment in CSF absorption (26). Risk factors for communicating hydrocephalus include leptomeningeal metastases and intraventricular hemorrhage.

When hydrocephalus develops acutely, the ventricles may reach 80% of maximal enlargement within six hours, thus necessitating quick intervention. A slower phase of enlargement follows the initial rapid expansion with continuous production of CSF, thus causing cerebral edema in the periventricular white matter. This interstitial edema, as described above, may resolve over time as the hydrocephalus stabilizes into a chronic phase. Accompanying atrophy may also occur in the chronically hydrocephalic white matter. As the rate of ventricular enlargement stabilizes in patients with incomplete ventricular obstruction, CSF pressure may also normalize. Although the hydrocephalus may appear to have stabilized or "arrested," the clinician must remain aware that these patients may still acutely decompensate.

Clinical Presentation: The clinical presentation of hydrocephalus depends on the acuity with which it develops (acute, subacute, or chronic) and the underlying etiology. Symptoms of acute hydrocephalus may include headaches, papilledema, diplopia, and changes in mental status. Brainstem signs, hemiparesis, or drowsiness may indicate compression of posterior fossa structures. Subacute or chronic hydrocephalus classically presents as the triad of dementia, incontinence, and gait failure. In these patients, signs of acute hydrocephalus may not be present. These symptoms are attributed to pressure on white matter tracts in the frontal lobe.

Diagnosis: A diagnosis of hydrocephalus is established by radiological imaging combined with ICP measurement. CT or MRI scanning reveals enlargement of the ventricular system out of proportion to the brain parenchyma. In obstructive hydrocephalus, the site of obstruction can usually be identified, although high-resolution images may be required to identify small lesions. Lumbar puncture with measurement of opening pressure serves to document ICP that typically exceeds 25 cm H_2O. As noted above, patients with chronic hydrocephalus may have normal ICP.

Treatment: Treatment of hydrocephalus involves shunting CSF to other spaces, including the peritoneum (ventriculoperitoneal shunt), heart (ventriculoatrial shunt), or subarachnoid space (third ventriculostomy). The choice of procedure depends on many variables and should be individualized. If there is concern for bleeding from the postoperative site, especially with intraventricular tumors, external ventricular drainage may help prevent hydrocephalus and an acute rise in ICP. Adverse events with shunts and ventriculostomies include infection, shunt malfunction, and misplacement of catheters.

Increased Blood Compartment

Increases in the blood compartment can occur for many reasons. Intratumoral hemorrhage, either spontaneous or related to anticoagulation, can cause a sudden increase in ICP. For small hemorrhages, conservative management with or without corticosteroids may be appropriate; for large hemorrhages, surgical intervention may be necessary to relieve dangerously elevated ICP. Venous sinus thrombosis can also increase ICP by reducing venous outflow from the brain (Fig. 4). Vascular congestion increases venous pressure, which reduces absorption of CSF at the arachnoid granulations. Patients with systemic cancer and other medical illnesses that are associated with venous thrombosis are at increased risk due to hypercoagulable states (27). Other patients at increased risk are those with dural-based lesions (e.g., metastases and meningiomas) that abut the venous system. Patients with venous sinus thromboses are treated with anticoagulation to minimize the extension of the thrombosis. In general, patients with impending venous occlusion due to rapidly expanding tumors should be treated either with surgery or with radiation to minimize the chance of venous sinus thrombosis. Finally, metabolic disturbances such as hypercapnia or hypoxia can increase blood volume and should be treated as indicated.

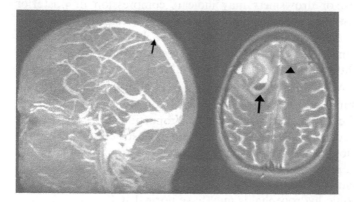

Figure 4 Magnetic resonance (MR) scan of a patient with esthesioneuroblastoma and venous sinus thrombosis. MR venogram (*left panel*) demonstrates lack of flow in the superior sagittal sinus (*arrow*). T2-weighted image (*right panel*) reveals hemorrhage in the right superior frontal gyrus (*arrow*) and contralateral infarct (*arrowhead*). A fluid–fluid layer is present within the hemorrhage.

PSEUDOTUMOR CEREBRI SYNDROMES

The presence of intracranial hypertension without focal neurologic signs or evidence of a brain tumor is known as pseudotumor cerebri syndrome. The diagnosis of primary pseudotumor cerebri, also known as idiopathic intracranial hypertension, is reserved for patients who fulfill the modified Dandy criteria (Table 1). In these patients, no cause for increased ICP such as venous sinus thrombosis can be identified. Patients with secondary pseudotumor cerebri fulfill the modified Dandy criteria but have an identifiable cause of increased ICP (28).

No clear cause for IIH has been identified although associations with other disorders abound. Obesity has been identified as a risk factor in multiple studies. The predominance of women with IIH (female:male ratio, 8 : 1) raises the possibility of an underlying endocrinologic cause. Hyperthyroidism, hypothyroidism, hypoparathyroidism, Cushing's disease, and pregnancy have been reported with IIH but these associations have not been substantiated in case-controlled studies. Similarly, tetracycline-type antibiotics, excess vitamin A, tamoxifen, cimetidine, corticosteroids, methylphenidate, lithium, nalidixic acid, nitrofurantoin, sulfonamides, and trimethoprim-sulfamethoxazole have been associated with IIH. The validity of these associations is difficult to prove because most of these medications are widely used in the general population. Finally, IIH has been reported in association with systemic lupus erythematosus, anemia, hypertension, uremia, multiple sclerosis, and nutrition. Using the modified Dandy criteria to rate the level of association, there appears to be a definite relationship with obesity and a probable relationship with chlordecone, lindane, hypervitaminosis A, and uremia. Other associations are thought to be either possible or unsupported at the present time (28).

Secondary pseudotumor cerebri has been documented in a variety of neurologic and medical conditions that either increase production or decrease absorption of CSF. Rarely, choroid plexus papillomas can results in overproduction of CSF in absence of significant mass effect. Processes that increase venous pressure reduce the absorption of CSF at the arachnoid

Table 1 Modified Dandy Criteria for Idiopathic Intracranial Hypertension

---

Signs and symptoms of increased intracranial pressure (papilledema and headache)
No other causes of increased intracranial pressure and
   No localizing findings on neurologic examination
   Normal magnetic resonance imaging/computed tomography scan without
      evidence of venous obstructive disease
   Intracranial pressure > 250 cm water; normal cerebrospinal fluid analysis
   Awake and alert patient

Source: From Ref. 28.

granulations. Possible causes include venous sinus disease (e.g., stenosis or thrombosis), arterialization of venous sinuses due to the presence of arteriovenous malformations, jugular outflow obstruction due to structural disease (e.g., radical neck dissection), and congenital heart disease.

Clinical Presentation

Headache is almost universal in patients with IIH. Headache is typically described as occurring daily and may worsen with eye movements or increases in intra-abdominal pressure (Valsalva maneuvers or coughing). Other common complaints include transient visual obscurations, tinnitus (either unilateral or bilateral), diplopia (usually horizontal), and dizziness. Papilledema is the cardinal feature of this disorder and is the cause of visual field loss in patients. Papilledema may be unilateral or asymmetric. Ocular motor abnormalities have been documented. Abducens palsies are the most common and have traditionally been ascribed to stretching of the intracranial portion of the sixth cranial nerve. Abnormalities of other cranial nerves have been reported in a minority of patients with IIH and should prompt a review of the diagnosis. Patients with secondary pseudotumor syndrome may present with similar symptoms and signs as patients with IIH. In addition, they may develop findings suggestive of the primary pathology involved in development of increased ICP (e.g., seizures in a patient with venous sinus thrombosis).

Diagnosis

Patients with compatible symptoms or signs should be imaged to exclude secondary causes of increased ICP such as tumor, thrombosed venous sinuses, or hydrocephalus. MRI has supplanted CT scanning as the imaging modality of choice. If a space-occupying lesion has been excluded, magnetic resonance venography should be considered as occult thromboses of the intracranial venous sinuses may be more common than previously thought (29). Lumbar puncture is essential for diagnosis of IIH as elevated ICP (>25 cm of water in adults, >20 cm in children) is one of the modified Dandy criteria. ICPs between 20 and 25 cm of water are considered nondiagnostic in adults. Patients with ICP in this range may need a repeat lumbar puncture at a separate time to confirm a diagnosis. Compatible laboratory findings on CSF analysis include normal, or rarely low, protein, normal glucose, and normal cell count. Cisternal puncture is not acceptable for diagnosis of IIH because there exists a concentration gradient of protein within the neuroaxis. CSF protein content is lowest in the ventricle (6–15 mg/dL), and highest in the lumbar subarachnoid space (20–50 mg/dL) (30).

Treatment

A complete review of the treatment options for pseudotumor cerebri syndromes is beyond the scope of this chapter. The goal of therapy for IIH is to reduce ICP. First-line therapy includes weight loss in obese patients and acetazolamide, which reduces CSF production in the choroid plexus. Second-line agents include other carbonic anhydrase inhibitors and loop diuretics such as furosemide. In general, corticosteroids should be avoided due to their ability to cause weight gain and to cause increases in ICP when the dose is tapered (i.e., rebound). In patients who do not respond to these interventions, serial lumbar punctures or shunting procedures constitute second-line therapy. In patients who present with significant visual loss or in those in whom visual loss progresses despite medical therapy, surgical intervention is warranted. Serial lumbar punctures may be effective for a minority of patients but ICP generally returns to baseline after a short period of time. Furthermore, lumbar punctures may be technically difficult and uncomfortable in obese patients. Lumboperitoneal shunting may be effective but carries the risk of infection and shunt malfunction. Alternatively, optic nerve fenestration can be performed to drain CSF through the optic nerve sheath and reduce ICP. Finally, bariatric surgery to promote weight loss has been shown to improve symptoms and signs of IIH.

COMPRESSION SYNDROMES

Skull and Dural Metastases

The brain is covered by the skull and the meninges, which can be divided into the pachymeninges (dura mater) and the delicate leptomeninges (arachnoid and pia mater). Any space-occupying lesion, whether primary or metastatic, arising from the skull or dura mater can produce extradural compression. Metastatic deposits are thought to reach the skull via Batson's venous complex. Involvement of the dura typically occurs by direct extension from a skull lesion after erosion of the bony plates. Less commonly, dura is the initial site of metastasis. Neoplastic involvement of the leptomeninges (i.e., leptomeningeal metastases) is discussed in Chapter 25.

Incidence

Primary skull lesions represent a fraction of the 8000 primary bone and soft-tissue malignancies diagnosed each year. In contrast, 50% of patients with metastatic carcinoma have evidence of skeletal metastases at autopsy (31). Meningiomas are the most common primary dural lesions, comprising 13% to 26% of all intracranial tumors (32). In an autopsy study of 2375 patients with metastatic disease, 9% of patients had evidence of dural metastases. In 52% of these cases (4% overall), dural metastases were the sole manifestation of intracranial disease (33). In this series, breast cancer accounted for the most common primary tumor (22%), followed by lymphoma (16%), prostate (12%), neuroblastoma (11%), and lung cancer (6%). A more recent autopsy and surgical series of dural metastases demonstrate a similar pattern with some notable differences. Similar to previous studies, the most common primary tumors encountered in autopsy cases were prostate (26%), breast (19%), hematologic (19%), and lung (11%). However, the surgical series revealed that among patients undergoing resection of their lesions, the most common tumors were melanoma (21%), breast (18%), and lung (9%) (34).

Clinical Presentation

The presentation of skull tumors depends on their size and location. Small calvarial tumors may be asymptomatic whereas large tumors or those located in the skull base or adjacent to dural sinuses may be symptomatic. Reported symptoms include local swelling and pain, headaches, cranial neuropathy, seizures, focal motor or sensory deficits, or increased ICP (35,36). In a retrospective review of 38 patients with skull tumors, patients with skull metastases presented less frequently with a neurological deficit, had a shorter history of symptoms, and were older than patients with primary skull tumors (36). Half of patients with skull metastases had infiltration of the dura noted intraoperatively. Patients with skull base lesions were more likely to present with neurological findings such as facial palsies. Increased ICP from skull metastases is not necessarily caused by compression of the venous sinuses. In a series of patients with metastases to the calvarium, increased ICP was noted in 14% of patients with lesions overlying the dural sinuses and in 14% of patients with lesions distant from the dural sinuses (35). In addition, benign and nontumor skull lesions can cause neurological symptoms and compression, although less frequently than with malignant tumors (37).

Like skull tumors, dural metastases may be asymptomatic or may cause severe disability due to compression of the dural sinuses and involvement of cranial nerves.

Diagnosis

Skull lesions may first be recognized on plain skull X-rays or radiolabeled bone scans, which are frequently performed as screening tools in cancer patients. CT scanning is the preferred method for determining the extent of bony involvement. Skull metastases typically appear as expansile, osteolytic, hypervascular lesions. MRI is the preferred method for detecting infiltration of the subcutaneous tissue, dura, or brain parenchyma (36).

Dural lesions are best visualized by MRI. The most common presentation consists of either solitary or multifocal nodules protruding into the subdural space. In case of a solitary lesion, dural metastases may be difficult to distinguish from other dural-based masses such as meningioma (38). Histopathological confirmation is necessary for definitive diagnosis of dural metastases. Less commonly, dural metastases present as diffuse dural enhancement on MRI scan, but caution is warranted as intracranial hypotension may have a similar appearance (39). Finally, dural metastases can present as subdural collections. Metastatic subdural fluid collections are radiographically indistinguishable from traumatic or spontaneous chronic subdural hematoma and must be suspected if the patient has cancer (34,40). Dural metastases may adhere to the arachnoid membrane but usually do not involve the underlying leptomeninges or brain parenchyma. This observation has led to the concept that the arachnoid membrane serves as a barrier against tumor invasion.

Treatment

The presence of skull and dural disease does not necessarily reflect end-stage cancer (34). After histopathological diagnosis has been confirmed, some patients will benefit from either surgery or radiation therapy. The goal of treatment is to relieve pain and to minimize neurologic disability. Radiation therapy is the treatment of choice for lesions that are not surgically accessible. For other lesions, the decision to proceed with surgery or radiation is made on a case-by-case basis.

Epidural Spinal Cord Compression

Spinal cord compression due to tumor constitutes a neuro-oncologic emergency. Both primary vertebral and metastatic spinal cord tumors can cause epidural spinal cord compression (ESCC). Neuropathologic studies of metastatic ESCC reveal evidence of demyelination and infarction in the adjacent spinal cord (41). Spinal cord injury in ESCC is multifactorial but likely related to venous engorgement, diminished arterial perfusion, and direct compression of spinal axons.

Incidence

ESCC by metastases is more common than compression by primary spinal tumors. Autopsy studies suggest that 5% of patients with cancer develop ESCC, representing over 25,000 cases annually (42). In 75% of these patients, metastases begin in the vertebrae and grow into the epidural space (41). Metastases from lung, breast, and prostate cancer or lymphoma, account for about half of cases of ESCC (42–44). Older data suggests that the likelihood of developing spinal metastases in multiple myeloma is 14%, in prostate cancer 10%, in breast cancer 5%, and in lung cancer 5% (42). Epidural metastases are the initial presentation of cancer in about 20% of cases. In this setting, the most common primary malignancies include lung cancer, cancer of unknown primary, multiple myeloma, or non-Hodgkin's lymphoma (45).

The distribution of metastases to the spine is a function of length, with involvement of the cervical cord in 8% of cases, the thoracic cord in 82%, and the lumbosacral spine in 10% (44). An important consideration when evaluating a patient with possible ESCC is that an involvement of multiple noncontiguous levels is by no means uncommon (46,47).

Clinical Presentation

Pain is the most common initial feature of vertebral metastasis or spinal cord compression and is reported by 95% of patients (44). The pain may be localized, radicular, unilateral, or bilateral. ESCC pain is characteristically aggravated by recumbency due to venous congestion, but may also worsen with Valsalva's maneuver, straight-leg raising, and neck flexion. In general, there is poor concordance between the level of pain and the level of ESCC. Other common symptoms at diagnosis include weakness (74%), autonomic dysfunction (52%), and sensory disturbances (52%) (44). The sensory complaints may consist of painful dysesthesias and, rarely, this may be the initial symptom without any evidence for other neurological involvement. In a large series from Scotland, 41% of patients were nonambulatory at diagnosis and an additional 34% could walk with assistance (46). Despite the presence of pain, weakness, or sensory changes, the typical patient is diagnosed two months after initial presentation to their primary-care physician (46). These statistics highlight the importance of prompt investigation of neurological signs in patients with cancer.

Diagnosis

Historically, myelography was the gold standard for diagnosis of spinal cord compression. Due to the invasive nature of the procedure and the risk of neurologic deterioration (48), it has been supplanted by contrast-enhanced MRI scan. At the present time, myelography is reserved for patients with metal implants that cause unacceptable distortion of MRI images or those unable to tolerate MRI scan. Advantages of MRI include superior visualization of the spinal cord and surrounding tissues. It allows for delineation of the extraspinal extent of the lesion and evaluation beyond the symptomatic level.

The current recommendation is to screen the entire spine with MRI since neurologic symptoms in the lower body can be caused by lesions in the thoracic and cervical spine and because up to 20% of patients with symptomatic lesions have additional lesions at other levels (46,47). The presence of multiple lesions is important for treatment planning with surgery or radiation therapy.

Spine X-rays or bone scans are inadequate to diagnosis spinal cord compression. Spine X-rays lack sensitivity because 30% to 50% of the vertebral body must be destroyed before changes will be visible (44). Furthermore, ESCC is present in only 10% of patients with vertebral metastases without vertebral collapse. Bone scans are limited by false-positive rates that exceed 20%.

Treatment

The standard treatment for ESCC continues to evolve as randomized studies are performed. For most patients, treatment includes corticosteroids and radiotherapy. A randomized trial of high-dose corticosteroids in patients with spinal cord compression demonstrated benefit for dexamethasone 96 mg daily compared with placebo (49). Since high dose steroids are associated with significant side effects, many clinicians treat to clinical benefit with lower doses. Thus, the loading dose of dexamethasone ranges from 10 to 100 mg intravenously followed by 4–24 mg every six hours. Corticosteroids should be tapered after 48 to 72 hours if possible but should be maintained through radiotherapy as edema may initially worsen with treatment.

Radiation therapy has been the primary treatment modality for patients with ESCC because they often harbor multiple symptomatic lesions and are poor surgical candidates. Radiation therapy should begin as soon as possible once the diagnosis of ESCC has been established. As noted above, the entire spine should be imaged before treatment to establish the rostral and caudal boundaries for the radiation ports.

In recent years, surgical management of ESCC has been reserved for selected patients on a case-by-case basis. In general, surgical decompression was performed in patients who had (i) no established diagnosis, (ii) progressive neurologic deterioration during or after radiation therapy, (iii) localized disease (who are good surgical candidates), or (iv) unstable spines. Recently, a randomized trial of surgical decompression with postoperative radiation versus radiation only was published (50). In this study, subjects were required to have a single contiguous lesion, displacement of the spinal cord from its usual position, at least one neurologic sign or symptom, and duration of paraplegia for less than 48 hours. Subjects in the surgery group had higher rates of posttreatment ambulation (84% vs. 57%) and retained the ability to walk for longer (122 days vs. 13 days) than subjects in the radiation group. It should be noted that 40% of subjects in each group had evidence of spinal instability. The influence of this factor on posttreatment ambulation, as opposed to tumor progression, in both groups remains unanswered. This study suggests that for a group of highly selected patients with ESCC, surgical decompression with postoperative radiation is superior to radiation alone. These results cannot be used to justify surgical decompression in all patients with ESCC because patients with radiosensitive tumors, multiple areas of spinal cord compression, and long-standing paraplegia were excluded.

FUTURE DIRECTIONS

Increased ICP is a major source of morbidity for patients with primary and metastatic CNS lesions. As the molecular basis of cerebral edema unravels, targeted drugs should help treat this complication of metastatic disease with fewer side effects than seen with corticosteroids. Because the majority of patients with ESCC present with neurologic dysfunction at the time of presentation, future studies are needed to screen for this complication before it becomes clinically apparent.

REFERENCES

1. Fishman RA. Intracranial pressure: physiology and pathophysiology. Cerebrospinal Fluid in Diseases of the Nervous System. Philadelphia: W.B. Saunders Company, 1992:71–101.
2. Fishman RA. Disorders of intracranial pressure: hydrocephalus, brain edema, pseudotumor, intracranial hypotension, and related disorders. Cerebrospinal Fluid in Diseases of the Nervous System. Philadelphia: W.B. Saunders Company, 1992:103–155.
3. Dean BL, Drayer BP, Bird CR, et al. Gliomas: classification with MR imaging. Radiology 1990; 174(2):411–415.
4. Pope WB, Sayre J, Perlina A, Villablanca JP, Mischel PS, Cloughesy TF. MR imaging correlates of survival in patients with high-grade gliomas. AJNR Am J Neuroradiol 2005; 26(10):2466–2474.
5. Ide M, Jimbo M, Yamamoto M, Umebara Y, Hagiwara S, Kubo O. MIB-1 staining index and peritumoral brain edema of meningiomas. Cancer 1996; 78(1):133–143.
6. Tamiya T, Ono Y, Matsumoto K, Ohmoto T. Peritumoral brain edema in intracranial meningiomas: effects of radiological histological factors. Neurosurgery 2001; 49(5):1046–1051.
7. Papadopoulos MC, Saadoun S, Binder DK, Manley GT, Krishna S, Verkman AS. Molecular mechanisms of brain tumor edema. Neuroscience 2004; 129(4): 1009–1018.
8. Machein MR, Plate KH. VEGF in brain tumors. J Neurooncol 2000; 50(1–2): 109–120.
9. Dvorak AM, Feng D. The vesiculo-vacuolar organelle (VVO). A new endothelial cell permeability organelle. J Histochem Cytochem 2001; 49(4):419–432.
10. d'Avella D, Cicciarello R, Angileri FF, Lucerna S, La Torre D, Tomasello F. Radiation-induced blood-brain barrier changes: pathophysiological mechanisms and clinical implications. Acta Neurochir Suppl 1998; 71:282–284.
11. Hong KS, Cho YJ, Lee SK, Jeong SW, Kim WK, Oh EJ. Diffusion changes suggesting predominant vasogenic oedema during partial status epilepticus. Seizure 2004; 13(5):317–321.
12. Tsao MN, Li YQ, Lu G, Xu Y, Wong CS. Upregulation of vascular endothelial growth factor is associated with radiation-induced blood-spinal cord barrier breakdown. J Neuropathol Exp Neurol 1999; 58(10):1051–1060.
13. Adair JC, Baldwin N, Kornfeld M, Rosenberg GA. Radiation-induced blood-brain barrier damage in astrocytoma: relation to elevated gelatinase B and urokinase. J Neuroconcol 1999; 44(3):283–289.
14. Forsyth PA, Posner JB. Headaches in patients with brain tumors: a study of 111 patients. Neurology 1993; 43(9):1678–1683.
15. Crevel HV. Absence of papilloedema in cerebral tumors. J Neurol Neurosurg Psychiatry 1975; 38(9):931–933.
16. Young DF, Posner JB, Chu F, Nisce L. Rapid-course radiation therapy of cerebral metastases: results and complications. Cancer 1974; 34(4):1069–1076.
17. Levin BE. The clinical significance of spontaneous pulsations of the retinal vein. Arch Neurol 1978; 35(l):37–40.

18. Koehler PJ. Use of corticosteroids in neuro-oncology. Anticancer Drugs 1995; 6(1):19–33.
19. Heiss JD, Papavassiliou E, Merrill MJ, et al. Mechanism of dexamethasone suppression of brain tumor-associated vascular permeability in rats. Involvement of the glucocorticoid receptor and vascular permeability factor. J Clin Invest 1996; 98(6):1400–1408.
20. Vecht CJ, Hovestadt A, Verbiest HB, van Vliet JJ, van Putten WL. Dose-effect relationship of dexamethasone on Karnofsky performance in metastatic brain tumors: a randomized study of doses of 4, 8, and 16 mg per day. Neurology 1994; 44(4):675–680.
21. Jubiz W, Meikle AW. Alterations of glucocorticoid actions by other drugs and disease states. Drugs 1979; 18(2):113–121.
22. Tankisi A, Rolighed LJ, Rasmussen M, Dahl B, Cold GE. The effects of 10 degrees reverse trendelenburg position on ICP and CPP in prone positioned patients subjected to craniotomy for occipital or cerebellar tumours. Acta Neurochir (Wien) 2002; 144(7):665–670.
23. Durward QJ, Amacher AL, Del Maestro RF, Sibbald WJ. Cerebral and cardiovascular responses to changes in head elevation in patients with intracranial hypertension. J Neurosurg 1983; 59(6):938–944.
24. Fujimura M, Onuma T, Kameyama M, et al. Hydrocephalus due to cerebrospinal fluid overproduction by bilateral choroid plexus papillomas. Childs Nerv Syst 2004; 20(7):485–488.
25. Schijman E, Peter JC, Rekate HL, Sgouros S, Wong TT. Management of hydrocephalus in posterior fossa tumors: how, what, when? Childs Nerv Syst 2004; 20(3):192–194.
26. Marquardt G, Setzer M, Lang J, Seifert V. Delayed hydrocephalus after resection of supratentorial malignant gliomas. Acta Neurochir (Wien) 2002; 144(3):227–231.
27. Renowden S. Cerebral venous sinus thrombosis. Eur Radiol 2004; 14(2):215–226.
28. Digre KB, Corbett JJ. Idiopathic intracranial hypertension (pseudotumor cerebri): a reappraisal. Neurologist 2001; 7(1):2–67.
29. Farb RL, Vanek I, Scott JN, et al. Idiopathic intracranial hypertension: the prevalence and morphology of sinovenous stenosis. Neurology 2003; 60(9):1418–1424.
30. Fishman RA. Composition of the cerebrospinal fluid. In: Cerebrospinal Fluid in diseases of the Nervous System. Philadelphia: W.B. Saunders Company, 1992: 183–252.
31. Hage WD, Aboulafia AJ, Aboulafia DM. Incidence, location, and diagnostic evaluation of metastatic bone disease. Orthop Clin North Am 2000; 31(4):515–528, vii.
32. Louis DN, Scheithauer BW, Budka H, von Deimling A, Kepes JJ. Meningeal tumours. In: Kleibues P, Cavenee WK, eds. Pathology & genetics: tumours of the nervous system. Lyon: IARC Press, 2000:176–184.
33. Posner JB, Chernik NL. Intracranial metastases from systemic cancer. Adv Neurol 1978; 19:579–592.
34. Kleinschmidt-DeMasters BK. Dural metastases. A retrospective surgical and autopsy series. Arch Pathol Lab Med 2001; 125(7):880–887.
35. Constans JP, Donzelli R. Surgical features of cranial metastases. Surg Neurol 1981; 15(1):35–38.

36. Stark AM, Eichmann T, Mehdorn HM. Skull metastases: clinical features, differential diagnosis, and review of the literature. Surg Neurol 2003; 60(3):219–225.
37. Wecht DA, Sawaya R. Lesions of the calvaria: surgical experience with 42 patients. Ann Surg Oncol 1997; 4(1):28–36.
38. Tagle P, Villanueva P, Torrealba G, Huete I. Intracranial metastasis or meningioma? An uncommon clinical diagnostic dilemma. Surg Neurol 2002; 58(3–4):241–245.
39. River Y, Schwartz A, Gomori JM, Soffer D, Siegal T. Clinical significance of diffuse dural enhancement detected by magnetic resonance imaging. J Neurosurg 1996; 85(5):777–783.
40. Fukino K, Terao T, Kojima T, Adachi K, Teramoto A. Chronic subdural hematoma following dural metastasis of gastric cancer: measurement of pre- and postoperative cerebral blood flow with N-isopropyl-p-[123I]iodoamphetamine—case report. Neurol Med Chir (Tokyo) 2004; 44(12):646–649.
41. McAlhany HJ, Netsky MG. Compression of the spinal cord by extramedullary neoplasms; a clinical and pathologic study. J Neuropathol Exp Neurol 1955; 14(3):276–287.
42. Barron KD, Hirano A, Araki S, Terry RD. Experiences with metastatic neoplasms involving the spinal cord. Neurology 1959; 9(2):91–106.
43. Stark RJ, Henson RA, Evans SJ. Spinal metastases. A retrospective survey from a general hospital. Brain 1982; 105(Pt 1):189–213.
44. Posner JB. Spinal metastases. In: Neurologic complications of cancer. Philadelphia: F.A. Davis Company, 1995:111–142.
45. Schiff D, O'Neill BP, Suman VJ. Spinal epidural metastasis as the initial manifestation of malignancy: clinical features and diagnostic approach. Neurology 1997; 49(2):452–456.
46. Levack P, Graham J, Collie D, et al. Don't wait for a sensory level—listen to the symptoms: a prospective audit of the delays in diagnosis of malignant cord compression. Clin Oncol (EL Cell Radiol) 2002; 14(6):472–480.
47. Gilbert RW, Kim JH, Posner JB. Epidural spinal cord compression from metastatic tumor: diagnosis and treatment. Ann Neurol 1978; 3(1):40–51.
48. Hollis PH, Malis LI, Zappulla RA. Neurological deterioration after lumbar puncture below complete spinal subarachnoid block. J Neurosurg 1986; 64(2):253–256.
49. Sorensen S, Helweg-Larsen S, Mouridsen H, Hansen HH. Effect of high-dose dexamethasone in carcinomatous metastatic spinal cord compression treated with radiotherapy; a randomised trial. Eur J Cancer 1994; 30A(1):22–27.
50. Patchell RA, Tibbs PA, Regine WF, et al. Direct decompressive surgical resection in the treatment of spinal cord compression caused by metastatic cancer: a randomised trial. Lancet 2005; 366(9486):643–648.

25

Leptomeningeal Cancer

Joachim M. Baehring
Yale University School of Medicine,
New Haven, Connecticut, U.S.A.

Serguei Bannykh
Department of Pathology and Laboratory Medicine, Yale University
School of Medicine, New Haven, Connecticut, U.S.A.

INTRODUCTION

Leptomeningeal metastasis (meningeal carcinomatosis, sarcomatosis, lymphomatosis, gliomatosis; "neoplastic meningitis") denotes seeding of malignant cells from systemic or intracranial neoplasms to pia, arachnoid, and ventricular spaces. This occurs in 5% to 15% of patients with systemic cancer (1,2). Adenocarcinomas predominate (usually of breast, lung or gastrointestinal origin), although melanoma, small cell lung cancer, the acute leukemias, and high-grade Non-Hodgkin lymphomas have the highest disease-specific incidence (up to 50% in Burkitt's and lymphoblastic lymphoma). Risk factors for neuraxis seeding in lymphoid neoplasms include involvement of testis, orbit, paranasal sinuses, skull base or bone marrow, nodal invasion, and elevated lactate dehydrogenase at presentation (3,4). The diagnosis of leptomeningeal involvement is most commonly made six months to three years after the primary tumor is discovered. The meningeal compartment serves as a sanctuary for cancer cells where systemic chemotherapy does not achieve sustained therapeutic levels. This problem has become more relevant with the availability of more effective treatment protocols for various types of systemic cancer with limited penetration across the blood–brain barrier (taxane- or trastuzumab-based therapy for breast cancer; imatinib mesylate therapy for chronic myelogenous leukemia; and transretinoic acid therapy for promyelocytic leukemia). Meningeal spread of primary brain tumors is mostly encountered in medulloblastoma, germ cell tumors, as well as tumors of the ependyma and the choroid plexus.

PATHOGENESIS

Tumor cells may enter the arachnoid space hematogenously through lepto-meningeal veins, the choroid plexus, veins draining the diploe of the skull or marrow of the spinal column; through perineural spread along cranial or spinal segmental nerves; or as a result of inadvertent shedding during neu-rosurgical procedures. Predominant involvement of the posterior fossa may be explained by spread of cells from mediastinal or pelvic tumors through the paravertebral venous system (Batson's plexus). Rarely, primary or secondary parenchymal tumors of brain or spinal cord seed into the cerebrospinal fluid (CSF), usually when there is involvement of subpial or subependymal areas (5). CSF circulation is frequently impaired as a result of meningeal cancer. Meningeal or parenchymal tumor deposits at the fora-men of Monro, aqueduct of Sylvius, or outflow of the fourth ventricle result in obstructive hydrocephalus. CSF reabsorption at the arachnoid granula-tions may be impaired by cancer cells or proteinaceous debris. Low CSF glucose concentrations are found, likely a result of a glucose transport dis-turbance as in meningeal infections, chronic inflammation, or hemorrhage.

CLINICAL PRESENTATION

An almost pathognomonic manifestation of neoplastic meningitis consists of asymmetric cranial neuropathies combined with progressive multifocal radi-culopathies in a patient with systemic cancer. However, the clinical syndrome is commonly elusive and 5% to 10% of patients lack a history of cancer. In patients with acute leukemia, meningeal involvement is encountered at the time of staging procedures in the absence of neurological symptoms. Classi-cal signs of meningeal irritation are frequently absent. Nonlocalizing signs and symptoms predominate. Headache, gait disturbance (apraxia, ataxia, or paresis), psychomotor decline, and micturition abnormalities reflect direct effects of cancer or hydrocephalus. A more fulminant presentation with headache, nausea, vomiting, and hiccoughs is seen with aggressive neoplasms or CSF flow obstruction. The cranial nerves are either compressed by infil-trates of tumor cells or rendered ischemic when tumor invades the feeding vessels. This results in impaired visual acuity, diplopia from oculomotor or abducens nerve involvement, facial numbness or atypical facial pain, Bell's palsy, sensorineural hearing loss, dysphagia, or hoarseness. The compro-mised spinal nerve roots induce radicular pain and paresthesias. Involvement of the cauda equina produces pain, foot drop, perineal dysesthesias, and incontinence. Acute focal neurological deficits resembling thrombotic small vessel occlusion arise from tumor progression in Virchow-Robin spaces and obstruction of blood flow in encased penetrating vessels. Metastatic meningeal nodules within the spinal canal can exert pressure on the spinal cord and give rise to transverse myelopathy. Aggressive neoplasms may penetrate the pial covering of the cord and cause partial cord syndromes.

DIAGNOSIS

The diagnosis of meningeal cancer is generally difficult. A single CSF examination reveals tumor cells in 50% of patients, rising to 80% after two procedures (2). It is recommended that at least 10 mL of fluid from both ventricular and lumbar areas be sampled if possible, especially when assessing the response to treatment. Sensitivity may be further increased if the sample is taken in proximity to a site involved clinically or radiographically (i.e., cisternal puncture in a patient with involvement of cranial nerves; lumbar puncture in a patient with cauda equina syndrome) (6,7). CSF cytology remains persistently negative on repeated fluid examinations in 20% of patients with leptomeningeal disease (2). The CSF specimen should be processed immediately as tumor cells are fragile (Fig. 1). Certain tumors, such as sarcomas or malignant gliomas, are seldom detected in CSF because their cells strongly adhere to the leptomeninges or occur as focal nodules rather than widespread leptomeningeal disease (8). Lymphatic neoplasms are an even bigger challenge; they may be indistinguishable from reactive infiltrates on morphological grounds. Cell numbers are commonly insufficient for flow cytometry characterization. Clonality assessment with immunoglobulin heavy chain—or T-cell receptor—gene rearrangement analysis is available but sensitivity and specificity of this test in CSF remains unknown (Fig. 1). Magnetic resonance imaging (MRI) is a valuable tool in the diagnosis of leptomeningeal metastasis (Figs. 2 and 3). Often gadolinium-enhanced MRI is definitive in the absence of CSF cytological abnormalities. MRI delineates leptomeningeal or subependymal enhancement, superficial cerebral lesions, enhancement of cranial nerves, or communicating hydrocephalus, the latter occurring most often in patients with solid, rather than hematological, tumors (9,10). The single most characteristic finding is the appearance of thickened, often nodular enhancing lumbar nerve roots within the subarachnoid space. Increased sulcal signal on fluid-attenuated inversion recovery sequences may be of diagnostic value in the correct clinical setting. The notion that intracranial hypotension after a lumbar puncture may mimic the findings of neoplastic meningitis is a myth. Intracranial hypotension results in diffuse pachymeningeal enhancement that is easily distinguished from the typically multifocal, leptomeningeal abnormalities of carcinomatosis. Nonetheless, an imaging study is preferably obtained prior to lumbar puncture, especially if obstruction of CSF flow is suspected.

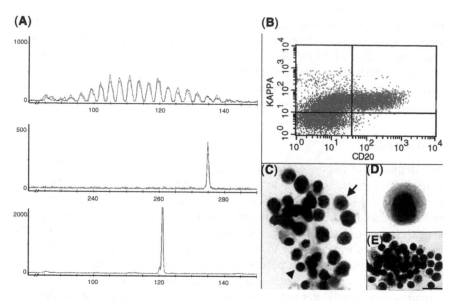

Figure 1 Spinal fluid analysis in patients with leptomeningeal cancer. (**A**) Immunoglobulin heavy chain gene (IgH) rearrangement analysis of DNA isolated from cerebrospinal fluid (CSF) of a patient with lymphomatous seeding of the leptomeninges [diffuse large B-cell lymphoma (DLBCL)]. Polymerase chain reaction (PCR) using DNA isolated from CSF, and degenerate primers for the complementarity determining regions II (*middle*) and III (*bottom*) of IgH yielded a single product of 275 and 121 base pairs in length, respectively, which were reproducible in duplicate assays (middle and bottom capillary electropherogram: two superimposed curves; x-axis: length of PCR product in base pairs, y-axis: relative concentration of PCR product; upper graph: "polyclonal control" using DNA isolated from a human tonsil as a template). (**B**) Automated fluorescent cell sorting using kappa light chain and CD20 antibodies identifies a clonal B-cell population (right upper quadrant of this scatter plot) in this patient with leptomeningeal metastasis from DLBCL. (**C–E**) Cytopathological evaluation of CSF sediment obtained from patients with various types of cancer. (**C**) Systemic DLBCL. There is a mixed population of normal (*black arrow head*; size approximately 8 μm) and malignant lymphocytes (*black arrow*). (**D**) Non–small-cell lung cancer (cell diameter approximately 10 μm). (**E**) Central neurocytoma. A sample of cerebrospinal fluid was obtained from a ventriculostomy catheter after subtotal tumor resection. The specimen consists of small clumps of round cells. The cell nuclei have a "salt and pepper" chromatin pattern and are surrounded by moderate amount of cytoplasm (Papanicolaou stain). Bar: 25 μm.

Biochemical markers such as vascular endothelial growth factor or carcinoembryonic antigen have not improved the diagnosis of leptomeningeal cancer. Exceptions are α-fetoprotein and β-human chorionic gonadotropin, which given in an adequate clinical setting and imaging findings, may be diagnostic for nongerminomatous germ cell tumors of the CNS (11).

(A) **(B)** **(C)**

(D) **(E)** **(F)**

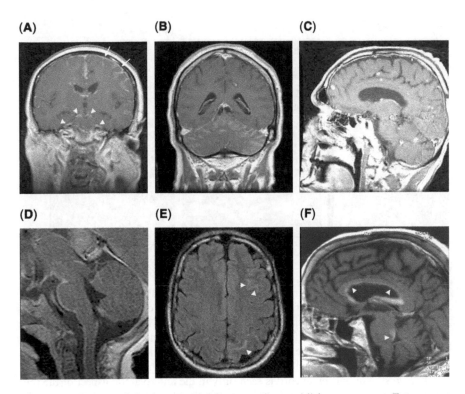

Figure 2 Cancer of the intracranial leptomeninges. All images except E represent T1-weighted magnetic resonance image (MRI) after gadolinium administration. (A) Primary leptomeningeal Non-Hodgkin lymphoma. This coronal image shows linear enhancement of the pia predominantly overlying the left frontal lobe (*arrows*). There is also infiltration of the oculomotor and trigeminal nerves on both sides (*arrow heads*). (B) Extensive leptomeningeal seeding to the posterior fossa is demonstrated in this patient with esophageal cancer. The cerebellar foliae are outlined by contrast-enhancing material. (C) This sagittal image reveals multiple enhancing meningeal metastatic nodules in a patient with alveolar cell carcinoma. (D) Sagittal MRI of a newborn with choroid plexus carcinoma of the right lateral ventricle. Meningeal carcinomatosis is recognized as linear enhancement on the surface of midbrain, pons, medulla oblongata, and cervical spinal cord. (E) Axial fluid attenuated inversion recovery image of a patient with acute myelogenous leukemia. There is increased signal following a sulcal pattern indicative of leukemic infiltration of leptomeninges (*arrow heads*). (F) Sagittal off-midline view of a patient with meningeal spread from intravascular Non-Hodgkin lymphoma. There is linear enhancement consistent with subependymal infiltration by tumor cells outlining the walls of the lateral and fourth ventricle (*arrow heads*).

In patients without the diagnosis of systemic cancer or in the absence of imaging or CSF findings, a meningeal biopsy may be indicated. It is advisable to withhold the use of corticosteroids until appropriate diagnostic material has been retrieved, if leptomeningeal lymphomatosis or leukemia is suspected.

(A) **(B)** **(C)**

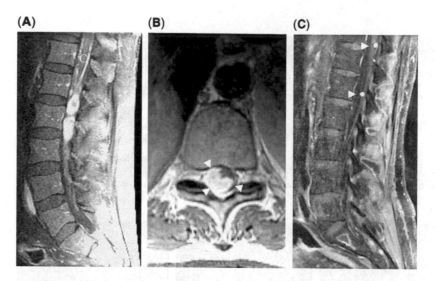

Figure 3 Leptomeningeal cancer of the spinal canal. All images are T1-weighted images after administration of gadolinium with (**A, C**) and without (**B**) fat suppression. (**A**) Meningeal gliomatosis. This sagittal image of the lumbar spine shows linear enhancement on the surface of the conus medullaris (c) and large, centrally necrotic nodular lesions attached to the cauda equina. (**B**) Meningeal metastasis invading and compressing the thoracic spinal cord in a patient with a pineal region yolk sac tumor (*arrow heads*). Normal spinal cord is seen only in the anterolateral aspect of the thecal sac to the left of the midline. (**C**) Enhancing nodules attached to the roots of the cauda equina in a patient with post-transplant lymphoproliferative disorder (PTLD); sagittal magnetic resonance imaging (MRI) of the lumbar spine. The patient complained of worsening chronic low back and leg pain. Repeated lumbar punctures were unrevealing. He had had a neurofibroma removed from his left arm years prior to diagnosis of PTLD. MRI of his legs revealed an enhancing tumor of the tibial nerve on the right and two similarly appearing lesions on the left suggestive of benign nerve sheath tumors. The cauda equina lesions have not changed over the course of two years and likely represent benign nerve sheath tumors as well.

Prior to initiation of therapy, many clinicians perform CSF flow studies using [111]Indium-,[99]Tc-diethylenetriamine penta-acetic acid, or ^{99}Tc-macroaggregated albumin, which is injected into the lumbar CSF. Sequential scans may reveal obstruction at the level of the basal cisterns, the spinal canal, within the ventricular system, or over the cerebral convexities (12).

DIFFERENTIAL DIAGNOSIS

Opportunistic meningeal infections such as bacterial, varicella zoster or cryptococcal meningitis and herpes simplex meningoencephalitis can resemble meningeal carcinomatosis. In the absence of systemic cancer, chronic meningitis of infectious (Borrelia) or noninfectious etiology has to be considered. Cranial neuropathies in cancer patients can result from dural tumor growth, leukemic obstruction of vasa nervorum (leukostasis), or hyperviscosity. Benign nerve sheath tumors are occasionally found when a patient with cancer undergoes MR imaging for back pain. They are difficult to distinguish from carcinomatous nodules attached to the cauda equina. Surveillance imaging usually reveals their benign growth behavior, but lumbar puncture or biopsy may be warranted in selected cases. Recipients of whole or partial brain radiotherapy may develop communicating hydrocephalus.

MANAGEMENT

As a general rule, symptomatic or nodular foci of tumor require irradiation, whereas chemotherapy is provided to patients without these findings. Symptomatic intracranial disease is usually treated with whole brain radiotherapy. For disease involving the spinal canal, involved field irradiation is used. Radiation to the entire neuraxis is generally avoided except for patients with isolated meningeal disease, excellent performance status, and bone marrow reserve.

Chemotherapy can be administered either systemically or intrathecally; in most instances, intrathecal chemotherapy via an Ommaya device is the preferable route of administration. This titanium-based reservoir covered by a Silastic membrane is implanted beneath the galea aponeurotica in communication with the ventricle, and serves as a painless delivery port (13). Complications from its use occur in 5% to 20% of patients and include infection, failure, bleeding, or drug toxicities to white matter (14).

Commonly employed chemotherapeutic agents include methotrexate (MTX; 12 mg twice a week), cytarabine (50 mg twice a week or liposomal cytarabine every two weeks), and thiotepa (10 mg twice a week). Remission induction is followed by variable consolidation and maintenance schedules. Combination of these drugs or the addition of corticosteroids does not appear to improve outcome compared to single agents (15,16). Myelosuppression can occur after intrathecal chemotherapy. If MTX is chosen, this complication can be prevented by using folinic acid (10 mg every six hours for 24 hours after administration of MTX). Use of the extended-release preparation of cytarabine results in prolonged neurological progression-free survival and an increased complete response rate but does not prolong survival (17–19). Intrathecal rituximab may be an alternative for patients with meningeal seeding from B-cell lymphoma (20,21). Intensive treatment regimens are required in adults with CSF seeding by leukemia. Early whole brain radiation therapy (WBXRT) is provided with intrathecal MTX or triple therapy (22). However, the appearance of neurocognitive sequelae without improved survival has prompted investigators to delay or defer WBXRT in favor of high-dose MTX or cytarabine (23). The most common adverse reaction to intrathecal administration of chemotherapy is chemical meningitis. This is most common after liposomal cytarabine but can effectively be treated with corticosteroids. A stroke-like syndrome is a rare complication of intrathecal MTX injection occurring 7 to 10 days after treatment. Symptoms are transient and re-exposure without recurrence of the syndrome has been described (24,25). Even more unusual are transverse myelopathies after intrathecal chemotherapy administration, and in most cases, the etiology remains obscure. A calcific leukoencephalopathy with devastating cognitive sequelae follows the combination of whole brain radiotherapy with high daily fractions and subsequent intrathecal MTX. When spinal fluid flow is obstructed by a meningeal or parenchymal deposit at a "bottle neck" such as the Foramen of Monro or the aqueduct, intrathecal administration of chemotherapy rostrally to the level of flow impairment is contraindicated. Only after successful treatment with irradiation can such treatment be reconsidered.

A few systemic chemotherapy options for leptomeningeal cancer exist. High-dose MTX (exceeding $3 \, g/m^2$) or cytarabine ($3 \, g/m^2$) given intravenously penetrate into the CSF at therapeutic concentrations, and the pharmacokinetic profile appears even better than with direct intrathecal administration. However, incorporation in chemotherapy regimens targeting the systemic component of the disease is difficult and thus, these regimens are usually reserved for patients with isolated meningeal disease (26). Responses of leptomeningeal carcinomatosis from breast cancer to systemic hormonal therapy (antiestrogens and aromatase inhibitors) have been reported.

Patients with Non-Hodgkin lymphoma (NHL) at high risk of nervous system involvement commonly receive prophylactic intrathecal chemotherapy or cranial irradiation. Prophylactic treatment of brain or meninges is provided for lymphoma of testicular, eye, or cranial sinus origin as well as lymphoblastic histologies or Burkitt lymphoma (3). Intrathecal MTX (12 mg weekly for five doses) may be combined with cytarabine or hydrocortisone.

MTX-based regimens are provided as prophylaxis of and treatment for CNS involvement in children with acute lymphoblastic leukemia (ALL). These therapies include intrathecal MTX, or MTX in combination with cytarabine and corticosteroids (triple intrathecal therapy: MTX $15 \, mg/m^2$ to a maximum of 15 mg, cytarabine $30 \, mg/m^2$ to a maximum of 60 mg, and hydrocortisone $60 \, mg/m^2$). In addition, systemic MTX is often included in the consolidation phase of treatment followed by WBXRT (27). Intrathecal chemotherapy is sufficient for patients with standard risk. High-dose systemic MTX is used in patients at intermediate risk who are not radiated. Adults are prophylaxed with WBXRT [with inclusion of the posterior retina and orbital apex (optic nerve sheath; 24 Gy at 2 Gy/day in 12 fractions)]. High-risk children receive 18 Gy at 1.8 Gy/day in 10 fractions. Lower radiation doses may be possible with intensification of systemic chemotherapy. As CNS involvement is rare at initial presentation in patients with acute myeloid leukemia, CNS prophylaxis is not generally provided. New management strategies are likely to concentrate on utilization of monoclonal antibodies, slow-release chemotherapy agents, or those with high penetrance into CSF after systemic administration. New drugs being evaluated for neoplastic meningitis include topotecan (28), gemcitabine (29), mafosfamide (30), diaziquone (31), cytokines, a microcrystalline formulation of temozolomide (32), and radioactively labeled monoclonal antibodies.

PROGNOSIS

Without treatment, patients with meningeal cancer succumb within six weeks. A fraction of patients with leukemia, lymphoma, and breast cancer, especially the few with isolated meningeal disease, respond to treatment, and progression-free survival exceeding one year is possible. The prognosis for patients with non–small-cell lung cancer, other adenocarcinomas, and melanoma is extremely poor both quoad vitam and in regards to functional recovery. The survival extends to three to six months with radiation therapy targeting symptomatic sites and intrathecal chemotherapy (10).

REFERENCES

1. Grossman SA, Krab MJ. Leptomeningeal carcinomatosis. Cancer Treat Rev 1999; 25(2):103–119.
2. Wasserstrom WR, Glass JP, Posner JB. Diagnosis and treatment of leptomeningeal metastases from solid tumors: experience with 90 patients. Cancer 1982; 49(4):759–772.
3. van Besien K, Ha CS, Murphy S, et al. Risk factors, treatment, and outcome of central nervous system recurrence in adults with intermediate-grade and immunoblastic lymphoma. Blood 1998; 91(4):1178–1184.
4. Hollender A, Kvaloy S, Nome O, Skovlund E, Lote K, Holte H. Central nervous system involvement following diagnosis of non-Hodgkin's lymphoma: a risk model. Ann Oncol 2002; 13(7):1099–1107.
5. Olson ME, Chernik NL, Posner JB. Leptomeningeal metastasis from systemic cancer: a report of 47 cases. Trans Am Neurol Assoc 1971; 96:291–293.
6. Glantz MJ, Cole BF, Glantz LK, et al. Cerebrospinal fluid cytology in patients with cancer: minimizing false-negative results. Cancer 1998; 82(4):733–739.
7. Chamberlain MC, Kormanik PA, Glantz MJ. A comparison between ventricular and lumbar cerebrospinal fluid cytology in adult patients with leptomeningeal metastases. Neuro-oncology 2001; 3(1):42–45.
8. Glass JP, Melamed M, Chernik NL, Posner JB. Malignant cells in cerebrospinal fluid (CSF): the meaning of a positive CSF cytology. Neurology 1979; 29(10):1369–1375.
9. Freilich RJ, Krol G, DeAngelis LM. Neuroimaging and cerebrospinal fluid cytology in the diagnosis of leptomeningeal metastasis. Ann Neurol 1995; 38(1):51–57.
10. Chamberlain MC. Neoplastic meningitis. J Clin Oncol 2005; 23(15):3605–3613.
11. Matsutani M. Clinical management of primary central nervous system germ cell tumors. Semin Oncol 2004; 31(5):676–683.
12. Glantz MJ, Hall WA, Cole BF, et al. Diagnosis, management, and survival of patients with leptomeningeal cancer based on cerebrospinal fluid-flow status. Cancer 1995; 75(12):2919–2931.
13. Ratcheson RA, Ommaya AK. Experience with the subcutaneous cerebrospinal-fluid reservoir Preliminary report of 60 cases. N Engl J Med 1968; 279(19):1025–1031.
14. Chamberlain MC, Kormanik PA, Barba D. Complications associated with intraventricular chemotherapy in patients with leptomeningeal metastases. J Neurosurg 1997; 87(5):694–699.

15. Hitchins RN, Bell DR, Woods RL, Levi JA. A prospective randomized trial of single-agent versus combination chemotherapy in meningeal carcinomatosis. J Clin Oncol 1987; 5(10):1655–1662.
16. Grossman SA, Finkelstein DM, Ruckdeschel JC, Trump DL, Moynihan T, Ettinger DS. Randomized prospective comparison of intraventricular methotrexate and thiotepa in patients with previously untreated neoplastic meningitis Eastern Cooperative Oncology Group. J Clin Oncol 1993; 11(3):561–569.
17. Glantz MJ, Jaeckle KA, Chamberlain MC, et al. A randomized controlled trial comparing intrathecal sustained-release cytarabine (DepoCyt) to intrathecal methotrexate in patients with neoplastic meningitis from solid tumors. Clin Cancer Res 1999; 5(11):3394–3402.
18. Glantz MJ, LaFollette S, Jaeckle KA, et al. Randomized trial of a slow-release versus a standard formulation of cytarabine for the intrathecal treatment of lymphomatous meningitis. J Clin Oncol 1999; 17(10):3110–3116.
19. Jaeckle KA, Batchelor T, O'Day SJ, et al. An open label trial of sustained-release cytarabine (DepoCyt) for the intrathecal treatment of solid tumor neoplastic meningitis. J Neurooncol 2002; 57(3):231–239.
20. Rubenstein JL, Combs D, Rosenberg J, et al. Rituximab therapy for CNS lymphomas: targeting the leptomeningeal compartment. Blood 2003; 101(2):466–468.
21. Schulz H, Pels H, Schmidt-Wolf I, Zeelen U, Germing U, Engert A. Intraventricular treatment of relapsed central nervous system lymphoma with the anti-CD20 antibody rituximab. Haematologica 2004; 89(6):753–754.
22. Larson RA, Dodge RK, Burns CP, et al. A five-drug remission induction regimen with intensive consolidation for adults with acute lymphoblastic leukemia: cancer and leukemia group B study 8811. Blood 1995; 85(8):2025–2037.
23. Gokbuget N, Hoelzer D. Meningeosis leukaemica in adult acute lymphoblastic leukaemia. J Neurooncol 1998; 38(2–3):167–180.
24. Haykin ME, Gorman M, van Hoff J, Fulbright RK, Baehring JM. Diffusion-weighted MRI correlates of subacute methotrexate-related neurotoxicity. J Neurooncol 2006; 76(2):153–157.
25. Fisher MJ, Khademian ZP, Simon EM, Zimmerman RA, Bilaniuk LT. Diffusion-weighted MR imaging of early methotrexate-related neurotoxicity in children. AJNR Am J Neuroradiol 2005; 26(7):1686–1689.
26. Lassman AB, Abrey LE, Shah GG, et al. Systemic high-dose intravenous methotrexate for central nervous system metastases. J Neurooncol 2005:1–6.
27. Schrappe M, Reiter A, Riehm H. Prophylaxis and treatment of neoplastic meningeosis in childhood acute lymphoblastic leukemia. J Neurooncol 1998; 38(2–3):159–165.
28. Blaney SM, Heideman R, Berg S, et al. Phase I clinical trial of intrathecal topotecan in patients with neoplastic meningitis. J Clin Oncol 2003; 21(1):143–147.
29. Egorin MJ, Zuhowski EG, McCully CM, et al. Pharmacokinetics of intrathecal gemcitabine in nonhuman primates. Clin Cancer Res 2002; 8(7):2437–2442.
30. Blaney SM, Balis FM, Berg S, et al. Intrathecal mafosfamide: a preclinical pharmacology and phase I trial. J Clin Oncol 2005; 23(7):1555–1563.
31. Berg SL, Balis FM, Zimm S, et al. Phase I/II trial and pharmacokinetics of intrathecal diaziquone in refractory meningeal malignancies. J Clin Oncol 1992; 10(1):143–148.
32. Sampson JH, Archer GE, Villavicencio AT, et al. Treatment of neoplastic meningitis with intrathecal temozolomide. Clin Cancer Res 1999; 5(5):1183–1188.

26

Neurovascular Complications of Cancer

Vineeta Singh and Terry Neill

*Department of Neurology, University of California at San Francisco,
San Francisco, California, U.S.A.*

INTRODUCTION

Neurovascular disorders are not uncommon in cancer patients and usually arise from mechanisms unique to malignancy. These disorders can be caused by one or a combination of factors present in cancer patients, e.g., direct tumor effect, complication of cancer therapy, hypercoagulability, and immuno-compromised state. The neurovascular disorders in cancer patients can be broadly categorized into ischemic strokes, hemorrhagic strokes, cerebral venous thrombosis (CVT), and microangiopathic disorders. In this chapter, we have discussed various possible etiological factors of these neurovascular syndromes in cancer patients, and their clinical characteristics, management, and prognosis.

ISCHEMIC STROKE

Ischemic stroke is one of the several neurological complications in cancer patients. Atherosclerotic risk factors, e.g., hypertension and diabetes, may be present in some cases. More commonly, however, the hypercoagulable state and tumor-related inflammation that in turn activates the coagulation system predispose these patients to stroke (Table 1). In some cases, ischemic stroke from leptomeningeal metastasis may be the first clinical evidence of an underlying solid tumor. The local infiltration or compression of a cerebral artery

Table 1 Mechanisms of Ischemic Stroke in Cancer

Cerebral embolization	*Cerebral thrombosis*
Solid tumor in the lung or heart	Cisplatin
Aortic arch tumor	*Carotid artery disease*
Thoracotomy for the removal of	Radiation therapy for childhood
lung tumor	lymphoma
Nonbacterial thrombotic	Radiation therapy for head and neck
endocarditis	cancer
Septic emboli from fungal	
infection	

with resultant vessel occlusion from a tumor or vessel occlusion from tumor emboli in rarer cases can cause a stroke. Patients with intravascular lymphoma generally present with signs of stroke with or without systemic evidence of tumor (1). In a female patient, recurrent cerebral embolism might be the first clinical sign of occult ovarian neoplasm (2).

Nonbacterial thrombotic endocarditis (NBTE) is usually a complication of advanced or terminal malignancies. The high incidence of multiple emboli and its association with malignant neoplasms and with a variety of cardiovascular, pulmonary, renal, and gastrointestinal disorders should provide clues for recognition of this serious disorder. Adenocarcinoma, mostly lung and pancreas, comprise more than 50% of associated malignancies. However, hematopoietic malignancies, including acute leukemia, multiple myeloma, and Hodgkin's and non-Hodgkin's lymphoma have also been implicated (3). The pathophysiology of NBTE involves coagulopathy resulting in an increased propensity of platelets and fibrin to deposit on the cardiac valves.

Cerebral thrombosis is reported with some chemotherapy treatments. Endothelial injury, venous stasis, vasculitis, vasospasm, or coagulation activation have been implicated as mechanisms for thrombosis in these cases (4). Cerebral infarction, particularly involving cortical blindness, has been widely reported with the use of cisplatin (5). A small risk of cerebral thrombosis exists with combination of chemotherapy and hormonal therapy for women with breast cancer (6). A stroke-like syndrome occasionally follows systemic high-dose methotrexate infusion (7). The disorder usually follows the second or third treatment by five or six days and is characterized by alternating hemiparesis associated with aphasia and sometimes encephalopathy and coma. Patients recover spontaneously in two to three days. Radiation therapy to the neck, often performed to treat lymphoma and head and neck cancer, can result in thrombosis and subsequent stenosis of the carotid arteries. Accelerated atherosclerosis from radiation is thought to be the etiology for thrombosis. The interval from radiation to infarction varies and is usually more than five years (8). The diagnosis of radiation-induced vasculopathy, to a great degree, is a diagnosis by exclusion coupled with any relevant history of radiation therapy to the affected vessels.

Neurovascular complications are among the many neurological complications that can occur as a result of bone marrow transplantation (BMT). The incidence of stroke after BMT has been reported near 3% in one study (9).

Fungal infections are one of the more common and unfortunately serious infections associated with cancer that can lead to neurovascular compromise. Fungal sepsis occurs most commonly in patients with leukemia or patients who have undergone bone marrow transplant and are immunosuppressed (9).

Clinical Features

Ischemic strokes in a cancer patient are usually accompanied by a global encephalopathy due to the diffuse nature of cerebral thromboses. The course of encephalopathy in patients with NBTE is fluctuating and progressive, eventually resulting in coma in some cases. The presence of concomitant systemic vascular thrombosis is often a clue to an underlying hypercoagulable state. The clinical diagnosis of NBTE can also be suspected from coexistent ischemic involvement of extremities, myocardial infarction, pulmonary embolism, or systemic bleeding. Of note, stroke or encephalopathy may be the first and in many cases the only sign of systemic thromboembolism.

In an immunocompromised patient, symptoms like fever, seizures, and headache imply an infective etiology. Fungal septic infarction may produce cranial neuropathies, cortical signs, seizures, or encephalopathy. In these cases, signs often progress rapidly.

Diagnosis and Treatment

Once a stroke or transient ischemic attack is suspected in a cancer patient, clinical history and exam data should be synthesized and a list of potential localizations generated before neuroimaging studies are ordered or interpreted. This prevents one from being misled by preexisting or unrelated abnormalities on computed tomography (CT) or magnetic resonance imaging (MRI). In ischemic stroke associated with leptomeningeal metastasis, CT and MRI can reveal focal or multifocal infarctions as well as leptomeningeal enhancement. With evolving techniques like CT perfusion studies, the entire neurovascular axis, the brain parenchyma, and the arteries can be screened promptly with minimum discomfort to the patient. A conventional angiogram can be performed for more thorough evaluation of the vasculature.

When a stroke is believed to be caused by tumor emboli, neuroimaging should be repeated in several weeks to determine if a tumor has developed. Therapy should be directed to the primary tumor to prevent further embolization.

A transesophageal echocardiogram can be diagnostic in patients with suspected NBTE. The vegetations are usually less than 2 mm in size and invariably present on aortic or mitral valve. Anticoagulation with heparin appears to help some patients and does not promote brain hemorrhage. Early diagnosis and vigorous treatment of nonbacterial endocarditis may prevent severe neurologic disability.

Intracranial tumors are considered an absolute contraindication for thrombolysis because of their association with spontaneous intracranial hemorrhage, although no such cases have been reported in connection with lytic treatment. Local catheter thrombolysis has been used routinely in this population, but systemic thrombolysis is not recommended for the treatment of acute stroke in patients with symptomatic malignancy.

In radiation-induced carotid disease, angiography usually reveals the extent of stenosis. Depending on the extent of disease, antiplatelet therapy may prove effective for stroke prevention. Revascularization procedures, such as angioplasty and stenting, and endarterectomy have been successfully performed in more severe cases of radiation-induced carotid disease (10,11). Treatment must be determined on an individual basis with comorbid conditions being taken into account. Cerebrospinal fluid (CSF) analysis in septic embolization is often nondiagnostic and CSF cultures can be negative. Antifungal therapy is often unsuccessful and the prognosis is poor (3).

Hemorrhagic Stroke

Intraparenchymal hemorrhage related to an underlying neoplasm is relatively uncommon. Tumor-related hemorrhage is more common in metastatic than primary brain tumors (Table 2). Four main factors are involved in the pathophysiology of tumor-related hemorrhage: (i) rapid tumor necrosis, (ii) rupture of newly formed vessels, (iii) tumor invasion of vessel wall, and (iv) associated coagulation defects (12).

Neoplastic cerebral aneurysms are a rare but known cause of intracerebral hemorrhage (13). Leukemias have also been reported to cause hemorrhagic brain metastases. The mechanism is thought to be indirect due to leukostasis resulting in local hypoxia and vessel destruction, or direct due to invasion of blood vessels by leukemic infiltrates.

Table 2 Tumors Presenting with Hemorrhagic Stroke

Primary brain tumors	*Metastatic brain tumors*
Glioblastoma	Melanoma
Oligodendroglioma	Choriocarcinoma
Astrocytoma	Renal cell carcinoma
	Thyroid carcinoma
	Bronchogenic carcinoma
	Breast cancer
	Retinoblastoma

Chemotherapy, particularly, mitomycin C as well as bleomycin, cisplatin, and gemcitabine may precipitate microangiopathic hemolytic anemia and hemolytic uremic-like syndrome with thrombocytopenia (3). The hematological abnormalities, which also include coagulopathies, may be responsible for some cerebral hemorrhages during chemotherapy. Intracerebral hemorrhages secondary to radiation-induced angiomatous malformation have also been well documented in the literature. The pathogenesis of angiomatous changes in irradiated vessels is unclear.

Studies have also noted a higher than expected incidence of cerebral hemorrhages in patients after bone marrow transplant (3). This could be explained by a relatively high incidence of strokes caused by infectious causes, particularly fungal infections such as aspergillosis (3). Neurological outcome from these severe infections can be difficult to predict, particularly when stroke has occurred and unfortunately is frequently fatal.

Clinical Features

Parenchymal hemorrhage associated with brain metastasis usually produces acute symptoms of headache, obtundation, or seizure that may be accompanied by focal signs.

Diagnosis and Treatment

Brain hemorrhages associated with metastasis are more often multiple than single and are easily visible on CT or MRI. Early edema, enhancement adjacent to the hemorrhage, and the presence of distant enhancing lesions suggest hemorrhage that is associated with brain metastasis (Table 3). If there is no known cancer and tumor-related hemorrhage is suspected, resection or biopsy of the hematoma should be performed to search for tumor. The hemorrhages of hyperleukocytosis are usually multiple and located in the white matter. Lowering of the peripheral blast cell count in hyperleukocytosis by

Table 3 Imaging Characteristics of Tumor-Related Hemorrhage

Computed tomography brain
 Multiple hemorrhages
 Located at gray-white junction
 Unusual location with extensive edema
 Perihematoma enhancement after 8–12 wks

Magnetic resonance imaging brain
 Marked signal heterogeneity in the mass
 Contrast enhancement of nonhemorrhagic portion
 Diminished, faint or absent hemosiderin rim
 Pronounced and persistent edema
 Delayed hematoma evolution

emergency administration of antimetabolites and leucopheresis reduces the risk of brain hemorrhage. When parenchymal intratumoral hemorrhage is acute and life threatening, resection of the hematoma may be beneficial. Radiation or chemotherapy should be directed to the underlying tumor.

SUBDURAL HEMATOMA

Tumor-related subdural hemorrhages can result from dural metastasis or from skull metastasis that invades the dura. The mechanism of subdural hemorrhage is speculated to be rupture of vessels within the metastatic tumor, erosion of adjacent vessels by the tumor, or rupture of the inner dural vessels because of congestion of the outer vessels. Head trauma or coagulopathy contributes to the risk of subdural hemorrhage in some patients. Subdural hemorrhage occurs most often with dural or skull metastasis from carcinoma, especially breast, prostate, or gastric carcinoma, but it is also reported with lymphoblastic leukemia and lymphoma (3).

Clinical Features

Clinical signs of tumor-related subdural hemorrhage can develop acutely or subacutely. Headache, confusion, and lethargy are characteristic and these may be accompanied by focal cerebral signs.

Diagnosis and Treatment

In tumor-related subdural hemorrhage, the CT or MRI may show prominent dural enhancement from the tumor and, in the case of skull metastasis, enhancement and destruction or expansion of the adjacent skull in addition to the subdural fluid. When dural metastasis is microscopic, it is necessary to histologically examine the dural membrane and subdural fluid to identify cancer. Drainage of subdural fluid may be necessary if tumor-related subdural hematoma is symptomatic, and drainage should be followed by brain radiation to prevent recurrence.

CEREBRAL VENOUS THROMBOSIS

CVT occurs most commonly in patients with hematological malignancies, especially leukemia following the administration of L-asparaginase. There are a few less clearly identified risk factors that might play a role in the development of CVT in these patients, for example, repeated lumbar puncture with a potential CSF leak, headache, and nausea causing dehydration. Administration of estrogen and erythropoietin in some cases also increases the hypercoagulability.

This has also been reported in patients with solid tumors following the administration of chemotherapy or tamoxifen. The true incidence of venous thrombosis is unknown, as the sinus can recanalize and thus is not present at autopsy.

Clinical Features

CVT is extremely variable in its clinical presentation and mode of onset. Headache is the earliest symptom of CVT. Presence of other neurologic signs, such as papilledema, focal neurologic deficits, and seizures, distinguishes it from more benign causes of headache.

Diagnosis and Treatment

A high index of clinical suspicion is required to diagnose this challenging condition, so that appropriate therapy can be instituted in timely fashion. Thrombosis of a venous sinus from L-asparaginase or other cancer-related causes can be detected on MRI or magnetic resonance venogram (MRV). Despite the presence of intraparenchymal hemorrhage and the general perception of increased risk of intracranial hemorrhage in this population, heparin is the recommended treatment of established CVT. Optimal dosing of low-molecular-weight heparin therapy has not been established for cancer patients who are at particular risk of venous thromboembolism and generally require escalated or prolonged anticoagulation with intense monitoring of therapy (14).

DISSEMINATED INTRAVASCULAR COAGULATION

In hematologic malignancies like leukemia, intracranial hemorrhage usually occurs at presentation or during relapse. In these individuals, thrombocytopenia is almost always associated with intracranial hemorrhage. At least in some cases, it is the result of platelet consumption due to disseminated intravascular coagulation (DIC) rather than reduced platelet production. DIC is characterized by a propensity for both fibrin deposition and increased fibrinolysis. In the absence of any other abnormality of coagulation, intracranial hemorrhage is unusual if the platelet count is greater than $20,000/mm^3$. Characteristically, the hemorrhages are multiple, and vary in size from multiple petechial hemorrhages to large confluent ones. The diffuse nature of these hemorrhages results in rapid neurologic decline. If the bleeding is localized and not multicentric, the stroke syndromes depend on the vascular territory involved. Both acute and chronic subdural hematomas may occur.

Clinical Features

These patients present with acute or subacute onset of headache, vomiting, confusion, and, in some cases, focal seizures. In acute DIC and in severe thrombocytopenia, there may also be evidence of spontaneous bleeding from the mucosal surfaces, and at the sites of venipuncture or bone marrow aspiration. In a substantial number of cases, there are signs of systemic thrombosis, in the form of deep venous thrombosis, pulmonary embolism, mesenteric ischemia, or myocardial infarction.

Diagnosis and Treatment

The diagnosis can be suspected by the clinical setting and by systemic thrombosis, hemorrhage, or both. The presence of microangiopathic changes on peripheral smear, thrombocytopenia, increased fibrinogen degradation product, and D-dimer confirm the diagnosis. Therapy of acute DIC is controversial and should be individualized for the clinical setting. Judicious blood product support with red blood corpuscles, platelets, fresh frozen plasma, and cryoprecipitate may protect the patient from hemorrhagic complications. In cases of massive thromboembolism in the setting of acute promyelocytic leukemia, where the pace of the process can be fast and fatal, heparin therapy is appropriate along with blood product support.

An astute clinician can usually establish the cause of neurovascular complication in the cancer patient by having a high index of suspicion and carefully evaluating the clinical background—including the nature and severity of cancer and the modality of antineoplastic therapy—in which the event occurred. The identification and management of one of these unusual neurovascular disorders that leads to the detection of an occult and treatable cancer can be particularly rewarding.

REFERENCES

1. Anghel G, Pettinato G, Severino A, et al. Intravascular B-cell lymphoma: report of two cases with different clinical presentation but rapid central nervous system involvement. Leuk Lymphoma 2003; 44:1353–1359.
2. Borowski A, Ghodsizad A, Gams E. Stroke as a first manifestation of ovarian cancer. J Neurooncol 2005; 71(3):267–269.
3. Rogers LR. Cerebrovascular complications in patients with cancer. Semin Neurol 2004; 24:453–460.
4. Lee AY, Levine MN. The thrombophilic state induced by therapeutic agents in the cancer patient. Semin Thromb Hemost 1999; 25:137–145.
5. El Amrani M, Heinzlef O, Debroucker T, et al. Brain infarction following 5-fluorouracil and cisplatin therapy. Neurology 1998; 51:899–901.
6. Pritchard KI, Paterson AH, Paul NA, Zee B, Fine S, Pater J. (For the NCI of Canada Clinical Trials Group Breast Cancer Site Group) Increased thromboembolic complications with concurrent tamoxifen and chemotherapy in a randomized trial of adjuvant therapy for women with breast cancer. J Clin Oncol 1996; 14:2731–2737.
7. Walker RW, Allen JC, Rosen G, Caparros B. Transient cerebral dysfunction secondary to high-dose methotrexate. J Clin Oncol 1986; 4(12):1845–1850.
8. Lam WW, Leung SF, So NM. Incidence of carotid stenosis in nasopharyngeal carcinoma patients after radiotherapy. Cancer 2001; 92:2357–2363.

9. Coplin WM, Cochran MS, Levine SR, Crawford. Stroke after bone marrow transplantation-frequency, aetiology, and outcome. Brain 2001; 124:1043–1051.
10. Kashyap VS, Moore WS, Quinones B, Baldrich WJ. Carotid surgery repair for radiation-associated atherosclerosis is a safe and durable procedure. J Vasc Surg 1999; 29:90–96.
11. Leseche G, Castier Y, Chataigner O. Carotid artery revascularization through a radiated field. J Vasc Surg 2003; 38:244–250.
12. Nutt SH, Patchell RA. Intracranial hemorrhage associated with primary and secondary tumor. Neurosurg Clin N Am 1992; 3(3):591–599. (Review).
13. Cohen NR, Tan TS, Barker CS. Intracerebral haemorrhage secondary to metastasis from presumed non-small cell lung carcinoma. Neuropathol Appl Neurobiol 2004; 30(4):419–422.
14. Michota F, Merli G. Anticoagulation in special patient populations: are special dosing considerations required? Cleve Clin J Med 2005; 72(suppl 1):S37–S42.

27

Symptomatic Epilepsy

Lawrence M. Cher

Department of Oncology, Austin Health, Heidelberg, Victoria, Australia

INTRODUCTION

Seizures are an important source of morbidity in patients with neurologic involvement in cancer. Seizures may lead to the diagnosis of a primary or secondary brain tumor, malignant leptomeningeal infiltration, neurologic paraneoplastic disorder, or metabolic dysfunction, or complication of immunosuppression such as an abscess or meningitis.

EPIDEMIOLOGY

In a study of patients from the community presenting with first seizure investigated with early EEG and magnetic resonance imaging (MRI), 17 tumors were found out of 300 patients. These included nine astrocytomas, one neuroectodermal tumor, two meningiomas, one ganglioglioma, and four dysembryoplastic neuroepithelial tumors (1).

Incidence of Seizures in Patients with CNS Malignancy

In patients with glioma, seizures are common. They are more common in low-grade gliomas (up to 80%), and in high-grade gliomas are associated with a better prognosis. They may occur in 20% to 40% of brain metastases, 15% of leptomeningeal metastases, 20% of meningiomas, and 10% of Primary Central Nervous System Lymphomas. In patients with tumors and intractable seizures 75% involve the temporal lobe. In addition, patients with primary brain tumors who present with epilepsy generally have a better prognosis (2).

However, seizures can have a significant effect on patients' quality of life, and many patients will have ongoing seizures despite the use of anticonvulsants (3).

SPECIFIC CLINICAL FEATURES

Seizures are classified as partial if they are localized to a specific region of cortex, or generalized if they involve the whole of the cortex. In the symptomatic epilepsies, the seizure always begins as a partial seizure even if the history is that of generalized tonic-clonic seizure, unless there is underlying primary generalized epilepsy aggravated by metabolic factors.

Simple partial seizures do not affect consciousness whereas complex partial seizures will interfere with awareness of the environment. The individual appears to be awake but does not respond to his or her environment and this may be accompanied by automatisms such as lip smacking or rubbing of the nose. In seizures originating in the temporal lobe, it is not uncommon that the patient will develop contralateral aversive head turning, which can be a useful localizing sign.

Seizures may be heralded by an aura, which may help characterize the onset of the seizure. Temporal lobe auras, for example, are characterized by a sensation of déjà vu, and may be accompanied by a sense of dread, or a gustatory component. Involvement of the primary motor cortex leads to Jacksonian seizures with clonic movements that move up the limb. Similarly, sensory symptoms may move up the limb if the tumor is in the primary sensory cortex. Seizures originating from the language cortex are often associated with speech arrest. An occipital focus will be associated with a variety of visual auras.

It is helpful to question *both* the patient and the observer specifically as to such symptoms.

Nonconvulsive Status Epilepticus

Nonconvulsive status epilepticus is difficult to diagnose unless the possibility is considered. It may present with confusion, and fluctuating level of consciousness. In patients with brain tumors, a progressive focal neurologic deficit may develop that mimics tumor progression. One clue is that it may occur without radiologic evidence of tumor progression. EEG will generally show continuous focal epileptiform discharges, often in the form of periodic lateralizing epileptiform discharges. MRI may show an increased signal on T2 and fluid-attenuated inversion recovery imaging associated with continuous epileptiform activity that is usually reversible (4).

ETIOLOGY

The pathophysiology of seizures in patients with primary brain tumors is not well understood, but it is likely that the seizures arise from the periphery of the tumor where the cells infiltrate around neurons and interfere with neuronal connections. There is evidence to suggest that inhibitory synapses on neurons in the peritumoral regions were significantly reduced, but that excitatory inputs were still present (5). There is also intriguing data on glutamate production by glial tumors, inducing seizures and neuronal death (6).

In patients with systemic cancer, cerebral metastases are the most common cause of seizures, but other causes include paraneoplastic syndromes such as limbic encephalitis, leptomeningeal carcinomatosis, radiation necrosis, infectious diseases and metabolic disorders such as syndrome of inappropriate antidiuretic hormone secretion or hypomagnesemia (7). Chemotherapy can cause seizures. Ifosfamide is well recognized as a cause of encephalopathy and seizures. It is more common in patients with pleural or peritoneal effusions. Methylene Blue has been shown to be effective for the encephalopathy and may prevent this complication in subsequent cycles (8).

DIAGNOSIS

Obtaining a diagnosis of epilepsy is often straightforward and requires an integration of the clinical history and description of the event, combined with supportive tests.

Electroencephalography

EEG is important, but a normal EEG does not "rule out" a seizure as the cause of symptoms. In patients with known brain lesions, nonspecific findings such as focal slowing of the brain rhythms may occur in the absence of seizures. Nevertheless, in a patient presenting with a first seizure, theta or delta activity localized to one brain region is very suggestive of an underlying lesion causing the seizure, and warrants urgent neuroimaging.

Neuroimaging

Computed tomography (CT) is useful in an urgent situation, but is less detailed than MRI and, in particular, less sensitive in detecting lesions in the temporal lobe, a region that is more "epileptogenic" than other regions of the brain (9). Therefore in almost all circumstances, MRI is required, especially if the CT is normal. In a patient with known systemic malignancy and a normal MRI, leptomeningeal disease or a paraneoplastic syndrome should be considered (see the relevant chapters for appropriate diagnostic approaches).

THERAPY

Effective therapy requires an understanding of the cause of the seizure. Thus treatment of the underlying condition is important. In patients with a first seizure and a cerebral malignancy, the likelihood of further seizures is high and therefore anticonvulsant therapy is usually indicated.

Antiepileptic Drugs

Antiepileptic Drugs (AEDs) are important in controlling seizures. The number of available agents has markedly increased over the last decade.

When deciding to start anticonvulsants, it appears that most anticonvulsants are equivalent in efficacy in monotherapy. Approximately 40% will achieve seizure freedom on the initial drug, and therefore the initial drug should be chosen with care. It is important therefore to look at potential side effects. The newer anticonvulsants are likely to have lower side effects, overall, although there is less data on the long-term effects of these newer drugs. In addition, many of the newer drugs require a gradual titration of dose to reach a therapeutic level, and this may limit their utility in newly diagnosed patients. Availability and cost are also relevant considerations in choosing the newer drugs.

There are a number of principles in the use of anticonvulsants:

1. Monotherapy is the preferred approach.
2. Drug dose should be individualized.
3. Drug dosages should be increased if seizures are not controlled initially. Exceptions to this include topiramate and levetiracetam. With these two drugs, increased doses above recommended levels, only increase toxicity with little improvement in seizure control.
4. Compliance is a common problem and may be a cause of poor seizure control. Drug levels can be helpful particularly for phenytoin, carbamazepine, and valproate.

Previously, the commonest anticonvulsant used was phenytoin, because initial dosing was relatively straightforward, and patients could be loaded rapidly with intravenous (IV) drug if required. It still has an important place in the setting of status epilepticus as a result. However, it may not be the ideal first-line drug now because of its side effect profile and complex pharmacology. The raft of new drugs available can be confusing for the non-neurologist, and each drug has it's own advantages and disadvantages. The individual issues are detailed in the two tables.

Drug interactions are increasingly important. Many of the older drugs activate the P450 cytochrome system and are known as enzyme-inducing AEDs (EIAEDs), which may affect the metabolism of concomitant drugs including chemotherapy. This list comprises phenytoin, carbamazepine, the barbiturates, and oxcarbazepine.

Changes in drug metabolism are particularly important for a range of chemotherapy drugs including the taxanes, irinotecan, and many of the newer molecular therapies (10). Fortunately, this is not a problem with temozozlomide, which has become the first line drug in gliomas.

However, for trials of new drugs, this issue complicates trial design. Phase I studies need to stratify patients on EIAEDs separately from those not on such drugs. This has been important in the large number of targeted therapies coming on line such as imatinib.

It has been suggested therefore that patients who may be enrolled in trials and require AEDs should preferentially be placed on non-EIAEDs, or switched over to such drugs prior to entry into such trials to more rapidly assess efficacy without the need to be concerned with complex drug interactions and pharmacokinetic studies. If a drug is found to be active, then these studies can be performed secondarily. Paradoxically, recent retrospective trial data reported by Jaeckle (reported in abstract form), showed *improved* survival and progression-free survival in patients taking EIAEDs (11). Almost 70% of patients were on EIAEDs and confidence intervals were not available from the abstract. Prospective studies may be required. Valproate in comparison may inhibit the break down of certain active metabolites such as with the chemotherapy drug, irinotecan, leading to *increased* toxicity.

It is often not appreciated that phenytoin and dexamethasone interact in a complex fashion, such that the increasing dose of one drug increases the metabolism of the other therefore reducing the serum level. This may lead to underdosing of phenytoin and result in seizures, or lead to increased intracranial pressure due to inappropriately low dexamethasone dosing. It is a reasonable rule of thumb to expect that the required dexamethasone dose will be doubled for patients on Phenytoin. This is not an issue with other EIAEDs.

A number of authors describe an increased incidence of Stevens–Johnson syndrome in patients on Phenytoin, which may occur during radiotherapy or as corticosteroids are tapered (12).

In addition, the neurocognitive effects of AEDs need to be recognized. This tends to be more common with the older drugs such as the barbiturates and phenytoin, but some of the newer drugs can also have specific effects. Topiramate, for example, may affect language function, perhaps more commonly in those with a seizure focus in the dominant hemisphere.

Carbamazepine may cause hyponatremia, and anecdotally this may be more problematic in patients who are predisposed to syndrome of inappropriate diuretic hormone secretion (SIADH) because of intracranial malignancy. Thrombocytopenia can occur with valproate and even occasionally with clonazepam. Leukopenia has been described in carbamazepine as well. These effects can complicate the myelosuppression associated with chemotherapy.

Which Drug to Use?

There is no perfect anticonvulsant. Table 1 gives an overview of the most commonly used anticonvulsants, while Table 2 summarizes potential drug interactions. Of the older drugs, carbamazepine is an effective and convenient-to-use drug, particularly using the prolonged release format for twice daily dosing. In patients who may go on to drug trials in which drug metabolism could be of concern, levetiracetam is a good choice, because it has a rapid onset and no drug interactions. However awareness of the risk of agitation and behavioural disorders is important (14). Lamotrigine is a useful drug and well tolerated. It could be given as an initial therapy in patients, or when switching from an alternative drug.

Anticonvulsant Prophylaxis

The role of prophylactic anticonvulsant therapy remains controversial. Many neurosurgeons put patients on prophylactic AEDs, but a metanalysis has recently made the following recommendations (15):

1. In patients with newly diagnosed brain tumors, anticonvulsant medications are not effective in preventing first seizures. Because of their lack of efficacy and their potential side effects, prophylactic anticonvulsants should not be used routinely in patients with newly diagnosed brain tumors (standard).
2. In patients with brain tumors who have not had a seizure, tapering and discontinuing anticonvulsants after the first postoperative week is appropriate, particularly in those patients who are medically stable and who are experiencing anticonvulsant-related side effects. Whether the newer drugs may be more effective or cause less toxicity is undetermined.

Status Epilepticus

Status epilepticus is a medical emergency, and requires urgent attention and untreated has a high mortality or morbidity. It may be defined either as a single epileptic seizure lasting at least 30 minutes or two or more seizures in a 30-minute period without return to baseline mental state in between. It is important to educate patients and families to recognize when they need to come to the hospital. For some patients with an aura, sublingual clobazam tablets or clonazepam drops can be useful for rapid resolution of seizures.

A detailed management strategy is beyond the scope of this article. Initial therapy should include IV benzodiazepines in the first instance; IV loading with phenytoin can be useful. If seizure activity is not terminated, intubation and the use of thiopental or propofol are required (16).

Table 1 Antiepileptic Drugs: Enzyme-Inducing and Non–Enzyme-Inducing Drugs

Drug	Advantages	Serious disadvantages	Nonserious disadvantages	Approximate adult doses
Enzyme-inducing antiepileptic drugs				
Phenytoin	Rapid loading IV	Hypersensitivity, Stevens–Johnson syndrome, pseudolymphoma, cognitive impairment, osteomalacia	Osteoporosis, corticosteroid interaction, complex pharmacokinetics, gingival hyperplasia	300–500 mg directed by drug levels
Carbamazepine	First-line therapy	Neutropenia, SIADH, rash, aplasticanemia, hepatotoxicity	Dizziness, ataxia, diplopia, rash, hyponatremia	600–1200 mg
Phenobarbital	–	Stevens–Johnson syndrome, hepatotoxicity, connective tissue disorders, sedation, dependence	Ataxia, nystagmus, depression	–
Oxcarbazepine	–	SIADH, rash, hepatitis	Nausea, headache, dizziness, fatigue	600–2400 mg
Non–enzyme-inducing antiepileptic drugs				
Valproate	–	Hepatotoxicity, encephalopathy, hyperammonemia, pancreatitis	Tremor, weight gain, thrombocytopenia	600–3000 mg with gradual titration
Lamotrigine	Minimal cognitive effect	Rash, hypersensitivity (reduced slow titration)	Tremor, slow titration, insomnia	50 mg daily for 2 wk, b.i.d. for 2 wk, 100 mg b.i.d. Increase to 400 mg/day (slower and lower doses for patients on valproate)

(Continued)

AQ4

Table 1 Antiepileptic Drugs: Enzyme-Inducing and Non–Enzyme-Inducing Drugs (*Continued*)

Drug	Advantages	Serious disadvantages	Nonserious disadvantages	Approximate adult doses
Topiramate	?Increased seizure control	Nephrolithiasis, open angle glaucoma, slow titration	Language disturbance, metabolic acidosis, weight loss	25–50 mg daily increase by 25 mg weekly, usually not above 400 mg
Levetiracetam	Rapid onset	None	Behavioural reaction	500 mg b.i.d. initially, up to 1.5 gm b.i.d.
Gabapentin	Mild side effects	None	Drowsiness, weight gain, peripheral edema	600–1800, up to 3600 mg
Tiagabine	–	Stupor, spike-wave stupor	Weakness, nausea, headache, dizziness	4 mg daily, then 4 mg b.i.d.; increase gradually to 32 mg in divided doses
Clonazepam	Rapid onset of effect, useful in status epilepticus	Sedation, thrombocytopenia (rare)	Tolerance	1–6 mg
Zonisamide	–	Rash, renal calculi	Irritability, photosensitivity, weight loss	Initial 100 mg daily, then increase 100 mg every 2 wk; usually not >400 mg

Note: Approximate adult dosing is included. Brief comments are included on potential advantages and known side effects.
Abbreviations: IV, intravenous; SIADH, syndrome of inappropriate antidiuretic hormone secretion; b.i.d., twice daily.

Table 2 Common Drug–Drug Interactions Associated with the New Antiepileptic Drugs

Antiepileptic drugs	Oral contraceptive	Warfarin	Other agents	Enzyme inducer	Enzyme inhibitor	Clinical notes
Gabapentin	–	–	None	–	–	No known interactions with other AEDs
Lamotrigine	+ ↓ [L]	–		+/–	–	Modest ↑glucuronidation and ↓ (valproate)
Levetiracetam	–	–		–	–	No known interactions with other AEDs
Topiramate	+ ↓ [Ethinylestradiol] if dose > 200 mg/d	–	Modest ↑ [haloperidol] ↓ [lithium] ↓ [digoxin]	+/–	+	Modest induction CYP 3A4 ↓ CYP 2C19 → ↑ (phenytoin)
Tiagabine	–	–	Nil	–	–	Potential for protein binding displacement
Oxcarbazepine	+ ↓ [Ethinylestradiol]	–	Modest ↓ [felodipine]; no interaction with erythromycin	+/–	+	Modest induction CYP 3A4; Possible ↓ [lamotrigine]; ↓ CYP 2C19 → ↑ [phenytoin]
Zonisamide	–	–		–	–	↑ Clearance with EIAEDs

Note: [] refers to drug concentration.
Abbreviations: AEDs, antiepileptic drugs; EIAEDs, enzyme-inducing AEDs.
Source: From Ref. 13.

Surgery

Surgery is important in patients with intractable seizures, and is particularly important in patients with low-grade tumors for which surgery may be curative. In patients with intractable partial seizures, epilepsy surgery is now well established in improving seizure-freedom rates. In low-grade glioneuronal tumors, gross total resection may be possible, although for many patients, the tumor is diffusely infiltrative and not amenable to surgery. In high-grade gliomas, seizure freedom is less likely (5).

Radiotherapy and Chemotherapy

Radiotherapy anecdotally may reduce the frequency of seizures. In patients with low-grade gliomas, this may be an indication for therapy if seizures are difficult to control (17). In chemosensitive tumors such as oligodendrogliomas, chemotherapy may likewise result in improvement of seizure control (18).

CONCLUSION

Seizures remain a common problem, and better management may improve the quality of life for our patients. It is an area in which there has been a patchy research effort, and studies directed at the neuro-oncology population should be considered.

REFERENCES

1. King MA, Newton MR, Jackson GD, et al. Epileptology of the first-seizure presentation: a clinical, electroencephalographic, and magnetic resonance imaging study of 300 consecutive patients. Lancet 1998; 352(9133):1007–1011.
2. Lote K, Stenwig AE, Skullerud K, Hirschberg H. Prevalence and prognostic significance of epilepsy in patients with gliomas. Eur J Cancer 1998; 34(1):98–102.
3. Moots PL, Maciunas RJ, Eisert DR, Parker RA, Laporte K, Abou-Khalil B. The course of seizure disorders in patients with malignant gliomas. Arch Neurol 1995; 52(7):717–724.
4. Hormigo A, Liberato B, Lis E, DeAngelis LM. Nonconvulsive status epilepticus in patients with cancer: imaging abnormalities. Arch Neurol 2004; 61(3): 362–365.
5. Wetjen NM, Radhakrishnan K, Cohen-Gadol AA, Cascino G. Resective surgery of neoplastic lesions for epilepsy. In: Shorvon SD, Fish DR, Perrucca E, Dodson WE, eds. The Treatment of Epilepsy. 2nd ed. Malden: Blackwell Science, 2004:728–741.
6. Sontheimer H. Malignant gliomas: perverting glutamate and ion homeostasis for selective advantage. Trends Neurosci 2003; 26(10):543–549.
7. Glantz M, Recht LD. Epilepsy in the cancer patient. In: Vecht CJ, ed. Handbook of Clinical Neurology: Neuro-Oncology, Part III. Amsterdam: Elselvier Science BV, 1997:9–18.

8. Pelgrims J, De Vos F, Van den Brande J, Schrijvers D, Prove A, Vermorken JB. Methylene blue in the treatment and prevention of ifosfamide-induced encephalopathy: report of 12 cases and a review of the literature. Br J Cancer 2000; 82(2):291–294.
9. Briellmann RS, Pell GS, Wellard RM, Mitchell LA, Abbott DF, Jackson GD. MR imaging of epilepsy: state of the art at 1.5T and potential of 3T. Epileptic Disord 2003; 5(1):3–20.
10. Grossman SA, Batara JF. Current management of glioblastoma multiforme. Semin Oncol 2004; 31(5):635–644.
11. Jaeckle KBK, Uhm J, O'Fallon J, et al. Ta-27. Relationship of administration of enzyme-inducing anticonvulsants (EIAC) to survival patients with glioblastoma: a North Central Cancer Treatment Group (NCCTG) study. Neuro-oncology 2004; 6(4):376.
12. Delattre JY, Safai B, Posner JB. Erythema multiforme and Stevens-Johnson syndrome in patients receiving cranial irradiation and phenytoin. Neurology 1988; 38(2):194–198.
13. French JA, Kanner AM, Bautista J, et al. Efficacy and tolerability of the new antiepileptic drugs I: treatment of new onset epilepsy: report of the Therapeutics and Technology Assessment Subcommittee and Quality Standards Subcommittee of the American Academy of Neurology and the American Epilepsy Society. Neurology 2004; 62(8):1252–1260.
14. White JR, Walczak TS, Leppik IE, et al. Discontinuation of levetiracetam because of behavioral side effects: a case-control study. Neurology 2003; 61(9):1218–1221.
15. Glantz MJ, Cole BF, Forsyth PA, et al. Practice parameter: anticonvulsant prophylaxis in patients with newly diagnosed brain tumors. Report of the Quality Standards Subcommittee of the American Academy of Neurology. Neurology 2000; 54(10):1886–1893.
16. Gaitanis JN, Drislane FW. Status epilepticus: a review of different syndromes, their current evaluation, and treatment. Neurologist 2003; 9(2):61–76.
17. Rogers LR, Morris HH, Lupica K. Effect of cranial irradiation on seizure frequency in adults with low-grade astrocytoma and medically intractable epilepsy. Neurology 1993; 43(8):1599–1601.
18. Hoang-Xuan K, Capelle L, Kujas M, et al. Temozozlomide as initial treatment for adults with low-grade oligodendrogliomas or oligoastrocytomas and correlation with chromosome 1p deletions. J Clin Oncol 2004; 22(15):3133–3138.

28

Cancer and the Peripheral Nervous System

Kleopas A. Kleopa and Theodoros Kyriakides

Department of Clinical Neurosciences, The Cyprus Institute of Neurology and Genetics, Nicosia, Cyprus

DIRECT EFFECTS OF MALIGNANCY

Cancer can directly involve any part of the neuromuscular system, including the spinal neurons and nerve roots, the brachial and lumbosacral plexus, the peripheral nerves, and muscles.

Brachial Plexopathy

Brachial plexopathy can result from metastases to the axillary or supraclavicular nodes, from primary tumor invasion or rarely, in the case of breast carcinoma, from hematogenous spread. About 4% of lung and 2% of breast cancers cause symptomatic tumor infiltration of the brachial plexus followed in frequency by lymphomas. Relentlessly progressive pain is the presenting feature in most patients, usually in the shoulder and axilla radiating to the medial arm, forearm, and the fourth and fifth fingers (1). Weakness and sensory loss follows after a variable period, involving the C8/T1 roots in most patients. In the remaining cases, there is diffuse and often patchy plexus infiltration. Carcinomatous involvement of more than one root is almost always the case and should help in the distinction from degenerative disc disease. Almost half of patients have unilateral Horner's syndrome as well as tumor spread to the adjacent epidural space, both features helping to distinguish tumor involvement of the plexus from radiotherapy-induced damage. The differential diagnosis includes, besides radiation plexopathy (Table 1), rare entities such as paraneoplastic plexopathy associated with lymphomas and toxicity from chemotherapy (2).

Electrodiagnostic studies usually reveal severe axonal loss with absent sensory responses of the ulnar and medial antebrachial nerves (thus ruling out radiculopathy) and reduced ulnar and median nerve compound motor action potentials (CMAP). An important aspect is the absence of myokymia in electromyography (EMG), which is frequently present in radiation plexopathy. Gadolinium-enhanced magnetic resonance imaging (MRI) demonstrates a soft-tissue mass or diffuse enhancement in 80% to 90% of cases and is more sensitive than computed tomography (CT). Prognosis depends on systemic tumor load, and whether the patient presents early after the appearance of pain and before weakness and sensory loss set in. Treatment is palliative and consists of local radiotherapy, which can relieve pain in up to 50% of patients. Other measures include transcutaneous nerve stimulation, local nerve blocks, and even cordotomy.

Lumbosacral Plexopathy

Lumbosacral plexopathy (LSP) can arise either as a result of direct extension from a primary pelvic tumor, such as colorectal and gynecological cancers, or by spreading from adjacent lymph nodes or bone metastases. Breast and prostatic cancer, lymphomas, and sarcomas are also common malignancies causing LSP. Pain is the presenting symptom in 75% of patients, and may initially involve the low back, hip region, and thigh. Nocturnal

Table 1 Differential Diagnosis of Radiation vs. Tumor Plexopathy

	Radiation plexopathy	Tumor plexopathy
Presenting symptoms	Paresthesias, weakness	Severe pain (75–98%)
Edema	Common	Often absent
Brachial plexus involvement	Usually upper	Usually lower (lower trunk, medial cord)
Lumbosacral plexus involvement	Extensive, often bilateral	Lower, commonly unilateral
Horner's syndrome	Usually absent	Found in up to 50%
Rectal mass	Absent	Often present
Myokymia in electromyography	Common (50–70%)	Usually absent
Magnetic resonance imaging enhancement of plexus	Infrequent	Generally present, with circumscribed mass in 80%
Positron emission tomography scan	Negative	Often positive

radicular pain involving more than one root is common, often with a positive stretch sign, followed by weakness and sensory loss. Bladder dysfunction is not an early sign unless the tumor directly invades the bladder or the coccygeal plexus.

LSP involves the lower part of the plexus (L4-S1 roots) in 50% of cases, the upper (L1-L4) part in 30%, or both in 20%. Lower plexus involvement may be confused with degenerative disc disease, although multiple root involvement and the relentlessly progressive, often nocturnal pain should raise suspicion (3). Upper lumbar plexopathy presents with pain and paresthesias in the groin and low abdominal wall and is less likely to be attributed to degenerative disc disease, but may mimic diabetic truncal neuropathy. Clinical findings in favor of tumor involvement include a rectal mass, hydronephrosis, and leg edema, helping to distinguish from radiation-induced LSP (Table 1) (4).

Electrodiagnostic studies in LSP often show bilateral, acute, and chronic denervation even in patients with unilateral symptoms. MRI and CT scan show a mass or lymphadenopathy in about 75% of cases while in 30% the abnormalities are bilateral. Radionuclide scans are positive in 65% showing uptake in pelvis, sacrum, or vertebrae. Treatment is aimed mainly at relieving pain with radiotherapy, steroids, cordotomy, and epidural or intrathecal opiates.

Peripheral Neuropathy

Direct peripheral nerve involvement due to cancer occurs through invasion along the perineurial space. Cutaneous squamous and basal cell carcinoma of the head and neck, and sometimes malignant melanoma can spread to involve the fifth and seventh cranial nerves, presenting with facial pain, hypesthesia, and facial palsy (5). More commonly, involvement is due to diffuse infiltration by hematological malignancies giving rise to a generalized neuropathy. In the case of lymphoma, this is also known as neurolymphomatosis. The lymphoma is usually high grade and in 50% of the cases, the patient is not known to suffer from systemic disease. Even at autopsy in up to one-third of patients, lymphoma is restricted to the nervous system, but systemic manifestations may occur as late as three years following the neuropathy (6). Neurolymphomatosis can be acute, mimicking Guillain-Barre syndrome (GBS), relapsing, remitting, or chronic progressive. Nocturnal pain, paresthesias, distal sensory loss, weakness, and hyporeflexia are characteristic. Asymmetric distribution and associated mononeuropathies or cranial neuropathies are common and may help distinguish lymphomatous involvement from other causes of neuropathy such as drug toxicity (7).

Electrodiagnostic evaluation shows features of axonal or demyelinating sensorimotor neuropathy. Fasciculations may be seen in the EMG, perhaps indicating proximal root involvement. MRI may reveal enlarged nerves, which are hyperintense on T2, isointense on T1 and enhancing with gadolinium. Gallium and positron emission tomography scan may also be usefully employed for diagnosis. Cerebrospinal fluid (CSF) examination shows elevated protein and cell count in most patients, with malignant cells found in about 50%. Nerve biopsy shows differential fascicular involvement, with lymphomatous tissue mainly in the epineurium. There may be perivascular cuffing and even vessel infiltration but no fibrinoid necrosis, in contrast to vasculitic neuropathy. Mitotic figures and pleomorphism suggest the diagnosis while immunocytochemistry may confirm clonality. There is mainly axonal degeneration and rarely segmental demyelination. Treatment is against the primary disease and symptomatic for the pain.

Clinically relevant infiltration of peripheral nerves occurs less frequently in leukemia as compared to lymphoma. It has been described in chronic lymphocytic leukemia, but also in association with other acute and chronic forms of leukemia. A symmetrical sensorimotor axonopathy, at times painful, is the most common presentation, but asymmetrical polyneuropathy and multiple mononeuropathies have also been reported. Pathologically, there is preferential perineurial invasion and features of axonal degeneration and demyelination. Infiltration of peripheral nerve by myeloma cells is extremely rare and causes a symmetrical sensorimotor neuropathy. Nerve biopsy shows demyelination and axonal degeneration in juxtaposition to foci of malignant cells. Treatment is symptomatic and against the primary disease.

REMOTE EFFECTS OF MALIGNANCY

Neuromuscular Paraneoplastic Syndromes

While paraneoplastic syndromes are rare, occurring in only about 1% of patients with cancer, they are more frequent with certain types of malignancy such as small cell lung cancer (SCLC) (8). Expression of antigenic determinants in malignant cells, mimicking those of neural tissues, is thought to give rise to an immune response directed against the nervous system. Often neurological manifestations precede the diagnosis of tumor by as much as two years, emphasizing the importance of early recognition. Aggressive search for cancer is imperative once the diagnosis of a paraneoplastic syndrome has been made, including at least a thorough physical examination, CT scans of the chest, abdomen, and pelvis, mammograms in women, upper or lower gastrointestinal endoscopy, and fecal occult blood testing. If the initial investigations are negative, this workup should be repeated periodically (9).

Paraneoplastic Sensory Neuronopathy

Paraneoplastic sensory neuronopathy (PSN) presents with painful dysesthesias and numbness, often beginning in the arms asymmetrically. The onset can be acute or insidiously progressive, and PSN can involve the lower limbs, the trunk, and sometimes the cranial nerves causing facial numbness or sensorineural hearing loss. There is prominent loss of proprioception leading to sensory ataxia and pseudoathetosis. Reflexes are decreased or abolished while muscle strength is usually preserved. Only about 20% of sensory neuronopathy cases are paraneoplastic, half of which have SCLC, and, less commonly, carcinoma of the breast and kidney, chondrosarcoma, seminoma, or lymphoma. PSN is more common in women and frequently coexists with paraneoplastic encephalomyelitis (PEM), especially in patients with SCLC and anti-Hu antibodies (10).

PSN affects primarily the dorsal root ganglia (DRG) neurons. Pathologic features include inflammation and degeneration of the DRG and dorsal nerve roots with secondary degeneration of peripheral sensory axons and dorsal columns. Nerve conduction studies (NCS) reveal low-amplitude or absent sensory responses with normal CMAP. The reduction of sensory responses in PSN can be asymmetric and, in contrast to the more common length-dependent axonopathies, it is more prominent in the upper than in the lower extremities. EMG may show evidence of denervation in cases with overlapping PEM (11).

Detection of anti-Hu antibody in serum and CSF helps to confirm the diagnosis but is not found in all cases with PSN. CSF may be normal or may demonstrate mild lymphocytic pleocytosis and elevated protein. Patients should be screened for other treatable disorders with similar presentation including vitamin deficiencies, especially of B12 and E, infections (HIV, tabes dorsalis, and diphtheria), autoimmune disorders, especially Sjögren syndrome, and toxicity of medications. PSN is relentlessly progressive in most cases leading to severe disability within six to nine months. Patients occasionally improve with immunosuppression, but response to treatment is usually disappointing and they may succumb from complications of the neurological syndrome rather than from the primary cancer.

Motor Neuron Syndromes

Bulbar or spinal motor neuron involvement occurs in up to 20% to 25% of patients with the anti-Hu syndrome of PSN and PEM (10). In rare patients, motor neuron involvement predominates. EMG shows segmental denervation, and autopsy cases revealed neuronal loss in the anterior horns, sometimes with inflammation (12). In each of these patients, nonmotor involvement was evident. The existence of paraneoplastic pure motor neuronopathy has been controversial. Hematologic malignancies have been reported in patients with progressive, asymmetric lower motor neuron dysfunction, affecting predominantly the lower extremities, with minor sensory symptoms. Evidence of chronic active denervation is found in EMG, with essentially normal NCS. Neuronal degeneration is evident in the anterior horns but also mild demyelination of posterior columns and anterior roots. The illness is rather benign and the etiology has not been proven, with effects of radiation and opportunistic infections possibly being involved.

Lymphoproliferative disorders have also been reported in patients with amyotrophic lateral sclerosis (ALS), paraproteinemia and increased protein content or oligoclonal bands in the CSF (13). However, the temporal relationship between the two disorders is variable, and many patients received potentially neurotoxic treatment for the malignancy including radiation prior to neurological manifestations. Neurological improvement after treatment of the malignancy occurred rarely, usually in patients with lower motor neuron syndrome. Because there is no epidemiological evidence to suggest an association with malignancy, extensive screening is not recommended in patients with typical ALS. However, patients with pure lower motor neuron syndromes should be screened for the presence of paraproteinemia and CSF abnormalities. When nonmotor manifestations are also present, testing for anti-Hu antibodies and screening for SCLC is appropriate. A predominantly upper motor neuron syndrome, presenting as primary lateral sclerosis, has been reported in a series of patients with breast cancer (12). Although a causal relationship has not been established, a basic screening for this malignancy is justified in affected women, especially those with progressive disease.

Stiff-Person Syndrome

Stiff-person syndrome (SPS) occurs in association with diabetes, polyendocrinopathy, and antibodies to glutamic acid decarboxylase. An underlying malignancy, especially cancer of the breast and lung, thymoma, or lymphoma, is found in the minority of patients, who may also have antibodies to amphiphysin. Fluctuating muscle stiffness and painful spasms triggered by sudden noise, voluntary movement, or emotion are characteristic and result from continuous motor unit activity and simultaneous activation of agonist and antagonist muscles. The symptoms may begin asymmetrically, disappear during sleep, and involve thoracic, abdominal, lumbar paraspinal, and lower limb muscles. Autonomic abnormalities may occur (14). EMG reveals involuntary continuous activity of morphologically normal motor unit potentials (MUPs). Both the myographic and the clinical manifestations of SPS may improve after treatment of the tumor and with benzodiazepines, dantrolene, antiepileptic agents, intravenous immunoglobulin (IVIG), or plasma exchange.

Sensorimotor Polyneuropathy

Polyneuropathy is a frequent complication in patients with advanced cancer. Contributing factors include toxic effects of chemotherapy, weight loss, malnutrition, infectious complications, and organ failure. Paraneoplastic etiology is much more rare and can precede the diagnosis of malignancy by as much as five years. Patients usually present with subacute onset of distal weakness and/or sensory disturbances with reduced or absent reflexes. Autonomic involvement is common. In contrast to PSN, NCS show length-dependent axonopathy with reduced motor and sensory amplitudes. EMG reveals variable degrees of active denervation. Pathological studies show axonal degeneration and, in some cases, segmental demyelination or sparse lymphocytic infiltration. DRG neurons are not affected. A mixed axonal-demyelinating polyneuropathy has been associated with anti-CV2 antibodies, which react with peripheral nerve antigens and occur with SCLC, thymoma and neuroendocrine tumors (15). Some of these patients also harbor anti-Hu antibodies and may have superimposed PSN with underlying SCLC.

Neuropathies Associated with Malignant Paraproteinemic Disorders

Nonmalignant monoclonal gammopathies of "undetermined significance" (MGUS) are the most common cause of paraproteinemic neuropathies. Despite negative initial screening, 6% to 25% of MGUS patients eventually develop a hematologic malignancy, even several years after the onset of neuropathy. Paraproteinemic neuropathy occurs in about 10% of patients with multiple myeloma, usually preceding the discovery of the malignancy (16). The neuropathy is primarily axonal but rarely patients may have chronic inflammatory demyelinating polyneuropathy (CIDP). In about one-third of cases, amyloid deposition may be found. Although osteosclerotic myeloma is seen in less than 3% of all patients with myeloma, more than half of the affected patients develop polyneuropathy, which resembles CIDP (17). Prominent loss of vibration sensation and proprioception, high CSF protein, and nerve conduction slowing are characteristic. Most of these patients have monoclonal serum proteins at low concentration, usually immunoglobulin G or immunoglobulin A with lambda light chains. Their detection requires serum immunofixation, emphasizing the importance of this test in the workup of CIDP. Systemic features of the polyneuropathy, organomegaly, endocrinopathy, M spike, and skin changes syndrome are frequently associated, but patients may manifest only some of them. Deposition of the paraprotein in the endoneurium and elevation of proinflammatory cytokines have been implicated in the pathogenesis of the neuropathy, which may improve or stabilize with treatment of the underlying tumor. Plasma exchange is generally ineffective, whereas CIDP cases may respond to corticosteroids.

Peripheral neuropathy occurs in about 5% to 10% of patients with Waldenström's macroglobulinemia. Patients present with distal sensory symptoms, gait ataxia, and reduced fine motor coordination of the hands, followed by weakness and distal muscle atrophy. A large monoclonal Immunoglobulin M (IgM) protein is typically detected. Electrodiagnostic studies reveal a demyelinating but, rarely, also an axonal neuropathy. Plasma exchange may slow the progression while some patients respond to prednisone, melphalan, and chlorambucil.

Subacute or chronic paraproteinemic neuropathies also occur in patients with lymphoma, Castleman's disease, and leukemia. Sensory or motor variants of CIDP or GBS, as well as multiple mononeuropathies have been reported. GBS in association with Hodgkin's lymphoma may develop during active disease or in the phase of remission (18). Inflammatory brachial plexopathy also occurred in a few patients lacking evidence of direct infiltration. Peripheral nerve biopsy shows segmental demyelination with perivascular mononuclear cell infiltration and endoneurial deposition of IgM kappa or lambda. However, epidemiologic studies showing a higher incidence of GBS or CIDP in lymphoma patients compared to the general population are lacking.

Patients with lymphoma, SCLC, and other cancers may develop vasculitic neuropathy. This is usually a symmetric sensorimotor axonal polyneuropathy, but it may also present asymmetrically or as multiple mononeuropathies (19). Nerve biopsies show microvasculitis that is rarely necrotizing and may respond to cyclophosphamide. Distal symmetric painful sensorimotor neuropathy may also occur in the setting of hematologic malignancies with cryoglobulinemia and immune-mediated vasculitis. Associated vascular signs such as purpura and Raynaud's phenomenon may be absent or discrete. Some patients improve with immunosuppression.

Acquired Neuromyotonia

Neuromyotonia (NMT) is characterized by peripheral nerve hyperexcitability presenting with muscle stiffness and cramps, as well as muscle twitching in the form of fasciculations or myokymia. The muscle stiffness worsens with activity, and in contrast to the SPS it may persist during rest and sleep. Some patients also develop autonomic and sensory symptoms such as hyperhidrosis, laryngeal spasms, paresthesias, and numbness. CNS involvement may occur, causing agitation, confusion, anxiety, and delirium, known as Morvan's syndrome. Only about 20% of NMT cases are paraneoplastic, usually associated with thymoma, SCLC, lymphoma, or plasmocytoma (20).

Motor NCS in patients with NMT may sometimes demonstrate "after-discharges." Needle EMG shows spontaneous firing of morphologically normal MUP in different patterns, including fasciculations, doublets, triplets, and multiplets, myokymic discharges, and irregular bursts reaching a frequency of over 50 and up to 300 Hz. The neuromyotonic discharges disappear with neuromuscular blockade, and sometimes with nerve block, indicating that the origin of hyperexcitability is in the peripheral nerve, especially its distal part. Antibodies directed against voltage-gated potassium channels (VGKC) can be detected in most patients and reduce potassium currents probably by increasing channel turnover. NMT improves with plasma exchange or IVIG. Symptomatic treatment with phenytoin or carbamazepine may reduce hyperexcitability.

Lambert-Eaton Myasthenic Syndrome

Lambert-Eaton myasthenic syndrome (LEMS) is associated with SCLC in up to 60% of cases and rarely with other tumors. Paraneoplastic LEMS may coexist with PEM, cerebellar degeneration, and PSN, especially in cases with SCLC (11). Nonparaneoplastic cases tend to have a slower symptom progression and associate with other autoimmune conditions (21). LEMS usually precedes tumor diagnosis by several months to years, presenting with progressive proximal weakness, affecting the legs more than the arms. There is less fatigability than in myasthenia gravis (MG), but often muscle stiffness or pain after exertion. Autonomic dysfunction is prominent with dry mouth, dry eyes, impotence, orthostatic hypotension, and hyperhidrosis. Neurological examination shows proximal weakness and waddling gait, with characteristic improvement in muscle power after brief maximal voluntary muscle activity. Reflexes are diminished but may improve after forceful exercise of the corresponding muscles. Respiratory and craniobulbar involvement is uncommon in LEMS and is generally mild when present (21). Ptosis is not uncommon in LEMS, but ophthalmoplegia should raise suspicion for superimposed PEM.

LEMS is a disorder of neuromuscular transmission associated with antibodies to presynaptic P/Q-type voltage-gated calcium channels (VGCC), found in over 90% of cases. The autoimmune process results in depletion of VGCC and reduced calcium influx into the nerve terminal, leading to impaired quantal release of acetylcholine at the synaptic junction (22). Antibodies to N-type VGCC and acetylcholine-receptor (AchR) may also be found. NCS typically show reduced CMAP amplitudes recorded from rested muscle, which increase by at least 100% or more after brief voluntary isometric contraction of the muscle (23). A similar CMAP increment occurs with high-frequency repetitive stimulation of 20 to 50 Hz (Fig. 1), but this

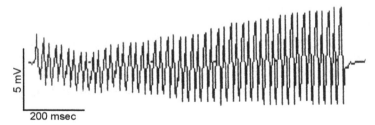

Figure 1 Repetitive stimulation of the ulnar nerve (50 Hz, train of 50 stimulations) and recording at the abductor digiti minimi muscle in a 70-year-old patient with Lambert-Eaton myasthenic syndrome. There is a ~100% increase in the compound muscle action potential amplitude (from 2.09 mV at the beginning to 4.04 mV at the end of the stimulation), characteristic of presynaptic neuromuscular junction dysfunction.

is uncomfortable and should be used only when patients are unable to voluntarily exercise. The CMAP increment likely results from facilitation of acetylcholine release mediated by calcium influx. In contrast, routine low-frequency stimulation (2–3 Hz) results in decremental motor response, as in MG. Needle EMG shows variability in amplitude and configuration of the recruited MUP. When neuromuscular dysfunction is severe, MUP may appear myopathic due to complete block of transmission to individual muscle fibers within each motor unit (21). Single fiber EMG shows very high jitter values and blocking, both of which decrease as the MUP firing frequency increases, in contrast to MG.

The most important aspect of LEMS management is the early identification and treatment of the underlying malignancy, which may also improve the neuromuscular manifestations. Symptomatic therapy includes 3,4-diaminopyridine (3,4-DAP) and pyridostigmine. 3,4-DAP inhibits presynaptic VGKC and improves acetylcholine release. It has a narrow therapeutic window with doses of 20 to 60 mg daily, above which seizures could occur, but may also cause perioral and acral paresthesias, epigastric discomfort, and insomnia. 3,4-DAP has not been approved by the Food and Drug Administration but can be obtained on a compassionate-use basis for LEMS patients. Patients with aggressive disease may need immunosuppressive treatment, including corticosteroids, azathioprine, plasma exchange, and IVIG (24).

Myasthenia Gravis

MG is a postsynaptic disorder of the neuromuscular junction associated with antibodies to muscle AchR in the majority of cases and, unlike LEMS, it is usually not a paraneoplastic condition. However, all patients diagnosed with MG should undergo imaging of the mediastinum, because a thymoma is found in about 10% of cases, mostly in the age group between 50 and 70 years. Thymectomy is indicated in patients with thymoma, but the disease does not always improve after tumor removal, and further treatment may be necessary as for MG patients without thymoma. About 50% of all patients with thymoma eventually develop MG, which may coexist with other paraneoplastic syndromes, including inflammatory myopathy, myocarditis, or NMT. These patients may have antibodies to various antigens in addition to AchR, including the muscle protein titin and the ryanodine receptor, as well as VGKC, perhaps reflecting differences in the underlying thymic malignancy (25).

Myopathies Associated with Cancer

Leukemia, lymphoma, and, more rarely, solid tumors can metastasize into muscle directly causing either a discrete or diffuse enlargement, with or without weakness (26). However, myopathy usually occurs as a remote effect of malignancy.

Paraneoplastic Inflammatory Myopathies

Dermatomyositis (DM), especially in those over 40 years of age and in contrast to childhood DM, may be associated with malignancy in 6% to 45% of cases, including cancer of the lung, breast, ovary, and others (27). Cancer may precede but more often follows the diagnosis of DM by 2 to 5 years. The association of malignancy with polymyositis (PM) is less robust but is probably higher than age-matched controls. Clinical and histological features do not reliably distinguish between idiopathic and paraneoplastic inflammatory myopathies. The skin manifestations of DM include purplish discoloration of the eyelids (heliotrope rash) and erythematous scaly lesions over the knuckles and elbows. Onset of proximal weakness is usually subacute over weeks, although it can develop abruptly over days or insidiously over months. The myopathy may involve oropharyngeal and esophageal muscles in about 30%, resulting in dysphagia.

Creatine kinase (CK) is often elevated but can be normal. Muscle biopsy in DM reveals perivascular inflammation, perifascicular atrophy, complement deposition and CD4+ T cells and B-cells. PM is characterized by endomysial inflammation and invasion of non-necrotic muscle fibers by CD8+ T-cells. The myopathy may improve with treatment of the tumor but steroids and/or IVIG treatment are often needed. Patients diagnosed with DM over the age of 40 should be screened for malignancy at presentation and, if negative, at least for the next five years.

Acute Necrotizing Myopathy

Paraneoplastic acute necrotizing myopathy is extremely rare and presents with painful proximal weakness prior to the diagnosis of cancer, usually of the lung, breast, and bladder. There is often involvement of respiratory and bulbar muscles. In contrast to inflammatory myopathies, there is widespread necrosis in skeletal muscle with scant inflammation. Chemotherapy and cytokines may be some of the causative factors. Patients improve after tumor resection and occasionally with steroid treatment (28).

Carcinoid and Amyloid Myopathies

Carcinoid myopathy is associated with increased serotonin secretion by carcinoid tumors, and presents after the diagnosis of carcinoid syndrome with proximal muscle weakness and cramps. CK may be mildly elevated, and muscle biopsy shows type-2 fiber atrophy without much necrosis or inflammation. Muscle weakness and other symptoms of the carcinoid syndrome may improve with cyproheptadine or the somatostatin analog octreotide. Amyloid deposition in muscle is rare and sometimes is associated with myeloma, malignant carcinoid tumor, and melanoma. The clinical features include pseudohypertrophy of the muscles, weakness, and fatigue. Autonomic and peripheral nerve involvement coexists in most cases (29).

Cachectic Myopathy

Tumor-derived proteolytic peptides and cytokines [tumor necrosis factor-α, Interferone-γ, Interleukin (IL)-6, IL-1β] are some of the molecules implicated in the wasting and weakness caused by chronic debilitating disease including cancer. Pathologically there are atrophic fibers some of which are in groups, implying a neurogenic component, and there is noninflammatory fiber degeneration. Cachectic myopathy may improve with treatment of the underlying neoplasm.

IATROGENIC EFFECTS IN CANCER PATIENTS

Complications of Radiation Therapy

Radiation-Induced Brachial Plexopathy

Radiation-induced brachial plexopathy develops with total doses over 6000 cGy in one-third of patients with breast cancer, and these patients make the majority of cases presenting with this complication, followed by patients with lung cancer. The plexopathy can take three forms: A rare, acute type occurs during or shortly after radiotherapy of patients with Hodgkin's disease, perhaps on a dysimmune basis. The clinical picture resembles neuralgic amyotrophy: severe unilateral pain followed by weakness, especially affecting the deltoid and supraspinatus (30). "Early" delayed plexopathy usually presents within six months of completion of radiotherapy with paresthesias in the hand and forearm, as well as mild weakness. It is due to reversible damage to myelin and axons, and prognosis is good (31). "Late" delayed plexopathy is the most serious type and presents on average 1.5 years, and as late as 10 years or more after radiation, possibly a result of progressive vascular damage and fibrosis of the brachial plexus. Patients have numbness and paresthesias in the hand and forearm, followed by progressive distal or diffuse arm weakness (32). Pain eventually occurs in up to 60% of patients but it is not an early feature, in contrast to direct cancer invasion (Table 1).

Electrophysiologic abnormalities include reduced sensory responses and prolonged F waves, but initial NCS may be normal. There is diffuse denervation in the arm, especially in the distribution of the upper trunk. The most useful distinguishing EMG feature is myokymia, which is present in at least one muscle in at least 50% of patients (33). MRI and high-contrast CT scan are useful in distinguishing metastases to the brachial plexus from radiation-induced plexopathy. Two-thirds of cases with "late" delayed radiation plexopathy progress over several years while a third stabilize. Management consists of symptomatic relief of pain. Neurolysis to remove fibrous tissue and anticoagulation have been used with success in uncontrolled studies.

Radiation-Induced Lumbosacral Radiculopathy

This complication may occur after a mean of six years (up to 25 years) following radiation with 4000 to 6000 cGy encompassing the cauda equina and the low spinal cord, typically for the treatment of testicular cancer, lymphoma, and vertebral metastases. Patients develop flaccid weakness in one or two limbs asymmetrically, especially in the distribution of the L5/S1 myotomes and minimal, if any, sensory symptoms. There may be a continuous progression or stabilization after one to two years, and treatment is symptomatic. MRI may show gadolinium nodular enhancement of the cauda equina and conus. EMG usually does not show myokymia. Neuropathological studies reveal clusters of dilated, thickened, and hyalinized blood vessels on nerve roots, which exhibited demyelination and axonal loss (34).

Complications of Chemotherapy

Peripheral neuropathy is a common complication of many chemotherapeutic agents. The type and degree of neuropathy depend on the chemotherapeutic agent, the individual as well as the cumulative dose.

Vinca Alkaloids

Vincristine and other vinca alkaloids cause a dose-dependent symmetric axonal length-dependent sensorimotor polyneuropathy. Numbness and paresthesias in the hands or feet begin within weeks of treatment. Pain and temperature sensation is impaired more than vibration and proprioception. Distal weakness may occur with continuation of treatment. Autonomic neuropathy develops in up to 30% of patients, causing constipation, urinary retention, impotence, and postural hypotension. Vincristine may rarely cause isolated cranial neuropathies, typically involving the oculomotor, abducens, or facial nerves, as well as optic neuropathy, hearing loss, and laryngeal nerve palsy (35).

NCS show sensorimotor length-dependent axonal polyneuropathy. Patients usually recover from vincristine-induced neuropathy except in severe cases. Improvement is more rapid if the drug is stopped at an early stage of the neuropathy, but mild residual distal sensory loss is common. The drug can be reintroduced at a lower dose without recurrence of symptoms. Vincristine is believed to cause neuropathy by disrupting axonal transport, because it binds to tubulin and prevents microtubule formation. Although toxicity is dose related, individual susceptibility may vary and patients with preexisting neuropathy may develop acute quadriplegia after vincristine treatment with prolonged and incomplete recovery.

Platinum Compounds

Cisplatin typically causes sensory neuropathy at cumulative doses above 300 to 400 mg/m^2. There is preferential loss of large fiber sensation, not necessarily in a length-dependent manner, with subsequent development of sensory ataxia and pseudoathetosis. Reflexes are diminished or absent, but weakness is rare. Lhermitte sign may occur in up to 40% of patients, probably related to dorsal column involvement. NCS show low amplitude or diffusely absent sensory responses with normal motor responses, suggesting selective damage to the DRG neurons. Nerve biopsies reveal selective loss of large myelinated nerve fibers. As with other chemotherapeutic agents, the neuropathy may continue to deteriorate for weeks or months after discontinuation of cisplatin. Improvement may be slow and incomplete with significant functional disability in severe cases (36).

Oxaliplatin causes both acute and chronic neuropathy (37). The acute form occurs in the majority of patients and may begin during the infusion or within hours of completion. It is typically aggravated by exposure to cold. The presentation is usually self-limited and rapidly reversible. Chronic sensory neuropathy is similar to the cisplatin-induced, occurs with cumulative doses over $540 \, mg/m^2$, and may cause functional disability. Acute oxaliplatin-induced neuropathy may be prevented by calcium and magnesium solutions, antiepileptic drugs, glutathione, and alpha-lipoic acid. There is no proven prophylaxis for the chronic form.

Paclitaxel and Docetaxel

Both paclitaxel and to a lesser degree docetaxel cause a predominantly sensory distal neuropathy. Incidence and severity are related to both individual and cumulative dose. In patients treated with 250 to $350 \, mg/m^2$ per cycle, neuropathy develops after the first or second cycle and sometimes within 24 hours of the first infusion. Neurotoxicity is less likely with 24-hour infusions compared to bolus injection. Patients usually present with paresthesias, pain, and distal numbness. Large fiber modalities, autonomic and motor function may be impaired in severe cases. Cumulative doses above $1500 \, mg/m^2$, preexisting neuropathy, and previous or concurrent exposure to other neurotoxic agents predispose to the development of a severe sensory neuropathy (38). After discontinuation of the drug, most patients improve but, in severe cases, sensory loss and ataxia may persist. Taxanes are microtubular toxins, but unlike vincristine, they promote polymerisation of tubulin and inhibit microtubule disassembly. Disruption of various cell functions, including axonal transport, affects both the distal axon and the neuronal cell body.

Suramin

Suramin is associated with two forms of peripheral neuropathy: a mild, dose-dependent distal axonal sensorimotor polyneuropathy; and a more severe, subacute demyelinating polyradiculoneuropathy resembling GBS (39). The more common distal axonopathy presents with length-dependent sensory loss, paresthesias, mild weakness, and diminished ankle reflexes.

These deficits are reversible after discontinuation of the drug. The subacute demyelinating form is associated with higher suramin doses, evolves over a period of two to nine weeks, and causes diffuse proximal more than distal weakness and sensory loss. Bulbar and respiratory dysfunction may occur, and some patients require ventilatory assistance. NCS reveal demyelination, and CSF protein may be elevated. Nerve biopsy shows variable loss of myelinated fibers, segmental demyelination, and sometimes inflammation.

Etoposide (VP-16), Procarbazine, and Cytosine Arabinoside

Treatment with high-dose etoposide causes a predominantly sensory distal axonal polyneuropathy, often in patients previously treated with vincristine. Severe autonomic dysfunction can occasionally result in orthostatic hypotension and gastroparesis. The clinical course is chronic with slow improvement over months after discontinuation of the drug. Procarbazine, which is believed to interfere with DNA synthesis, is given orally due to unacceptable neurotoxicity with intravenous administration. Even in the oral form, besides encephalopathy, 10% to 20% of treated patients develop reversible peripheral neuropathy with distal paresthesias, decreased reflexes, and myalgias. About 1% of patients treated with high-dose Arabinoside (Ara-C) develop a severe sensorimotor polyneuropathy, resembling GBS. Patients may present two to three 3 weeks after chemotherapy with generalized weakness usually progressing to quadriparesis requiring ventilatory support. Increased CSF protein, slowing of nerve conduction velocities with conduction block, and predominantly demyelinating pathology have been reported (40).

Complications of Bone Marrow Transplantation

Peripheral neuropathy is commonly associated with bone marrow transplantation (BMT) and has multiple etiologies, including toxic effects of chemotherapy, radiation, or opportunistic infections, particularly with Herpes zoster virus. BMT recipients may also develop autoimmune neuromuscular complications after allogenic transplantation in the setting of graft-versus-host disease (GVHD). Inflammatory myopathies including PM and DM can be a manifestation of GVHD, along with fasciitis or synovitis, resulting in joint contractures. CK is normal or mildly elevated. Muscle biopsy shows degenerating fibers, inflammation, and, sometimes, fibrosis. These complications occasionally improve with corticosteroid treatment, sometimes in combination with other immunosuppressing drugs, although recovery may be incomplete (41). MG has been diagnosed in several cases with chronic GVHD following BMT. The clinical and laboratory findings are similar to the cases of idiopathic MG, and patients respond to the standard immunosuppressive treatments. MG may result from antigenic differences in AchR between donor- and recipient-triggering antibody production by the donor B-lymphocytes. CIDP or GBS also occur in GVHD and have the same features as the idiopathic forms. They improve with immunosuppressive treatment and resolution of the GVHD.

ACKNOWLEDGMENTS

The research of Kleopas A. Kleopa is supported by the National Multiple Sclerosis Society (USA) and Telethon. The research of Theodoros Kyriakides is supported by Telethon.

REFERENCES

1. Kori S, Foley K, Posner J. Brachial plexus lesions in patients with cancer: 100 cases. Neurology 1981; 31:45–50.
2. Lederman RJ, Wilbourn AJ. Brachial plexopathy: recurrent cancer or radiation? Neurology 1984; 34:1331–1335.
3. Jaeckle K, Young D, Foley K. The natural history of lumbosacral plexopathy in cancer. Neurology 1985; 35:8–15.
4. Thomas JE, Cascino TL, Earle JD. Differential diagnosis between radiation and tumor plexopathy of the pelvis. Neurology 1985; 35:1–7.
5. Catalano PJ, Sen C, Biller HF. Cranial neuropathy secondary to perineural spread of cutaneous malignancies. Am J Otol 1995; 16:772–777.
6. Diaz-Arrastia R, Younger DS, Hair L, et al. Neurolymphomatosis: a clinicopathologic syndrome re-emerges. Neurology 1992; 42:1136–1141.
7. Kelly JJ, Karcher DS. Lymphoma and peripheral neuropathy: a clinical review. Muscle Nerve 2005; 31:301–313.
8. Clouston PD, DeAngelis LM, Posner JB. The spectrum of neurological disease in patients with systemic cancer. Ann Neurol 1992; 31:268–273.
9. Levin KH. Paraneoplastic neuromuscular syndromes. Neurol Clin 1997; 15:597–614.
10. Dalmau J, Graus F, Rosenblum MK, et al. Anti-Hu-associated paraneoplastic encephalomyelitis/sensory neuronopathy. A clinical study of 71 patients. Medicine 1992; 71:59–72.
11. Kleopa KA, Teener JW, Scherer SS, et al. Chronic multiple paraneoplastic syndromes. Muscle Nerve 2000; 23:1767–1772.
12. Forsyth PA, Dalmau J, Graus F, et al. Motor neuron syndromes in cancer patients. Ann Neurol 1997; 41:722–730.
13. Gordon P, Rowland LP, Younger DS, et al. Lymphoproliferative disorders and motor neuron disease: an update. Neurology 1997; 48:1671–1678.
14. Brown P, Marsden CD. The stiff man and stiff man plus syndromes. J Neurol 1999; 246:648–652.
15. Antoine JC, Honnorat J, Camdessanche JP, et al. Paraneoplastic anti-CV2 antibodies react with peripheral nerve and are associated with a mixed axonal and demyelinating peripheral neuropathy. Ann Neurol 2001; 49:214–221.
16. Kelly JJ Jr., Kyle RA, Miles JM, et al. The spectrum of peripheral neuropathy in myeloma. Neurology 1981; 31:24–31.
17. Kelly JJ Jr., Kyle RA, Miles JM, et al. Osteosclerotic myeloma and peripheral neuropathy. Neurology 1983; 33:202–210.

18. Lisak RP, Mitchell M, Zweiman B, et al. Guillain-Barre syndrome and Hodgkin's disease: three cases with immunological studies. Ann Neurol 1977; 1:72–78.
19. Oh SJ, Slaughter R, Harrell L. Paraneoplastic vasculitic neuropathy: a treatable neuropathy. Muscle Nerve 1991; 14:152–156.
20. Newsom-Davis J. Autoimmune neuromyotonia (Isaac's syndrome): an anti-body-mediated potassium channelopathy. Ann NY Acad Sci 1997; 835:111–119.
21. O'Neill JH, Murray NM, Newsom-Davis J. The Lambert-Eaton myasthenic syndrome. A review of 50 cases. Brain 1988; 111:577–596.
22. Lennon VA, Kryzer TJ, Griesmann GE, et al. Calcium-channel antibodies in the Lambert-Eaton syndrome and other paraneoplastic syndromes. N Engl J Med 1995; 332:1467–1474.
23. Tim RW, Massey JM, Sanders DB. Lambert-Eaton myasthenic syndrome: electro-diagnostic findings and response to treatment. Neurology 2000; 54:2176–2178.
24. Newsom-Davis J. A treatment algorithm for Lambert-Eaton myasthenic syndrome. Ann N Y Acad Sci 1998; 841:817–822.
25. Mygland A, Vincent A, Newsom-Davis J, et al. Autoantibodies in thymoma-associated myasthenia gravis with myositis or neuromyotonia. Arch Neurol 2000; 57:527–531.
26. Koike Y, Hatori M, Kokubun S. Skeletal muscle metastasis secondary to cancer-a report of seven cases. Ups J Med Sci 2005; 110:75–83.
27. Sigurgeirsson B, Lindelof B, Edhag O, et al. Risk of cancer in patients with der-matomyositis or polymyositis. A population-based study. N Engl J Med 1992; 326:363–367.
28. Levin MI, Mozaffar T, Al-Lozi MT, et al. Paraneoplastic necrotizing myopathy: clinical and pathological features. Neurology 1998; 50:764–767.
29. Prayson RA. Amyloid myopathy: clinicopathologic study of 16 cases. Hum Pathol 1998; 29:463–468.
30. Malow BA, Dawson DM. Neuralgic amyotrophy in association with radiation therapy for Hodgkin's disease. Neurology 1991; 41:440–441.
31. Pierce SM, Recht A, Lingos T, et al. Long-term radiation complications follow-ing conservative surgery (CS) and radiation therapy (RT) in patients with early stage breast cancer. Int J Radiat Oncol Biol Phys 1992; 23:915–923.
32. Fathers E, Thrush D, Huson SM, et al. Radiation-induced brachial plexopathy in women treated for carcinoma of the breast. Clin Rehabil 2002; 16:160–165.
33. Harper CM Jr, Thomas JE, Cascino TL, et al. Distinction between neoplastic and radiation-induced brachial plexopathy, with emphasis on the role of EMG. Neurology 1989; 39:502–506.
34. Bowen J, Gregory R, Squier M, et al. The post-irradiation lower motor neuron syndrome neuronopathy or radiculopathy. Brain 1996; 119:1429–1439.
35. MacDonald D. Neurologic complications of chemotherapy. Neurol Clin 1991; 9:955–967.
36. Roelofs R, Hrushesky W, Rogin J, et al. Peripheral sensory neuropathy and cisplatin chemotherapy. Neurology 1984; 34:934–938.
37. Cersosimo R. Oxaliplatin-associated neuropathy: a review. Ann Pharmacother 2005; 39:128–135.
38. Postma T, Vermorken J, Liefting A, et al. Paclitaxel-induced neuropathy. Ann Oncol 1995; 6:489–494.

39. Chaudhry V, Eisenberger M, Sinibaldi V, et al. A prospective study of suramin-induced peripheral neuropathy. Brain 1996; 119:2039–2052.
40. Openshaw H, Slatkin N, Stein A, et al. Acute polyneuropathy after high dose cytosine arabinoside in patients with leukemia. Cancer 1996; 78:1899–1905.
41. Adams C, August CS, Maguire H, et al. Neuromuscular complications of bone marrow transplantation. Pediatr Neurol 1995; 12:58–61.

29

Neurological Complications of Cancer Therapy

Jerzy Hildebrand and Antony Béhin

Service de Neurologie Mazarin, Hôpital de la Salpêtrière, Paris, France and Service de Médecine Interne, Institut Jules Bordet, ULB, Bruxelles, Belgium

INTRODUCTION

Complications of antineoplastic treatments are, next to malignant spread, the most common cause of neurological lesion in cancer patients. We will consider the complications of surgery, radiation therapy, and various medical treatments including cytotoxic chemotherapy, cytokines, adjuvant treatments, and cell grafts, and infections.

COMPLICATIONS OF SURGERY

The incidence of transient or persisting neurological deficits following neurosurgery is declining, thanks to the progress made in tumor localization and delineation, functional imaging, and operative techniques. Despite these advances, posterior fossa surgery remains a common cause of cranial nerve injury, particularly in patients with meningioma, as these structures are often wrapped by the tumor. All cranial nerves from the sixth to twelfth are at risk during resection of petroclival tumor (1). Removal of foramen magnum meningioma may cause lesion of the IXth to XIIth nerves. In cerebellopontine angle tumors (meningioma and schwannoma) the facioacoustic complex is at risk.

The most common neurological complications of surgery performed for systemic tumors are traumatic cranial and peripheral nerve lesions.

The deficits are usually diagnosed shortly after the operation. They are either reversible or permanent. Nerve lesions may occasionally result from compression during anesthesia or be caused by hematoma, and such deficits usually recover. Cranial nerve lesions are common after extensive resection of head and neck tumors (2). The most frequently involved nerves are the XIth, causing shoulder drooping, the mandibular branch of the Vth nerve, and the XIIth nerve causing tongue hemiatrophy. Lesion of the sympathetic innervation causes Horner's syndrome. Head and neck surgery may also damage the cutaneous branches of the cervical plexus, causing dysesthesia and pain in pre- and postauricular areas, over the anterior shoulder and neck, and the supraclavicular nerves causing a sensory deficit extending from the jaw to the anterior and posterior aspect of the chest.

Radical mastectomy is followed by hypoesthesia of the axilla and the upper median and posterior aspect of the arm resulting from damage of the cutaneous branch of the second and third intercostal nerves. Pain may develop in these areas within weeks of surgery and is usually not associated with recurrent tumor (3). The long thoracic nerve is injured in 5% to 10% of the patients causing scapular winging.

Thoracotomy results in section of intercostal nerves causing segmental thoracic sensory loss and painful dysesthesia, which usually resolve within two to three months. Persistent or recurrent pain around the thoracic scare is often associated with malignant infiltration (4).

An Ommaya reservoir is commonly used in the treatment of leptomeningeal malignant disease to allow an easy access to the cerebrospinal fluid (CSF), and a more uniform and predictable drug distribution compared to lumbar puncture. Complications have been reported after its placement in up to 10% of patients, and include intracranial bleeding, bacterial meningitis, and seizures.

COMPLICATIONS OF RADIOTHERAPY

All modalities of radiotherapy may injure the central nervous system (CNS) and peripheral nervous system. These complications are classified according to the interval between treatment initiation and symptom onset (Table 1). Early acute toxicity develops mainly within two weeks, and early delayed toxicity after a few weeks to a few months. Both are usually reversible. Late delayed toxicity appears after an interval of six months to several years and is irreversible. Radiotherapy may induce secondary tumors, usually after a delay superior to 10 years.

Brain and Spinal Cord Lesions

Early Acute Toxicity

This complication is mainly seen in patients irradiated for brain tumor. It is uncommon when the conventional schedule of 1.8 to 2 Gy/day in five

Table 1 Neurologic Toxicity of Radiation Therapy

Lesion site	Early acute toxicity	Early-delayed toxicity	Late-delayed toxicity
Brain	Acute encephalopathy	Somnolence syndrome	Focal radionecrosis
		Worsening of preexisting signs	Diffuse leukoencephalopathy
		Mental impairment	
		Brain stem and cerebellar signs	Large vessel thrombosis
			Endocrine disorders
			Radiation-induced tumor
Spinal cord and motor roots		Lhermitte's sign	Progressive myelopathy
			Lower motor neuron syndrome
Visual apparatus and cranial nerves		Smell and hearing changes	Keratoconjunctivitis
			Cataract
			Retinopathy
			Optic nerve atrophy
			Mainly, last cranial nerve palsy
Plexus and peripheral nerves			Brachial and lumbosacral plexopathy
			Radiation-mononeuritis
			Radiation-induced tumor

weekly fractions is used, but is more likely to occur with hyperfractionated schedule. Clinical manifestations consist in an acute, usually mild, encephalopathy with headaches, nausea, and drowsiness or in worsening of deficits caused by the underlying tumor. Brain herniation may occur in patients with overt or impending intracranial hypertension. These manifestations are attributed to vasogenic edema and respond to glucocorticosteroids.

Early Delayed Toxicity

This group of miscellaneous and self-limiting diseases has been attributed to demyelination. Somnolence syndrome of various severities associated with anorexia and irritability has been reported in children with acute leukemia six to eight weeks after prophylactic irradiation with 18 to 24 Gy even without methotrexate (MTX) administration. The incidence varies from

8% to up to 80%. Younger age is the main risk factor. A similar syndrome characterized by a biphasic pattern has been observed in adults irradiated for brain tumor (5). The benefit of glucocorticoid administration is debatable.

Worsening of preexisting focal deficits with or without increased somnolence or mental changes, affecting mainly attention and memory, may be observed up to six months following brain tumor irradiation. Neuroimaging is either stable or shows progressive contrast enhancement (6), which may be mistaken for tumor progression. The diagnosis of this condition is often retrospective and based on spontaneous regression of clinical and radiological manifestations. The use of glucocorticosteroids is uncertain, but they are often used because tumor progression is suspected. Brainstem and cerebellar signs have been observed about 10 weeks after irradiation for extracranial lesions, or tumors not involving the posterior fossa. These disorders are reversible, but may be occasionally fatal (7). Pathologic examination shows scattered demyelination.

Lhermitte's sign consists of an unpleasant sensation, often described as an electric shock irradiating along the spine into limbs, elicited by neck flexion. It has been reported in up to 15% of the patients, mainly with lymphoma, two to four months after irradiation of the cervical cord with a total dose of about 45 Gy. The incidence is related to the dose per fraction. Lhermitte's sign caused by irradiation is self-limited, and it does not predict the occurrence of late-delayed radiation myelopathy.

Late-Delayed Toxicity

This group of irreversible and life-threatening diseases includes focal radionecrosis, diffuse leukoencephalopathy, progressive myelopathy, lesion of large blood vessels, endocrine disorders, lesions of visual apparatus, and radiation-induced tumors.

Focal brain radionecrosis: Focal brain radionecrosis (FBRN) generally appears during the second year following irradiation (range 6 months to 10 years) with a total dose more than 55 Gy. The risk of FBRN is related to total dose and inversely proportional to the number of fractions used to reach a given total dose. However, its occurrence cannot be entirely explained by radiation characteristics; an idiosyncratic sensitivity seems to play a role. FBRN is largely confined to the white matter. Early pathological changes include foci formed by eosinophilic exudates of fibrin, necrosis of small vessels with fibrin exudation (fibrinoid necrosis), and vascular proliferation. Subsequent vascular thickening and obstruction may develop, with formation of necrotic lesions, small and large cysts, and occasional calcium deposits. Clinical and radiological features (Fig. 1), and response to glucocorticosteroids mimic tumor progression. Positron emission tomography allows to differentiate a hypometabolic FBRN lesion from a hypermetabolic high-grade glioma in most patients. Magnetic resonance (MR) spectroscopy is also useful in differential diagnosis (8). Nowadays, FBRN is seen in less

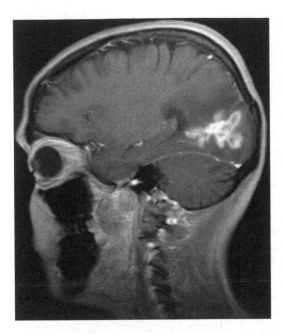

Figure 1 Sagittal postcontrast T1-weighted magnetic resonance (MR) imaging showing an occipital focal necrosis surrounded by edema in a 33-year-old woman. The lesion was diagnosed 18 months after a first and eight months after a second external stereotactic irradiation with gamma knife of a breast cancer metastasis. The lesion was hypometabolic on fluorodeoxyglucose-positron emission tomography scan. MR spectroscopy was characterized by low *N*-acetyl aspartate (NAA), choline and creatine peaks, and low choline/NAA ratio.

than 1% of patients irradiated for brain tumor with 55 to 60 Gy given in 30 daily fractions. The precise incidence, however, is difficult to assess even by pathological examination because radionecrotic changes are common in the bed of irradiated tumors. FBRN incidence is higher with hypofractionated doses. It occurs in 40% to 50% of patients treated with brachytherapy (interstitial implantation of iridium-192 or iodine-125 seeds) and in about 5% of the patients treated with external stereotactic irradiation using either gamma knife or linear accelerator. FBRN is treated symptomatically with glucocorticosteroids. Surgical resection may be necessary in patients with mass effect, who no longer respond to medical treatment. A second operation aiming to remove the radionecrotic mass has to be performed in up to 40% of patients treated with brachytherapy. The occurrence of FBRN is exceptional in the brain stem and the cerebellum. However, multiple lesions characterized by axonal and myelin loss without inflammatory reaction have been observed in basis pontis after irradiation combined with chemotherapy (9).

Late-delayed leukoencephalopathy: It represents nowadays the most common complication due to irradiation of large brain volume or of the whole brain (10). Concomitant chemotherapy contributes to its pathogenesis. Demonstration of diffuse white matter lesions has been made possible by computed tomography (CT) scan and by T2W, Fluid attenuation inversion recovery, and proton density MR imaging (MRI) (Fig. 2). White matter involvement is usually symmetrical, and varies from foci limited to the angles of frontal and occipital horns to lesion extending from ventricular lining to the cortex. These lesions correspond to axonal and myelin loss, reactive astrocytosis, vascular changes, and edema. In late stages, leukoencephalopathy is often accompanied by cortical and subcortical atrophy. Leukoencephalopathy mainly occurs during the two years following irradiation. Its most prominent clinical feature is dementia of subcortical type. Unsteady gait is common, but seizures and focal deficits are not. There is a fair correlation between cognitive impairment and the degree of leukoencephalopathy in patients with severe MRI changes, but the correlation between cognitive deficits and mild-to-moderate white matter change or cortical atrophy is poor. In addition to concomitant chemotherapy, the risk factors for leukoencephalopathy are irradiation dose and volume, and vascular risk factors including age. The combination of several risk factors may cause an unacceptable neurotoxicity. For example, (i) children with acute leukemia treated with prophylactic 24 Gy, whole brain irradiation (WBRT), and intrathecal and systemic MTX, the incidence of necrotic leukoencephalopathy was considerably higher in patients treated with systemic MTX 50 to 80 mg/m^2 than those who received only 20 to 30 mg/m^2. (ii) A severe dementia occurs in up to 50% of patients over 60 years treated for primary CNS lymphoma with WBRT (54 Gy) and chemotherapy based on high-dose MTX. (iii) A high rate of symptomatic leukoencephalopathy is observed in patients with brain metastases surviving 18 to 24 months after being treated with WBRT and chemotherapy. There is no treatment for postirradiation leukoencephalopathy, but its incidence can be substantially reduced by minimizing irradiation dose and avoiding concomitant administration of chemo- and radiation therapy, especially in high-risk patients.

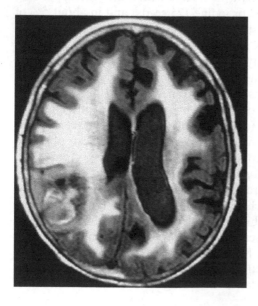

Figure 2 Axial fluid attenuation inversion recovery magnetic resonance imaging showing a diffuse late delayed leukoencephalopathy in a 78-year-old woman treated with hyperfractionated brain irradiation for a right parietal glioblastoma.

Progressive myelopathy: It is caused by a necrotic lesion pathologically similar to late FBRN, with prominent demyelination and small-vessel occlusion. Clinical manifestations (11) often appear in the beginning of the second year following irradiation with at least 45 Gy, but the range of the delay is wide (three months to over five years). In the past, overlap of adjacent fields causing localized overdose, high total irradiation dose, and dose per fraction favored focal spinal necrosis. Nowadays this complication is rare. First symptoms usually involve the lower limbs, with sensation of numbness or painful burning and follow an ascending course up to the level of the damaged spinal segment. Radicular-like pain is uncommon. Patients may complain of inability to perceive pain or temperature. Weakness is rarely the presenting feature, and also tends to follow an ascending course, causing progressive paraplegia or quadriplegia. Sphincter abnormalities are common. Brown-Séquard syndrome is a transient stage. Delayed myelopathy is irreversible, although in some patients a partial deficit may stabilize. There is no specific treatment.

Pure lower-motor neuron signs with preserved sphincter function have been observed after irradiation of pelvic and para-aortic region, especially in patients with testicular tumor. Although the deficit suggests injury to anterior horn neurons, the lesions may also involve spinal roots and cauda equina (12).

Lesion of large vessels: Thickening and occlusion of small- and medium-sized arteries is a prominent component in all late-delayed radiation complications. In addition, delayed lesion of large vessels including accelerated atherosclerosis, particularly of cervical internal or common carotid, may cause transient ischemic attacks and stroke. Carotid endarterectomy may be useful, but is technically more difficult than in common atherosclerosis.

Endocrine disorders: These are attributed to the irradiation of hypothalamus; anterior pituitary is considered much more radioresistant. Potentiating effect of chemotherapy is not established. These complications are probably underdiagnosed (13). Endocrine complications of surgery are less common and may be transient. Postirradiation endocrine changes are mainly seen after treatment of hypothalamic–pituitary axis tumors. In such patients, however, the issue of radiation-induced endocrine disorders is complicated by endocrine abnormalities due to tumor growth and surgery. In addition, the significance of gonadotropin changes is difficult to assess in patients with hyperprolactinemia. Endocrine disorders have been also observed after irradiation of nasopharyngeal carcinoma, of distant brain tumors, and prophylaxis of acute leukemia. Endocrine dysfunctions are usually diagnosed after a delay greater than two years, but may occur within few months. Their incidence is related to irradiation dose and volume, and to the dose per fraction. Growth hormone is first affected, followed by deficiency in gonadotropins and adrenocorticotropin hormone (ACTH). Thyroid stimulating hormone is the least likely and the last affected, but may cause significant disability. Thyroid function may also be affected by irradiation of the thyroid gland. Hyperprolactinemia is often observed after hypothalamus irradiation, causing galactorrhea and amenorrhea in women, gynecomastia in men, and decreased libido in both genders. Other features such as precocious puberty and growth deficiency (also due to bone irradiation) are particularly worrisome, because they have been occasionally observed in leukemic children treated with only 18 to 24 Gy. Endocrine disorders need to be detected early as they may be corrected by the administration of the deficient hormone. Hyperprolactinemia responds to dopaminergic drugs.

Lesions of visual apparatus following conventional radiation therapy may affect the visual system anywhere along its path. Keratoconjunctivitis sicca, due to impaired tear production, may be prevented by early and regular eye lubrication with substitute tears. Postradiation cataract is common even after low-dose treatment. The most serious and untreatable complications occurring after a delay ranging from six months to six years involve the retina and the optic nerve. The delay is inversely proportional to the total irradiation dose. Radiation retinopathy is dose related and has been observed for a total dose beyond 50 Gy given in 1.8 to 2.0/Gy fraction. After a period of normal sight, painless vision loss occurs insidiously and progresses over months. Small vessels are the primary target of injury. Their obliteration causes ischemia, edema, cotton-wool exudates, microaneurysms, and retinal hemorrhage leading to blindness. These changes can be demonstrated by ophthalmoscopy or fluorescein angiography. Optic nerve atrophy is also due to ischemia resulting from small-vessel occlusion. It causes decreased visual acuity or visual-field defect, and is detected as pallor of the optic disc on fundoscopy. In anterior optic nerve lesions, disc pallor may be preceded by swelling and hemorrhage.

Radiation induced tumor: The diagnosis of radiation-induced tumor requires three criteria: (i) pathology different from that of the primary tumor, (ii) long delay from irradiation, usually over 10 years, and (iii) development within or at the margin of radiation portal. Irradiation threshold may be low, because an increased incidence of radiation-induced brain tumors was found after low-dose irradiation for Tinea capitis, and in leukemia prophylaxis. Secondary brain tumors are mostly meningiomas followed by gliomas and sarcomas.

Peripheral Nervous System Lesions

Late-delayed lesions of cranial nerves, plexus, and peripheral nerves result from direct neuronal damage, and secondary fibrosis, and ischemia. Peripheral nervous structures are fairly radioresistant, and the respective contribution of the two mechanisms is unclear. Regardless of the mechanism, all late-delayed complications are related to the total irradiation dose, dose per fraction, and the size of irradiation field. A potentiating effect of, even highly neurotoxic, chemotherapeutic drugs has not been clearly demonstrated. Radiation-induced lesions of the peripheral nervous system are rare, and a metastatic lesion must be ruled out before considering this diagnosis.

Cranial nerve lesions: Reversible changes in the sense of smell may occur during or shortly after irradiation, but late anosmia is exceptional. Involvement of the third, fourth, fifth, sixth and seventh nerve due to irradiation is very rare with the possible exception of the sixth nerve. Neuromyotonia, which corresponds to delayed muscle relaxation after voluntary contraction, has been observed after irradiation of the fifth (14) and sixth nerves (15). Hearing loss and tinnitus due to otitis media are common during or shortly after head irradiation. The deficit slowly resolves in most patients, but may lead to sensorineural hearing loss months to years later.

Lower cranial nerve palsy has been mainly reported after irradiation of head and neck tumors with 60 Gy or more. In a series of 25 patients with 35 cranial nerve palsies (16), the XIIth nerve was involved in 19 patients, the recurrent laryngeal in nine, the XIth in five cases, and the fifth nerve in only one case. Radiosurgery may be followed by a mostly transient trigeminal or facial palsy (17).

Plexopathies and peripheral nerve lesions: Brachial plexopathy occurs mainly in patients treated for lung and breast tumor. Its first symptoms are dysesthesia and paresthesia. Unlike in cancerous plexopathy, pain is initially seen in only about 20% of the patients. The disease progresses insidiously and is sometimes self-limiting. Radiological diagnosis is based on the absence of neoplastic lesions around the plexus and the loss of definition of muscle planes on MRI. Presence of myokymia on Electromyogram (EMG) favors the diagnosis of postradiation plexopathy.

Lumbar plexopathy is most frequently seen in patients with cervical, ovary, rectal, and prostate cancer. Clinical and radiological features are similar to those reported for brachial plexopathy. Because of radiation field location, lumbar plexopathy is bilateral in about 80% of cases. Treatment of radiation plexopathy is limited to physiotherapy combined with analgesic drugs. Surgery aiming at the release of nervous structures from fibrosis is not recommended because it may put at risk the already compromised blood supply of the nerve trunks.

Progressive mononeuritis occurring within radiation portals suggests postradiation fibrosis or radiation-induced tumor. MRI and ultrasound may help in the differential diagnosis. Peripheral nerve sheath tumors have been observed after irradiation with 20 to 54 Gy. The majority are neurofibromas, and about half of the patients have type 1 neurofibromatosis.

COMPLICATIONS OF MEDICAL TREATMENTS

Dysfunction of brain, spinal cord, and peripheral nervous structures may occur after administration of cytotoxic chemotherapy and cytokines [alfa interferon and interleukin (IL)-2], adjuvant treatments (glucocorticosteroids, antiepileptics, and opioids), and bone marrow grafts. These treatments also favor opportunistic infections, and probably cerebrovascular diseases. As mentioned above, several disorders are caused by the combined effect of radio- and chemotherapy, and the respective pathogenetic role of each treatment is often difficult to determine. Toxicity related to chemotherapy usually starts during or shortly after drug administration, in contrast to radiation toxicity, which is often delayed.

Brain Lesions

Cytotoxic Chemotherapy

Chemotherapeutic drugs are neurotoxic. However, the CNS is usually spared, because most of these agents do not readily cross an intact blood–brain barrier. Therefore signs of encephalopathy such as headaches, altered cognition, or arousal with or without seizures are rare after systemic administration of conventional chemotherapy doses. Nevertheless encephalopathy is occasionally observed during treatment with MTX, vincristine, cytosine arabinoside (Ara-C), cisplatin, etoposide, nitrosourea derivatives, thiotepa, and capecitabine. In most patients, the occurrence of this complication is unpredictable, and the pathogenesis remains speculative. However, there are exceptions.

Ifosfamide encephalopathy (18) develops in 10% to up to 50% of patients 12 to 16 hours after treatment initiation. Clinical manifestations include confusion, stupor or coma, asterixis, extrapyramidal signs, cranial nerve palsy, psychotic behavior, hallucinations, and seizures. The risk factors include oral versus intravenous administration, short infusion time, total dose, underlying CNS lesion, age, history of psychosis, concurrent high-dose emetics, pelvic tumor location, low serum albumin, liver insufficiency, and high serum creatinine. The symptoms usually clear three to four days following drug discontinuation, but fatal outcome has been reported. The efficacy of methylene blue treatment is based on case reports and small series of patients (19). Oral administration of $50 \, mg \times 3/day$ is often used for prophylaxis. Intravenous route ($50 \, mg \times 3$ to $6/day$) is preferred to treat symptomatic patients.

Acute encephalopathy, possibly followed by a pancerebellar syndrome characterized by gait ataxia, limb dysmetria, nystagmus and dysarthria, may occur after administration of conventional doses of 5-fluorouracil (5-FU) (20). The toxicity of 5-FU is dose dependent, and patients with constitutionally low serum levels of dihydropyrimidine dehydrogenase are more likely to develop neurotoxic side effects.

Encephalopathy used to occur in 30% to 60% of patients with acute leukemia treated with L-asparaginase, but has become rare because much lower doses (about 10,000 units/day) are used. L-asparaginase does not cross the blood–brain barrier, and the encephalopathy is attributed to hepatic toxicity.

Acute encephalopathy was observed after intravenous administration of procarbazine preventing this modality of drug administration.

High-dose systemic chemotherapy may overwhelm the blood–brain barrier resulting in neurotoxic effects. MTX, used alone, may cause acute diffuse leukoencephalopathy (21). It also exacerbates the delayed effect of irradiation (late-delayed leukoencephalopathy). Ara-C at $3 \, \text{g/m}^2$ given every 24 hours may produce within five days an acute encephalopathy followed by cerebellar signs. Imaging studies may show white matter changes (22). Later, cerebellar atrophy corresponding to loss of Purkinje cells may be seen.

Intrathecal chemotherapy circumvents the blood–brain barrier. MTX and Ara-C are the main drugs used for intrathecal injection. Their neurotoxic effects are fairly similar, but have been best characterized for MTX. Acute aseptic meningitis causing headaches, nausea, vomiting, and neck rigidity develops 24 hours to a few days after drug administration in up to 50% of patients. CSF examination usually shows lymphocytic pleocytosis and elevated protein, but its composition may also mimic infectious meningitis. The presence of fever is frequent, and may be misleading by suggesting infection. The disease is self-limiting and requires no specific treatment.

Intrathecal MTX also contributes to late-delayed leukoencephalopathy. In addition, a fatal necrotic periventricular leukoencephalopathy has been reported in children operated for posterior fossa tumor and treated with intrathecal MTX.

Over a 1000 brain tumor patients have received intracarotid chemotherapy using nitrosoureas, cisplatin, or etoposide. This treatment modality has been largely abandoned, at least for these drugs, due to focal encephalopathy and retinal damage, which occurs when the tip of the catheter is placed below the origin of the ophthalmic artery.

Cytokines

Systemic administration of alpha interferon causes a flu-like syndrome, which tends to be more severe with higher dose and in older patients. The syndrome includes headaches, lethargy, hallucinations, and seizures (23). Manifestations of emotional instability have been observed with recombinant interferon alpha 2b especially in patients with psychiatric history. The neurotoxicity of interferon is reversible, and tends to decrease with time.

Confusion of varying severity with hallucinations, seizures, and altered arousal occurs in up to 30% to 50% of patients treated by IL-2 (24). Sensory motor deficits have been occasionally observed with abnormal focal signs on T2W-MRI.

Glucocorticosteroid, Antiepileptics, and Opioids

Glucocorticosteroids may produce behavioral and mental changes. Anxiety, nervousness, insomnia, or euphoria are common, but serious psychiatric manifestations such as depression or acute psychosis associated with hallucinations occur in less than 3% of cases, and are less frequent with methylprednisolone and dexamethasone than with natural corticoids or ACTH. These complications may occur in early stages of therapy or during drug tapering, and usually resolve after the drug is discontinued. "Steroid dementia" including disturbances in memory (25) and attention is a reversible, and possibly underestimated, disorder (26). Epidural lipoma is a rare manifestation of fat redistribution caused by chronic glucocorticosteroid administration. It may cause a progressive spinal cord compression, which occasionally requires surgical decompression. Myopathy, corresponding to type-2 muscle fibre atrophy, is a disabling disorder occurring in up to 20% of patients on high-dose glucocorticosteroids (27). Its main feature is pelvic weakness, which may impair gait and mimic tumor progression. Weakness of neck flexion and reduction of ventilatory capacity are less well-recognized symptoms. EMG is usually normal. Corticosteroid myopathy slowly improves after drug discontinuation. Its severity may be reduced by physical training.

Most antiepileptic drugs produce some degree of fatigability, somnolence, or dizziness. Others may cause more specific CNS toxicity, and mimic brain tumor progression. The complications tend to be more severe in the elderly, and during rapid drug escalation. Cognitive changes have been observed mainly with phenobarbital, benzodiazepines, and more recently with topiramate. Levetiracetam and topiramate may cause aggressive behavior. Patients treated with valproic acid frequently develop dose-related postural tremor, and, occasionally, an encephalopathy with or without hyperammonemia. Diplopia and instability may be caused by carbamazepine, oxcarbazepine, lamotrigine, and topiramate. Nystagmus, ataxia, and rarely cerebellar atrophy may occur in patients on phenytoin. Concentric narrowing of visual fields has greatly reduced the use of vigabatrin.

CNS side effects of opioids range from sedation to confusion. In our experience, opioid administration often contributes to acute confusion in patients with systemic cancer.

Spinal Cord and Spinal Root Lesions

Acute or subacute paresis or quadriparesis has been observed after intrathecal administration of MTX, Ara-C, and thiotepa. Three clinical presentations have been described, based on the time of onset following drug administration and the extent of neurologic deficit (28). Group 1 and 2 present, within 48 hours of intrathecal therapy, a severe radicular pain in the legs, followed by ascending paraplegia or quadriplegia. The distinctive sign of Group 1 is a rapid progression to respiratory distress and coma. In Group 2, the neurological disorders are restricted to spinal cord and spinal roots. They may recover within hours to a few days, but death due to acute pulmonary edema may occur. Scant pathological data indicate that spinal cord and roots may be involved. The pathogenesis is putative, and may involve neurotoxicity of the drugs or drug preservatives, or a hypersensitivity reaction. Group 3 patients develop a progressive paraparesis or quadriparesis with hyper-reflexia, Babinski's sign, and sphincter dysfunction weeks to months after intrathecal therapy. Pathological lesions are restricted to the spinal cord, and are probably caused by drug toxicity.

Peripheral Nerve Lesions

Chemotherapy is the leading cause of peripheral neuropathy in cancer patients. A barrier, similar to the blood–brain barrier, surrounds peripheral nerves but does not protect their proximal and distal portions. Vinca alkaloids (29), platinum derivatives (30), and taxanes (31) cause severe peripheral neuropathy.

Symptoms and signs suggesting peripheral nerve toxicity have been reported for a series of other agents. Features of distal dying-back neuropathy have been observed after the administration of etoposide, procarbazine, hexamethylmelamine, 5-azacytidine, and mitotane.

Suramin and Ara-C tend to produce a Guillain-Barré–like polyradiculoneuritis. All these drugs usually cause mild-to-moderate neurotoxic manifestations, and are seldom the limiting factor of drug administration. But they are potential aggravating factors when other neurotoxic drugs are used, either concomitantly or shortly after their administration. Other risk factors for chemotherapy-induced peripheral neuropathy include preexisting acquired or congenital nerve lesions, diabetes mellitus, liver dysfunction, and advanced age. The severity of peripheral neuropathy increases with total dose, and shorter interval of drug administration. Clinical manifestations usually appear during drug administration, but may progress for weeks to months after its discontinuation (32,33). The clinical presentation is often evocative of the nature of the neurotoxic agent.

Vinca alkaloids cause a dying-back peripheral neuropathy through inhibition of fast axonal transport by preventing microtubule polymerization. Vincristine is the most neurotoxic, vinblastine is only mildly neurotoxic, and vindesine and vinorelbine have an intermediate neurotoxicity. Early manifestations are tingling, burning, and prickling sensations, or numbness in feet, hands, and perioral area. Ankle jerks disappear during early stages followed by patellar and upper limb tendon reflexes. Distal symmetrical weakness is usually seen for a cumulative dose exceeding 15 mg of vincristine. In contrast to sensory symptoms and motor deficit, sensory signs are mild. Autonomic neuropathy is common and may cause severe constipation, paralytic ileus, bladder atony, impotence, and orthostatic hypotension.

Sensory neuronopathy is the main limiting factor for the use of two platinum compounds: cisplatin (CDDP) and oxaliplatin, whereas carboplatin is very mildly neurotoxic. The mechanism of CDDP neurotoxicity is unclear. Postmortem studies have shown that platinum accumulates in the dorsal root ganglia cells. Large sensory fibres are predominantly affected, leading to loss of proprioception and depression of tendon reflexes. Motor function is preserved. CDDP causes tinnitus and dose-related hearing loss. Oxaliplatin causes two different types of peripheral neuropathy. The most characteristic is the acute neurotoxicity, which consists of paresthesia, cold hypersensitivity, jaw and eye pain, and cramps starting 30 to 60 minutes after the administration and lasting for a few days. Acute oxaliplatin neuropathy may respond to calcium and magnesium infusion (34). The late oxaliplatin neurotoxicity resembles CDDP neuronopathy.

Paclitaxel and docetaxel promote the formation of microtubules and prevent their depolymerization thus inhibiting axonal transport and causing a sensory-motor neuropathy. Sensory symptoms (paresthesia and numbness) and signs (decreased vibratory sensation) are predominant. Weakness is usually mild. Several agents including glutamate, Org-2677 (a corticotropin analogue), amifostine, mesna, BNP-7787 (a mesna precursor), glutathione, vitamin E, and neurotropic factors have shown protective activity in vitro, in experimental models, and even in some clinical trials, but none has gained routine clinical use so far.

Cerebrovascular Lesions

Cancer and stroke are common diseases and may occur concomitantly by chance. In addition they share common risk factors such as smoking, alcohol abuse, and advanced age. However, several mechanisms favor stroke in cancer patients, and anticancer drug is one of them. Chemotherapy-induced thrombopenia favors brain and subdural hemorrhage, and spinal subdural hematoma following lumbar puncture. Anticancer drugs have also been implicated in the pathogenesis of ischemic lesions, although the evidence is based on small patient's series or single case reports. The pathogenic role of L-asparaginase has been best established in a relatively large number of strokes observed in children without other risk factor (35,36). L-asparaginase also causes thrombosis of cerebral veins and sinuses. Ischemic stroke was reported in young adults, without other risk factors, shortly after the administration of cisplatin used alone or combined with 5-FU (37). Multiple strokes and livedo have been observed in cancer patients treated with IL-2 and interferon alpha (38).

BONE MARROW TRANSPLANTATION AND INFECTIONS

Complications of hematopoietic stem cell transplantation are more common after allogeneic than autologous graft. Neurological complications mainly include encephalopathy, with or without seizures, cerebrovascular disorders, and infections. Encephalopathy may result from drug toxicity (ifosfamide,

MTX, Ara-C, and busulfan) or vital organ dysfunction. The most characteristic, but not specific, presentation is posterior leukoencephalopathy appearing on CT scan and MRI, and clinically characterized by headaches, seizures, cortical blindness, and systemic hypertension. High doses of cyclosporine A may play a key pathogenic role (39). The disease is reversible, and has been attributed to vasospasm. Subarachnoid hemorrhage is more common than cerebral bleeding or ischemia, in grafted patients and is mainly attributed to platelet dysfunction. The microbial spectrum causing CNS infections in patients with bone marrow transplantation is similar to those found in the general cancer population (40). Opportunistic pathogens predominate, and their proliferation is facilitated by immunosuppression, neutropenia, and neurosurgery. The overall incidence of CNS infections in cancer patients is low (around 0.01%), but they are more common in certain malignancies such as lymphomas and leukemias.

Reactivation of Herpes zoster virus in cranial nerve and spinal root ganglia is the most common neurological infection in cancer. It occurs in 9% to 25% of patients with myeloma, lymphoma, or leukemia. Disseminated varicella may follow localized disease in immunosuppressed patients. Postherpetic neuralgia is a troublesome, age-related, complication.

Meningitis (and meningoencephalitis) is the second most common CNS infection in cancer patients. Its manifestations—headache, fever, and neck rigidity—may be milder than those seen in the general population. Listeria monocytogenes *and Cryptococcus neoformans* (favored by T-lymphocyte and mononuclear defect) are the most common causes. Other agents include *candida* (neutropenia), enteric bacilli, *Staphylococcus aureus* (head and spine surgery, and neutropenia), *S. epidermidis* (CSF shunt and neurosurgery), and *Streptococcus pneumonie* (splenectomy and B lymphocyte defect).

The main agents causing cerebral abscess are enteric bacilli and *S. aureus* (neutropenia and neurosurgery), *Aspergillus, candida* (neutropenia, and bone marrow transplantation), *Nocardia asteroides, Cryptococcus neoformans* and *Toxoplasma gondii* (T-lymphocyte and mononuclear defect). Diffuse encephalitis may be caused by Papova JC virus (progressive multifocal leukoencephalopathy), Herpes simplex, and *Toxoplasma gondii.*

REFERENCES

1. Samii M, Ammirati M, Mahran A, et al. Surgery of petroclival meningiomas: report of 24 cases. Neurosurgery 1989; 24:12–17.
2. Swift TR. Involvement of peripheral nerves in radical neck dissection. Am J Surg 1970; 199:694–698.
3. Delmar AR, Milton JP. Complications associated with mastectomy. Surg Clin North Am 1983; 63:1332–1352.
4. Foley KM. Pain syndromes in patients with cancer. Med Clin North Am 1984; 71:169–184.

5. Faithfull S, Brada M. Somnolence syndrome in adults following cranial irradiation for primary tumour. Clin Oncol 1998; 10:250–254.
6. De Wit MCY, de Bruin HG, Eijkenboom W, et al. Immediate post-radiation changes in malignant glioma can mimic tumor progression. Neurology 2004; 63:535–537.
7. Lampert P, Tom MI, Rider WD. Disseminated demyelination of the brain following Co 60 radiation. Arch Pathol 1959; 68:322–330.
8. Galanaud D, Chinot O, Metellus Ph, Cazzone P. Apports de la spectroscopie par résonance magnetique dans l'exploration des gliomes. Bull Cancer 2005; 92: 327–331.
9. Breuer AC, Blank NK, Schoene WC. Multifocal pontine lesions in cancer patients treated with chemotherapy and CNS radiotherapy. Cancer 1978; 41:2112–2120.
10. Vigliani MC, Duyckaert C, Dellatre JY. Radiation-induced cognitive dysfunction in adults. In: Vecht, ed. Handbook of Clinical Neurology. Vol. 2. 67th ed. Science Elsevier, Amsterdam 1997; 371–388.
11. Pallis CA, Louis S, Morgan RI. Radiation myelopathy. Brain 1961; 84:460–479.
12. Bowen J, Gregory R, Squier M, Donaghy M. The post-irradiation lower motor neuron syndrome neuronopathy or radiculopathy. Brain 1996; 119: 1429–1439.
13. Arlt W, Hove U, Muller B, et al. Frequent and overlooked treatment induced endocrine dysfunction in adults long-term survivors of primary brain tumors. Neurology 1997; 49:545–552.
14. Diaz JM, Urban ES, Schiffman JS, Peterson AC. Post-irradiation neuromyotonia affecting trigeminal nerve distribution: an unusual presentation. Neurology 1992; 42:1102–1104.
15. Lessel S, Lessel IM, Rizzo JF. Ocular neuromyotonia after radiation therapy. Am J Ophthalmology 1986; 102:766–770.
16. Berger PS, Bataini JP. Radiation-induced cranial nerve palsy. Cancer 1977; 40: 152–155.
17. Foote RL, Coffey RJ, Swanson JW, et al. Stereotactic radiosurgery using the gamma knife for acoustic neurinoma. Int J Radiat Oncol Biol Phys 1995; 32:1153–1160.
18. Merimski O, Inbar M, Reider-Groswasser I, et al. Ifosfamide-related acute encephalopathy clinical and radiological aspects. Eur J Cancer 1991; 27:1188–1189.
19. Pelgrims J, De Vos F, Van den Brande J, et al. Methylene blue in the treatment of ifosfamide-induced encephalopathy: report of 12 cases and a review of literature. Br J Cancer 2000; 82:598–599.
20. Lynch HT, Droszcz CP, Albano WA, Lynch JF. Organic brain syndrome secondary to 5-fluorouracil toxicity. Dis Colon Rectum 1981; 24:130–131.
21. Walker RW, Allen JC, Rosen G, Caparros B. Transient cerebral dysfunction secondary to high-dose methotrexate. J Clin Oncol 1986; 4:189–195.
22. Hwang TL, Yung WK, Estey EH, Fields WS. Central nervous system toxicity with high-dose Ara-C. Neurology 1985; 35:1475–1479.
23. Adams F, Fernandez F, Mavligit G. Interferon-induced organic mental disorders associated with unsuspected pre-existing neurologic abnormalities. J Neurooncol 1988; 6:32–35.

24. Ilowsky Karp B, Yang JC, Khorsand M, et al. Multiple cerebral lesions complicating therapy with interleukin-2. Neurology 1996; 47:417–424.
25. Uttner I, Müller BA, Zinser C, et al. Reversible impaired memory induced by pulsed methylprednisolone in patients with MS. Neurology 2005; 64:1971–1973.
26. Sacks O, Shulman M. Steroid dementia: an overlooked diagnosis? Neurology 2005; 64:707–709.
27. Weissman DE, Dufer D, Vogel V, Abeloff MD. Corticosteroid toxicity in neurooncology patients. J Neurooncol 1987; 5:125–128.
28. Grauss F. Acute meningospinal syndromes: acute myelopathy and radiculopathy. In: Hildebrand J, ed. Neurological Adverse Reactions to Anticancer Drugs. Berlin: Springer-Verlag, 1990:87–92.
29. Slander SG, Tobin W, Henderson ES. Vincristine-induced neuropathy. Neurology 1969; 19:367–374.
30. Standefer JC. Cisplatin neuropathy, clinical, electrophysiologic, morphologic and toxicologic studies. Cancer 1984; 54:1269–1275.
31. Hilkens PHE, Verweij J, Stoter G, et al. Peripheral neurotoxicity induced by docetaxel. Neurology 1996; 46:104–106.
32. Vanderstappen CCP, Koeppen S, Heimans JJ, et al. Dose-related vincristine-induced peripheral neuropathy with unexpected off-therapy worsening. Neurology 2005; 64:1076–1077.
33. Siegal T, Haim N. Cisplatin–induced peripheral neuropathy: frequent off-therapy deterioration, demyelinating syndromes, and muscle cramps. Cancer 1990; 15: 1117–1123.
34. Gamelin L, Boisdron-Celle M, Delva R, et al. Prevention of Oxaliplatin-related neurotoxicity by calcium and magnesium infusions: a retrospective study of 161 patients receiving oxaliplatin combined with 5-fluorouracil and leucovorin for advanced colorectal cancer. Clin Cancer Research 2004; 10:4055–4061.
35. Ott N, Ramsey NKC, Priest JR, et al. Sequelae of thrombotic or hemorrhagic complications following L-asparaginase therapy for childhood lymphoblastic leukaemia. Am J Pediatric Hematol Oncol 1988; 10:191–195.
36. Feinberg WM, Swenson MR. Cerebrovascular complications of L-asparaginase therapy. Neurology 1988; 38:127–133.
37. El Amrani M, Heinzlef O, Debroucker T, et al. Brain infarction following 5-fluoro-uracil and cisplatin therapy. Neurology 1998; 51:899–901.
38. Drapier S, Kassiotis P, Moutarda I, et al. Infarctus cérébraux multiples associés à un livedo secondaires à un traitement anticancéreux par intr-erleukine 2 et interferon alpha. Rev Neurol (Paris) 2000; 156:789–791.
39. Ghany AM, Tutschka PJ, Mc GheeRB Jr., et al. Cyclosporine-associated seizures in bone marrow transplantation recipients given busulfan and cyclosporine. Transplantation 1991; 52:310–315.
40. Bleggi-Torres LF, de Madeiros BC, Werner B, et al. Neuropathological findings after bone marrow transplantation: an autopsy study of 180 cases. Bone Marrow Trasplant 2000; 25:301–307.

30

Paraneoplastic Autoimmunity Affecting the Nervous System

Sean J. Pittock

Departments of Neurology and Laboratory Medicine and Pathology, Mayo Clinic College of Medicine, Rochester, Minnesota, U.S.A.

Vanda A. Lennon

Departments of Immunology, Neurology and Laboratory Medicine and Pathology, Mayo Clinic College of Medicine, Rochester, Minnesota, U.S.A.

INTRODUCTION

Paraneoplastic autoimmune neurological disorders are caused by a targeted immune attack on the nervous system, as the consequence of a potentially effective tumor immune response initiated by antigens derived from a systemic cancer, either new or recurrent. These disorders affect women twice as frequently than men. The neurological symptoms are not due to metastases and, in fact, metastases beyond regional lymph nodes are uncommon. Neurological symptoms precede the identification of a cancer in the majority of patients. The neoplasms encountered most frequently are lung (small-cell), breast and gynecologic (mullerian) carcinomas, seminoma, thymoma, Hodgkin's lymphoma and neuroblastoma (in children). A coexisting and usually unrelated neoplasm is found in approximately 15% of patients [e.g., carcinomas of prostate, colon, rectum, or kidney, skin (basal cell and squamous cell), melanoma, chronic lymphocytic leukemia, and non-Hodgkin's lymphoma].

Autoantibodies directed against onconeural antigens are frequently detectable in serum or spinal fluid of patients with paraneoplastic neurological disorders. These autoantibodies reflect a multifaceted immune response mounted against a non-obvious systemic cancer. Numerous autoantibody markers of cancer have been defined in the past two decades. Their specificities are classifiable generically as reactive with antigens in the nucleus (neurons and glia), cytoplasm (neurons, glia, and muscle), or plasma membrane (neurons and muscle). Their clinical and oncological associations are shown in Tables 1 and 2. Intracellular neural tissue proteins corresponding to the originally immunizing tumor antigen are not displayed on the surface of viable neural or muscle cells except under the influence of proinflammatory cytokines that upregulate surface expression of major histocompatibility complex (MHC) class 1 molecules bearing peptides derived from the intracellular compartment. Only then are these antigens accessible to tumor-activated peptide-specific CD8+ cytotoxic T cells that permeate all tissues in the course of immune surveillance. In contrast, autoantibodies

(*Text continues on p. 523*)

Table 1 Cancers and Their Autoantibody Markers

Cancer	Marker autoantibodies recognized to date
Lung carcinoma, small-cell type	ANNA-1 (1,2), ANNA-2 (3,4), ANNA-3 (5), AGNA (6), CRMP-5 (7), amphiphysin (8,9), PCA-2 (10), striational (11), recoverin (12), Zic4 (13), VGCC (N-type and P/Q-type) (11), VGKC (14,15), ganglionic AChR (16), muscle AChR (11)
Lung carcinoma, non-small-cell type	VGCC (N-type), striational, muscle AChR (11)
Thymoma	Muscle AChR, striational, GAD65, CRMP-5, VGKC, ganglionic AChR ANNA-1 (17)
Breast carcinoma	ANNA-2 (3,4), amphiphysin (8,9), PCA-1 (18–20), VGCC (N-type), muscle AChR (11)
Ovarian/mullerian duct carcinoma	PCA-1 (18–20), VGCC (N-type > P/Q type), muscle AChR,(11,19) EFA6A (teratoma) (21)
Testicular	Ma2 (22)
Hodgkin's lymphoma	PCA-Tr (10,23); mGluR1 (24)
Neuroblastoma	ANNA-1, muscle AChR, VGCC (N-type), striational (11)

Abbreviations: ANNA, anti-neuronal nuclear autoantibody; AGNA, anti-glial nuclear antibody; CRMP, collapsin response-mediator protein; VGCC, neuronal voltage-gated calcium channel; VGKC, neuronal voltage-gated potassium channel; PCA, Purkinje cell cytoplasmic autoantibody; GAD65, glutamic acid decarboxylase (65 kDa isoform); AChR, acetylcholine receptor.

Table 2 Oncological, Serological, and Neurological Accompaniments of Currently Recognized Paraneoplastic Autoantibodies and Anecdotal Treatment Responses

Autoantibody	Associated cancers	Coexisting autoantibody frequency	Neurological accompaniments	Response to therapy
Anti-neuronal nuclear				
ANNA-1 (1,2,19,25,26)	SCLC, rarely thymoma; children: neuroblastoma or no detectable tumor	43% (CRMP-5 > VGCC > muscle AChR = ganglionic AChR > striational = VGKC)	Neuropathies (80%; mixed sensorimotor, pure sensory, predominantly autonomic, rarely motor) > GI dysmotilities (25%) > limbic encephalitis > subacute cerebellar degeneration, myelopathy, radiculopathy	Generally poor. Patients with limbic encephalitis more likely to improve after tumor treatment, with or without corticosteroids, IVIg
ANNA-2 (3,4,19,27)	Lung and breast	35% (ANNA-1 > CRMP-5 (both lung cancer-related) > VGCC > ganglionic AChR)	Brainstem syndrome (opsoclonus/myoclonus > cranial neuropathy, laryngospasm and trismus), cerebellar syndrome, myelopathy, neuropathy (sensorimotor > polyradiculopathy > cauda equina syndrome), movement disorder, encephalopathy, seizures	Variable. Outcome of tumor treatment and immunotherapy more favorable than for ANNA-1-related syndromes

(Continued)

Table 2 Oncological, Serological, and Neurological Accompaniments of Currently Recognized Paraneoplastic Autoantibodies and Anecdotal Treatment Responses (*Continued*)

Autoantibody	Associated cancers	Coexisting autoantibody frequency	Neurological accompaniments	Response to therapy
ANNA-3 (5,19)	SCLC	30% (CRMP-5 > ANNA-1 = PCA-2 = VGCC)	Sensory and sensorimotor neuropathies, cerebellar ataxia, myelopathy, brainstem and limbic encephalopathy	Variable
Zic4 (13)	SCLC	82% (ANNA-1 > CRMP-5)	Pure or predominant cerebellar syndrome	Unknown
Anti-Ma (22,28)	Testicular, breast, lung adenocarcinoma	Unknown	Limbic and brainstem encephalitides. A minority exhibit narcolepsy (with low CSF hypocretin attributed to autoimmune hypothalamitis), cerebellar symptoms	Improvement after tumor treatment, with or without corticosteroids, plasmapheresis, or IVIg
Anti-glial nuclear AGNA (6; D-Lachance and VA-Lennon, unpublished)	SCLC	43% with VGCC	Lambert-Eaton myasthenic syndrome, cerebellar syndrome, limbic encephalitis, sensorimotor neuropathy	Unknown

Antineuronal, glial, and muscle cytoplasmic antibodies

Amphiphysin-IgG (8,9,19)	SCLC and breast	38% (CRMP-5 > VGCC > ANNA-1 = PCA-2 > VGKC = ganglionic AChR = muscle AChR = striational)	Peripheral neuropathy, encephalopathy, myelopathy, encephalomyelitis with rigidity, cerebellar syndrome, myoclonus, focal pain, pruritis. A minority exhibit stiff-person phenomena	Variable. Best outcomes with early treatment
CRMP-5-IgG (7,19,29,30)	SCLC, Thymoma, Thyroid or Renal carcinoma, lymphoma	57% (ANNA-1 > VGCC > PCA-2 > muscle AChR > VGKC = striational > amphiphysin = ganglionic AChR)	Peripheral neuropathy > autonomic neuropathy, cerebellar ataxia, cerebrocortical disorders, basal ganglionitis (chorea > Parkinsonism > hemiballismus), cranial neuropathies (particularly loss of vision, smell, and taste), myelopathy and radiculoplexo-pathy≫neuromuscular junction disorders	Variable responses to tumor treatment, Corticosteroids cyclophosphamide, IVIg, Plasmapheresis
PCA-1 (anti-Yo) (18–20,31)	Ovarian, fallopian tubal, serous surface papillary or endometrial > breast adenocarcinoma	9% (ganglionic AChR > VGCC = muscle AChR > VGKC)	Cerebellar dysfunction predominates in 90%; 10% have isolated upper motor neuron or peripheral nerve disorder (sensorimotor > motor > autonomic neuropathy)	Generally poor or none

(Continued)

Table 2 Oncological, Serological, and Neurological Accompaniments of Currently Recognized Paraneoplastic Autoantibodies and Anecdotal Treatment Responses (*Continued*)

Autoantibody	Associated cancers	Coexisting autoantibody frequency	Neurological accompaniments	Response to therapy
PCA-2 (10,19)	SCLC	63% (CRMP-5 > VGCC > ANNA-1 > VGKC > amphiphysin > ANNA 3 = muscle AChR = striational)	Brainstem or limbic encephalitis, cerebellar ataxia, and neuropathy	Variable; generally poor
PCA-Tr (23)	Hodgkin's lymphoma	Unknown	Cerebellar dysfunction	Favorable with corticosteroids or IVIg
Anti-mGluR1 (24)	Hodgkin's lymphoma	Unknown	Cerebellar dysfunction	Favorable with corticosteroids or IVIg
Recoverin (anti-CAR) (12,32)	SCLC, also endometrial, cervical, ovarian, and breast	Unknown	Painless and progressive vision loss, loss of rod and cone function (demonstrated by electroretinography)	Variable
Striational (sarcomeric proteins) (11)	SCLC, thymoma, breast carcinoma	Not determined	Most common with, but not restricted to, paraneoplastic myasthenia gravis. Also encephalomyeloradiculopathies, autonomic, sensory and motor neuropathies	Variable

Cation channel antibodies				
VGCC, P/Q-type (11,33–35)	SCLC, breast, ovarian	Not determined	LES > encephalo-myeloneuropathies	Improvements reported with corticosteroids, azathioprine, cyclosporine, IVIg and plasmapheresis
VGCC, N-type (11,34)	Lung, ovarian, breast	Not determined	LES with lung cancer > LES with no cancer > LES with other types of cancer. Also encephalomy-eloneuropathies, acquired cerebellar ataxia and autonomic neuropathy (including gastrointestinal dysmotilities)	Variable response
VGKC (14,15,36)	SCLC, thymoma	Not determined	Encephalopathy and limbic encephalitis > neuromyotonia. Insomnia prominent. Morvan syndrome includes additionally myotonia, hypersalivation, excess sweating	Favorable responses: limbic encephalitis with plasmapheresis or corticosteroids; neuromyotonia with plasmapheresis, corticosteroids, or azathioprine

(Continued)

Table 2 Oncological, Serological, and Neurological Accompaniments of Currently Recognized Paraneoplastic Autoantibodies and Anecdotal Treatment Responses (*Continued*)

Autoantibody	Associated cancers	Coexisting autoantibody frequency	Neurological accompaniments	Response to therapy
Muscle AChR (11,33,37)	Thymoma, SCLC	Not determined	MG, LES, autoimmune dysautonomias, peripheral neuropathies and encephalomyelitides. Patients with autoimmune liver disease are frequently seropositive	LES and MG: favorable responses with corticosteroids, azathioprine, cyclosporine, IVIg and plasmapheresis. Symptomatic improvement with edrophonium (both), 3,4 diaminopyridine (LES)
Neuronal (ganglionic) AChR (16)	SCLC, thymoma	Not determined	Limited dysautonomia > encephalopathies > pandysautonomia (highest titers) > acquired neuromuscular hyperexcitability	Favorable response with corticosteroids, plasmapheresis, and IVIg

Abbreviations: ANNA, anti-neuronal nuclear autoantibody; CRMP, collapsin response-mediator protein; VGCC, neuronal voltage-gated calcium channel; VGKC, neuronal voltage-gated potassium channel; PCA, Purkinje cell cytoplasmic autoantibody; AChR, Acetylcholine receptor; SCLC, Small-cell carcinoma of the lung; IgG, immunoglobulin G; IVIg, intravenous immune globulin G; LES, Lambert-Eaton syndrome; MG, myasthenia gravis.

reactive with the extracellular domains of intrinsic plasma membrane proteins have potential to bind to native protein antigens in vivo. In the setting of unexplained subacute neurological symptoms, serum autoantibody profiles can predict an underlying neoplasm as the initiator of an autoimmune response targeting the nervous system.

Historically, paraneoplastic disorders were considered to have syndromic presentations such as sensory neuronopathy or subacute cerebellar ataxia. In the mid-1980s, it was thought, erroneously, that distinctive paraneoplastic autoantibodies accompanied specific neurological syndromes. Subsequent studies revealed that syndromic presentations account for only a minority of paraneoplastic disorders. Most are multifocal, commonly mistaken at onset for vascular, inflammatory, or degenerative disorders, and are associated with high morbidity, especially when diagnosis is delayed. Prompt serological evaluation facilitates early diagnosis and thus favors a better outcome by permitting early initiation of immunomodulatory therapy and identification and treatment of a non-obvious neoplasm. Despite rapid advances in the serological and radiological evaluation of these disorders in the past two decades, guidelines for efficacious immunotherapy are lacking. Therapeutic reports so far are anecdotal and retrospective.

NEOPLASMS COMMONLY ENCOUNTERED WITH AUTOIMMUNE NEUROLOGICAL PRESENTATIONS

The autoantibody profiles that predict specific cancer types are shown in Table 1. The neurological accompaniments of these autoantibodies often involve multiple levels of the nervous system. Small-cell carcinoma, usually of the lung (SCLC), is the most commonly identified cancer in men and women. In men, thymic epithelial neoplasia and Hodgkin's lymphoma are recognized more commonly than testicular carcinoma. In women, breast carcinoma follows SCLC in frequency; epithelial thymoma, ovarian and mullerian ductal carcinomas and ovarian teratomas are less common. Lymphoproliferative neoplasms are sometimes encountered in men and women. In children, neuroblastomas are the most common neoplasms associated with neurological autoimmunity. Paraneoplastic disorders with predominant peripheral nerve involvement have been described in patients with multiple myeloma and Waldenström macroglobulinemia.

CLINICAL PRESENTATIONS

Most patients lack symptoms or signs of cancer and present to a neurologist or internist, and sometimes to a rheumatologist, gastroenterologist, psychiatrist, physiatrist, or ophthalmologist. Neurological symptom onset is generally subacute and there is frequently a delay of months before tumor diagnosis. Sometimes several years elapse before the pertinent cancer is diagnosed.

Important clues to the diagnosis include a past history or family history of cancer or autoimmunity, and a history of smoking, social or occupational exposure to tobacco smoke, or exposure to other carcinogens, particularly asbestos. Table 1 summarizes the autoantibodies that are characteristically recognized with cancers that are identified most frequently in patients presenting with neurological autoimmunity.

The traditional view that paraneoplastic neurological disorders are syndromic led neurologists to accept the false concept that each syndrome has a specific autoantibody marker. For example, the antineuronal nuclear autoantibody-type 1, ANNA-1, (also known as anti-Hu) was initially reported in patients who had sensory neuronopathy related to SCLC (1), the Purkinje cell cytoplasmic autoantibody-type 1, PCA-1, (also known as anti-Yo) was first recognized in women who had cerebellar ataxia related to ovarian carcinoma (17), ANNA-2 (also known as anti-Ri) was first reported in women who had opsoclonus/myoclonus related to breast carcinoma (3), and amphiphysin autoantibody was first reported in women with "stiff-man" syndrome related to breast carcinoma (8). It is now recognized that most paraneoplastic autoantibodies are associated with multifocal and variable neurological presentations (Table 2) (2,4,9,19). Because symptoms involve more than one level of the neuroaxis in 70% of patients, we have tabulated the neurological symptoms and signs of paraneoplastic autoimmunity according to the level affected clinically. Table 3 summarizes the serological accompaniments of various neurological manifestations.

Cerebral Cortex and Limbic System

Paraneoplastic limbic encephalitis is characterized clinically by memory impairment, seizures, and psychiatric manifestations. The most commonly associated neoplasm is SCLC (70% of cases) and the serum autoantibody profile is variable (Table 3). Although underrecognized and reported infrequently, a neuropsychiatric presentation with mental status change and behavioral abnormalities is not rare. Some patients present with subacute dementia. It has recently been recognized that women with cerebral cortical presentations sometimes have ovarian teratoma. An autoantibody specific for the ARF6 exchange factor (EFA6A) aids its diagnosis (21).

Diencephalon

Hypothalamic dysfunction with narcolepsy-like excessive daytime sleepiness, and sometimes cataplexy and hypnagogic hallucinations occur in about 30% of patients with Ma2 autoantibody (22). Patients with paraneoplastic narcolepsy differ from patients with idiopathic narcolepsy by having accompanying limbic, brainstem, or endocrine deficits. Low (or undetectable) cerebrospinal fluid (CSF) hypocretin levels attest to hypothalamic involvement (28).

Table 3 Neurological Manifestations According to the Nervous System Level Involved; Serological Associations

Level	Disorder	Serological associations (see Table 2)
Cerebral cortex (2,4,6,8,13,14,21,24,37)	Limbic encephalitis	CRMP-5 > ANNA-1 > VGCC > Ma2 (>) amphiphysin > muscle AChR = ganglionic AchR
	Neuropsychiatric disorder	VGKC, VGCC, muscle AChR, ganglionic AChR, striational, CRMP-5-IgG > amphiphysin > ANNA-2 > ANNA-1 > PCA-1
Diencephalon (21,27)	Hypothalamic dysfunction	Ma2 > ANNA-1
Basal ganglia (6,28)	Chorea	Syndromic association with CRMP-5 IgG; multiple coexisting Abs
	Myoclonus	Multiple
Cerebellum (2,4,6,8,10,17,19,22,30,38,6)	Cerebellar ataxia	PCA-1 and PCA-Tr Predominant symptoms usually confined to cerebellum or connections. Symptoms usually multifocal with CRMP-5, VGCC (P/Q-type or N-type), PCA-2, ganglionic AChR, muscle AChR, and ANNA-1
Brainstem (2,4,6–8)	Brainstem encephalitis	VGCC (P/Q-type and N-type), CRMP-5, PCA-2, ANNA-1, muscle AChR, ganglionic AChR, ANNA-2, amphiphysin, Ma2
	Stiff-person phenomena	Amphiphysin IgG (39% of women and 12% of men)
Cranial nerves (2,6,29)	Special senses, bulbar, motor neuropathies	CRMP-5-IgG > ANNA-1 = VGCC (N-type > P/Q-type) > muscle and ganglionic AChR and striational
Spinal cord (4,6,8,39)	Myelopathy	VGCC = CRMP-5 > amphiphysin > ganglionic AChR > VGKC > ANNA-2 = ANNA-1
	Myoclonus	Multiple

(Continued)

Table 3 Neurological Manifestations According to the Nervous System Level Involved; Serological Associations (*Continued*)

Level	Disorder	Serological associations (see Table 2)
Peripheral somatic nerves and ganglia (2,16,24,39,58)	Sensory neuronopathy and sensorimotor neuropathies	ANNA-1 > CRMP-5 > VGCC > ganglionic AChR, AGNA, amphiphysin, muscle AChR, striational
Neuromuscular junction (4,8,10,16,32,33,39,40)	Lambert-Eaton Syndrome	VGCC (P/Q-type > N-type) > muscle AChR or striational = ganglionic AChR. Neuronal nuclear and cytoplasmic antibodies are rare unless other neurological accompaniments, AGNA detected in 43% of LES patients with SCLC (6)
	Myasthenia gravis	Muscle AChR > striational > CRMP-5 = ganglionic AChR = VGKC
Muscle (39,41)	Polymyositis/dermatomyositis	Anti-Jo
Autonomic and enteric nervous system (2,6,10,15,42,43)	Dysautonomias	VGCC (N-type≫P/Q-type), ganglionic AChR, muscle AChR > ANNA 1 > CRMP-5
	Gastrointestinal dysmotilities	Ganglionic AChR, muscle AChR, VGCC (N-type), VGKC, striational > ANNA-1 > CRMP-5 > VGCC (P/Q-type)

Abbreviations: ANNA, anti-neuronal nuclear autoantibody; AGNA, anti-glial nuclear antibody; CRMP, collapsin response-mediator protein; VGCC, neuronal voltage-gated calcium channel; VGKC, neuronal voltage-gated potassium channel; PCA, Purkinje cell cytoplasmic autoantibody; AChR, Acetylcholine receptor; IgG, immunoglobulin G; IVIg, intravenous immune globulin G.

Basal Ganglia and Extrapyramidal System

Paraneoplastic chorea, with accompanying imaging abnormalities in the caudate and putamen, occurs most commonly with SCLC and is recognized as a syndromic manifestation of CRMP-5 autoimmunity (7,29). Commonly coexisting neurological manifestations include loss of vision, smell and taste, peripheral neuropathy, and limbic encephalitis. Myoclonus is perhaps the most common of paraneoplastic movement disorders. Also reported are athetosis, Parkinsonism, hemiballismus, tremor, dystonia, and blepharospasm.

Cerebellum

Subacute cerebellar ataxia frequently dominates a multifocal paraneoplastic neurological presentation. In this context, however, sensory ataxia may be mistaken for cerebellar ataxia. Cerebellar ataxia is the most common presentation of patients seropositive for PCA-1 (18,20) (99% are women) or PCA-Tr (23). Although symptoms and signs predominate in the cerebellum and its connections, ~10% of PCA-1–positive patients exhibit neuropathic symptoms and signs as the sole neurological manifestation (motor more than sensory, and rarely autonomic; VA Lennon, unpublished observations). PCA-1 (a marker of ovarian or breast carcinoma) is rarely if ever accompanied by neuronal nuclear or cytoplasmic autoantibodies (19). In contrast, numerous neuronal nuclear and cytoplasmic autoantibodies (as well as cation channel and striational antibodies) aid the diagnosis of paraneoplastic cerebellar ataxia related to SCLC and breast carcinoma (Tables 1 and 3).

Brainstem

Manifestations of midbrain and pons involvement by encephalitis include ophthalmoplegia or a movement disorder with a variable admixture of parkinsonian tremor and rigidity, dystonia (contraction of agonist and antagonist musculature), and opsoclonus or myoclonus. Nausea, vomiting, vertigo, nystagmus, ataxia, and bulbar palsy may indicate medullary involvement. Brainstem phenomena occur in 71% of patients with ANNA-2 autoimmunity (4), 73% of patients with Ma2 autoimmunity (22), and in lower frequency with other paraneoplastic autoantibodies (Table 3). Paraneoplastic "stiff-man" (or, more correctly, stiff-person) syndrome is characterized by severe, painful, and progressive muscle rigidity or stiffness that prominently affects the spine and lower extremities. Variants of stiff-person syndrome are encountered most frequently with breast carcinoma and SCLC (8,9). Amphiphysin antibody is the most distinctive marker of stiff-person syndrome, but low titers of GAD65 antibody (<20 nmol/L) coexist with amphiphysin in 27% of patients (9). A high serum level of GAD65 autoantibody (usually >20 nmol/L) aids the diagnosis of classical stiff-man (Moersch-Woltmann) syndrome. This disorder is usually idiopathic but it may accompany thymoma. It is noteworthy that GAD65 antibody is the most frequent neuronal autoantibody recognized with thymoma (17). Progressive encephalomyelitis with rigidity is a rare and usually fatal syndrome that is associated with SCLC. It is characterized by diffuse inflammation of the brain and brainstem (40).

Cranial Nerves and Ganglia

Optic Nerve and Retina

CRMP-5-immune globulin G (IgG) is the most common marker of paraneo-plastic autoimmune vision loss related to SCLC. The characteristic ophthalmologic presentation is a combination of optic neuritis and retinitis associated with vitreous and intrathecal inflammation (30). Other paraneoplastic disorders of vision loss that are reported more commonly, but encountered less frequently, include cancer (SCLC)-associated retinopathy (CAR) (30) and melanoma-associated retinopathy (45). The autoantibody marker reported for CAR binds to recoverin, a 23 kDa retinal protein. Bilateral diffuse uveal melanocytic proliferation has been described, but lacks a defined autoantibody marker.

Other Cranial Neuropathies

Paraneoplastic cranial neuropathies are more commonly multiple than isolated. Common symptoms include abnormalities of smell [cranial nerve (CN) I], taste (CN V and VII), eye movement (CN III, IV, and VI), facial weakness (CN VII), numbness and pain (CN V), deafness, tinnitus and vestibular dysfunction (CN VIII) and dysphagia (CN X). CRMP-5-IgG is the most frequent marker autoantibody of these disorders (Table 3). Although seldom reported in a paraneoplastic context, subacute hearing loss was the most commonly encountered cranial neuropathy in a Mayo Clinic review of 162 ANNA-1–seropositive patients (2), and it was also reported with thymoma (17).

Spinal Cord

Myelopathies are a common manifestation of paraneoplastic autoimmunity, and a variety of neuronal nuclear and cytoplasmic autoantibodies serve as markers (Tables 2 and 3). The presentation is usually subacute with prominent motor involvement. It is critical to distinguish paraneoplastic myelopathies from myelopathies due to metastasis or radiation and from idiopathic cases. Concurrent optic neuritis (manifestations of CRMP-5 autoimmunity) may lead to misdiagnosis of neuromyelitis optica (30). Symptoms and signs of motor neuron disease may resemble amyotrophic lateral sclerosis (40). The involvement of multiple levels of the neuroaxis by paraneoplastic motor neuro-pathy may be a helpful distinguishing feature.

Peripheral Somatic and Autonomic Nervous System

Roots, Ganglia, and Nerves

Peripheral neuropathy is the most common manifestation of paraneoplastic neurological autoimmunity (40). Although subacute sensory neuronopathy is the most readily recognized presentation of autoimmunity related to SCLC, sensorimotor neuropathies are most common (2,25). Sensory neuronopathy affects 40% of ANNA-1–positive patients and is considered a syndromic manifestation of ANNA-1 autoimmunity (2). Other common autoantibody markers include CRMP-5-IgG, N-type Ca^{2+} channel, and ganglionic acetylcholine receptor (AChR) antibodies (Table 3). Motor and autonomic neurons (including synapses) may also be involved, either in isolation or in association with a sensory neuronopathy. A sensory neuropathy accompanies approximately 10% of Waldenström macroglobulinemia cases.

Mononeuropathies, plexopathies, polyradiculopathies, and small-fiber neuropathies are encountered in isolation or in a multifocal presentation. An acute, rapidly progressive, sensorimotor polyneuropathy similar to Guillain-Barré syndrome (or its Miller-Fisher variant, VA Lennon, unpublished observation) is encountered with SCLC and has been described with Hodgkin's lymphoma. A slowly progressive sensorimotor neuropathy occurs in about 10% of patients with multiple myeloma, and a predominantly motor neuropathy similar to chronic inflammatory demyelinating polyneuropathy develops in approximately 50% of patients with osteoclerotic myeloma. Vasculitis restricted to nerve or muscle has been reported with lymphoma, leukemia, and carcinoma of the prostate, kidney, lung, and endometrium. It presents as a symmetric or asymmetric, painful, sensorimotor neuropathy, and proximal muscle weakness. The diagnosis is confirmed by biopsy of muscle (microvasculitis) or nerve (intramural and perivascular inflammatory infiltrates).

Neuromuscular Junction and Muscle

The Lambert-Eaton syndrome (LES) is a presynaptic disorder of peripheral cholinergic neuromuscular transmission with limited dysautonomia (33). It presents as an insidious proximal limb weakness, with strength improving after several seconds of sustained voluntary contraction. Electromyographic characteristics and seropositivity for neuronal Ca^{2+} channel autoantibodies distinguish LES from myasthenia gravis (MG) (34,37). The P/Q-type Ca^{2+} channel antibody is the putative effector of LES (90% positive), and is not detected in patients with MG except in rare nonthymomatous paraneoplastic cases. Approximately 60% of LES patients have SCLC, and this disorder is estimated to affect 1% to 2% of patients with SCLC. Dysautonomia in LES characteristically impairs tearing, salivation, sweating, and penile erection. When other autonomic manifestations (e.g., gastrointestinal [GI] dysmotility or orthostatic hypotension) or sensory phenomena are present (e.g., pain in the low back, buttocks, and thighs), the autoantibody profile usually indicates that paraneoplastic autonomic neuropathy or radiculoneuropathy coexists with LES. For example, ANNA-1, amphiphysin-AGNA (6) or CRMP-5-IgG may be positive in addition to P/Q-type Ca^{2+} channel antibody, with or without N-type Ca^{2+} channel antibody.

MG is a postsynaptic disorder of neuromuscular transmission caused by antibodies directed at the extracellular domain of muscle AChR (37). Common symptoms are fatigable weakness of extremities and oculobulbar muscles. Thymoma is identified in about 15% of MG patients. The association of MG with other neoplasms is documented infrequently (46). Autoantibody profiles that predict thymoma (Table 1) are distinct from SCLC profiles by lacking Ca^{2+} channel antibodies (17). Neuromyotonia, rippling muscle disease, and cramp-fasciculation syndrome represent a continuum of acquired presynaptic disorders of continuous muscle fiber activity associated most commonly with thymoma or SCLC (47).

Muscle

About 9% to 15% of patients with polymyositis or dermatomyositis are reported to have visceral neoplasia (40). Symptoms and signs of both paraneoplastic and nonparaneoplastic dermatomyositis include a purplish discoloration of the eyelids with edema, red and scaly lesions over the knuckles, and necrotic skin ulceration. Skin symptoms usually precede muscle weakness. Interstitial lung disease sometimes occurs. Serum creatinine kinase (CK) elevation, detection of Jo-1 antibody, and EMG findings aid the diagnosis (42).

Acute necrotizing myopathy presents as painful proximal muscle weakness and is reported with carcinoma of the lung, breast, kidney, stomach, colon, pancreas, or prostate. Weakness of pharyngeal and respiratory muscles is usually fatal. Serum CK is elevated, and biopsy demonstrates muscle necrosis with minor inflammation. Rarer myopathies are reported with carcinoid tumors (0.5% of cases) and cachexia (40).

Autonomic Nervous System

Autoimmune autonomic neuropathy or ganglionopathy is usually a component of a multifocal neurological disorder associated with SCLC or thymoma (16). Less commonly reported cancers include pancreatic, testicular, ovarian, carcinoid, and lymphoma. Signs of sympathetic failure include severe orthostatic hypotension and anhidrosis. Parasympathetic failure includes dry mouth, erectile dysfunction, impaired pupillary response to light and accommodation, and a fixed heart rate. Symptoms and signs of autoimmune GI dysmotility are common, but underappreciated, often being attributed to "cancer cachexia." Anorexia, early satiety, postprandial abdominal pain, and vomiting are clues to gastroparesis. Constipation may progress to pseudo-obstruction. Diarrhea is sometimes prominent. Isolated achalasia, dysphagia, pyloric stenosis, and anal spasticity have been encountered (2). Motor and sensory nerve dysfunction may be minimal or absent. Currently recognized autoantibody markers of paraneoplastic GI dysmotility are shown in Table 3.

An informative autoantibody profile greatly facilitates the diagnosis of paraneoplastic autoimmune dysautonomia. The only proven effectors of autoimmune dysautonomia to date are antibodies specific for neuronal ganglionic-type AChR (16,43). Paraneoplastic GI dysmotility may occur in isolation, but it often coexists with a multifocal neurological presentation. The enteric nervous system is typically infiltrated by T-cells (44). Additional autoantibodies aiding this diagnosis are muscle AChR and striational antibodies (11), neuronal nuclear and neuronal cytoplasmic antibodies (e.g., ANNA-1 (2) or CRMP-5 IgG (7)], neuronal voltage-gated Ca^{2+} channel antibodies [usually N-type (11,34)] and voltage-gated K^+ channel antibody (48).

DIAGNOSTIC EVALUATION

Autoantibody Profiles

Autoimmune serology is an important first step in investigating a subacute, multifocal, neurological disorder without obvious cause, especially in a patient with personal or family history of cancer or smoking. Optimal serological evaluation requires broad screening for immunoglobulins of defined reactivity with onconeural antigens shared by cancer cells, neurons, glia, or muscle (11,19). Diagnostically important autoantibodies are frequently missed when testing is limited to a single or nominal number of individual antibodies driven by market advertising. Paraneoplastic autoantibodies are not detected in healthy subjects or in patients with neurodegenerative or inflammatory neurologic disorders (e.g., Lewy body disease, Alzheimer dementia, or multiple sclerosis) or, with the exception of muscle AChR and striational antibodies, rheumatologic disorders or other non-neurologic autoimmune disorders (unpublished observations, SJ Pittock and VA Lennon; 45,000 patients tested annually). For example, both ANNA-2 and amphiphysin-IgG were thought initially to be restricted to women with breast carcinoma, but when accompanied by ANNA-1, CRMP-5-IgG, or PCA-2, the serological profile has high specificity for SCLC (19).

An informative autoantibody profile is useful for: (i) establishing an autoimmune etiology, (ii) focusing the search for cancer in the context of the patient's risk factors, (iii) explaining neurological symptoms that appear in the course or wake of cancer therapy and are not latrogenic or explained by metastasis, (iv) differentiating autoimmune neuropathies from neurotoxic effects of chemotherapy, (v) monitoring the immune response of seropositive patients in the course of cancer therapy, and (vi) detecting early evidence of cancer recurrence in previously seropositive patients. However, a negative autoantibody profile does not exclude paraneoplastic autoimmunity. Novel autoantibodies continue to be discovered. Furthermore, initially seronegative patients may convert to seropositive with time. When suspicion for a paraneoplastic disorder remains high and no cancer is found, we currently recommend repeating serological evaluation at four to six months.

The autoantibody profile is also useful for evaluating non-neurological patients in whom lung cancer or thymoma is suspected. Among 21 asymptomatic patients presenting with an anterior mediastinal mass that was proven surgically to be thymoma, more than 70% had one or more neuronal or muscle autoantibodies consistent with thymoma (17). Among 58 non-neurological patients with newly diagnosed SCLC, a limited repertoire of tests revealed one or more autoantibodies predictive of SCLC in 28% (49). Among those with SCLC limited to the chest at diagnosis, 41% had one or more SCLC-predictive autoantibodies. Among those with extensive metastatic disease at diagnosis, only 17% had an SCLC-predictive autoantibody and, in all cases, it was a Ca^{2+} channel antibody (N-type or P/Q-type). The restriction of neuronal nuclear and cytoplasmic antibodies to patients with limited or no metastatic disease is consistent with our hypothesis that antibodies directed at intracellular antigens reflect an effective (cytotoxic CD8+ T-cell mediated) antitumor response.

Other Laboratory Investigations

It is beyond the scope of this chapter to discuss all laboratory investigations required to narrow the differential diagnosis in a patient who may have paraneoplastic neurological autoimmunity. These patients characteristically lack usual signs of malignancy, such as anemia, high erythrocyte sedimentation rate, tumor mass, ascites, pleural effusion, or abnormal liver function tests (reflecting metastasis). Patients with paraneoplastic autoimmunity related to SCLC are often hyponatremic. This is generally considered a manifestation of ectopic antidiuretic hormone secretion by the neoplasm, but, in some cases, hyponatremia may reflect autoimmune hypothalamitis. Hypothyroidism, type-1 diabetes, and non-neurological autoantibodies (both organ-specific and non-organ-specific) are all valuable indicators of predisposition to autoimmunity.

Electroencephalography, nerve conduction studies, electromyography, and magnetic resonance imaging (MRI) of the brain and spinal cord should be performed where appropriate. An inflammatory spinal fluid with leukocytosis (usually <50 cells/µL with predominant lymphocytosis) and elevated protein (with or without oligoclonal IgG bands) supports an inflammatory disorder of the central nervous system. Autoantibodies are sometimes detectable in the spinal fluid and not in the serum (7).

Cancer Search

If the patient's clinical evaluation reveals a neoplasm other than that predicted by the autoantibody profile, the search for cancer should not stop. More than one cancer is encountered in ~15% of patients with paraneoplastic autoimmunity related to SCLC (2,7). Because neoplasms associated with autoimmunity are usually limited, they are difficult to find by conventional imaging. Subtle imaging abnormalities should be investigated further. For chest evaluation, computed tomography (CT) is recommended in the first instance. Positron emission tomography (PET) is an alternative diagnostic tool to evaluate mediastinal lymph nodes. CT of the abdomen and pelvis is helpful in identifying primary visceral malignancies and metastases. If radiological investigation fails to indicate an abnormality suspicious for cancer, whole body PET (rather than thorax-restricted PET) can be helpful in identifying cancers, such as extrapulmonary SCLC.

Tissue diagnosis should be pursued aggressively if a thoracic lesion or lymphadenopathy is identified. Fine-needle aspiration biopsy guided by transesophageal ultrasonography, transbronchial endoscopy, or CT yields tissue confirmation with varying success and complications (50). If mediastinoscopy or less invasive approaches do not yield cancer tissue in the face of imaging evidence of neoplasia, exploratory thoracotomy should be considered.

Mammograms are the gold standard for breast cancer detection. Subtle abnormalities should be biopsied. The importance of regular self-examination in surveillance of patients without breast imaging abnormality warrants emphasis. Breast MRI or sonography is helpful in some cases. Evaluation of gynecological cancer status may require sonography of the pelvis in addition to CT and manual pelvic examination. For PCA-1–positive patients whose breast evaluation, pelvic imaging and examination, and serum CA-125 levels are all normal, exploratory laparotomy often reveals pelvic carcinoma (ovarian, fallopian tubal, or serous surface papillary adenocarcinoma) (20). Testicular ultrasonography is the most important test for men with subacute brainstem encephalitis, whether or not Ma2 antibody is detected (22).

PATHOGENESIS

Tumor-targeted immune responses are initiated by onconeural proteins expressed in the plasma membrane, nucleus, or cytoplasm of certain neoplasms. Corresponding antigens expressed in neurons, glia, or muscle are coincidental targets (11). Autoantibodies directed at neural and muscle plasma membrane antigens have potential to cause disease, as exemplified by MG, LES (33,41), and autonomic neuropathy (16,43). Intracellular antigens are not accessible to immune attack in situ, but peptides derived from intracellular proteins are displayed on upregulated MHC class I molecules in a proinflammatory cytokine milieu, and are thus accessible to peptide-specific CD8+cytotoxic T-cells (51). Tumor spread is limited by these effector cells (39).

Two disorders with contrasting immune mechanisms illustrate principles accounting for a spectrum of autoimmune neurological disorders. The LES related to SCLC has a characteristic presynaptic neurotransmission defect caused by neuronal P/Q-type Ca^{2+} channel IgG (33,41). This disorder is not inflammatory, and the pathogenicity of P/Q-type Ca^{2+} channel IgG for motor nerve terminals does not require complement activation (41). In contrast, cerebellar degeneration related to ovarian carcinoma exemplifies an inflammatory response mediated by peptide-specific CD8+ effector T-cells (51). The PCA-1 (or "anti-Yo") marker autoantibody is predominantly of the complement-activating IgG_1 subclass. Although not cytotoxic to cerebellar neurons in vivo, the presence of PCA-1 of IgG_1 subclass correlates significantly with neurological morbidity (52). This implies that the cytokine milieu prevailing at the tumor site of initial CD4+ helper T-cell activation favored a proinflammatory (T_{H1}) response. Proliferation of antigen-specific cytotoxic CD8+ cells (53), and the differentiation of B-cells secreting complement-activating IgG subclasses depend on continued antigen-driven activation of and cytokine secretion by T_{H1} helper cells. Albert et al. (51) demonstrated that a patient with recent onset paraneoplastic cerebellar degeneration had circulating CD8+ cytotoxic T-cells specific for a synthetic peptide of PCA-1 sequence (selected by computer algorithm to match the patient's MHC class 1). In patients with chronic paraneoplastic cerebellar degeneration, the authors demonstrated circulating peptide-specific CD4+ memory T-cells that yielded antigen-specific CD8+ cytotoxic T-cells following in vitro activation by appropriate PCA-1 peptide presentation. A potential role for cytotoxic T-cells in the pathogenesis of other inflammatory parenchymal neurological disorders is supported by demonstrations of parenchymal CD8+ T-cell infiltrates contacting neurons, in patients seropositive for amphiphysin-IgG and ANNA-2 (4,9).

THERAPY

The therapeutic approach for patients with paraneoplastic neurological autoimmunity has three important components: (i) Tumor ablation. Current opinion favors treating the tumor with standard chemotherapeutic medications and surgery/radiation. (ii) Immunomodulatory therapies, and (iii) Supportive care, symptom relief and prevention and management of complications.

Tumor treatment alone is effective for some patients (38). This likely reflects the efficacy of the residual tumor immune response. In ANNA-1-positive patients without a neurological syndrome (i.e., without a lead time bias) SCLC was reported to be of limited stage more frequently than in seronegative patients, the response to chemotherapy more favorable, and survival longer (54). Based on personal observations, we suspect that ablation of an efficacious tumor immune response by myelosuppressive agents (e.g., cisplatin and etoposide) may adversely affect tumor outcome in seropositive patients. In support of this hypothesis, Galanis et al. (49) found that non-neurological patients with limited SCLC had an impressive 41% frequency of neuronal autoantibodies at outset. In contrast, the frequency was 17% in patients with extensive cancer at outset. However, survival following standard chemotherapy did not differ in the two groups. In unpublished observations, we have encountered striking cases of cancer growth and dissemination following initiation of severely immunosuppressing chemotherapies after years of stable imaging evidence of cancer. Less immunosuppressant agents, such as cyclophosphamide, appear to be more beneficial in patients with paraneoplastic autoimmunity (55). The question of optimal antitumor therapy for patients with serological evidence of a protective immune response needs to be addressed in future therapeutic trials.

For most paraneoplastic syndromes, established immunotherapeutic protocols are lacking and reports are anecdotal (Table 2). Agents used most commonly for acute treatment include corticosteroids (1 g methylprednisolone intravenously daily for five days followed by a gradual taper of oral prednisone) and/or intravenous immune globulin (IVIg). In our experience, repeated courses of either steroid or IVIg are not indicated, if initial benefit is not observed. Plasmapheresis sometimes yields dramatic improvement, presumably when the neurological disability is antibody mediated. Benefit from acute treatment justifies consideration of maintenance immunosuppression with oral azathioprine, mycophenolate mofetil, or cyclophosphamide. Newer therapies such as rituximab (a humanized monoclonal antibody against B-cells expressing the CD20 antigen) or tacrolimus (directed at activated T-cells) hold therapeutic promise. Immunomodulatory therapy is generally not effective for inflammatory parenchymal syndromes such as encephalomyelitis or sensory neuronopathy (with ANNA-1) and cerebellar degeneration (with PCA-1) (18,26,31). Nevertheless, variable and sometimes dramatic improvements have been reported anecdotally (4,9,22,56). Syndromes thought to be mediated by IgG, such as limbic encephalitis associated with K^+ channel antibody, LES associated with P/Q-type Ca^{2+} channel antibody, and cerebellar ataxia associated with various cation channel antibodies, are more likely to respond to steroid, IVIg (35) or plasmapheresis than disorders accompanied by ANNA-1, CRMP-5 and PCA-1 autoantibodies, presumably due to their mediation by cytotoxic effector T-cells (2,25,26,31,57). The high frequency of multiple paraneoplastic autoantibodies makes it difficult to predict therapeutic outcome in patients with multifocal paraneoplastic disorders (19).

The third component of the treatment approach includes rehabilitation (physiotherapy, occupational therapy, and speech therapy), supportive care (respiratory and nutritional), and medical management of neurological symptoms [e.g., pyridostigmine or 3,4-diaminopyridine for LES (33,58); high doses of benzodiazepines for stiff-man syndrome or stiff-person phenomena and antiepileptic medications such as sodium valproate or clonazepam, for opsoclonus myoclonus]. The benefit of antiepileptic medications in the management of paraneoplastic seizures in the setting of limbic encephalitis is well recognized. Neuropsychiatric manifestations of paraneoplastic disorders can be difficult to manage, but may respond remarkably to corticosteroid therapy or neuroleptic medications. Pain, both central and peripheral, is a frequent and largely intractable complaint, but may respond to low-dose tricyclic antidepressants, gabapentin, or opiates.

REFERENCES

1. Graus F, Cordon-Cardo C, Posner JB. Neuronal antinuclear antibody in sensory neuronopathy from lung cancer. Neurology 1985; 35(4):538–543.
2. Lucchinetti CF, Kimmel DW, Lennon VA. Paraneoplastic and oncological profiles of patients seropositive for type 1 anti-neuronal nuclear autoantibodies. Neurology 1998; 50(3):652–657.
3. Luque FA, Furneaux HM, Ferziger R, et al. Anti-Ri: an antibody associated with paraneoplastic opsoclonus and breast cancer. Ann Neurol 1991; 29(3): 241–251.
4. Pittock SJ, Lucchinetti CF, Lennon VA. Anti-neuronal nuclear autoantibody type 2; Paraneoplastic accompaniments. Ann Neurol 2003; 53(5):580–597.
5. Chan KH, Vernino S, Lennon VA. ANNA-3 anti-neuronal nuclear antibody: Marker of lung cancer-related autoimmunity. Ann Neurol 2001; 50(3):301–311.
6. Graus F, Vincent A, Pozo-Rosich P, et al. Anti-glial nuclear antibody: Marker of lung cancer-related paraneoplastic neurological syndromes. J Neuroimmuno 2005; 165:166–171.
7. Yu Z, Kryzer TJ, Griesmann GE, et al. CRMP-5 neuronal autoantibody: marker of lung cancer and thymoma-related autoimmunity. Ann Neurol 2001; 49(2):146–154.
8. Folli F. Solimena M, Cofiell R, et al. Autoantibodies to a 128-kd synaptic protein in three women with the stiff-man syndrome and breast cancer. N Engl J Med 1993; 328(8):546–551.
9. Pittock SJ, Lucchinetti CF, Parisi JE, et al. Amphiphysin autoimmunity: Paraneoplastic accompaniments. Ann Neurol 2005; 58(1):96–107.
10. Vernino S, Lennon VA. New Purkinje cell antibody (PCA-2): Marker of lung cancer-related neurological autoimmunity. Ann Neurol 2000; 47(3):297–305.
11. Lennon VL. Calcium channel and related paraneoplastic disease autoantibodies. In: Peter JB, Schoenfeld Y, eds. Textbook of Autoantibodies. BV, The Netherlands: Elsevier Science Publishers, 1996:139–147.
12. Thirkill CE, Fitzgerald P, Sergott RC, et al. Cancer-associated retinopatiiy (CAR syndrome) with antibodies reacting with retinal, optic-nerve, and cancer cells. N Engl J Med 1989; 321(23):1589–1594.
13. Bataller L, Wade DF, Graus F, et al. Antibodies to Zic4 in paraneoplastic neurological disorders and small-cell lung cancer. Neurology 2004; 62(5):778–782.

14. Thieben MJ, Lennon VA, Boeve BF, et al. Potentially reversible autoimmune limbic encephalitis with neuronal potassium channel antibody. Neurology 2004; 62(7):1177–1182.
15. Pozo-Rosich P, Clover L, Saiz A, et al. Voltage-gated potassium channel antibodies in limbic encephalitis. Ann Neurol 2003; 54(4):530–533.
16. Vernino S, Low PA, Fealey RD, et al. Autoantibodies to ganglionic acetylcholine receptors in autoimmune autonomic neuropathies. N Engl J Med 2000; 343(12):847–855.
17. Vernino S, Lennon VA. Autoantibody profiles and neurological correlations of thymoma. Clin Can Res 2004; 10:7270–7275.
18. Peterson K, Rosenblum MK, Kotanides H, et al. Paraneoplastic cerebellar degeneration. A clinical, analysis of 55 anti-Yo antibody-positive patients. Neurology 1992; 42(10):1931–1937.
19. Pittock SJ, Kryzer TJ, Lennon VA. Paraneoplastic antibodies coexist and predict cancer, not neurological syndrome. Ann Neurol 2004; 56(5):715–719.
20. Hetzel D, Stanhope CR, O'Neill BP, et al. Gynecologic cancer in patients with subacute cerebellar degeneration predicted by anti-Purkinje cell antibodies and limited in metastatic volume. Mayo Clin Proc 1990; 65(12):1558–1623.
21. Vitaliani R, Mason W, Ances B, et al. Paraneoplastic encephalitis, psychiatric symptoms, and hypoventilation in ovarian teratomas. Ann Neurol 2005; 58(4):594–604.
22. Dalmau J, Graus F, Villarejo A, et al. Clinical analysis of anti-Ma2-associated encephalitis. Brain 2004; 127(Pt 8):1831–1844.
23. Bernal F, Shams'ili S, Rogas I, et al. Anti-Tr antibodies as markers of paraneoplastic cerebellar degeneration and Hodgkin's disease. Neurology 2003; 60(2):230–234.
24. Sillevis-Smitt P, Kinoshita A, De Leeuw B, et al. Paraneoplastic cerebellar ataxia due to autoantibodies against a glutamate receptor. N Engl J Med 2000; 342(1):21–27.
25. Graus F, Keime-Guibert F, Rene R, et al. Anti-Hu-associated paraneoplastic encephalomyelitis: analysis of 200 patients. Brain 2001; 124(Pt 6):1138–1148.
26. Sillevis Smitt P, Grefkens J, De Leeuw B, et al. Survival and outcome in 73 anti-Hu positive patients with paraneoplastic encephalomyelitis/sensory neuronopathy. J Neurol 2002; 249(6):745–753.
27. Dropcho EJ, Kline LB, Riser J. Antineuronal (anti-Ri) antibodies in a patient with steroid-responsive opsoclonus-myoclonus. Neurology 1993; 43(1):207–211.
28. Overeem S, Dalmau J, Bataller L, et al. Hypocretin-1 CSF levels in anti-Ma2 associated encephalitis. Neurology 2004; 62(1):138–140.
29. Vernino S, Tuite P. Adler CH, et al. Paraneoplastic chorea associated with CRMP-5 neuronal antibody and lung cancer. Ann Neurol 2002; 51(5):625–630.
30. Cross SA, Salomao DR, Parisi JE, et al. Paraneoplastic autoimmune optic neuritis with retinitis defined by CRMP-5-IgG. Ann Neurol 2003; 54(1):38–50.
31. Shams'ili S, Grefkens J, De Leeuw B, et al. Paraneoplastic cerebellar degeneration associated with antineuronal antibodies: analysis of 50 patients. Brain 2003; 126(Pt 6):1409–1418.
32. Guy J, Aptsiauri N. Treatment of paraneoplastic visual loss with intravenous immunoglobulin: a report of 3 cases. Arch Ophthalmol 1999; 117(4):471–477.

33. Harper CM, Lennon VA. Chapter: Lambert-Eaton syndrome. In: Kaminski HJ, ed. Current Clinical Neurology: Myasthenia Gravis and Related Disorders. Totowa, NJ: Humana Press, Inc., 2003:269–291.
34. Lennon VA, Kryzer TJ, Griesmann GE, et al. Calcium-channel antibodies in the Lambert-Eaton syndrome and other paraneoplastic syndromes. N Engl J Med 1995; 332(22):1467–1474.
35. Bain PG, Motomura M, Newsom-Davis J, et al. Effects of intravenous immuno-globulin on muscle weakness and calcium-channel autoantibodies in the Lambert-Eaton myasthenic syndrome. Neurology 1996; 47(3):678–683.
36. Vincent A, Buckley C, Schott J, et al. Potassium channel antibody-associated encephalopathy: a potentially immunotherapy-responsive form of limbic ence-phalitis. Brain 2004; 127(Pt3):701–712.
37. Lennon VA. Serological profile of myasthenia gravis and distinction from the Lambert-Eaton myasthenic syndrome. Neurology 1997; 48(Suppl 5):S23–S27.
38. Gultekin SH, Rosenfeld MR, Voltz R, et al. Paraneoplastic limbic encephalitis: neurological symptoms, immunological findings and tumour association in 50 patients. Brain 2000; 123(Pt7):1481–1494.
39. Darnell RB, Posner JB. Paraneoplastic syndromes involving the nervous system. N Engl J Med 2003; 349(16):1543–1554.
40. Rudnicki SA, Dalmau J. Paraneoplastic syndromes of the spinal cord, nerve, and muscle. Muscle Nerve 2000; 23(12):1800–1818.
41. Lambert EH, Lennon VA. Selected IgG rapidly induces Lambert-Eaton, myasthenic syndrome in mice: Complement independence and EMG abnormal-ities. Muscle Nerve 1988; 11(11):1133–1145.
42. Dalakas MC. Immunopathogenesis of inflammatory myopathies. Ann Neurol 1995; 37(Suppl 1):S74–S75.
43. Vernino S, Ermilov LG, Sha L, et al. Passive transfer of autoimmune antonomic neuropathy to mice. J Neurosci 2004; 24(32):7037–7042.
44. Lennon VA, Sas DF, Busk MF, et al. Enteric neuronal autoantibodies in pseudo-obstruction with small cell lung carcinoma. Gastroenterol 1991; 100(1):137–142.
45. Ling CP, Pavesio C. Paraneoplastic syndromes associated with visual loss. Curr Opin Ophthalmol 2003; 14(6):426–432.
46. Griesmann GE, Harper CM, Lennon VA. Paraneoplastic myasthenia gravis and lung carcinoma: distinction from Lambert-Eaton syndrome and hypothesis of aberrant muscle acetylcholine receptor (AChR) expression. Muscle Nerve Suppl 1998; 7:S122.
47. Vernino S, Auger RG, Emslie-Smith, AM, et al. Myasthenia, thymoma, presynaptic antibodies and a continuum of neuromuscular hyperexcitability. Neurology 1999; 53(6):1233–1239.
48. Knowles CH, Lang B, Clover L, et al. A role for autoantibodies in some cases of acquired non-paraneoplastic gut dysmotility. Scan J Gastroenterol 2002; 37(2): 166–170.
49. Galanis E, Frytak S, Rowland KM, et al. Neuronal autoantibody titers in the course of small cell lung carcinoma and platinum associated neuropathy. Cancer Immunol Immunother 1999; 48(2–3):85–90.
50. Verschakelen JA, De Wever W, Bogaert J. Role of computed tomography in lung cancer staging. Curr Opin Pulm Med 2004; 10(4):248–255.

51. Albert ML, Darnell JC, Bender A, et al. Tumor-specific killer cells in paraneoplastic cerebellar degeneration. Nat Med 1998; 4(11):1321–1324.
52. Tavee J, Yu Z, O'Neill BP, et al. PCA-1 autoantibody of IgGl subclass predominates in patients with most severe paraneoplastic cerebellar degeneration. Neurology 2001; 56(S3):A415–416.
53. Giuntoli RL. Lu J, Kobayashi H, et al. Direct costimulation of tumor-reactive CTL by helper T cells potentiate their proliferation, survival, and effector function. Clin Cancer Res 2002; 8(3):922–931.
54. Graus F, Dalmau J, Rene R, et al. Anti-Hu antibodies in patients with small-cell lung cancer: association with complete response to therapy and improved survival. J Clin Oncol 1997; 15(8):2866–2872.
55. Vernino S, O'Neill BP, Marks RS, et al. Immunomodulatory treatment trial for paraneoplastic neurological disorders. Neuro-Oncology 2003; 6:55–62.
56. Stark E, Wurster U, Patzold U, et al. Immunological and clinical response to immunosuppressive treatment in paraneoplastic cerebellar degeneration. Arch Neurol 1995; 52(8):814–818.
57. Uchuya M, Graus F, Vega F, et al. Intravenous immunoglobulin treatment in paraneoplastic neurological syndromes with antineuronal autoantibodies. J Neurol Neurosurg Psychiatr 1996; 60(4):388–392.
58. Lundh H, Nilsson O, Rosen I. et al. Practical aspects of 3,4-diaminopyridine treatment of the Lambert-Eaton myasthenic syndrome. Acta Neurol Scand 1993; 88(2):136–140.

Index

About the Editors

JOACHIM M. BAEHRING is Director of the Yale Brain Tumor Center, New Haven, Connecticut, and Assistant Professor, Departments of Neurology and Neurosurgery, Yale University School of Medicine, New Haven, Connecticut. His research interests include the development of molecular markers and treatment protocols for primary CNS lymphoma. Dr. Baehring received his M.D. degree from Johannes Gutenberg University School of Medicine, Mainz, Germany, and completed neurology training at Hahnemann University, Philadelphia, Pennsylvania. He completed post-doctoral fellowships in molecular oncology at Ruprecht Karls University, Heidelberg, Germany, and neuro-oncology at Massachusetts General Hospital, Boston, Massachusetts.

JOSEPH M. PIEPMEIER is the Nixdorff-German Professor and Vice-Chair in the Department of Neurosurgery, Yale University School of Medicine, New Haven, Connecticut. He is the Director of the Yale Brain Tumor Center, Yale Brain Tumor Center, New Haven, Connecticut. Dr. Piepmeier previously served as the Chairman for the Joint Section Tumors for the AANS/CNS. In addition, he is Editor -in-Chief of the *Journal of Neuro-oncology*. Dr. Piepmeier is a recipient of the Allied Services Award and the Wakeman Award for work in clinical neurosurgery. Dr. Piepmeier received the B.A. degree from Duke University, Durham, North Carolina, and the M.D. degree from the University of Tennessee School of Medicine, Nashville. He completed his internship and residency training in neurosurgery at Yale University School of Medicine, New Haven, Connecticut.